**W9-BWL-441**

# Ryan's Ballistic Trauma

Adam J. Brooks • Jon Clasper
Mark J. Midwinter • Timothy J. Hodgetts
Peter F. Mahoney
(Editors)

# Ryan's Ballistic Trauma

## A Practical Guide

**Third Edition**

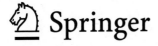

Springer

*Editors*

Adam J. Brooks, FRCS (Gen Surg),
DMCC RAMC (V)
Emergency Surgery and Major Trauma
Nottingham University NHS Trust
Nottingham
UK
and
Academic Department of Military
Surgery and Trauma, Royal Centre
for Defence Medicine
Birmingham
UK

Mark J. Midwinter, BMedSci (Hons),
MB, BS, Dip App Stats, MD,
FRCS (Eng), FRCS (Gen)
Academic Department of Military
Surgery and Trauma, Royal Centre for
Defence Medicine, University Hospital
Birmingham
UK

Peter F. Mahoney, OBE, TD,
MSc FRCA L/RAMC
Defence Professor Anaesthesia
and Critical Care
Royal Centre for Defence Medicine
Birmingham
UK

Jon Clasper, MBA, DPhil, DM,
FRCSEd (Orth), FIMC RCSEd, DMCC
Academic Department of Military
Surgery and Trauma
Frimley Park Foundation Trust
Frimley, Surrey
UK

Timothy J. Hodgetts, CBE, MMEd,
MBA, CMgr, FRCP, FRCSEd,
FCEM, FIMC RCSEd, FIHM,
FCMI, FRGS L/RAMC
Academic Department of Military
Emergency Medicine
Royal Centre for Defence Medicine
Vincent Drive, Edgbaston
Birmingham Research Park
Birmingham
UK

*Associate Editor*

John-Joe Reilly, BSc (Hons), GIBiol, PhD,
DIC, BMedSci (Hons), BM, BS
Academic Department of Military Surgery
and Trauma, Royal Centre for Defence
Medicine, University Hospital
Birmingham
UK

7/11
$239.00
MATT

ISBN 978-1-84882-123-1 3rd Edition          e-ISBN 978-1-84882-124-8 3rd Edition
ISBN 1-85233-678-1 (hardcover) 2nd edition     ISBN 1-85233-679X (softcover)

First edition, Ballistic Trauma: Clinical Relevance in Peace and War (0340581144),
published by Arnold, 1997.

DOI 10.1007/978-1-84882-124-8
Springer London Dordrecht Heidelberg New York

British Library Cataloguing in Publication Data
A catalogue record for this book is available from the British Library

Library of Congress Control Number: 2011922047

*Cover design*: eStudioCalamar Figueres/Berlin

Printed on acid-free paper

Springer is part of Springer Science+Business Media (www.springer.com)

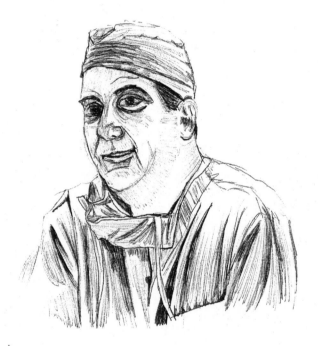

John P. Pryor[†]

*This book is dedicated to John Pryor, trauma surgeon, mentor and friend.*
*John died in a rocket attack during his second tour of duty as a Combat Surgeon in Iraq on Christmas Day 2008.*
*He is missed.*

*Adam J. Brooks*

# Preface

This Preface is being written at the joint UK–US Hospital in Helmand Province, Southern Afghanistan.

Over the last few weeks the Hospital has received casualties from gunshot, burns, mines and improvised explosive devices (IEDs). Adults, children, soldiers and civilians have all been received and cared for according to clinical need.

The lessons from the third edition of Ballistic Trauma are being used here on a daily basis. The third edition represents a blend of experience, best evidence and cutting edge scientific research from DSTL. The Royal Centre for Defence Medicine is a focal point where the three strands are blended and turned into practical guidance.

We hope that readers working in similar (and less extreme) circumstances will find the book helpful and to the benefit of all their patients.

Adam J. Brooks
Peter F. Mahoney

# Preface to the Second Edition

Why this book, why now?

In 1997 Prof JM Ryan and others produced the reference work "Ballistic Trauma: Clinical Relevance in Peace and War" (Arnold 1997). Much of this is still valid but a number of concepts in care of the ballistic casualty have changed. These include developing ideas on fluid resuscitation and refinement of field protocols based on operational experience.

Authors, editors and colleagues expressed the view that there was a need for a practical guide encompassing these developments, along the lines of Conflict and Catastrophe Medicine (Springer 2002). The aim was to distill 'real life' practice and try to capture that which is often lost or diluted in traditional texts.

Then with "9/11" the world changed. Since then major conflicts have occurred in Afghanistan and Iraq and operations are still on going. Many of the authors and editors deployed to these conflicts with NGOs, Aid Agencies and the military.

Others are working with these injuries on a day to day basis at one of the USA's busiest trauma centres.

This has delayed the production of "Ballistic Trauma-a practical guide" but means that people are writing with recent experience of managing ballistic injury. Colleagues returning from deployment have emphasised the need for clear guidance on managing ballistic injury, especially as more and more military reservists are being deployed and their day to day work may not include managing these types of injury.

Authors have been given a relatively free hand in structuring their chapters so they would be unconstrained by the book's style and able to pass on their lessons unhindered.

Finally our request is that this be a "living" document. Give us feedback. Record what treatment works and what doesn't. Use this knowledge to improve the care of the ballistic casualty.

Peter F. Mahoney
James M. Ryan
Adam J. Brooks
C. William Schwab

Ballistic Trauma: Clinical Relevance in Peace and War

This book aims to bring together the science behind and the management of ballistic trauma. It is directed at the surgeon, though perhaps not an expert, who might find him or herself having to deal with patients suffering from penetrating trauma in environments as diffuse as a late twentieth-century hospital or the arduous conditions of a battlefield.

The also brings together the views of UK and US experts from military and civilian backgrounds. This composite view was deliberate as it was recognized that these potentially diverse views reflected the complexity of an international problem that increasingly impinges on the practice of surgery in today's world.

The UK editors were the joint professors of military surgery to the three armed services and the Royal College of Surgeons of England along with a medical scientist with an international reputation in the field of ballistic science. The US editor is professor and chairman of the Department of Surgery at the Uniformed Services University of the health Sciences and has extensive experience in the management of ballistic trauma.

Though the book is heavily influenced by the military background of many of the authors, it is directed at a much wider audience, particularly those who may unexpectedly have to deal with the consequences of the trauma seen in an urban environment. It compares and contrasts the differing civil and military management viewpoints and goes on, where relevant, to debate the areas of controversy in the specialized fields of the relevant authors.

The subject of ballistic trauma is controversial in part because its management depends so much upon the situation in which it occurs. There is thus often confusion and a misunderstanding that emanates from the failure to recognize that the location of surgical facilities, the numbers of injured and whether the injuries are sustained during peace or war may have a profound effect on the way patients are treated. The lesson of history is that you cannot take the experience of an urban hospital on to the battlefield. It can also be said that you cannot do the reverse and nowadays there is further confusion from the deployment of troops to "peace-keeping" duties performed under the scrutiny of the media. The latter is not the same as war.

The book has four sections: the first is on the science behind understanding ballistic trauma; it also adds to its declared remit by including a chapter on blast injury; a second section is on general principles of assessment and initial management; a third section deals with management from a regional perspective; the fourth section is on more specific but general problems. The intention is to provide surgeons with an understanding of the fundamentals of ballistic trauma, the mechanisms and some insight into the significance of new weapons, as well as the variations on the principles of management.

The book acknowledges that no single viewpoint can address the management of patients sustaining ballistic injuries and does not fall into the trap of recommending rigid and single guides unless there is a convergence of opinion. Its approach has been to provide a greater understanding so that the clinician facing the clinical problem feels sufficiently informed as to make coherent choices appropriate to the circumstances.

James M. Ryan
N.M. Rich
R.F. Dale
B.T. Morgans
G.J. Cooper

# Acknowledgements

Illustrations provided by Corporal Anthony W. Green.

Corporal Green studied Art at North Oxfordshire College of Art and Design, after which he studied Journalism at University of Derby. He has written a number of books including the history of his own Territorial Army medical unit entitled "A Jolly Good Show". He has served with the Territorial Army for 10 years. This service has included tours in both Iraq and Afghanistan.

All illustrations contained within this book were made while he was serving with the UK JF Med Group Role 3 Hospital at Camp Bastion on 2009.

Jillian Staruch is a student at The Pennsylvania State University. She will graduate with an Architectural degree in 2012. As the youngest of five, she enjoys spending time with her family and freelances in graphic design.

Figure 18.3 and 28.2 drawn by Dan Miller. He works as a freelance graphic artist in the UK.

# Contents

## Part VI  Clinical Care

# Contributors

Dominic J. Aldington, B.Sc (Hons), MBBS, FRCA, FFPMRCA
Pain Relief Unit, Churchill Hospital, Oxford, UK

Steven R. Allen, MD
Surgery Department, Traumatology and Surgical Critical Care, Hospital of the University of Pennsylvania, Philadelphia, PA, USA

Toney W. Baskin, MD, BS
Trauma and Critical Care Service, Brooke Army Medical Center, United States Army Institute of Surgical Research, San Antonio, TX, USA

Tracy R. Bilski, MD
Surgery Department, Trauma/Surgical Critical Care/Acute Care Surgery Division, Mary Washington Hospital, Fredericksburg VA, USA

Matthew J. Borkon, MD
Department of Surgery, Division of Trauma and Emergency Surgery, Vanderbilt University Medical Center, Nashville, TN, USA

Benjamin Braslow, MD
Division of Traumatology and Surgical Critical Care, Department of Surgery, University of Pennsylvania School of Medicine, Philadelphia, PA, USA

Lt Col Adam J. Brooks, FRCS (Gen Surg), DMCC RAMC (V)
Emergency Surgery and Major Trauma, Nottingham University NHS Trust, Nottingham, UK and
Academic Department of Military Surgery and Trauma, Royal Centre for Defence Medicine, Birmingham, UK

Kate Brown, MA, BM, BCh MRCS (lon), DipSEM
Trauma and Orthopaedics, Royal College of Defence Medicine, Birmingham, UK

Chester C. Buckenmaier, III MD
Surgery Department, Anesthesiology Division, Anesthesiology, Uniformed Services University, Walter Reed Army Medical Center, Washington, DC, USA

Neil Buxton, MBChB, FRCS (NeuroSurg)
Neurosurgery Department, Walton Centre Liverpool, Liverpool, UK

Mark Byers, MBBS, MSc, MCEM, MFSEM, MRCGP
Ministry of Defence, Longlands, Lees Hill, Brampton, UK

Jon Clasper, MBA, DPhil,
DM, FRCSEd (Orth),
FIMC RCSEd, DMCC
Academic Department of Military
Surgery and Trauma, Frimley Park
Foundation Trust, Frimley, Surrey, UK

Dan Connor, BMedSci, BM,
BS, FRCA
Anaesthetic Department, MDHU
Portsmouth, Queen Alexandra Hospital,
Portsmouth, Hampshire, UK

Graham Cooper, OBE, PhD
Biomedical Sciences, Defence Science
and Technology Laboratory,
Porton Down, Salisbury,
Wiltshire, UK

Bryan A. Cotton, MD, MPH
Department of Surgery and Center for
Translational Injury Research,
University of Texas Health Science Center,
Houston, Texas, USA

Jay J. Doucet, CD, MD, FRCSC, FACS
Division of Trauma, Burns and Critical
Care, University of California Medical
Center, San Diego, CA, USA

Henry Dowlen, MD, MSc, BM, BS
45 Commando Royal Marines, Royal
Navy, Arbroath,
Angus, UK

Susan Duff, BSc (Hons)
Nutrition and Dietetic Department,
University Hospitals Birmingham
NHS Foundation Trust,
Birmingham, UK

Clare Dutton, RN, MBE
Critical Care Division, MDHU (N),
Friarage Hospital, Northallerton, UK

James M. Ecklund, MD
National Capital Consortium (Walter Reed
Army Medical Center, National Naval
Medical Center), Washington DC, USA
and Division of Neurosurgery,
Uniformed Services University of the
Health Sciences, Bethesda, MD, USA

John Etherington, MB, ChB, MSc,
FFSEM (UK), FRCP
Defence Medical Rehabilitation Centre,
Headley Court, Epsom, Surrey, UK

Philip Gotts, BSc
Formerly Defence Clothing, Research
and Project Support, Defence Logistics
Organisation now Ordnance Test
Solutions, Ridsdale, Hexham
Northumberland, UK

Jennifer Gray, BSc (Hons)
Nutrition and Dietetic Department,
Warrington and Halton NHS
Foundation Trust, Warrington, UK

Ian Greaves, L/RAMC, MB, ChB,
FRCP, FCEM, FIMC RCSEd,
DipMedEd, DMCC, DTM&H,
MIHM
Emergency Department, James Cook
University Hospital Middlesborough,
Middlesborough, UK

Stuart Harrisson, MB, BS, MRCS
Academic Department of Military
Surgery and Trauma, Royal Centre
for Defence Medicine,
Birmingham, UK

Alan Hepper, OBE, BEng, CEng,
FIMechE, MRAeS, ACGI
Biomedical Sciences, Defence Science
and Technology Laboratory,
Porton Down, Salisbury, Wiltshire, UK

**David E. Hinsley, MB, ChB,**
**FRCS (Tr&Orth)**
Trauma and Orthopaedics,
Frimley Park Hospital,
Wakefords Park,
Church Crookham, Fleet,
Surrey, UK

**Timothy J. Hodgetts, CBE, MMEd,**
**MBA, CMgr, FRCP, FRCSEd,**
**FCEM, FIMC RCSEd, FIHM,**
**FCMI, FRGS L/RAMC**
Academic Department of Military
Emergency Medicine,
Royal Centre for Defence Medicine,
Vincent Drive, Edgbaston,
Birmingham Research Park,
Birmingham, UK

**John B. Holcomb, MD**
Surgery Department, Acute Care Surgery,
Center for Translational Injury Research,
University of Texas Health Science
Center at Houston, Houston TX, USA

**David B. Hoyt, MD, FACS**
Division of Trauma, Burns and Critical
Care, University of California Medical
Center, San Diego, CA, USA

**Neal Jacobs, BSc (Hons),**
**MB, ChB, MRCS**
Academic Department of Military Surgery
and Trauma, Royal Centre for Defence
Medicine (RCDM), Salisbury, UK

**Lt Col Steven L.A. Jeffery, BSc, MB,**
**ChB, FRCS, EBOPRAS, FRCS (Plast)**
Burns and Plastic Surgery,
The Royal Centre for Defence Medicine,
Birmingham, UK

**Donald H. Jenkins, MD,**
**FACS, DMCC**
Surgery Department, Trauma, Critical
Care and General Surgery, Mayo Clinic,
Rochester, MN, USA

**Alan Kay, MB, BS, FRCS,**
**FRCS (Plast)**
Academic Department of Military Surgery
and Trauma, Royal Centre for Defence
Medicine, Birmingham, UK

**Damian Douglas Keene, MB, ChB,**
**BMedSc (Hons)**
Anaesthetics Department, Defence
Medical Services, Anaesthetics and
Intensive Care, University Hospitals
Birmingham, Birmingham, UK

**Emrys Kirkman, PhD**
Biomedical Sciences, Defence Science
and Technology Laboratory,
Porton Down, Salisbury,
Wiltshire, UK

**Ari K. Leppäniemi, MD, PhD**
Department of Surgery, Emergency
Surgery Division, Helsinki University,
Meilahti Hospital, Helsinki, Finland

**Geoffrey S.F. Ling, MD, PhD**
Medical Corps, US Army,
University of the Health Sciences,
MD, Bethesda, USA

**Daniel Longhurst**
Home Office Scientific Development Branch,
St. Albans Hertfordshire, UK

**Craig C. McFarland, MD**
Department of Anesthesia and Operative
Services, Brooke Army Medical Center
Fort Sam Houston, TX, USA and
Uniformed Services University for the
Health Sciences, Department of
Anesthesiology, Fort Sam Houston,
TX, USA

**Peter F. Mahoney, OBE, TD,**
**MSc FRCA L/RAMC**
Defence Professor Anaesthesia and
Critical Care, Royal Centre for Defence
Medicine, Birmingham, UK

**Mark J. Midwinter, BMedSci (Hons),
MB, BS, Dip App Stats, MD,
FRCS (Eng), FRCS (Gen)**
Academic Department of Military Surgery
and Trauma, Royal Centre for Defence
Medicine, University Hospital,
Birmingham, UK

**Andrew Martin Monaghan, BDS,
FDSRCS (Eng), MB, BS, FRCS (Eng),
FRCS (Max Fac)**
Maxillofacial Surgery, Royal Centre for
Defence Medicine, University Hospital
Birmingham Foundation Trust, Edgbaston,
Birmingham, UK

**Jonathan Morrison, MB, ChB,
MRCS (Glas) RAMC, (V)**
Surgical Intensive Care Unit, Southern
General Hospital, Glasgow, UK

**Chris J. Neal, MD**
Department of Neurosurgery,
Walter Reed Army Medical Center,
Washington DC, USA

**Aaron D. Nelson, CPT (Dr.)
MC, USA, DO**
Department of Anesthesiology and
Operative Services, Anesthesiology
and Pain Management Division,
Brooke Army Medical Center,
Fort Sam Houston, TX, USA

**Peter E. Nielsen, MD Col.**
Obstetrics and Gynecology,
Maternal-Fetal Medicine,
Madigan Army Medical Center,
Tacoma, WA, USA

**Giles R. Nordmann, BSc (Hons),
MBChB, FRCA, RAMC**
Department of Anaesthetics, Derriford
Hospital, Plymouth and Department of
Military Anaesthesia and Critical Care,
Royal Centre for Defence Medicine,
Birmingham, UK

**Tim Nutbeam, MB, ChB,
DipIMC RCS (Ed)**
Intensive Care, University Hospital
Birmingham, Birmingham, UK

**Piers R.J. Page, MBBS**
Department of Orthopaedics
and Trauma, Frimley Park Hospital,
Frimley, Surrey, UK

**Graeme Pitcher, MBBCh, FCS (SA)**
General Surgery Department,
Division of Pediatric Surgery,
University of Iowa Hospitals and Clinics,
Iowa, IA, USA

**Sir Keith Porter, MBBS, FRCSEng,
FRCSEd, FIMC RCSEd, FCEM,
FSSEM, FRSA**
Royal Centre for Defence Medicine,
Trauma and Orthopedic Surgery,
University Hospitals Birmingham,
Birmingham, UK

**Susan Price, BSc (Hons), M.Sc.**
Nutrition and Dietetic Department,
University Hospitals Birmingham NHS
Foundation Trust, Birmingham, UK

**John P. Pryor[†], MD**
Division of Traumatology and Surgical
Critical Care, Department of Surgery,
University of Pennsylvania Medical
Center, Philadelphia, PA, USA

**John-Joe Reilly, BSc (Hons), GIBiol, PhD,
DIC, BMedSci (Hons), BM, BS**
Academic Department of Military
Surgery and Trauma, Royal Centre
for Defence Medicine, University Hospital
Birmingham, UK

**Patrick M. Reilly, MD, FACS**
Department of Surgery, Traumatology,
Surgical Critical Care and Emergency
Surgery, University of Pennsylvania School
of Medicine, Philadelphia, PA, USA

**Rob Russell, MB, BS, MRCP (UK), FCEM, DipIMC RCSEd**
Academic Department Military Emergency Medicine, Royal Centre for Defence Medicine and University of Birmingham, Birmingham, UK and Emergency and Critical Care, Peterborough and Stamford Hospitals NHS Foundation Trust, Peterborough, UK

**James M. Ryan, OstJ, MCh, FRCS**
Conflict and Catastrophe Medicine, Cardiac, Thoracic and Vascular Sciences, St. George's University of London, London, UK

**Hendrik Scholtz, MB, ChB, MMedPath (Forens) CapeTown**
Forensic Medicine, School of Pathology, University of the Witwatersrand, Johannesburg, South Africa

**C. William Schwab, MD FACS, FRCS (Glasg)**
Division of Traumatology and Surgical Critical Care, University Hospital Pennsylvania Medical Center, Philadelphia, PA, USA

**Robert A.H. Scott, MBBS, FRCS (Ed), FRCOphth, DM (RAF)**
Vitreoretinal Surgery Service, Ophthalmology, Royal Centre for Defence Medicine, Birmingham Research Park, Birmingham, UK

**Jon David Simmons, MD**
General Surgery Department, Trauma and Critical Care Surgery Division, University of Mississippi Medical Center, Jackson, MS, USA

**Jason Smith, MBBS, MSc, MRCP, FCEM**
Academic Department of Military Emergency Medicine, Royal Centre for Defence Medicine Birmingham Research Park, Vincent Drive, Birmingham, UK

**Michael J. Socher, MD**
Obstetrics and Gynecology, Uniformed Services University of the Health Sciences, Walter Reed Army Medical Center, Washington DC, USA

**Kerry Starkey, PhD, RAMC**
Academic Department of Military Emergency Medicine, Institute of Research and Development, Royal Centre for Defence Medicine, Edgbaston, Birmingham, UK

**Christian B. Swift, MAJ AN ARNP MSN ACNP-BC FNP-BC**
Internal Medicine Division, Department of Medicine, Madigan Army Medical Center, Tacoma, WA, USA

**Nigel Tai, MBBS, MS, FRCS (Gen Surg)**
Academic Department of Military Surgery and Trauma, Trauma Clinical Academic Unit, Royal Centre for Defence Medicine, Royal London Hospital, London, UK

**Robert D. Tipping, MB, BS, FRCA, RAF**
Department of Anaesthetics and Critical Care, Royal Centre for Defence Medicine, Birmingham, UK

**Jeanine Vellema, MBBCh, FCPath**
Division of Forensic Medicine, School of Pathology, University of the Witwatersrand, Johannesburg, South Africa

**Jonathan Vollam, BA (Hons) Adult Nursing PMRAFNS**
Critical Care Air Support Team, Tactical Medical Wing, Royal Air Force Lyncham, Chippenham, Wiltshire, UK

**Sarah Watts, PhD, B.VET.MED**
Biomedical Sciences, Defence Science and Technology Laboratory, Porton Down, Salisbury Wiltshire, UK

# Part I

## Personal Views

# A Personal View

**1**

James M. Ryan

## 1.1
## Introduction

The period 1982–2010 covers nearly 30 years and has seen an exponential growth and global spread of war and conflict. Terrorist attacks and revolutionary wars remain a constant threat affecting the world from the United States, Europe, the Middle East, and Africa to Asia. When the 1st Edition of this book was published in 1997 Professor Howard Champion and his colleagues wrote the Foreword and emphasized that intentional injury had reached pandemic proportions of which the most lethal expression was ballistic injury. Although they recognized the existence then of war and insurrection they felt that the risk of mass armed force combat at close quarters seemed to be diminishing and that the greater risk of ballistic injury was within civil society, particularly in the United States. In the Preface to the first edition the editors noted: "The lesson of history is that you cannot take the experience of an urban hospital onto the battlefield. It can also be said that you cannot do the reverse, and nowadays there is further confusion from the deployment of troops to peacekeeping duties performed under the scrutiny of the media. The latter is not the same as war." The events of the following decade have called these beliefs into question. None could have foreseen the world shaking events that were to occur during the opening years of the twenty-first century – the terrorist attacks in the United States on 9 September 2001, the invasion of Afghanistan the same year by a US led coalition, the invasion of Iraq by a US led coalition in 2003, terrorist bombings in Madrid in 2004, terrorist bombings in London in July 2005, and countless other terrorist and insurgency events on every continent. It is sobering to visit Wikipedia and to note the seemingly endless list of terrorist events recorded for the period 1982–2009. War and terror have come to our streets, towns, and cities causing civilian urban hospitals to take on the mantle of field hospitals in war.

J.M. Ryan
Conflict and Catastrophe Medicine, Cardiac, Thoracic and Vascular Sciences,
St. George's University of London, London, UK
e-mail: jryan@sgul.ac.uk

A.J. Brooks et al. (eds.), *Ryan's Ballistic Trauma*,
DOI: 10.1007/978-1-84882-124-8_1, © Springer-Verlag London Limited 2011

3

## 1.2
## Changing Patterns in War and Conflict

It is useful to start by reproducing a few paragraphs from an article this author wrote on the 25th anniversary of the 1982 Falklands war. It gives a sense of a war that had more in common with those of the late nineteenth and early twentieth centuries but also hinted at the change that was taking place in the conduct of war.

> ….It is strange to look back over a quarter of a century to a war that we never anticipated. In 1982 the Cold War still occupied our thoughts – and planning. The RAMC were exercised for a major conventional, and possibly a nuclear and chemical war, in Europe. All worked to a strict military doctrine, which defined how medical support would unfold and was based around mass casualties and numerous huge Field and General Hospitals. There was little flexibility in our thinking. Principles of War Courses, run annually, were run by the book. Directors and Professors of Military Medicine and Surgery would baulk no discussions. These courses were exercises in Doctrine and debate was not encouraged. This author remembers discussion concerning Field Hospital with upwards of 600 beds – unheard of today. Doctrine defined what would be attempted at each Role – then called echelons. Mortality would have been appalling and the approach would have been "the most for the most," hoping to get as many as possible home to UK based hospitals using all means including cross channel ferries.

> What was faced in 1982 was unexpected and appeared to be outside planning. This was the first campaign of what would become the norm – expeditionary warfare with new doctrines and new methods of working – and new expectations. Mrs Thatcher's statement in the House of Commons some years later that wounded soldiers in war would get the same treatment as the injured in NHS hospitals had not yet been voiced. The first Gulf war was undreamt of and later expeditionary wars in the Balkans, Iraq and Afghanistan beyond our wildest imagination. ….[1]

Until the last quarter of the twentieth century many viewed war as a set piece activity between two massed armies facing each other in the field to do battle with rifle, machine gun, and artillery– in a word - symmetric warfare. The war in the Falklands in 1982 was such a war, although on a small scale. The massed armies of the American civil war and World War I also come to mind. Of course this view is quite wrong and risks viewing war through rose colored spectacles. In fact the nature of war had begun to change with the pace accelerating in the early twentieth century with advent of air warfare and strategic bombing of cities. Harris, who conducted strategic bombing between 1939 and 1945 in Northern Europe, had used aerial bombardment in Kurdistan in the 1920s. The Luftwaffe advanced further this method of warfare during the Spanish civil war – the destruction of Guernica in April 1937 was a watershed and pointed to what would follow in the decades ahead. The later destruction of German and Japanese cities, the carpet bombing of Vietnam and Cambodia put paid to any illusion that war was an event to be fought by standing armies in the field with sparing of the civilian population. We have now reached a point where military casualties, although appalling, pale when the civilian cost is considered. Prior to World War I military casualties far exceeded civilian losses – some reports suggest an 80% to 20% ratio. That ratio has now reversed. Key observations on changes in warfare are summarised in Table 1.1.

**Table 1.1** What can influence the way wars are fought and the wounds that result?

| Factor | | Examples from History |
|---|---|---|
| 1. General Health and Disease | In many campaigns the losses through illness have exceeded those from enemy action. Many examples of disease adversely affecting an army can be found throughout history, often related to the conditions in which the war or campaign was being waged. The pre-existing level of fitness, nutrition, hydration, health and hygiene or disease will influence the extent to which a soldier is able to mount an effective physiologic response to a wound, this may be markedly different in the civilian setting compared with that of war. | **1795** - Former Director General of the Army Medical Department, James McGrigor (regimental surgeon), was on Abercrombie's expedition to fight the French in the Caribbean. He reported those dying from yellow fever outnumbered four-fold those who fell from bullet or bayonet wounds.<br><br>**1806** - James McGrigor joined the British expeditionary forces in the Netherlands which was decimated by malaria, typhus and dysentery. Less than 1 per cent died of wounds sustained in action on that campaign but 10 per cent died of fever. |
| 2. Wound contamination | The conditions may influence the degree of contamination in a wound. Wounds inflicted on a soldier on the battlefield may differ in both contamination and severity from a wound sustained from the same weapon in a civilian setting. | **1899 – 1902** - South Africa, fighting occurred on the veld in a hot, dry climate. Uniforms were made of lightweight materials and wounds had little material carried in; soil contamination was minimal.<br><br>**1914 – 1918** - Flanders. Heavy clothing covered in manure from the fields meant soldier's wounds were deeply contaminated. |
| 3. The range that forces engage one another | The exact nature of the campaign can alter the severity of wounds inflicted. | **18th – 19th Century** - The effective range of the musket was about 100 – 200m, so forces front lines tended to separate at this distance.<br><br>**1899 – 1900** - South African War. This conflict was characterised by rifle fire ranges beyond 500m in many instances with sniping at even greater distances.<br><br>**1914–1918** - In comparison, in the early stages of the 1st World War rifle engagements were at much closer range than in South Africa, though with similar weapons; bullet wounds were reported as far more severe in WW1. |

(continued)

**Table 1.1** (continued)

| Factor | | Examples from History |
|---|---|---|
| 4. Overwhelming Technology | **1898** - Battle of Omdurman in the Sudan. The British employed 20 Maxim machine guns and artillery pieces to devastating effect. The Sudanese lost 11000 men, the British 48. | New technology is not always a guarantee of success, on many occasions guerrilla or irregular forces have defeated a technologically superior enemy, particularly in the low-intensity conflicts of the 20th century. |

Adapted by Starkey from Ryan et al.[2]

## 1.3
## War and Conflict in the Twenty-First Century

We now appear to have entered an era characterized by world wide terrorism waged by state and non-state actors and on an unprecedented scale. Terrorist war is being waged on every continent. Many of the terrorist groups have emerged from failed and rogue states – most notable are Taliban and Al-Qaeda and countless allied groups. They have a worldwide reach as is evident from earlier discussions. The response from countries targeted by these groups, the USA and UK in particular, has been an upsurge in what is best described as expeditionary warfare waged by invading countries and regions harboring the terrorist groups. But there is a sting in the tail. Iraq is an example. The purpose of the invasion was to depose a despot and prevent the proliferation and use of chemical and biological weapons. The result was a failed state (although now recovering) which then became a haven for the very people the expeditionary war was meant to destroy – in the case of Iraq, Al-Qaeda infiltrated the region and this led to on-going instability and asymmetric warfare. The invading coalition won the symmetric battle against the Iraqi army but has yet to achieve victory in the asymmetric battles that followed and continues albeit much reduced.

What does this mean for the readers of this new 3rd edition of Ballistic Trauma? The implications are many but two are paramount – the advent of asymmetric warfare carried out in the midst of civilian populations and the spiraling cost to civilian bystanders. The most startling consequence is that the clear and distinct separation between trauma surgery on the battlefield and in civilian hospitals has been blurred to point of irrelevance. Civilian surgeons in Europe and North America now face wounds caused by terrorist explosions which are indistinguishable from battlefield wounds and war surgeons are being required to treat civilians, particularly in failed and rogue states, where they may be the only effective health care providers – East Timor is a vivid recent example where humanitarian and military medical teams were faced with a population quite without any form of medical care. Clearly there has been a paradigm shift in this new and globalized world of the twenty-first century. Equally a radical change in outlook is needed by both civilian and military health care providers. This change has particularly resonance for surgeons and their teams – it seems that both sides have, not least, new training and educational needs and this is an important driver for this new 3rd edition of Ballistic Trauma.

One of the most worrying problems is the changing nature of surgical training. In 1982, when this author deployed to war, surgical training was long, arduous, and truly general.

Most of the deployed were senior registrars and were in the final year of a training program lasting at least 10 years. A further extract from the paper quoted earlier is illuminating.

...In 1982 the author was a 37 year old Senior Specialist in Surgery (in modern parlance – a Specialist Registrar) in the sixth and final year of higher professional training programme and seconded to St Peter's Hospital in Chertsey. It is worth pausing for a moment to reflect on this old and discarded training programme. Three years of general professional training, followed by six years of higher training had resulted in exposure to the generality of surgery. It included postings to nine separate hospitals including three NHS secondments to St Bartholomew's, Hackney and St Peters Hospitals with training in general, orthopaedic, plastic, neurosurgical, thoracic and vascular surgery – an unimaginable variety today. All military surgeons in training at that time had very similar training programmes. The aim was to produce a surgeon trained in the generality of surgery ready to work alone or in small groups in field surgical facilities. This system of training probably gave the surgeons who would deploy a training edge not available to civilian trainees of the period

This was also the age before war surgery workshops, Definitive Surgical Trauma Skills (DSTS) courses and the myriad of other training opportunities, including overseas secondments, available to today's military surgeons and their teams. Training in the art and science of war surgery prior to 1982 was not easy. Military surgeons "cut their teeth" during secondments to the Military Wing, Musgrave Park hospital in Northern Ireland. The "Troubles" were in full swing and a generation of surgical trainees worked with an earlier generation of military surgery consultants such as Bill McGregor, Bill Thompson and Brian Mayes who had learnt their trade during a myriad of post colonial conflicts in far flung places like Cyprus, Aden, Malaya and Borneo. There was, in short, an institutional memory for the surgery of war which would become evident as the Falkland Islands war progressed. The military surgeon's bible and almanac at that time was the latest edition of the Field Surgery Pocket book edited by Kirby and Blackburn and would become essential reading for all deployed military surgeons, irrespective of previous experience or colour of cloth...[1]

Clearly there were, and still are problems in training facing both groups.

## 1.3.1
### Training and Education Problems for Civilian Surgeons

Civilian surgeons and their supporting teams are now exposed (and will continue to be exposed) to battlefield ballistic and blast injuries and this exposure happens in three quite different scenarios –

- Terrorist attacks on the civilian populations in our cities and while traveling in countries with home grown terrorist groups – Bali in Indonesia for example.
- During deployments to war zones as a result of reserve service or volunteer commitment (In the UK The Territorial Army)
- During deployments as volunteers with non-governmental organizations (NGOs) in conflict and disaster environments

There seem to be irreconcilable difficulties here. The training environment has changed radically over the last 30 years. This is, and quite rightly, the age of shorter but intense training in sub-specialty fields such as colo-rectal or upper GI. Further, the European Working Time Directive is striving to achieve shorter and shorter working hours resulting in one Royal Medical College President calling the directive *"sheer lunacy."* Possible solutions will be discussed later but a personal communication with one of the editors of this 3rd edition heralds a warning. He was deployed with a leading humanitarian organization in a totally failed state – two surgeons were deployed, one orthopedic, the other a general surgeon. Perhaps not quite so general! On being told by the command that there was a need to provide a full surgical service, the general surgeon said he was a sub specialty trained, in particular, he was not trained or prepared to operate on children. In this setting – a disaster in the making is hardy an understatement.

### 1.3.2
### Training and Education Problems for Deployed Civil and Military Surgeons

Deployed surgeons, whether civilian or military face unique problems compared to civilian counterparts working in city hospitals. Deployed surgeons, while having to gain expertise in trauma and war surgery, are now faced with new difficulties. They have to take on the mantle of the old fashioned general surgeon. In the new operational environment, characterized by the failed state there is typically a collapse of the institutions of a functioning state, including health care. As a result deployed surgical (and medical teams), military and NGO, may be the only health care providers. This poses problems for all, but particularly for surgeons who, increasingly are trained within narrow specialty and sub-speciality fields. This is leading to what an eminent colleague of this author calls ".... deployed surgeons hunting in teams." Working in teams helps but is not always possible or feasible.

So in summary, we have the curious situation in which the civilian surgeon working at home has little or no trauma and war injury experience and on the other hand we are faced with a new generation of deployed military and NGO surgeons, who will probably be competent in trauma but who do not have the broad based general experience to provide care for a local population in need. A curious paradox.

### 1.4
### Towards a Solution

There is no single solution to deal with these complex problems. However, solutions, some of them novel, can be found. Based on this author's own experience some or all of the following might be considered by prospective volunteer surgeons, depending on the likely mission.

### 1.4.1
### General and Trauma Training

For civilian surgeons wishing to widen their day to day skills in general surgery and to improve their skills in trauma care there are a number of options. These options might also be useful for deployments to natural and man made disaster settings where the focus will be on old fashioned general surgery and major trauma. These include:

### 1.4.1.1
### Visits and Attachments to Leading International Trauma Centers

Increasingly health care providers and deploying agencies are turning to secondments to busy trauma center in the USA and South Africa to expose surgeons and their teams to the skills needed to manage major trauma. Johannesburg, with a very high incidence of penetrating ballistic and knife injury, is a popular destination for both civilian and military surgeons and their teams (Fig. 1.1).

### 1.4.1.2
### Courses and Workshops

Craft workshops and courses abound. Some of these such as ATLS© and DSTC©/DSTS© are particularly popular and regarded by some as mandatory. Most of these courses have supporting Web sites and provide details on course provision (Fig. 1.2).

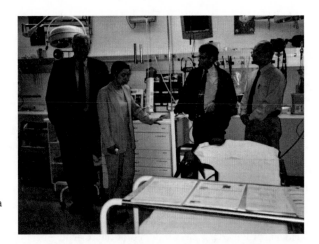

**Fig. 1.1** A UK team visiting a trauma center in Johannesburg

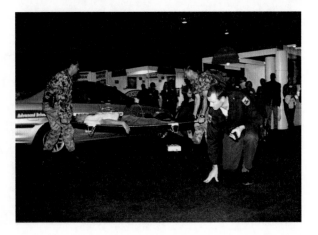

**Fig. 1.2** A pre-hospital trauma exercise in South Africa

### 1.4.1.3
### Secondments to Austere/Post Conflict Environments

These can be useful, particularly for civilian surgeons considering an austere overseas mission. The author ran a university based conflict and catastrophe center at University College London tasked with assessing health needs in post conflict and post disaster settings. While the main tasks were data gathering these missions allowed an exposure to austere environments and gave useful pointers to clinical practice in a variety of post conflict and post disaster environments. In this author's view these type of mission provide a reality check for potential volunteers prior to the real thing! One of these missions was to the former Soviet republic of Azerbaijan.

#### *Azerbaijan Assessment Mission 1997–2003*

Azerbaijan, a former Soviet Republic, now independent state, serves as a good case example. Although now a recovering state, in 1997 it fitted the definition of a failed state. The background to the crisis in Azerbaijan can be summarized as

- 70 years of control by the former Soviet Union
- Devastation of the territory's agricultural and industrial base.
- Breakdown of the national health system.
- All major hospitals, although geographically distant from the conflict zone, suffered from the consequences of financial ruin and loss of social cohesion.
- Major teaching hospitals fared better retaining staff and supported by a growing private practice
- Creation of dozens of refugee and IDP camps accommodating up to one million men, women, and children.

Deployment to Azerbaijan of UK NHS volunteer health care professionals, particularly surgeons, anesthetists, and emergency physicians, gave an unparalleled exposure to the practice of medicine in all its generality well away from the "ivory tower" of the modern NHS and provided priceless training for future deployment (Figs. 1.3 and 1.4).

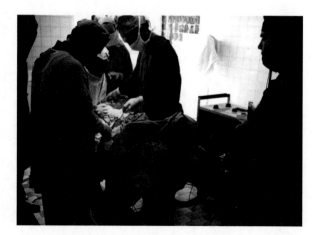

**Fig. 1.3** Expatriate and local surgeons operate in an Azeri university hospital in the capital Baku

**Fig. 1.4** Professor
P Mahoney, mentoring
theater staff in an Azeri
hospital

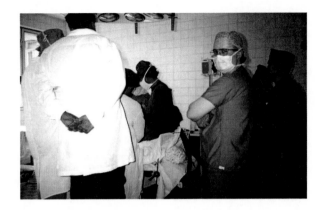

## 1.4.2
## War and Conflict Surgery Training

Visits or detachments to zones of conflict are not an option – these environments are not for the novice and should not be seen as opportunities for training. Likewise, although secondments to major trauma center are useful they cannot reproduce the nature and range of injuries nor the working environment. It is interesting to consider what the UK Defence Medical Services do to prepare and inoculate their teams.

### 1.4.2.1
### Master – Apprentice Training

This is an on-going process in peacetime but requires two key elements – a reservoir of master war and trauma surgeons and a ready supply of materials – patients on which to practice. In the period of unrest in Northern Ireland 1969–2002 and at the time of the Falklands War of 1982 there were masters and patients aplenty (Fig. 1.5).

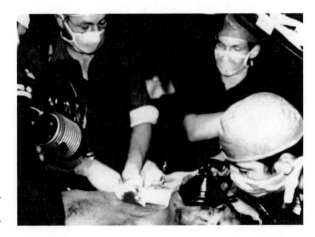

**Fig. 1.5** The Master –
Apprentice system at work
in the Falkland Islands 1982.
The Master Surgeon is the
late Colonel Bill McGreggor

Now there are few masters in war and trauma and new strategies are being tried. These include.

### 1.4.2.2
### Courses and Workshops in War and Conflict Surgery

These are run by military and humanitarian agencies. The ICRC and the Defence Medical Services in UK run regular principles of war surgery courses for deployed teams. Complimenting these is a series of specialist craft workshops covering maxillo-facial, neurosurgical, and vascular injury. Two relatively recent initiatives merit further comment.

### Definitive Surgical Trauma Skills ©

This is a tri-partite course run jointly by the Royal College of Surgeons of England, The Royal Centre for Defence Medicine and the United Services University of the Health Sciences in Bethesda, MD, USA. It is a 2 day hands on, master class cadaver based course covering abdominal, vascular, and thoracic injury with international military and civilian trauma surgeons as faculty. Military and civilian students from Europe are the main participants and feed back is very positive. Variants of this course are run in many countries in the world, many using a bleeding live animal model which is forbidden in the UK.

### Military Field Hospital Deployment Exercises (Hospexs)

These training exercises are held in Strensall, outside York, and are aimed at collective training for field hospital staff about to deploy. A modular field hospital with virtually full equipment scales and departments is used. Exercise casualties, based on actual casualty data from Iraq and Afghanistan, are fed into the hospital over a 3 day period. The aim is to facilitate collective team training covering all aspects of hospital activity, including command and control, communication, casualty evacuation as well as clinical activity covering A&E, ITU, Theater, wards, and all support functions.

This environment provides a highly realistic training tool as evidenced by feed back from deployed teams. Training is being enhanced by the addition of computer controlled simulators providing real time physiology and responses to interventions.

### 1.5
### Summary

This paper reviews war and conflict trauma over a near 30 year period – a period that has seen radical change both in society and in the way medical training is conducted. "May you live in interesting times" is a well-known Chinese aphorism attributed to Confucius. We do live

**Fig. 1.6** Troops in Helmand, Afghanistan 2009. Cpl Tony Green

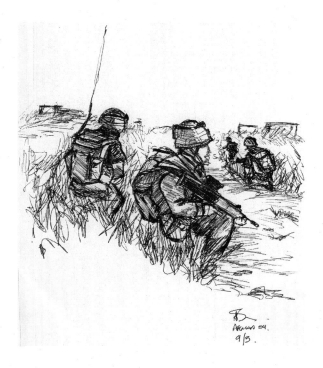

in interesting and changed times. As demand grows for wider skills in the deployed setting, our colleges and universities are producing ever more sub specialized hospital doctors, particularly surgeons. There are no easy answers – however novel solutions are being discussed and some of these are outlined in this paper. It is too early to say if these will be successful – the author and editors hope this new edition will be part of the wider solution.

## References

1. Ryan JM. A personal reflection on the Falklands Islands War of 1982. *J R Army Med Corps*. 2007;153:88-91.
2. Ryan JM, Rich NM, Dale RF, Morgans BT, Cooper GJ. *Ballistic Trauma: Clinical Relevance in Peace and War*. London: Hodder Arnold; 1997:18-20.

Quotes from reference 1 used with permission of the Editor. *J R Army Med Corps*.

# A Personal Experience

**2**

Damian Douglas Keene

## 2.1
## Background

For 7 months I was based in Helmand province, Afghanistan as a Medical Officer providing medical care to the deployed ISAF forces. Most of this care was provided from Combat outposts (COPs) or Forward Operating Bases (FOBs) which are isolated locations that combat troops use to push out patrols and secure areas of Helmand provinces "Green Zone," this is a band of fertile land that runs along the banks of the Helmand river.

This time was spent based in six different outposts, some more "mature" than others but the principals behind the way trauma care was delivered always fell back to the same system.

- Catastrophic Hemorrhage
- Airway
- Breathing
- Circulation

Word was received that an improvised explosive device (IED) had detonated next to an Afghan National Army (ANA) vehicle and that there were two casualties on route with unknown injuries.

On Arrival one walked up the steps so was directed towards a medic. The next casualty was brought in on his side on a stretcher, he was very agitated and struggling to breathe. The only injuries were to his face and once the interpreter had spoken to him it became clear his agitation was due to his difficulty breathing rather than a head injury.

In this instance his only life threatening injury was to his airway; he was bleeding heavily from his mouth, had loose teeth in his lower jaw, and it became apparent that his maxilla was fractured and hanging down into his mouth effectively mechanically obstructing his airway. Immediate thoughts were he was going to need a cricothyroidotomy.

D.D. Keene
Anaesthetics Department, Defence Medical Services, Anaesthetics and Intensive Care, University Hospitals Birmingham, Birmingham, UK
e-mail: damokeene@doctors.org.uk

A.J. Brooks et al. (eds.), *Ryan's Ballistic Trauma*,
DOI: 10.1007/978-1-84882-124-8_2, © Springer-Verlag London Limited 2011

First we sat him up and lent him forward to allow the blood to drain. The remaining loose teeth were removed to prevent aspiration. His maxilla was reduced back to its normal position manually and held in place. Despite the posture improving the airway the patient still had poor saturations and it was difficult to keep an oxygen mask on him as it filled with blood. A yankauer sucker was used to try to improve things leaving it in his mouth and a further effort to reduce the bleeding was made by packing the lower jaw where teeth had been dislodged. It was possible to keep him in this position as he understood what was happening and what we were doing.

The suction ran out of power after 10 min and he immediately struggled to breathe again; we had collected 200 mL of blood in this time as well as a significant amount on the stretcher. There was nothing else that could be done to reduce the bleeding further. When the suction was plugged in things improved again- this gave us another issue. The HLS was outside the building and we had only a 10 min window in which to move the casualty. He was kept and transferred sat up upon the arrival of the MERT, It was decided to wait for the helicopter to land before moving the casualty the 200 m to the HLS so that the suction would last until he was handed over.

This incident highlighted that simple things are best. Position was enough to improve the airway without any advanced interventions. It brought an acute awareness of the importance of communication, as blast injury can result both in hearing loss and loss of sight through direct injury.

At one stage, four casualties with unknown injuries/mechanism were received, they were all children-roughly 6 years old; two walked in and one was carried.

This was the first time I had really seen pediatric trauma let alone been responsible for their care.

The non walking casualty was assessed and had a broken ankle but was otherwise unhurt, a medic assessed the other two casualties. One had minor bruises. The other had an open depressed skull fracture but had no neurological deficit.

This left one casualty unaccounted for. After discussion through the interpreter it appeared that all had been involved in a tractor "roll over" and the driver of the vehicle was still to arrive. Ten minutes later he was brought in to the aid post. He was 14 years old and responsive but in severe pain.

Monitoring and intravenous access was obtained and a primary survey concurrently carried out. He was tachycardic at 150 and had a BP of 100/40 which was checked manually. Initial assessment of C<ABC picked up no external hemorrhage or penetrating injuries. It was apparent he had a deformity at his left hip and was very tender suprapubically. There was blood at the external urethral meatus indicating a likely pelvic fracture. The pelvis was not "sprung" as it was not going to change management. At this stage casevac was requested with a description of injuries.

He then lost his radial pulses and had dropped his GCS to 12. Fluid was given to maintain a radial pulse while the MERT was awaited, and they were informed over the radio of his deteriorating condition. It took an hour and a half for the MERT to arrive from the time he had been brought to the aid post; during this time he required 3 L of fluid to maintain a radial pulse.

The MERT arrived and the team disembarked as we were approaching the ramp so we moved the casualty away from the Chinnook. As they had had an update on his condition a decision had been made to stabilize him on the ground as much as possible. He was transferred to a vacuum mattress and given O neg blood and thawed plasma and then loaded on to the MERT for evacuation.

## 2.2
## Summary

Despite what are outwardly very significant injuries, basic care delivered well by often very junior medical personnel will keep casualties alive until more senior help arrives.

# The War in West Philadelphia

# 3

John P. Pryor[†]

> *Dr. John Pryor died on active duty in Iraq on Christmas Day 2008. He wrote this essay following his first tour of Iraq in 2006 and it was published in the Washington Post in 2007 (http://www.drjohnpryor.com/John_Pryor/War_in_Philadelphia.html). This book is dedicated to him.*

I didn't hear the cars screech to a halt, but one of the trauma nurses did. He ran outside with two emergency department medics to find several people in a car, all of their clothes soaked with blood. The passengers were screaming for someone to help the young man in the front seat, who was unresponsive. The team threw the limp victim onto a gurney, one of several that stand waiting for these types of scenarios, which occur almost nightly at our trauma center.

As the gurney rolled in, I saw a lifeless young man with more gunshot wounds than I could count. I was poised to start a resuscitation effort when a voice behind me announced that three more were coming in. As the team started CPR and checked for cardiac activity, the second and third victims were wheeled in.

A young girl had a gunshot wound to the abdomen that made her writhe in pain. Her movements were slow and her mental functioning was impaired, signaling to me that she was in profound shock – she was dying. I caught only a passing glance of the third patient, who had a gunshot wound to the neck and was coughing up blood. Those brief images were enough for me to sum up a desperate situation; I pronounced the first patient dead to concentrate resources on the other critically injured.

The nursing staff rolled the dead man's body into a bed and readied the stall for the fourth patient, who had three gunshot wounds to his right arm and two to his left. With the emergency medicine physicians, surgery residents, and medics working on the two critical patients, I assigned the fourth patient to a capable medical student who courageously accepted the battlefield promotion to intern.

In the swirl of screams and moving figures, my mind drifted to my recent experience in Iraq as an Army surgeon. There we dealt regularly with "mascals," or mass-casualty situations. In Iraq, ironically, I found myself drawing on my experience as a civilian trauma surgeon each time mascals would overrun the combat hospital. As nine or ten patients

J.P. Pryor[†]
Division of Traumatology and Surgical Critical Care, Department of Surgery,
University of Pennsylvania Medical Center, Philadelphia, PA, USA

A.J. Brooks et al. (eds.), *Ryan's Ballistic Trauma*,
DOI: 10.1007/978-1-84882-124-8_3, © Springer-Verlag London Limited 2011

from a firefight rolled in, I sometimes caught myself saying "just like another Friday night in West Philadelphia."

The wounds and nationalities of the patients are different, but the feelings of helplessness, despair, and loss are the same. In Iraq, soldiers die for freedom, for honor, for their country, and for their buddies. Here in Philadelphia, they die without honor, without purpose, for no country, for no one.

More young men are killed each day on the streets of America than on the worst days of carnage and loss in Iraq. There is a war at home raging every day, filling our trauma centers with so many wounded children that it sometimes makes Baghdad seem like a quiet city in Iowa.

Unlike the Iraq conflict, this war is not on the front pages of The Post or on CNN. You have heard of the Washington area sniper shootings and the massacre at Virginia Tech. I am sure you have not heard about the "Lex Street massacre," in which ten people ages 15–56 were lined up and shot, execution-style, in the winter of 2000. Seven were killed, three critically injured.

You haven't heard about this tragedy because it happened to inner-city poor people in a crack house in Philadelphia. Imagine, for a moment, if this had occurred in a suburban shopping mall or if a Marine unit in Iraq had been involved. There would be shock, outrage, 24-h news coverage, Senate hearings, and a new color of ribbon to wear. That double standard, that triage of compassion and empathy, is why the war on the streets continues unabated.

I am on call Wednesday night. The statistics indicate that then I will once again walk with the chaplain to a small room off the emergency room. I will open a heavy brown door and make eye contact with a room full of people; a mother, perhaps a father or a grandmother. They will look at me with tears welling up, their knees weak, and lean forward while watching my lips, bracing for news about their loved one. I will remain standing and reach out to hold the mother's hand. My announcement will be short and firm, the intonation polished from years of practice. The words will be simple for me to say, but sharp as a sword for them to hear; "I am sorry, your son has died."

# Part II

## Weapons, Blast and Ballistics

# How Guns Work

# 4

Mark Byers, Kerry Starkey, and Peter F. Mahoney

## 4.1
## Introduction

This chapter is written for clinical staff with little or no previous exposure to firearms. Although one must "treat the wound and not the weapon," acknowledgment of how firearms work should lead to a better understanding of how bullets and other projectiles cause injury.

## 4.2
## History

Nearly all firearms work the same way. An explosive force is applied to a projectile that is propelled down a tube to fly towards its target. The first guns were cannons, the first propellant was black powder, and the first projectiles were cannon balls. Gunpowder was placed in the barrel, the cannon ball rolled in, and then the gunpowder was ignited. The hot gases produced by the burning gunpowder pushed the cannon ball up and out of the barrel.

The nineteenth century saw the development of the cartridge. The cartridge packaged the bullet, propellant, and primer/detonator within a case. This allowed the development of repeating firearms, such as the bolt-action rifle (Table 4.1).

## 4.3
## Small Arms: Revolvers and Pistols

Some of the first modern small arms were revolvers (Fig. 4.2). Cartridges are loaded into a chamber, the chamber revolves, lines up with a fixed barrel, and then the cartridge's primer is struck by a hammer. The propellant ignites and the cartridge expands within the

P.F. Mahoney (✉)
Defence Professor Anaesthesia and Critical Care, Royal Centre for Defence Medicine, Birmingham, UK
e-mail: prof.dmacc@rcdm.bham.ac.uk

A.J. Brooks et al. (eds.), *Ryan's Ballistic Trauma*,
DOI: 10.1007/978-1-84882-124-8_4, © Springer-Verlag London Limited 2011

**Table 4.1** Major landmarks in the development of firearms

| Date | Development/event | Significance | Note/reference |
|---|---|---|---|
| Paleolithic times, BC | Use of bow to project a missile | Important step in ballistic weapon design, represented the use of stored mechanical energy from the bent bow being used to propel a projectile | |
| Mid thirteenth century | Explosive powder formulated | | |
| End of fourteenth century | Hand guns | | Had taken place on battlefield by early fifteenth century |
| 1324 | Firearms | | |
| 1326 | Earliest record of a firearm (man depicted firing a cannon) | Represents change from stored mechanical energy (the bow) to chemical energy as the means of propulsion | Walter's De Officiis Regnum |
| 1521 | First *effective* use of the Musket at the siege of Parma | | |
| 1530 | Trigger mechanisms improved and the means of igniting the charge in the gun changed | Weapons could be carried cocked and ready to fire | Pyrites applied to a serrated wheel produced a spark to ignite the powder charge |
| 1635 | Perfection of flintlock (French) | Reliable mechanism with durability, easy maintenance, and low cost, suitable for general use by whole armies of foot soldiers | Flintlock musket became the dominant battlefield weapon over the next 200 years |
| 1775–1783 | High muzzle velocity rifle used by colonists in the American War of independence | Up to 500 m/s and accurate to 400 m | |

| 1776 | British Armed Forces prototype high muzzle velocity rifle (Colonel Patrick Ferguson) | Breech loading with effective rate of fire of four shot's/min at 200 m, and hit the bull's eye at 100 m | |
| First half of nineteenth century | Military rifle replaced the musket | Breech loading allowed tighter fit of ball in barrel allowing the weapon to be loaded without standing. Reduced risk of user being hit by enemy fire | Seven Weeks War (1866), the Austrians used muzzle-loading and suffered greater numbers of casualties than the Prussians using the breech loader |
| Mid eighteenth century | Invention of the Minié bullet | | The base expanded to provide a tight fit between the bullet and rifling when the weapon was fired |
| 1850s | British modification of Minié bullet for the Enfield rifle | | Smaller caliber, 0.577 in. |
| 1870–1871 | Franco-Prussian War both sides used breech-loading rifles | Caused more than 90% of casualties from each side | |
| Mid eighteenth century | Invention of the percussion cap | Rifle no longer required priming to initiate the charge | |
| Last quarter of nineteenth century | Invention of magazine rifles | Faster re-loading permit increased rates of fire | The tubular magazine in the Winchester repeating rifle, used by the Turks defending Plevna against the Russians (1877) proved to be effective, rapid, and disciplined fire could be used to great effect |

(continued)

**Table 4.1** (continued)

| Date | Development/event | Significance | Note/reference |
|---|---|---|---|
| 1870s–1880s | Improvement in gunpowder and more powerful cartridges | Spin-stabilized rounds could be fired at muzzle velocities of around 600 m/s | Lead bullets had to be jacketed with copper or nickel due to closer fit and faster velocity |
| | Tubular magazine | Problems of the nose of one round firing the percussion cap of the adjacent round in the magazine as the rifle recoiled | The Lee bolt action overcame this problem |
| | Lee bolt action | Provided a clip of bullets and cartridges stacked side by side in a spring loaded metal box, bullets were pushed sequentially into the chamber, as the bolt extracted the spent cartridge | Lee bolt action coupled with Metford or Enfield barrel provided the standard British rifle from 1888 until the mid-twentieth century. Lee Enfield and German Mauser each fired a jacketed bullet weighing about 11 g at a muzzle velocity of 800 m/s, and were effective up to a distance of 1,000 m |
| 1870 | *Mitrailleuse* machine gun brought into service by French in Franco-Prussian War | Progression from rapid manual reloading to automatic reloading, firing, and cartridge ejection | 25 barrels fired sequentially by turning a crank producing a rate of fire approaching 300 rounds/min |
| 1860s | Gatling gun adopted by British Army and used in the Zulu War (1979) | | Also used a hand-cranking mechanism |
| 1883 | Gatling gun modified | Used a drum fed system | |
| 1893 | Gatling gun modified | Electric motor added | Rate of fire 3,000 rounds/min |
| 1880s | Hiram Maxim used recoil of the gun to extract the cartridge, reload, and fire | | Modified over the 1880s and adopted into the service of several European armies (1890), including the Vickers (0.303 in.) which was in service in the British Army until 1968 |

| | | | |
|---|---|---|---|
| 1895 | Machine gun using "Blow-back" technique pioneered by Browning was used by the US army | "Blow-back" technique is the basis of most of today's automatic weapons | Gas from the combustion of the charge, rather than recoil was used to provide the power for extraction, loading, and firing |
| Late 1960s–1970s | Development of the automatic rifle or *Sturmgewehr* (assault rifle) | Automatic weapons lighter and more available to the general infantry man | Germans appreciated that the standard infantry rifle of the Second World War was unnecessarily high powered and therefore selected an intermediate-powered cartridge, and adopted a cross between the lightweight submachine gun and the normal rifle |
| 1970s | Western forces changed to 5.56 mm ammunition<br>Former Soviet Union adopted 5.45 mm bullet for the AK74<br>Larger caliber ammunition was retained for snipers' rifles, some light support weapons, and heavier machine guns | | |

Adapted from Ryan by K Starkey[7]

**Fig. 4.1** Helmand Afghanistan 2009. Cpl Tony Green

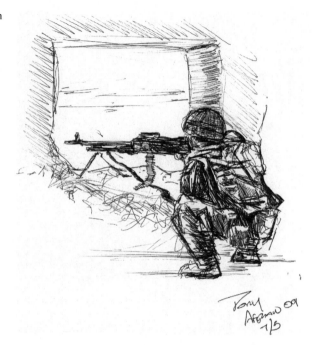

cylinder, forcing all the gases forward, which accelerates the bullet down the barrel. Grooves in the barrel spin the bullet, which imparts stability to the bullet in flight and improves accuracy.

The original revolvers needed to have their hammer manually pulled back until it caught. The trigger then could be pulled, and the hammer was released (the "single-action" revolver). "Double-action" revolvers can be used the same way. Alternatively, by exerting continued pressure on the trigger, the hammer moves back and compresses a spring housed in the handle. A lever attached to the trigger causes a ratchet to turn the cartridge cylinder to align the next bullet with the barrel. When the hammer is all the way back, further pressure on the trigger releases it and it is pushed forward by the spring.

Revolvers are robust, simple, and rarely malfunction. Revolvers do have disadvantages. They need frequent reloading, and the empty cases need to be ejected manually from the cylinder.

The modern pistol has a magazine that holds more cartridges than the revolver cylinder and is capable of self-loading as the magazine itself is spring loaded (Fig. 4.3). The magazine spring pushes a cartridge into place, which is loaded, fired, and then automatically ejected. There are two methods for self-loading. The simplest method employs the reaction forces of the fired cartridge to push back a heavy breech block against a breech spring. The empty casing is discarded and the breech block is pushed forward by the breech spring, collects the next bullet (forced into place by the magazine spring), and loads it into the barrel. The trigger then can be pulled; the cartridge is fired and the process repeats itself.

**Fig. 4.2** The mechanism of
the Colt "Frontier" revolver
(Reprinted from Wilkinson[3])

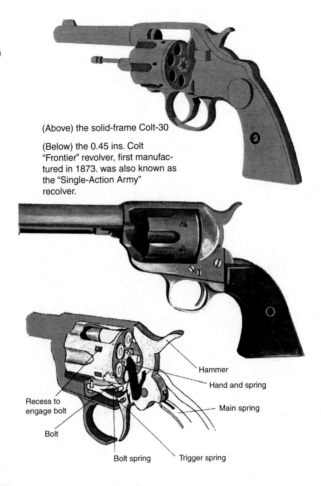

(Above) the solid-frame Colt-30

(Below) the 0.45 ins. Colt
"Frontier" revolver, first manufac-
tured in 1873. was also known as
the "Single-Action Army"
recolver.

Hammer

Hand and spring

Recess to
engage bolt

Main spring

Bolt

Bolt spring       Trigger spring

## 4.4
## Rifles and Carbines

Modern rifles have long barrels cut with a spiral groove to spin the bullet. The spin imparts stability to the bullet in flight. Carbines are shorter and lighter (Fig. 4.4). The first breech-loaded rifle appeared in the 1830s. Individual cartridges were loaded by a bolt, which cocked and housed the firing pin. By the 1880s, the Swiss, French, and Germans had developed a bolt-action rifle with a magazine using full metal-jacketed bullets. The more bullets that can be housed in the magazine, the more that can be individually loaded and fired using the bolt action before the magazine is empty and has to be changed.

Similar advances occurred in rifles as had occurred in pistols, and semiautomatic and automatic rifles were developed. Semiautomatic rifles work in a similar manner to semiautomatic pistols. Gases from firing a bullet are used to re-cock and reload the weapon with the next bullet from the magazine, but the trigger has to be pulled again to fire the next bullet.

To achieve higher rates of fire, manufacturers developed the machine gun.

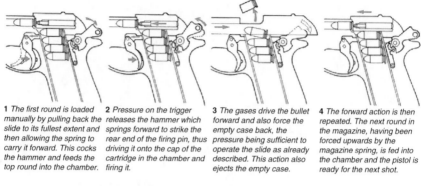

1 *The first round is loaded manually by pulling back the slide to its fullest extent and then allowing the spring to carry it forward. This cocks the hammer and feeds the top round into the chamber.*

2 *Pressure on the trigger releases the hammer which springs forward to strike the rear end of the firing pin, thus driving it onto the cap of the cartridge in the chamber and firing it.*

3 *The gases drive the bullet forward and also force the empty case back, the pressure being sufficient to operate the slide as already described. This action also ejects the empty case.*

4 *The forward action is then repeated. The next round in the magazine, having been forced upwards by the magazine spring, is fed into the chamber and the pistol is ready for the next shot.*

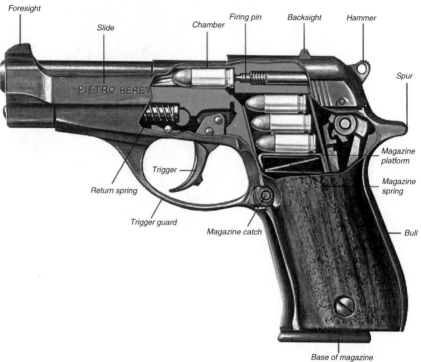

**Fig. 4.3** Diagram of semiautomatic pistol, Beretta Modello 84 (With permission, Myatt[4])

## 4.5
## Machine Guns

A machine gun (Fig. 4.5) is an automatic weapon. The term includes automatic rifles, "assault rifles," and submachine guns. They are belt or magazine fed, and theoretically keep firing for as long as the trigger is depressed or until the ammunition runs out.

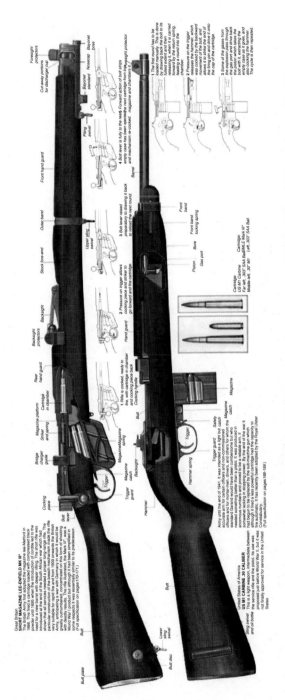

**Fig. 4.4** Upper picture shows the bolt action Lee enfield MK III rifle. Lower picture shows the US M1 carbine (With permission, Myatt[1])

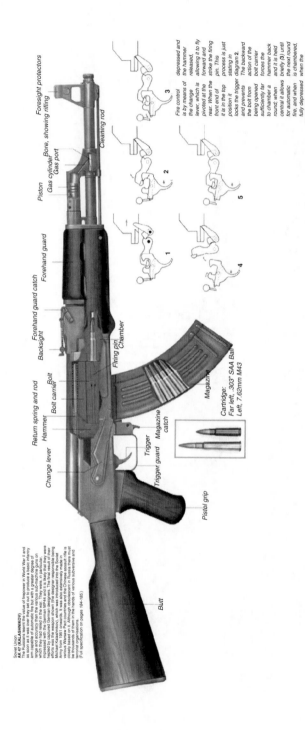

**Fig. 4.5** Diagram of AK47 (With permission, Myatt[1])

Foresight protectors

Cleaning rod

Bore, showing rifling

Gas cylinder

Gas port

Piston

Foresight protectors

Forehand guard

Forehand guard catch

Backsight

Firing pin

Chamber

Return spring and rod

Hammer

Bolt

Bolt carrier

Change lever

Trigger

Trigger guard

Magazine catch

Magazine

Cartridge:
Far left, .303" SAA Ball
Left, 7.62mm M43

Pistol grip

Butt

Fire control is by means of the change lever, which is pivoted at the rear. When the front end of it is in the top position it locks the trigger and prevents the bolt from being opened sufficiently far to chamber a round, when central it allows for automatic fire, and when fully depressed it gives single shot. Diagram **1** shows the weapon cocked and set for automatic, the hammer being held back by the sear. When the bolt is forward and locked and the trigger pressed, the sear is depressed and the hammer released, allowing it to fly forward and strike the firing pin. This process is just stating in diagram **2**. The backward action of the bolt carrier forces the hammer back and it is held briefly (3) until the next round is chambered, when the process is repeated. At single rounds the hammer, having been forced back in the normal way, is held back by an auxiliary sear and cannot be released until the trigger has again been pressed (**4** and **5**).

Soviet Union
AK 47 (KALASHNIKOV)
The Russians learnt the value of firepower in World War II and as soon as it was over they set out to produce a basic infantry arm capable of automatic fire but with a greater degree of range and accuracy than the various sub-machine guns on which they had relied in the war. They were, in particular, impressed with the German MP44 and it is likely that they were helped by captured German designers. The final result of their efforts was the weapon shown (the designer responsible being Michael Kalashnikov), which was introduced into the Soviet Army from 1951 onwards. It was also extensively made in various Warsaw Pact countries and the Chinese assault rifle is closely based on it. Although obsolescent in Russia there must be thousands of them in the hands of various subversive and terrorist organisations.
(Full specification on pages 184–185.)

## 4.6
## Shotguns

Shotguns, developed for sport or combat, fire a cartridge containing shot (Fig. 4.6). Shotguns may be single barreled or double barreled. If double barreled the barrels may be next to each other (side by side) or one on top of the other (under and over). Working mechanisms include semiautomatic and pump action (Fig. 4.7). Shotgun calibers are measured by the number of spherical lead balls, of the same diameter as the barrel, that make up a pound of lead.

For instance, an 8-bore has the same diameter as a 2-ounce ball of lead ($8 \times 2$ oz $= 16$ oz or 1 lb). The 12-bore has a diameter the same as a 1.33-ounce ball of lead ($12 \times 1.33$ oz $= 16$ oz or 1 lb). The smaller the bore number of the gun, the larger the diameter of the barrel and the cartridge.[1]

Cartridges contain primer, propellant, and shot. The choking of the gun determines how much the shot spreads on discharge. A fully choked gun has a narrower barrel than a gun with true cylinders. Choking gives constrictions ranging from 3- to 40-thousandths of an inch towards the muzzle end of the barrel. The constriction means that the shot is kept closer together as it leaves the end of the barrel. The other feature that affects the spread of shot is the length of the barrel. A short barrel allows the shot to spread out earlier after discharge than a long barrel. A "sawn-off" shotgun is a shotgun with its barrels cut off, thus shortening the weapon and allowing early and wide spread of the shot. In the US, the legal barrel limit is 20 in.

Combat shotguns are designed to be quick to load and relatively short barreled. They are commonly "slide-loaded" or pump action, have a magazine under the barrel, and gain their effect from the ammunition they use. Where as sporting shotguns use small loads with many hundreds of pellets per shell (e.g. No. 7 shot for a 12-bore shotgun has 361 pellets per shell), combat shotguns use shells such as the double 00 buck, which are loaded with nine balls each. Shotguns have an effective range of between 30 and 50 m. Beyond this distance, the velocity falls off and the spread increases markedly.

## 4.7
## Ammunition

There is a great deal of difference between pistol and rifle ammunition. Pistol ammunition is designed to be accurate to a range of around 40 m, whereas rifle rounds need to be capable of hitting a target up to 1,000 or more meters away (Fig. 4.8). Pistol ammunition usually is straight cased. Rifle ammunition is often "bottle necked," so it can contain a larger amount of propellant.

The distinction is not quite so clear, as there are pistols that fire rifle ammunition and long-barreled weapons (including some submachine guns) that fire pistol ammunition.

**Fig. 4.6** A modern Eley cartridge showing (**a**) crimp closure, (**b**) frangible waterproof seal, (**c**) plastic case, (**d**) under-shot card, (**e**) vegetable felt "Kleena" wad, (**f**) over-powder card, (**g**) doubled-based powder, (**h**) compressed paper base wad, and (**i**) cap or primer (With permission, Thomas[5])

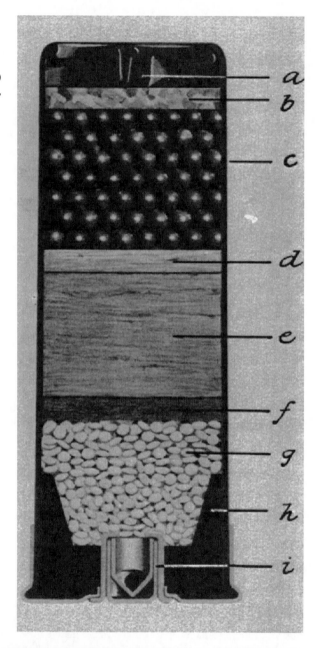

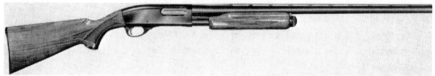

**Fig. 4.7** A typical American pump gun. The model shown is the popular Remington M 870 (With permission, Thomas[5])

**Fig. 4.8** A 5.56 mm modern, high-velocity assault rifle round is shown on the left. Note its slender, elongated shape and sharp, pointed nose. On the right is a short, squat, blunt-nosed 9 mm low-velocity handgun round (With permission, Ryan[6])

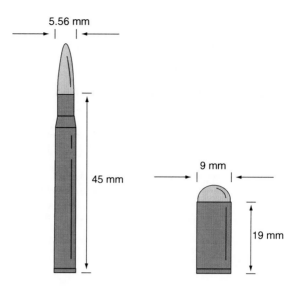

There are several different sorts of bullets, such as:

- *Full Metal Jacket*: A metal casing around a lead core. This produces a nonexpanding, deep-penetrating round that is considered very reliable.
- *Jacketed Hollow Point*: These bullets have an exposed, hollowed lead tip that allows expansion of the round on impact. They are likely to penetrate tissue less deeply than a full metal jacket bullet but more energy is transferred to the tissue.
- *Soft Point*: An exposed lead tip allows the bullet to expand rapidly on impact at lower velocities. A wide wound of up to 200% of original bullet diameter is produced from the round's rapid expansion.
- *Altered Ammunition*: People alter ammunition to increase the severity of the inflicted wounds. An example is the Dum Dum, produced by cutting a cross in the soft lead tip of the bullet to ensure it that it fragments on impact. The term Dum Dum comes from the Dum-Dum Arsenal in India, which produced soft-nosed bullets for the British Army in about 1890 for the Lee Metford rifle. British troops found their weapons did not have as much stopping power with the new full metal-jacketed bullets compared to the 0.45 ≤ Martini-Henry rifles, and this led them to modify the bullet design. An amendment to the The Geneva Convention banned such projectiles.
- *Rubber Bullets*: Rubber bullets first were used in Northern Ireland in 1970 by the British Army. The missiles are blunt-nosed, with a low muzzle velocity, and they are designed to inflict superficial injuries only, but they have caused death.[2]

In 1989, they were replaced by plastic bullets, which were considered less dangerous. There are several variants available in many countries, including rubber-coated metal bullets, rubber plugs, and beanbag rounds (a fabric beanbag full of lead pellets).

## References

1. Sedgwick NM. *The Young Shot*. 3rd ed. London, England: Adam and Charles Black Ltd; 1975.
2. Millar R, Rutherford WH, Johnston S, Malhotra VJ. Injuries caused by rubber bullets: a report on 90 patients. *Br J Surg*. 1975;62:480-486.
3. Wilkinson F. *Guns*. Hamlyn; 1970:121.
4. Myatt F. *Modern Small Arms*. London: Salamander Books; 1978:154-161.
5. Thomas G. *Shotguns & Cartridges for Game and Clays*. 4th ed. London, England: Adam and Charles Black; 1987:86.
6. Ryan JM, Biant L. Gunshot wounds and blast injury. In: Greaves I, Porter K, eds. *Pre-hospital Medicine: The Principles and Practice of Immediate Care*. London: Arnold; 1999:363-373.
7. Ryan JM, Rich NM, Dale RF, Morgans BT, Cooper GJ, eds. *Ballistic Trauma: Clinical Relevance in Peace and War*. London: Hodder Arnold; 1997:11-14.

# The Effects of Bullets

# 5

Donald H. Jenkins

*The opinions expressed herein are the private views of the authors and are not to be construed as official or reflecting the views of the US Department of the Army, or the US Department of the Air Force, or the US Department of Defense.*

## 5.1
## Introduction

Bullets cause wounds by interacting with body tissues. The kinetic energy (KE) of a bullet is given by the formula $KE = \frac{1}{2} MV^2$, where $M$ is the bullet's mass and $V$ is the velocity. While the formula indicates how much energy is available, it does not describe how this energy is used nor the surgical magnitude of the problem.

A number of factors influence the severity of the wound, including the diameter, shape, and composition of the projectile, its linear and rotational velocity, and the type of tissue struck, including intermediate targets (Fig. 5.1).

## 5.2
## Mechanism of Injury

There are two areas of projectile–tissue interaction in missile-caused wounds: the permanent and the temporary cavity. The *permanent* cavity is the localized area of cell necrosis, proportional to the size of the projectile as it passes through tissue. The *temporary* cavity is the transient lateral displacement of tissue, which occurs after passage of the projectile. *Elastic* tissue, such as skeletal muscle, blood vessels, and skin, may be pushed aside after

D.H. Jenkins
Surgery Department, Trauma, Critical Care and General Surgery,
Mayo Clinic, Rochester, MN, USA
e-mail: Jenkins.Donald@mayo.edu

A.J. Brooks et al. (eds.), *Ryan's Ballistic Trauma*,
DOI: 10.1007/978-1-84882-124-8_5, © Springer-Verlag London Limited 2011

**Fig. 5.1** The energy transferred to the tissues by a bullet depends upon the bullet's shape, how it impacts the tissue (point first, side first, or blunt end first) (Reprinted from *NATO Handbook*[1])

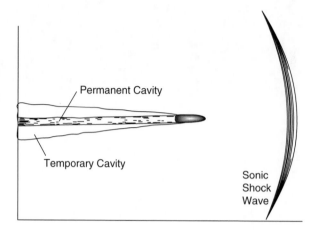

passage of the projectile, but then rebound. *Inelastic* tissue, such as bone or liver, may fracture.

Below are some examples of the characteristics of commonly encountered firearms seen throughout the world. The illustrations are of the entire path of missiles fired consistently at 5–10 m in range into ordnance gelatin tissue-simulant blocks. Variations of range and intermediate targets such as body armor and different body tissues will alter the wound seen.

## 5.3
## Examples of Different Bullet Effects

The AK-47 rifle is one of the most common weapons seen throughout the world. For this particular bullet (full metal jacketed or ball), there is a 25 cm path of relatively minimal tissue disruption before the projectile begins to yaw. This explains why relatively minimal tissue disruption may be seen with some wounds (Fig. 5.2).

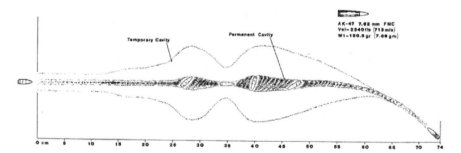

**Fig. 5.2** The AK-47 rifle is one of the most common weapons seen throughout the world (Reprinted from *NATO Handbook*[1])

The AK-74 rifle was an attempt to create a smaller-caliber assault rifle. The standard bullet does not deform in the tissue simulant, but does yaw relatively early (about 7 cm of penetration) (Fig. 5.3).

The M-16A1 rifle fires a 55-grain full metal-jacketed bullet (M-193) at approximately 950 m/s. The average point forward distance in tissue is about 12 cm, after which it yaws to about 90°, flattens, and then breaks at the cannalure (a groove placed around the middle section of the bullet). The slightly heavier M-855 bullet used with the M-16A2 rifle shows a similar pattern to the M-193 bullet (Fig. 5.4).

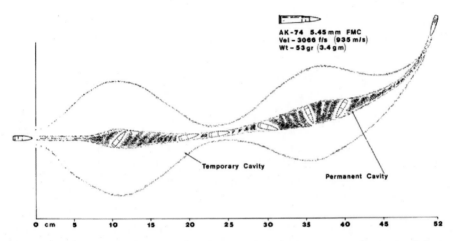

**Fig. 5.3** The AK-74 rifle was an attempt to create a smaller caliber assault rifle (Reprinted from *NATO Handbook*[1])

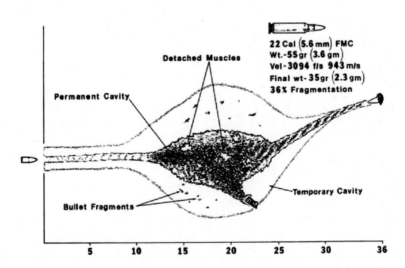

**Fig. 5.4** The M-16A1 rifle fires a 55-grain full metal-jacketed bullet (M-193) at approximately 950 m/s (Reprinted from *NATO Handbook*[1])

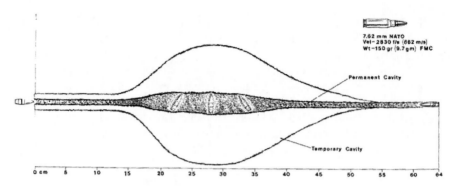

**Fig. 5.5** The 7.62 mm NATO rifle cartridge still is used in sniper rifles and machine guns (Reprinted from *NATO Handbook*[1])

The 7.62 mm NATO rifle cartridge still is used in sniper rifles and machine guns. After about 16 cm of penetration, this bullet yaws through 90° and then travels base forward. A large temporary cavity is formed and occurs at the point of maximum yaw (Fig. 5.5).

The wound created by a shotgun is created by the shot. The actual size and damage done is a function of the size of shot used and the range from which the gun is fired. As a rough guide, ranges over 10 m produce multiple superficial wounds; between 5 and 10 m, the pellets can penetrate deeply into the tissue; and below 5 m, the shot acts as a solid "slug." The slug can penetrate deeply, impart a great deal of energy, and produce a large high-energy transfer wound. Additionally, the wounds often are contaminated.

Bullet wounds and their different characteristics are considered further in Chapter 12, on "Forensic Aspects of Ballistic Injury."

## 5.4
## Summary

All small arms work in roughly the same way. An explosive imparts a force to a missile (bullet) that is directed along a tube towards its target.

Bullets cause wounds by interacting with tissue. The factors involved with the production of a missile wound are: projectile diameter, shape, and composition; linear and rotational velocity; and the type of tissue struck.

## Reference

1. *Emergency War Surgery: 2nd United States revision of the emergency war surgery. NATO Handbook*. US Government Printing Office: 1988.

# Bombs, Mines, and Fragmentation

# 6

Toney W. Baskin and John B. Holcomb

## 6.1
## Introduction

Once confined to the battlefield and the occasional industrial accident, the sequela of explosive force has now become all too commonplace and continues to increase as explosive weaponry proliferates. The chaos and "fog of war" no longer can be considered the sole province of the battlefield. The ubiquitous threat of terrorism places responsibility for the care of victims not only upon the military surgeon, but upon civilian counterparts as well. The medical system, military and civilian must understand the pathophysiology of injury induced from explosive devices, be they letter bombs, shaped warheads from a rocket propelled grenade (RPG), anti-personnel land mines, aerial-delivered cluster bombs, or enhanced blast weapons.

Urban warfare is becoming more widespread, providing both a rich environment for the bomber to strike and the ideal medium for enhanced blast weapons. The terrorist may employ pipe bombs, large high-energy car bombs, or the suicide bomber wearing several kilograms of explosive.

In the United States alone from 1990 to 1995, the FBI reported 15,700 bombings, with 3,176 injuries and 355 deaths, and these numbers only continue to increase.

Primary blast injury, secondary to conventional high explosives, is uncommon in surviving casualties. This is because they would have been close to the epicenter of the explosion and are likely to have suffered lethal fragment and heat injury. With the advent of enhanced blast weapons (already populating the arms market), primary blast injury will increase in frequency, placing extreme clinical and logistical stress on the medical system.

Although anti-personnel mines were banned by the Ottawa Convention in 1997, civilian mine injuries have become even more common than military mine injuries that occur during combat, with farmers, women, and children ten times more likely to encounter these abandoned weapons of war. The immense number of anti-personnel mines scattered

T.W. Baskin (✉)
Trauma and Critical Care Service, Brooke Army Medical Center,
United States Army Institute of Surgical Research, San Antonio, TX, USA
e-mail: toney.baskin@amedd.army.mil

A.J. Brooks et al. (eds.), *Ryan's Ballistic Trauma*,
DOI: 10.1007/978-1-84882-124-8_6, © Springer-Verlag London Limited 2011

throughout many parts of the world continues to plague civilization with horrible disabling injuries that, according to the International Committee of the Red Cross (ICRC), number 24,000 per year.[1]

## 6.2
## Explosions

An explosive is a chemical compound or mixture that, when subjected to heat, shock, friction, or other impulse, leads to a rapid chemical reaction or combustion and an equally rapid generation of heat and gases. The consequent combined volume is much larger than the original substance.

Explosives are classified as high or low, depending upon the rate at which this reaction takes place. Gunpowder, the first explosive used in military ordnance, is an example of a low explosive. Low explosives change relatively slowly from a solid to a gaseous state, generally less than 2,000 m/s.

By comparison, high explosives (HE) react almost instantaneously, causing sudden increases in pressures and a detonation wave that moves at supersonic speed (1,400–9,000 m/s). Common examples are 2,4,6-trinitrotoluene (TNT) and the more recent polymer-bonded explosives, such as Semtex and Gelignite, which have 1.5 times the power of TNT. High explosives are used commonly in military ordnance.

A detonator is a type of explosive that reacts very rapidly and is used to set off other more inert explosives. Fulminate of mercury mixed with potassium chlorate is the most commonly used detonator. Detonators also can be equipment, which by flame, spark, percussion, friction, or pressure are used to set off a chemical detonator. Detonation refers to the chemical and exothermic reaction that creates a pressure wave propagating throughout the explosive, creating rapid production of heat and gases, resulting in a "runaway" process and producing the resulting explosion.

The rapid release of enormous amounts of energy in a high explosion results in a primary blast wave, propulsion of fragments and environmental material or debris, and often generates intense thermal radiation. The initial explosion creates an instantaneous rise in pressure, resulting in a shock wave that travels outward at supersonic speed. The shock wave is the leading front and an integral component of the blast wave. The generation and propagation of blast waves are governed by nonlinear physics.

The response of structures, including human tissues, also may be nonlinear, as evidenced by the pathophysiology of blast injuries.

This sudden variation in air pressure creates a mass movement of air known as the dynamic overpressure or blast wave. The Friedlander Relationship (Fig. 6.1) illustrates the physical properties of an ideal blast wave in open air. With the arrival of the shock wave, the pressure instantly increases to a peak overpressure, then rapidly falls, and creates subatmospheric pressures before returning to normal ambient atmospheric pressure.

In reality, the reflection of the blast wave as it encounters environmental structures creates a very complex pattern of overpressures. These overpressures and an actual reversal of the blast wind in the negative phase may cause significant damage. For an in-depth

**Fig. 6.1** Friedlander relationship

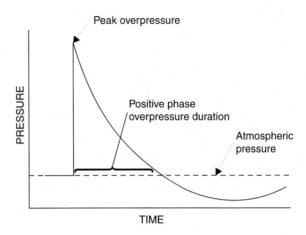

discussion of the creation and propagation of blast waves and how they interact with various structures, the reader is referred to an article by I.G. Cullis.[2]

## 6.3
## Enhanced-Blast Weapons

Ongoing research in the ordnance industry and recent technological advances in explosives and material has propagated the development of enhanced-blast weapons (EBW). There are four known types of enhanced-blast explosives:

1. metallized explosives,
2. reactive surround,
3. fuel-air,
4. thermobaric.

Once confined to fuel-air explosive (FAE) bombs, EBWs span the range of weapon systems from small grenades and handheld weapons to large-caliber rockets (Table 6.1).

Relatively few primary blast injuries have been seen, as there are few survivors with primary blast injury from conventional HEs. Most die immediately, but this may change with the increase of EBW usage. With conventional HEs, the blast wave decays very rapidly and is affected significantly by the environment. Enhanced-blast weapons produce a lower overpressure than conventional HE, but the period of overpressure lasts longer and reaches farther, thereby increasing the lethality zone and producing blast casualties further from the epicenter of the detonation (Fig. 6.2).

The classic EBW mechanism is illustrated best in the FAE, which has an initial small explosion that disperses a vapor cloud of ethylene oxide or other fuel. At a critical time and distance, the dispersed fuel is ignited by a second detonation, producing a uniform dynamic overpressure through the covered area. This may produce lethal overpressures as high as 2 Mpa, whereas a conventional HE would produce only 200 Kpa at a similar

**Table 6.1** EBWs currently in use

|  | Fuel-air explosives | Thermobaric |
|---|---|---|
| United States | Fuel-air warheads<br>• BLUE-64/B (200 kg fuel)<br>• BLUE-72B Pave Pat 2 | (1,202 kg ethylene oxide) |
| Former Soviet Union | ODAB-500 PM (193 kg) high-speed low-level attack, can be launched from vehicle<br>KAB-500Kr<br>S8-DM – 3.6 kg multiple-barrel rocket launcher<br>• SPLAV 220 mm<br><br>(Uragan) BM 9P140<br>• SPLAV 300 mm<br><br>(SMerch) BM 9A52 | Guided missiles<br>• AT-6-SPIRAL (helicopter launch)[a]<br>• AT-9 (vehicle launch)[a]<br>• AT-14<br>• METIS-M (crew-served weapon)<br>• Khrizantema (BMP)[a]<br><br>• TOS-1 (Burantino – mobile rocket launder)<br>S8 unguided air-launched rocket<br>TOS-1 Buratino – multiple-barrel rocket launcher<br>Flame thrower RPO-A (2.1 kg)<br>Grenade launcher GM-94<br>RShG-1 Multipurpose assault weapon<br>RPG (range 900 m)[a] |
| China | 250 kg with 2 bomblets<br>500 kg with 3 bomblets<br>(800 m²) | |

[a]Denotes FAE ability as well

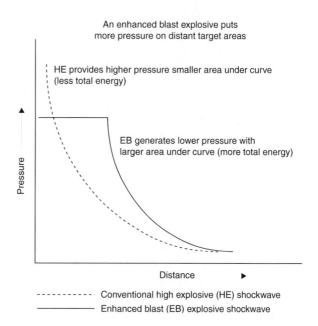

**Fig. 6.2** Enhanced blast wave

distance from the initiating explosion. The EBW also produces a longer-lasting fireball and may produce more energy [area beneath the curve (see Fig. 6.2)], resulting in more casualties with primary blast injuries combined with burns, crush, and penetrating-fragment injuries.

The blast wave from an EBW can diffract around corners, rapidly expanding and filling a structure, and is enhanced by reflection in enclosed spaces, making this an ideal weapon to defeat field defenses, soft unreinforced buildings, communication equipment, and low-flying aircraft. As an anti-personnel weapon, an EBW can be expected to rapidly produce large numbers of casualties with burns, blast injuries, fragment, translational injuries, and crush injuries from demolished buildings, placing a sudden and intense clinical and logistical strain on medical resources.

Several foreign studies have suggested that body armor enhances the effects of primary blast, creating a "behind armor blunt trauma" (BABT). Although studies by the US Army Soldier Systems Command, Natick, MA, indicated that the Interceptor Body Armor in use by US forces does not enhance the blast effect – and may actually reduce effects – when the ceramic plates are included in the armor, it is safe to say that most body armor currently in use will protect only marginally against primary blast injury and offer little, if any, protection against accompanying thermal injury. Armor-employing decouplers or layers of material with different acoustic and mechanical properties specifically designed to maximally attenuate the shock wave needs to be designed.

It is the combination of the shock wave or leading edge, the dynamic overpressure, the secondary and tertiary effects, and the associated thermal energy that result in the characteristic injuries seen following detonation of an explosive device. These injuries may be classified according to the mechanism by which they are produced (Table 6.2).

Both conventional and terrorist weapons are designed to produce multiple wounds with the maximum number of casualties. Indeed, on today's battlefield, up to 90% of casualties are secondary to fragmentation wounds, with wounding from small arms or bullets producing generally less than 15–20% of battlefield casualties. Modern fragmentation weapons have a high casing-to-explosive ratio designed to produce preformed fragments, which

**Table 6.2** Classification of injury by mechanism

| Class of injury | Mechanism |
| --- | --- |
| Primary | Interaction of blast wave (overpressure) with body, gas-filled structures being most at risk, complex stress and shear waves produce organ injury |
| Secondary | Wounds produced by fragments from weapon, environmental projectiles, and debris, with penetrating injury predominating |
| Tertiary | Displacement of body (translational) and structural collapse with acceleration–deceleration, crush, and blunt injuries |
| Quaternary | All other mechanisms producing injury, burns, toxidromes from fuel, metals, septic syndromes from soil and environmental contamination (*septic meliodosis*) |

**Table 6.3** Major weapon classification

| Conventional | Grenades, aerial bombs, artillery, RPG. See all types of injuries with fragment wounds from preformed fragments predominating along with environmental debris |
|---|---|
| Antipersonnel mines | Point detonating mine (5 kg), traumatic amputation of foot or lower extremity, dirty, contaminated with debris, clothing, footwear, body parts, and soil Triggered mine (Claymore, Bouncing Betty), upper extremity, chest, face, and ocular injury |
| Enhanced blast munition | Designed to injure by blast wave, dispersed by fuel vapor, pulmonary injury, may have delayed onset, destroy and damage "soft" targets and personnel |
| Terrorist bombs | Letter bomb to several hundred kilograms, low mortality, fragment wounds, debris and crushing injury, some primary blast injury, suicide bomber with human-tissue fragments as wounding agent |

significantly enhances the wounding radius and casualty probability. The major classes of available weapons are categorized in Table 6.3.

## 6.3.1
### Fragmentation Injury

There are a myriad of weapon systems and missiles, ranging from grenades to aerial-delivered bombs weighing several tons that depending on the size and design of the weapon may deliver several thousand fragments ranging in weight from a few milligrams to many grams with an initial velocity of greater than 1,500 m/s. These fragments decline in velocity rapidly generally producing multiple low velocity incapacitating wounds. Modern fragmentation weapons are designed with preformed fragments to optimize velocity, distance, and probability of hit producing multiple casualties with multiple wounds (Fig. 6.3). Body armor has altered the pattern of distribution of fragmentation injury so that the most common casualty seen on today's battlefield will have multiple extremity, head, and facial wounds (Table 6.4).

The use of anti-personnel bomblets or submunitions effectively has increased the probability of a hit and increased the lethality and wounding area of the munition. In the Israeli–Egyptian October War of 1973, each anti-personnel canister released 600 Guava bomblets (named from an Egyptian fruit with large numbers of seeds), with each bomblet containing 300 pellets. Each bomblet is released at 1-m intervals and can travel 150 m, with an explosive lethal radius of 5–8 m. Each pellet acts as a small missile of moderate velocity, striking from different angles within the lethal zone. This raised the incidence of multiple system injuries, with penetrating wounds of the extremities constituting 56% of injuries. There also was a 15% increase in head and neck injuries, with 14% of injuries to the chest and abdomen. Pellet paraplegia was a characteristic injury seen with the Guava bomblet in the Israeli–Egyptian conflict. Penetrating abdominal wounds with visceral

**Fig. 6.3** Preformed fragments from cluster bomblet (Major Scott Gering, Operation Iraqi Freedom)

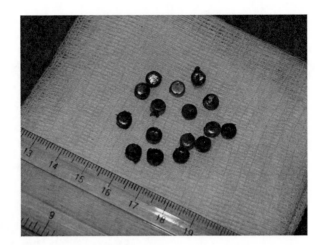

**Table 6.4** Anatomical distribution of penetrating wounds as a percent (80% fragment)

| Conflict | Head and neck | Thorax | Abdomen | Limbs |
|---|---|---|---|---|
| World War I | 17 | 4 | 2 | 70 |
| World War II | 4 | 8 | 4 | 75 |
| Korea | 17 | 7 | 7 | 67 |
| Vietnam | 14 | 7 | 5 | 74 |
| Northern Ireland | 20 | 15 | 15 | 50 |
| Israel 1975 | 13 | 5 | 7 | 40 |
| Israel 1982 | 14 | 4 | 5 | 41 |
| Falkland Island | 16 | 15 | 10 | 59 |
| Gulf War (UK) | 6 | 12 | 11 | 71 |
| Gulf War (US) | 11 | 8 | 7 | 56 |
| Afghanistan (US) | 16 | 12 | 11 | 61 |
| Chechnya (Russia) | 24 | 9 | 4 | 63 |
| Somolia | 20 | 8 | 5 | 65 |
| Average | 15 | 9.5 | 7.4 | 64.6 |

injury proved difficult, with frequently missed visceral injury due to the small pellet size (Fig. 6.4).

Improved grenade launchers with preformed fragments, laser-sighted accuracy, and precision fusing such as the US Objective Infantry Combat Weapon, with a 5.56 barrel combined with a 20-mm grenade launcher, will increase firepower and extend the killing range to 1,000 m. The use of flechettes, depleted uranium, and tungsten missiles capable

**Fig. 6.4** (**a**, **b**) Multiple
fragment wounds from
cluster bomblet (US) (Major
Scott Gering, Operation
Iraqi Freedom). (**c**) Multiple
fragment wounds from
cluster bomblet with
environmental fragments
(Major Scott Gering,
Operation Iraqi Freedom)

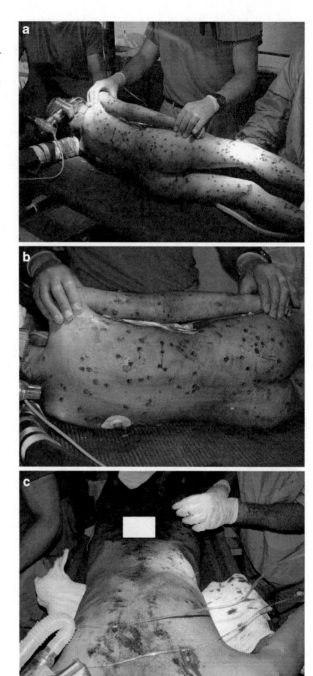

of penetrating body armor and conventional cover may further compound the complexity of wounding with toxicities that have yet to be defined, thus increasing the impact on the medical support system.

Many of the more modern fragment munitions are designed to produce multiple pre-formed fragments that weigh 100–200 mg and are 2–3 mm in diameter, whereas others may weigh as much as 20 g. Both have initial velocities of 1,500 m/s, which falls off rapidly, especially with the large, more irregular-shaped fragments. The mechanism of injury is related as much to energy transfer as to the velocity of the projectile, and the magnitude of injury is thought to depend more upon the inherent tissue characteristics of the organ involved than upon the projectile itself. The clinical impact and priority of treatment depends on the tissue or organ involved. Extremity wounds that may be innumerable usually are not life threatening and perhaps may not be immediately disabling. In contrast, wounds of the eyes or thorax are far more likely to be immediately disabling or life threatening, respectively.

Environmental debris such as glass, splinters, soil, and various structural particles are propelled with similar velocities by the blast wind and may well be the major cause of fragment wounding. The advent of the human suicide bomber brings a new dimension to fragment wounding, with human body parts acting as missile fragments and projectiles that may carry with them the specter of human immunodeficiency virus (HIV), hepatitis, and other serious and yet to be identified threats of unknown clinical consequence, thus presenting a rather complex therapeutic dilemma for the clinician.

Penetrating fragment wounds of the abdomen and thorax are no different than other penetrating wounds except that the number of pellets and the small size of visceral injuries demand meticulous attention to detail. Almost all penetrating fragment wounds of the abdomen can be closed primarily and 85% of penetrating thoracic wounds can be managed successfully by tube thoracostomy. Animal studies examining multiple colonic injuries found that colotomies closed by either one-layer interrupted absorbable suture or stainless steel skin staples were equivalent, except that the stapled anastomosis histologically healed more quickly than the sutured anastomosis, supporting definitive repair of intestinal low-velocity wounds.

All war wounds are contaminated by soil, clothing, and skin. High-velocity missiles have been shown to widely contaminate a wound track,[3] whereas low-velocity fragmentation wounds are minimally contaminated with debris. Bacterial contamination is ubiquitous in fragmentation wounds, with soil and skin organisms, *Clostridia*, *Streptococcus*, *Staphylococcus*, *Proteus*, *E Coli*, and *Enterococcus*,[4] although infection is uncommon in small low-velocity wounds of the extremity.

Although somewhat controversial, some reports in the literature support early antibiotics and nonoperative treatment of extremity wounds less than a centimeter in size in patients who show no evidence of neurovascular injury or compartment syndrome and also have a stable fracture pattern.[5] Operative debridement of these numerous wounds can lead to increased morbidity and, in general, is unnecessary.[6] However, in the authors' experience, small low-velocity wounds involving a major joint resulted in a higher incidence of infection when treated with early antibiotics and delayed operative treatment of more than 6 h (Operation Just Cause).

Small (less than 1 cm) low-velocity wounds with no evidence of contamination that can be cleaned and dressed with early administration of appropriate broad-spectrum antibiotics may be treated nonoperatively. However, when there is question, delay in treatment greater than 6 h, or evidence of cavitation and contamination in wounds greater than 1 cm, operative debridement should be the standard.

## 6.4
## Land Mine

Land mines currently are deployed in 64 countries around the world and number between 84 and 100 million. Two thousand victims a month fall prey to this indiscriminate forgotten remnant of war that are ten times more likely to injure a noncombatant than a soldier. Although banned by the Ottawa Convention of 1997 and prohibited by International Humanitarian Law, mines continue to be laid across the world. It is estimated that in countries with existing mine fields such as Cambodia, Angola, and Somalia, 1 in every 450 persons undergoes traumatic amputation compared to United States, where amputations only number 1/22,000. It is estimated that only half of these non-combatant victims even live to reach a hospital and undergo treatment for these devastating injuries.[7]

Mines can cost no more than $3.00 apiece and can be distributed by a plethora of weapon systems to include aerial delivery and Multiple Launch Rocket Systems (MLRS) that can deliver 8,000 bomblets and hundreds of mines in a matter of minutes. The American Gator mines (72 anti-tank and 22 anti-personnel) are delivered aerially in containers with one fighter aircraft able to deliver 600 mines in a single sortie. There is no reason to expect that the use of anti-personnel mines will cease or that the incidence of land-mine injuries will decline. Mines with increased blast radius and lethality, and with fuel-air–enhanced blast technology already are in development.[8]

There are essentially three classes of conventional anti-personnel land mines based on mechanism of action – static, bounding, and horizontal-spray mines.

Static mines are implanted in the ground and vary from 5 to 15 cm in diameter, contain 20–200 g of explosive, and most commonly are detonated by direct contact, although newer mines that detonate on motion and proximity motion are being developed.

Bounding mines, known as "Bouncing Betty," have the highest mortality. These mines propel a small explosive device 1–2 m above ground then explode, dispersing multiple small preformed fragments.

Horizontal-spray or directional fragmentation mines, of which the US M18A1 Claymore AP munition mine is the best known, can be command detonated or victim detonated by means of trip wires. The Claymore fires 700 steel spheres, each weighing 0.75 g in a 60° arc, resulting in multiple penetrating wounds dispersed throughout the body, creating multiple system injuries and multiple casualties. The horizontal spray and bounding mines essentially produce multiple penetrating injuries of both high and low velocity, depending on the range of the target, with a very high mortality. Thus, the mechanism of injury is no different than any other penetrating wound and surviving casualties are treated as such.

The static mine is most common throughout the world, and its mechanism of injury is unique to this weapon system. Upon contact and detonation, an instantaneous rise in pressure or shock wave is produced, which along with the products and heated air produce a blast wave or dynamic overpressure. Contact with the body produces stress waves that propagate proximally along with shear waves produced by the blast effect. These stress waves can propagate as far as the middle thigh with demyelination of nerves occurring 30 cm above the most proximal area of tissue injury. This, combined with fragments from the device, soil, and footwear, produces the classic land-mine injury of complete tissue destruction, distally associated with traumatic amputation at the midfoot or distal tibia (Figs. 6.5 and 6.6). Proximal to the variable level of amputation there is complete stripping of tissue from the bony structures and separation of fascial planes contaminated with soil debris, microorganisms, pieces of the device, footwear, and clothing. Associated penetrating injury to contralateral limb and perineum are common.

Injuries occur in three distinct patterns. Pattern 1 injuries occur with contact of a buried mine that produces severe lower-extremity, perineal, and genital injury. Pattern 2 injuries occur with a proximity device explosion that produces less severe lower-extremity injury with less traumatic amputation. Head, thoracic, and abdominal injuries are common. Pattern 3 injuries occur with handling or clearing that produce severe head, face, and upper-extremity injury.

Ocular injuries are not uncommon with all categories of mines. The products of detonation and environmental fragments and debris producing penetrating ocular wounds are the primary mechanism and were seen in 4.5% of all antipersonnel mine injuries in Afghanistan.

All lower-extremity injuries need debridement or completion of amputation and many may require laparotomy, with all wounds of perineum, buttocks, back, and abdomen having a low threshold for laparotomy. Every effort should be made to conserve the contralateral limb. The primary injury is treated with excision, lavage, and exploration and lavage of fascial planes with delayed closure. All casualties should receive broad-spectrum antibiotics to cover indigenous soil spore-forming microorganisms.

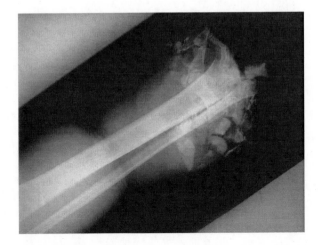

**Fig. 6.5** Boot and clothing debris from small anti-personnel land mine (Major Scott Gering, Operation Iraqi Freedom)

**Fig. 6.6** Injury from anti-personnel mine (Major Darryl Scales, Kosovo, 2000)

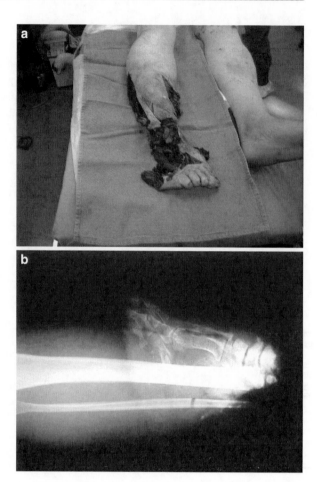

## 6.5
## Combined Injury

Combined injuries, including primary blast injury, penetrating fragment wounds, crush, burn, and inhalation injuries, are to be expected, especially in urban-warfare environments or urban terrorist bombings. With the advent of EBWs and handheld thermobaric weapons, these combined injuries are likely to become even more common, placing extreme stress on medical support systems, be they military or civilian. Triage and appropriate patient distribution may be the most critical piece of patient management. Combined blast and penetrating injuries are almost always the most life threatening and the basic principles of the <C>ABCs should always be adhered to. Blast lung may not present for 24–48 h; therefore, all patients requiring early mechanical ventilation or those going immediately to the operating room should be managed with low tidal volumes of 5–6 ml/kg of ideal body weight, peak inspiratory pressures of less than 25 cm $H_2O$, allowing for permissive hypercapnia. If associated TBI is present, hypercapnia should be avoided or minimized, if possible, due to the deleterious effects on intracranial hypertension. For a patient undergoing anesthesia with obvious signs of blast lung injury, there is an increased risk of barotrauma with resultant tension pneumothorax. The authors recommend consideration of bilateral prophylactic tube thoracostomy.

Patients without vascular compromise or evidence of compartment syndrome who have penetrating injuries of the extremities of 1 cm or less may be managed conservatively with early antibiotics and cleansing with frequent observation.

Penetrating injuries of the trunk associated with hemodynamic instability should undergo immediate operation. Most thoracic injuries can be managed with tube thoracostomy, and thoracotomy is rarely indicated in combined injury. Emergency Thoracotomy for penetrating thoracic injury in the presence of primary blast should be considered futile and be abandoned.

Abdominal wounds with associated hemodynamic instability require immediate laparotomy once the airway is controlled.

Management of truncal penetrating injuries combined with blast should undergo, at minimum, a focused abdominal sonogram for trauma (FAST) exam if available, but the decision to operate frequently must be based on clinical judgment and a high index of suspicion. Patients with blast injury and associated blunt abdominal trauma from tertiary and quaternary mechanisms who are hemodynamically unstable should undergo immediate laparotomy, as conservative management in this scenario is not indicated.

## 6.5.1
### Retained Ordnance

An injury that is truly unique to the military is the casualty presenting with retained and unexploded ordnance. Since World War II there have been 36 documented cases with only four deaths. The deaths occurred not from the detonation of the missile, but from the moribund condition of the casualty, usually due to hemorrhage. The M79 grenade launcher (40 mm), mortars, and RPG missiles have been the most commonly reported cause of retained ordnance. A fuse or detonator that can be triggered by impact, electromagnetic energy, or time and distance normally detonates this type of ordnance. There is often a safety built into the device requiring a defined number of revolutions or a required distance and time before the missile is armed to explode. The RPG round must travel a defined distance before the fuse is armed to trigger on impact. All missiles that have been fired must be considered armed, and a defined and predetermined algorithm for the care of the casualty and the safety of the medical personnel should be followed.

A casualty with unexploded ordnance should be transported in the position found so as not to change the missile orientation and should always be grounded to the airframe if evacuated by air. These patients should be isolated and, in a mass casualty situation, should be treated last as the removal of ordnance is time consuming and the surgeon must attend to other casualties before placing his or herself at risk. Closed chest massage or defibrillation should never be attempted, and during removal, any equipment emanating

**Table 6.5** Removal of unexploded ordnance

1. Notify EOD
2. No CPR or electric shock
3. Isolate to protected area (sandbagged bunker)
4. Protective equipment for medical personnel
5. Do not use cautery, power equipment, blood warmers
6. Avoid vibration, change in temperature, change in missile orientation
7. Do plain radiograph, no CT or ultrasound
8. Minimal anesthesia, anesthesia provider to leave after induction
9. Surgeon and assistant (EOD) only personnel present during removal
10. Remove without changing orientation and hand over to EOD
11. Move casualty to Operating theater for definitive procedure

*Source*: Lein et al.[9] Reprinted with kind permission from Association of Military Surgeons of the United States

electrical energy, heat, vibration, or sonic waves, such as the electrocautery, ultrasound, blood warmers, or power instruments, should be avoided. The patient should be placed in a protected area away from the main hospital, and all personnel in the immediate area should employ body armor or explosive ordnance disposal (EOD) equipment. Explosive ordnance disposal personnel should be involved prior to removal to help with identifying the round and fuse; a plain radiograph will help in planning the operative removal and will not cause the round to explode. The minimum anesthesia required should be used and in such a manner that the anesthesia provider need not be present during actual removal. The only personnel required during removal are surgeon and an assistant – ideally, EOD personnel. The round should be removed *en bloc* without touching the missile with metal instruments. Every effort should be employed to maintain the orientation of the missile until removed from the area by EOD. The basic guidelines for removal of ordnance are outlined in Table 6.5.

## References

1. International Committee of the Red Cross. Available at: http://www.icrc.org/eng. Accessed registry of mine incidents: From March 1996 until September 1996. April 23, 2003.
2. Cullis IG. Blast waves and how they interact with structure. *J R Army Med Corps*. 2001;147: 16-26.
3. Ryan J. *An Enquiry into the Nature of Infection in Fragment Wounds* [master's thesis]. Dublin: University College Dublin; 1990.
4. Hill PF, Edwards DP, Bowyer GN. Small fragment wounds: biophysics, pathophysiology and principles of management. *J R Army Med Corps*. 2001;147:41-51.
5. Coupland RM. *War Wounds of Limbs – Surgical Management*. Oxford, England: Butterworth-Heinemann Ltd; 1993.
6. Stein M, Hirschberg A. 9th Annual Brooke Army Medical Center San Antonio Trauma Symposium, August 18–19, 2003. Henry B. Gonzales Convention Center, San Antonio, Texas, Medical consequences of terrorism. The conventional weapon threat. *Surg Clin North Am*. 1999;79:1537-1552.

7. International Committee of the Red Cross. Five years on: anti-personnel mines remain a constant threat for millions. Available at: www.Icrc.org. April 25, 2003.
8. Trends in land mine warfare. London, England: Janes information group; July 1995. Special Report.
9. Lein B, Holcomb J, Brill S, Hetz S, McCrorey T. Removal of unexploded ordnance from patients: a 50-year military experience and current recommendations. *Mil Med.* 1999;164: 163-165.

# Cluster Munitions

# 7

Henry Dowlen

## 7.1
## Introduction

Cluster munitions have been used in at least 23 countries, produced in 33, and stockpiled in over 70; their submunitions number into the billions.[1] The year 2008 heralded an international agreement prohibiting the use, production, transfer, and stockpiling of cluster munitions due to the unacceptable harm they cause to civilians.[2]

The discussions leading to this agreement (known as the Oslo process), whilst not as high-profile as the Ottawa Convention relating to the ban of land mines, highlighted a wide difference in opinion on the legitimacy of cluster munitions. The Oslo process was launched by the Norwegian Government in February 2007 in order to negotiate a ban on cluster munitions (which throughout their history have been the subject of debate on their definitions) the post-conflict legacies they create and the legislation that might apply to them.

This chapter summarizes the history, utility, and legacy of cluster munitions before considering the legislation surrounding them and the outcome of the Oslo process.

## 7.2
## Technical Specifications

Cluster munitions can deploy large amounts of explosives over a wide area and can be ground- or air-launched. They are also multipurpose weapons with variants that target vehicles, personnel, roads, and electrical stations (the latter by deploying reels of conductive wire). They can also contain chemical weapons or lay landmines. Although modern variants are designed to break up concentrations of armored vehicles and infantry, they have evolved for a variety of uses. In general, they consist of a canister, which breaks open to release submunitions over an area known as a "footprint."

H. Dowlen
45 Commando Royal Marines, Royal Navy, Arbroath, Angus, UK
e-mail: henry.dowlen@btinternet.com

A.J. Brooks et al. (eds.), *Ryan's Ballistic Trauma*,
DOI: 10.1007/978-1-84882-124-8_7, © Springer-Verlag London Limited 2011

Older designs of cluster munitions are simpler and generally do not have guidance or self-destruct mechanisms. Some submunition fuses are armed through the spinning motion that occurs after they are jettisoned from the parent casing, and malfunction can occur during either of these processes. The "all-ways acting fuse" is designed to ensure the device explodes even if it does not land in the correct alignment; however, it also acts as an anti-handling device, making unexploded ordnance UXO much more likely to detonate with a small movement.[1]

Failure rates for cluster munitions are high enough that they are accounted for in the planning of military operations.[2] In the past 42 years, nine countries confirmed the use of at least 440 million cluster submunitions, with average failure rates between 5% and 30%. A minimum of 22–132 million would therefore have become Explosive Remnants of War (ERW).[3] Several operational factors influence the reliability of submunitions, including poor delivery technique, age of the submunition, weather, and terrain.[2] Recent tests in Norway have shown that self-destruct features are often not as reliable as manufacturers claim.

The vast stockpiles and multiple variants of cluster munitions would seem to indicate that the military viability of these weapons is beyond question, but this argument has not been made coherently to date.[4] Cluster munitions apply an area effect for a military advantage; therefore, the effects of any attack should be in proportion to the target and the importance of the military goal. Cluster munitions used in an area of civilian and military cohabitation, however, almost guarantee civilian casualties.[2] The military efficacy of cluster munitions has been further questioned as a result of U.S. troops being killed post-conflict by their own UXO, not to mention the impediment to mobility when operating in contaminated areas.

## 7.3
## History

Cluster munitions' first use dates back to World War II when German forces dropped "butterfly bombs." (Fig. 7.1) These air-deployed munitions held anti-personnel bomblets that could detonate on impact or be set for delayed and anti-handling settings. Civilians were specifically targeted (bomblets were camouflaged to kill farmers at harvest time), and unexploded bomblets were found too unstable to disarm. The disruption caused was significant enough to be kept secret by the British in order to avoid encouraging further use by the Germans. It is significant that butterfly bombs killed as many people after air raids as during them, and the bombs' last casualty occurred 11 years after being dropped, a bomb disposal expert trying to disarm the device (Fig. 7.2).

It was not until the Vietnam War that cluster munitions were used again – most notably in Laos – with any significance. Between 2 and 3 million tons of ordnance were dropped over Laos from 1964 to 1973, much of which was cluster munitions that subsequently failed to explode. In 2005, the recorded casualties increased from 100 a year to almost 200, an increase attributed to a rise in the price of scrap metal, which enticed people to take greater risks by trying to recover the metal from unexploded ordnance.

The more modern variants of cluster munitions were designed in the context of the Cold War to attack large military formations; furthermore, they act as force multipliers, reducing the logistics and manpower risked for a military goal.[1] The "footprint," or effective area, of a single cluster munition can be half a square kilometer (0.2 square miles), although this clearly varies between munitions. The rationale for cluster bomb use is important, as the military efficacy of them has been in some dispute: "No detailed military study of the military utility of these weapons…has ever been made public"[1].

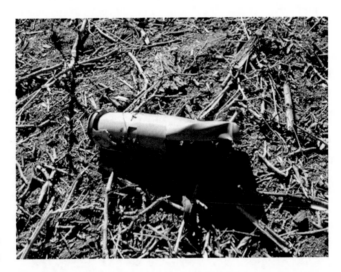

**Fig. 7.1** Close-up of a non-detonated cluster submunition (Courtesy of Mr. Steve Mannion)

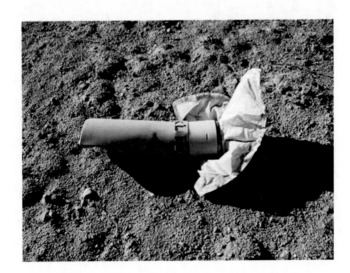

**Fig. 7.2** A non-detonated cluster submunition with parachute deployed, lying on the ground outside an Afghan village (Courtesy of Mr. Steve Mannion)

Indiscriminate use and high failure rates are cited as the two areas of concern giving grounds for humanitarian scrutiny of cluster weapons,[5] and according to research by the Cluster Munitions Coalition (a coalition working to ban cluster munitions internationally), at least 60% of casualties from unexploded cluster munitions are children. Also, clearance is hampered by a lack of access to and visibility of any unexploded ordnance.

During the first Gulf War in 1991, over 13 million submunitions were used, of which around 400,000 failed to detonate[1] due to factors such as poor manufacture, inappropriate use, and inclement weather conditions. With regard to this last factor, some cluster munitions' self-arming capacities are particularly susceptible to high winds or variations in altitude when dropped – for instance if conditions do not allow the munitions' subunits to attain the correct spin, they cannot arm and detonate as intended. During the post-Gulf War cleanup of unexploded ordnance, seven U.S. troops were killed in one incident (Fig. 7.3).

Records from Kosovo in 1999 suggest that cluster munitions were a weapon of convenience, while post-conflict studies concluded that the attacks had little immediate impact.[6] In 2003, Human Rights Watch criticized the number of cluster munition attacks by United States and United Kingdom forces that affected civilians. After the first Gulf War, however, the US military recorded that "Iraqi units were devastated and demoralized. ... The fact that the ground war lasted only four days…can be largely attributed to the effect of cluster munitions."[1]

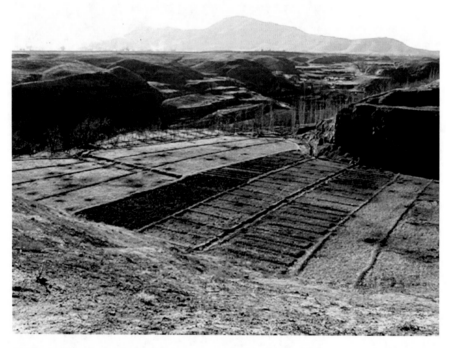

**Fig. 7.3** Aerial photograph showing craters over impact site of a cluster munition (Courtesy of Mr. Steve Mannion)

## 7.4
## Legacy

The main type of submunition that was dropped on Laos has a life expectancy in the soil of approximately 100 years, and while some are found badly corroded, others look almost new. There is growing interest in the effects of ERW on the natural environment and also the effects of removing them. [7] (Fig. 7.4).

Despite advances in clearance vehicles and the use of special detecting animals, clearance inevitably must be done manually. A recent environmental impact study undertaken by the United Nations Mine Action Service, however, found that removal operations significantly damage the environment, and long-term damage arises from destruction of flora, contamination of water systems, and damage to the natural habitats of wildlife.[8] Disposal of ERW by burning or detonation releases huge quantities of metal fragments, dust, and nitrogen oxides into the environment, although it is possible to incinerate ERW and reclaim the energy, or utilize the chemicals for other purposes. Richard Kidd, former Director of the Office of Weapons Removal and Abatement in the United States Department of State's Bureau of Political-Military Affairs, argues that "the problems associated with cluster munitions are not nearly as bad as other ERW… [and] there simply is no large-scale demand for financial resources to clear cluster munitions."[9]

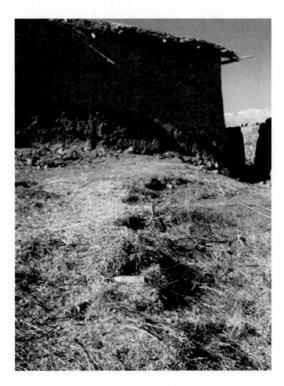

**Fig. 7.4** A non-detonated cluster submunition lying on the ground outside an Afghan village (Courtesy of Mr. Steve Mannion)

Laos farmers are gradually expanding the land they use, but this involves a risk of exploding UXO, serious injury, and death. In case studies carried out by Richard Moyes of Landmine Action and the Cluster Munitions Coalition, land is abandoned only if other economic options are available. People without options are forced to use contaminated land by necessity.[3] ERW degrade habitats by altering food chains, making conservation of protected areas difficult, and polluting the soil and water supplies. There are those, however, that argue that the very presence of ERW is protective of the natural environment, as it prevents human development, which may otherwise destroy natural ecosystems.

Some evidence from Afghanistan, Kosovo, and elsewhere shows there is a significantly greater risk of being killed by a submunition than by an anti-personnel landmine. In a 2006 study by Handicap International, casualties from cluster munitions were greater than the predicted value based on landmine data, as well as being disproportionately comprised of civilians (98%).[3] It should be noted however that Mr. Steve Mannion, in work for The HALO Trust, concluded that there is far less threat to civilians than from landmines, and that submunitions are unlikely to detonate unless handled or thrown.

Those most likely to disturb and detonate ERW are farmers or children, although there is a growing trend of collecting ERW for scrap metal. Injuries sustained include multiple traumatic amputations of limbs, burns, puncture by fragments, ruptured eardrums, and blindness.

The International Committee of the Red Cross observed that those killed or injured by submunitions in Kosovo were 4.9 times more likely to be under 14 years of age than victims of anti-personnel mines. According to the ICRC, "This may be due to the fact that such submunitions are often brightly coloured, lying on the ground and assumed to be duds."

There is a lack of accurate mortality and morbidity rates related to cluster munitions. As a consequence, the use of cluster munitions is likely to remain: "impulsive, crude and indiscriminate, with lip service paid to humanitarian laws."[10]

ERW pose a crippling threat to the development of a community. There are costs incurred not only in clearing land for use, but also in caring for those injured and a slow resumption of land use due to fear of ERW. Prioritization of clearance, focusing on the number of square kilometers of productive land that has been lost, is important where it is not possible to clear every square meter of contaminated land.

The U.S. donates about US$2.5 million per year for UXO removal, but this is compared to 2.5 million dollars per day for nine years spent on bombing Laos. The U.K. has contributed significant resources to understanding the extent of the problem, but many NGOs feel that the users of cluster munitions have done little to contribute to understanding the harm caused by these weapons.[11]

## 7.5
## Relevant Legislation

Recommendations based on existing legislation have been put forward to guide best practice when cluster munitions are deployed, including responsibilities to provide information and warnings to civilians both during and after conflict. Despite these recommendations, there is no agreement over which pre-existing rules of international humanitarian law are relevant, although legislation exists to cover indiscriminate weapons and obligations to clear landmines.

Additional Protocol I (1977) of the Geneva Conventions sets out rules regarding distinction, discrimination, proportionality, and feasibility in the use of weapons. Many feel cluster weapons violate the principles of proportionality, distinction, and discrimination, and that there is 40 years' worth of evidence concerning consistent civilian harm.[11]

In 1993, the 1980 U.N. Convention on Certain Conventional Weapons (CCW) was updated with a fifth protocol on ERW. Adopted in 2003 and entering into force in late 2006, it was criticized for not being strongly worded enough.[12] The weaknesses in the CCW catalyzed formation of the Oslo process, which takes a much harder line toward cluster munitions.

Other legislation of relevance is the Rio Declaration of 1992, principle 24 of which states that "warfare is inherently destructive of sustainable development. States shall therefore respect international law providing protection for the environment in times of armed conflict and cooperate in its further development."

Sections of the ISO 14000 Environmental Management Systems series, and the European Commission's Eco-Management and Audit Scheme are concerned with the "polluter pays" principle. When and how much the polluter should pay is often unclear, however, and compliance with both ISO 14000 and EMAS is voluntary.

Corporate social responsibility is also relevant, especially relating to companies producing cluster bombs. This, again, requires voluntary engagement, although the U.K. government believes this is how business should account for economic, social, and environmental impacts.

Although not specifically directed at cluster munitions, the Aarhus Convention links government accountability, human rights, and environmental protection. Still in the process of being adopted, it is intended for countries within the European community, but is open to non-European Commission's Eco-Management countries.

The Ottawa Convention, under which signatories agree to ban landmines, holds some parallels for cluster munitions, but the blurring of boundaries between the two types of weapons can be unhelpful as there are some distinct differences. For practical purposes, cluster munitions do not fall under the Ottawa Convention, and therefore require specific legislation.

One notable absentee from the Ottawa Convention and discussion relating to cluster munitions is the United States. The U.S. is the world's largest single financial contributor to mine and UXO clearance, and the only major military power that has pledged to leave no mine behind on any battlefield; yet many still feel it pays lip service to the two issues. The United States still produces, uses, and sells cluster munitions; however, in 2007 the United States placed restrictions on the sale or transfer of these weapons.

## 7.6
## The Oslo Process

The Cluster Munition Coalition was founded at The Hague in November 2003 to protect civilians from cluster munitions; it consists of some 200 civil-society organizations. It was partly a response to Norway's declaration in late 2006 that it would work toward an international ban on these weapons, following frustration with a perceived lack of effort by the CCW. In February 2007 the United Nations, CMC, ICRC, some interested countries, and other humanitarian organizations met in Oslo to discuss means of moving toward a ban. This became known as the Oslo process. Follow-up meetings occurred with the aim of concluding the process by the end of 2008.

Three distinct constituencies appeared to form in response to the Oslo process as it pursued a wholesale ban on all cluster bombs. First, the ban proponents who felt that these weapons will always cause unnecessary civilian harm without more fundamental changes to individual states' practices, and they advocated for nothing less than a total ban.[11] Second are opponents of the ban – most notable is the United States, whose stance hardened against any convention that specifically sought to ban cluster munitions in the run up to the February 2007 Oslo meeting. This is, however, an over-simplification; the U.S. Congress took steps to place controls on cluster munition stockpiles, design, manufacture, and exportation. Finally, there are moderates who see compromise as the only viable resolution for the issue. The Norwegian Minister of Foreign Affairs in 2006 stated that, "Today, no serious actors advocate a total prohibition against all...cluster munitions." Indeed, it was possible that pressure for the over-rigorous application of humanitarian principles in war to cluster munitions, without a realization that states will continue to use area-effect weapons, would weaken the Oslo process.

Definition of cluster munitions is important, as can be seen from that mentioned in the introduction and produced by the Oslo process. Some states felt that cluster munitions should have a minimum number of subunits, which would allow them to possess "area-effect weapons" that are not defined as cluster munitions. There is some logic to this argument as, below a certain number of submunitions, the problems associated with cluster munitions dwindle into insignificance, or to the significance of multiple single munitions with no subunits.

For instance, a German delegation proposed a definition of cluster munitions as having less than 10 submunitions that are sensor-fused. A more radical measure is using non-explosive "kinetic energy rods" in cluster munitions, which can pose no ERW threat as they mechanically destroy targets that they are guided to.[13] Finally, a move from mechanical to electrical fuses would reduce the likelihood of events in which failure might occur.[1]

Prior to the Oslo process agreement in Dublin in May 2008, the United Kingdom had agreed to withdraw munitions from service that could not self-neutralize, could not discriminate between targets, had explosive content or numerous submunitions. China and Russia indicated they would not replace all their submunitions. Russia claimed that modern cluster munitions are reliable, safe, and effective, and it would be better to concentrate on munition design rather than implement new legislation ([9]).

In the end, over one hundred countries adopted the treaty to ban cluster munitions at the cluster munitions conference held in Dublin, Ireland in May 2008. However, at the time of writing, the treaty had yet to be ratified in December 2008 in Oslo, which must be carried out by at least 30 countries. The scope of the ban exceeded many expectations, the exact terms of which were that each country would not;

- Use cluster munitions
- Develop, produce, otherwise acquire, stockpile, retain or transfer to anyone, directly or indirectly, cluster munitions
- Assist, encourage, or induce anyone to engage in any activity prohibited to a country under the convention

However, the all-important definition of a cluster munition sheds light on the discussion that took place to reach this agreement. A "cluster munition" is defined as a weapon designed to disperse or release explosive submunitions each weighing less than 20 kg, and includes the explosive submunitions.[14] Those for air defense or which produce electronic effects are not included, nor are those which fulfil all the following criteria;

- Each munition contains fewer than ten explosive submunitions
- Each explosive submunition weighs more than 4 kg
- Each explosive submunition is designed to detect and engage a single target object
- Each explosive submunition is equipped with an electronic self-destruction mechanism
- Each explosive submunition is equipped with an electronic self-deactivating feature

## 7.7
## Conclusion

It seems that cluster munitions are suited for a form of warfare unlikely in modern conflict. Those who would support their use are undermined by the lack of hard evidence of military efficacy and drowned out by those voices against cluster munitions that have growing evidence to support their point. Not only are cluster munitions viewed as an indiscriminate weapon in their mechanism of area effect, but they also have consistently been used in a seemingly indiscriminate manner, leaving a profound legacy.

With the success of ban proponents in Dublin, May 2008, it will be difficult for non-signatories of the Oslo process to rationalize use of munitions that fall outside the definition. However, it is worth noting that although 75% of the world's cluster munitions stockpilers were present in Dublin, and most of the producers and past users, the United States of America, Russia, Israel, and China have not yet adopted the Cluster Munitions Convention.

While there are strong opponents and proponents of the cluster-munition ban, it is only with due consideration of their military utility versus humanitarian imperatives that a realistic solution can be devised. As limited empirical data is currently available on either their military efficacy or the effects on human morbidity and mortality rates, a workable solution will require further research into these factors. Only then can appropriate technology be harnessed to ensure that future use is aligned with international humanitarian law.

Military forces that continue to use these weapons would do well to identify the circumstances where cluster munitions have conferred a real military advantage over other munitions, and to provide recommendations for the development of viable alternatives and better guidance for commanders on how and when to use such weapons. More rigorous restrictions on munitions' non-detonation rates and self-destruct features would also help.

**Acknowledgement**   An earlier version of this material was used for the author's dissertation for the Diploma in the Medical Care of Catastrophes, Society of Apothecaries of London.

## References

1. Hiznay M. Operational and technical aspects of cluster munitions. *Disarmament Forum.* 2006;4:15-23.
2. GICHD. *A Guide to Cluster Munitions First Edition.* Geneva: GICHD; 2007:14, 16, 24, 25, 27-28, 83.
3. Handicap International. *Circle of Impact: The Fatal Footprint of Cluster Munitions on People and Communities.* Brussels: Handicap International ASBL-VZW; 2007:41, 138-139.
4. ICRC. *Humanitarian, Military, Technical and Legal Challenges of Cluster Munitions.* Switzerland: Montreux; 2007:66-68, 74.
5. Landmine Action. *Out of Balance: The UK Government's Efforts to Understand Cluster Munitions and International Humanitarian Law.* London: Landmine Action; 2005:5.
6. Moyes R. *Cluster Munitions in Kosovo: Analysis of Use, Contamination and Casualties.* London: Landmine Action; 2007:2-3.
7. Pacific Centre for Military Law. Report on States' Parties' Responses to the Questionnaire on International Humanitarian Law & Explosive Remnants of War. Thirteenth Session, Geneva, 6–10 March, 2006, Item 7 of the Agenda, Explosive Remnants of War, Working Group on Explosive Remnants of War. Prepared by the Asia Pacific Centre for Military Law, presented at the request of the Coordinator on ERW; 2005.
8. UNMAS. Safety & occupational health – Protection of the environment. International Mine Action Standard. United Nations Mine Action Service; 2007.
9. Women's International League for Peace and Freedom – Meeting of the Group of Governmental Experts (GGE) of the Convention on Certain Conventional Weapons (CCW)19–22 June 2007 [Online]. Available at: http://www.wilpf.int.ch/disarmament/CCWGGE2007/GGEindex.html. Accessed 2 November 2007.
10. Editorial. Cluster bombs: measuring the human cost. *Lancet.* 2005;366:1904.
11. Rappert B. Moyes R. *Failure to Protect: A Case for the Prohibition of Cluster Munitions.* London: Landmine Action; 2006:8, 13, 22, 27.
12. Moyes R. *Explosive Remnants of War: Unexploded Ordnance and Post-Conflict Communities.* London: Landmine Action; 2002.
13. Garwin R, Worden S. Ballistic Missiles: Threat and Response [Online]. http://www.marshall.org/article.php?id=66. Accessed 14 October 2007.
14. Diplomatic Conference for the Adoption of a Convention on Cluster Munitions. Dublin Conference, May 2008 [Online]. Available at: www.clustermunitionsdublin.ie/pdf/ENGLISHfinaltext.pdf. Accessed 1 July 2008.

# Shaped Charges and Explosively Formed Projectiles

**8**

Jonathan Morrison and Peter F. Mahoney

## 8.1
## Introduction

Detonation of a high explosive (HE) material in air results in an omnidirectional blast wave. By confining the HE in a container and shaping the exposed end, the blast wave can be focused in a specific direction: this is generically referred to as a "shaped charge" (SC).[1-3] By inlaying a solid "liner" material into the shaped explosive, detonation results in the formation of a high-velocity projectile. In a SC, the liner shape is usually a cone, although that can vary depending on the desired projectile. Figure 8.1 is a typical construction of a shaped charge.

In a SC, the confined explosion collapses the liner into a projectile which can achieve a velocity of up to 10–15 km/s.[1] The projectile is not formed instantaneously, but the collapse takes place over a distance referred to as the "standoff distance." Equally, once formed, the projectile is not a stable entity and will only maintain its integrity dependent on several liner related factors (such as the grain and ductility of the liner material used).[4] By changing the confinement, explosive, liner material, and configuration, a spectrum of projectiles and behaviors can be obtained. An important sub-type of SCs are Explosively Formed Projectile's (EFP) which utilize a saucer liner configuration to create a slower but more stable projectile.

Shaped charges and their derivatives are utilized in a number of fields including mining, construction, demolition, and the military either as a primary anti-armor weapon or as components of a weapon sub-system (e.g., the initiation of nuclear weapons). Militarily, two important groups of shaped charge weapons (SCW) are High Explosive Anti-Tanks (HEAT) munitions and the EFP-Improvised Explosive Devices (EFP-IED) utilized by irregular forces.

A comprehensive understanding of SCs and their derivatives requires knowledge of mathematics, physics, chemistry, and engineering. Due to the complex subject matter, the mechanism of weapon function and injury may be poorly understood amongst clinicians. A number of inaccuracies have been perpetuated due to oversimplification in various media. This is further compounded by a confusing non-standardized vocabulary. This

J. Morrison (✉)
Surgical Intensive Care Unit, Southern General Hospital, 1345 Govan Road,
Glasgow, G51 4TF, UK
e-mail: jonny_morrison@doctors.org.uk

A.J. Brooks et al. (eds.), *Ryan's Ballistic Trauma*,
DOI: 10.1007/978-1-84882-124-8_8, © Springer-Verlag London Limited 2011

**Fig. 8.1** A line drawing of a generic shaped charge weapon (From Weickert.[2] Reprinted with kind permission of Springer Science and Business Media)

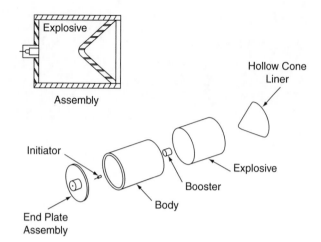

**Table 8.1** Glossary of shaped charge terminology

| Term | Definition |
|---|---|
| Explosively formed penetrator <br> Explosively formed perforator <br><br> Self forging fragment | Also known as explosively formed projectile |
| Miznay-Schardin plate | Large anti-tank EFP, often laid as a mine |
| Ballistic disk <br> Lense | Another term for liner |
| CD | Charge diameter, width of liner |

chapter is designed to provide the reader with a basic guide to the historical context, physics, and terminal ballistics involved in HEAT and EFP weapon systems. Table 8.1 is a glossary of terms used throughout this chapter.

## 8.2
## Historical Context

The history of the development of shaped charges is open to debate. It is generally accepted that the first published report was by von Baader in 1792 who discussed bore hole drilling and the behavior of confined explosives. The essence of his analysis was that one could focus the explosive power of a charge by forming a hollow in the explosive. He did not specifically use the term "hollow charge,"[1] although subsequent researchers used this in deference to his findings.

The hollow charge effect was more fully demonstrated by von Fœrster in 1883 who used shaped guncotton to propel a coin into a wrought-iron plate. This was repeated in 1888 by Charles Munroe in America who used this technique to engrave lettering into a steel plate. Munroe made detailed observations that for the same mass of non-shaped explosive, only minor indentation could be achieved in the same steel plate.[5] The phenomenon of a hollow charge is known in Europe as the von Fœrster Effect and in the UK and US as the Munroe Effect.

In 1910, Neuman of Germany used the first metal liner in conjunction with a hollow charge, creating the modern "explosively formed projectile." Neuman used a tin can with a hole in the top and filled with dynamite to punch a hole through a steel safe.

During the build-up to the Second World War, the Swiss chemical engineer Mohaupt experimented with Shaped Charge Weapons (SCW) while developing a hand held anti-tank weapon. He noted that when he tried to propel steel cones (the weapon liner) at a target using conically shaped explosives, the hole produced in the target was smaller than the liner. He also noted that penetration of the target was far greater than expected, with no evidence of liner fragmentation.

With these established principles, a number of countries began developing SCW for soldiers to defeat steel armor. Mohaupt initially lead research for the French, although later he worked for the Americans on the Bazooka Project. The likely first SCW was the British No. 68 rifle grenade which entered service May 1940. This could only penetrate up to 50 mm of steel armor, rendering it ineffective against the thickly armored German Panzer Tanks. Subsequent devices included the British PIAT spigot mortar and the German Panzerfaust.[5]

Following the end of the Second World War, it became apparent that SCs could be utilized by certain industries in addition to military applications. Mohaupt continued to lead the field, experimenting with bigger devices and different liner material. These types of devices are utilized extensively by the mining industry as a cutting tool to open up rock formations and in demolitions.[2] They are preferable to bulk charges as SCs are directional and thus more predictable in their behavior.

The warhead in a HEAT munition uses a shaped charge detonated at a precise standoff distance to penetrate vehicle armor. To achieve this precise detonation, the engineering requirements are significant. HEAT munitions have become one of the main munitions of choice for Main Battle Tank (MBT) combat. Figure 8.2 is a drawing of such a munition. HEAT munitions

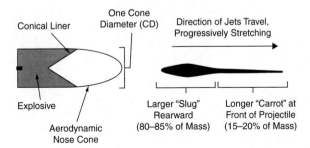

**Fig. 8.2** A drawing of a HEAT Munition (*left* image) and the resultant projectile (*right* image). The projectile will progressively stretch until it breaks up into small fragments (Reproduced from Morrison[6] by kind permission of the Editor)

accounted for around 20–25% of "hits" by Israeli MBTs against Arab armored units in the 1973 Arab-Israeli conflict.[7] In the 1991 Gulf War, this figure increased to 70% of "hits" by coalition forces based on the analysis of 308 recovered Iraqi MBTs.[8] Further examples of HEAT munitions include the missile based systems such as Maverick and Hellfire.

## 8.3
## Physics

A shaped charge is constructed from a robust casing filled with a high explosive (HE) – the shape of the casing is referred to as the *confinement*.[4] At one end of the casing there is an axis-symmetric geometric shape precisely indented in the HE in which a *liner* is inlayed. The configuration of the liner in a SC is usually conical; however, an ellipse, tulip or similar also work.[1] The liner material is usually metallic, although, ceramic and glass have been described.[9,10] A wide range of metals have been employed from simple copper and steel to complex alloys and depleted uranium.[4] At the opposite end to the liner lies the detonator. Figure 8.1 is an illustration of a generic SC device.

Upon detonation of the shaped charge, the rapidly expanding gaseous products push a high pressure wave along the axis of symmetry towards the liner at around 8 km/s, concentrating the power of the detonation along an axis (the Munroe Effect described previously). Upon reaching the liner, the detonation wave exerts enormous pressures, up to 200 GPa (30 million psi) for a few microseconds. This collapses and distorts the liner on its central axis, driving it into a jet shaped projectile with the tip traveling in excess of 10 km/s. About 80–85% of the jet mass is rearward and travels more slowly at around 1 km/s.[1,2] The penetration *potential* of a shaped charge is proportional to the penetrator length and the square root of the penetrator density.[10] While airborne the penetrator length is not constant due to the different speeds of the tip and the base and it will stretch until it eventually undergoes *particulation*. Particulation diminishes the ability to penetrate the target. The distance at which the projectile is formed so that it can "optimally" penetrate its target is the *standoff distance*. Figure 8.3 is a computer generated image of a liner collapse and subsequent projectile formation.

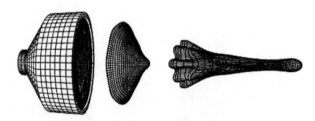

**Fig. 8.3** A computer generated image of the stages of formation of an explosively formed penetrator. *Left* image: liner prior to detonation. *Middle* image: liner collapse and distortion during detonation. *Right* image: the explosively formed penetrator in flight (From Florence,[11] Fig. 1. Reprinted with kind permission from Elsevier)

The real measure of a shaped charge is its capacity to penetrate the target material. On impact of the penetrator with its target, exceptionally high pressures are generated. These maybe from 100 to 200 GPa and the target metals temperature rises to between 25% and 50% of its melting point.[9] The penetrator creates a cavity and begins to propel through the target material. This effect is not a thermal phenomenon but related to the enormous pressures pushing the target metal aside. The overall mass of the target should theoretically remain stable throughout impact, although some will be lost through vaporization and spall (debris from the internal surface of the vehicles armor). A well engineered shaped charge with a standard copper liner of charge diameter CD will make a hole about CD/6 in diameter and about 5–10 CD deep in steel.[2] The small diameter of the hole is crucial to the penetration potential; the energy of the jet is concentrated in a very small area.

The penetration characteristics and standoff performance of a SC will need to differ depending on the task to be accomplished. For example, in mining, a cutting jet with a precise and predictable penetrating depth is essential. In a HEAT munition, a very short standoff performance is important otherwise the projectile would not be fully formed prior to "engaging" the enemy armor. Additionally, as the HEAT warhead detonates at a known distance, the jet needs only to maintain its integrity for a short period of time. This requires very precise initiation of the HEAT round.

These characteristics are the opposite requirement to the EFP-IEDs used by irregular forces to defeat armor.[6] As the distance between the EFP-IED and target is more variable, a long standoff distance is essential. This is achieved by using a saucer shaped liner producing a larger, slower, more stable projectile, albeit with a reduced penetration potential. A typical single piece EFP can travel at around 2–3 km/s achieving a penetration depth of 0.8–1 CD.[2] Additionally, the initial hole will be much greater in size. Figure 8.4 is a drawing of an EFP and Fig. 8.5 is a photograph of a captured insurgent EFP-IED.

A further issue is the precise engineering requirement. Successful liner collapse, jet formation, and penetration depend upon the maintenance of axisymmetrical flow. Any uneven radial force will interrupt the process and impair jet function. To illustrate the requirements, a typical 81 mm copper cone requires the liner thickness to vary no more than $\pm 0.001$ inch. As the cone diameter decreases, the tolerances become yet more precise.[4] This has implications for irregular forces constructing EFP-IEDs and thus such

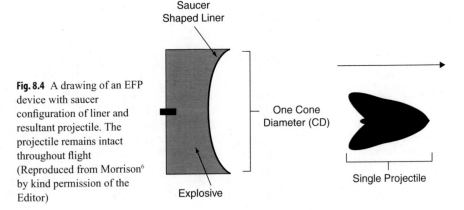

**Fig. 8.4** A drawing of an EFP device with saucer configuration of liner and resultant projectile. The projectile remains intact throughout flight (Reproduced from Morrison[6] by kind permission of the Editor)

**Fig. 8.5** A drawing of shaped charge using a "Tandem" liner to deliver a hypervelocity jet followed by a slower, larger projectile

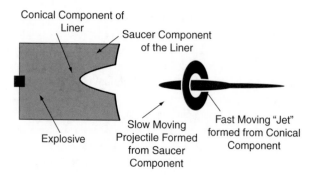

Conical Component of Liner

Saucer Component of the Liner

Explosive

Slow Moving Projectile Formed from Saucer Component

Fast Moving "Jet" formed from Conical Component

devices may not function efficiently. It has to be understood however, that while an EFP-IED may not function efficiently, it still functions delivering a high-velocity projectile.

Conical and saucer shapes are not the only liner configuration utilized. Stability of the projectile is crucial if the target is to be engaged accurately. A spinning projectile is inherently more stable as illustrated by a round traveling through a rifled barrel. In an effort to duplicate this, fluted lines have been developed which provide angular momentum providing a degree of stability.[1] Figure 8.6 is a line drawing of a conical and saucer fluted liners. A more effective strategy is to change the confinement of the explosive from cylindrical to a geometric shape with straight sides such as hexagonal.[2] This creates a "finned" appearance of the projectile enhancing the aerodynamic properties.

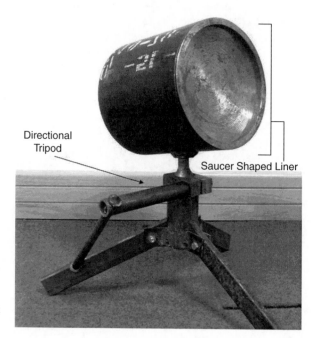

Directional Tripod

Saucer Shaped Liner

**Fig. 8.6** A captured Iraqi insurgent IED-EFP. Note the saucer configured liner and directional tripod (Courtesy of SSgt Chris Hewitt of Joint (UK) EOD Group)

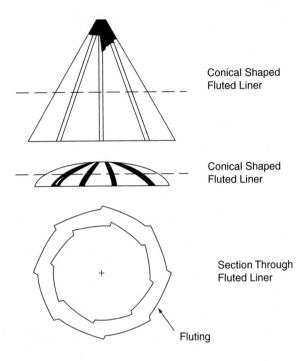

**Fig. 8.7** A line drawing of a conical and saucer shaped fluted liner. The *bottom* image is a cross-section illustrating the fluting (Modified from Walter.[1] With kind permission from Springer Science + Business Media)

Conical Shaped Fluted Liner

Conical Shaped Fluted Liner

Section Through Fluted Liner

Fluting

As described above, HEAT munitions have short standoff distances yet large penetrating potential. EFP have longer standoff distances but less penetrating power. In certain military circumstances, such as "bunker-busting" or defeating Explosive Reactive Armour, a munition with both properties is desirable. By using a "Tandem" liner which incorporates both a saucer and conical liner component that effect can be achieved.[12] The conical liner fires a fast jet into the target which is then followed up a slower larger projectile formed from the saucer. Figure 8.7 illustrates such a configured liner.

## 8.4
## Clinical Aspects

HEAT munitions have been used in conventional war fighting since the Second World War and there is a large volume of open source material assessing injury patterns.[5,7] The widespread use of EFP-IED is a relatively new phenomenon and has been largely confined to the Iraq conflict. Open source data specific to EFP-IED is available, although limited in patient numbers.[13,14]

Past experience of injuries sustained by armored vehicle crew has identified ballistic (fragment) and burns as major mechanisms. Ballistic injury has accounted for around 75% of all injuries.[7,15-17] Burns made up about 26% of injuries incurred by crews in the 1982 Lebanon War.[17] Vehicle design improvements to protect crews against fragment and fire include spall-suppression linings, compartmentalizing fuel and munitions, flame resistant clothing, and automatic fire suppression systems.[18]

Toxic fumes and blunt trauma depend upon the construction material and strength of the vehicle under attack. Blunt trauma is also influenced by the shape of the passenger compartments and whether there are exposed bolts and other structures for crew members to be thrown against.

Primary blast injury (PBI) is common in fatalities.[19] The effect of a blast wave is exaggerated by the "confined" nature of vehicles compared with "open-air" explosions.[20] The exact incidence of primary blast injury in survivors is uncertain. Ripple and Phillips [18] quote closed source US Army Medical Research and Developmental Command (USA MRDC) studies indicating a probable incidence of between 1% and 20% PBI in survivors from a large warhead penetrating an armored vehicle (in addition to their other injuries).

While there are numerous studies analyzing casualty data from the Iraq theater, few specifically include EFP-IED as a mechanism of injury (MOI) as it is a relatively recent development. Most currently available data pertains to the combat and occupation phases of operations in Iraq, 2003, i.e., Operation Telic I and II (UK) and Operation Iraqi Freedom I and II (US).[21-27] EFP-IEDs have only become prevalent post-invasion.[28-30] Many studies include the term IED; however, by definition this encompasses all manner of hostile explosions from modified convention munitions to homemade bulk explosives. Table 8.2 is an amalgam of open source

**Table 8.2** Location of penetrating wounds and mechanism

| Reference | Anatomical location (%) | | | | | | Mechanism (%) | | |
|---|---|---|---|---|---|---|---|---|---|
| | Head | Neck | Chest | Back | Abdo | Limb | IED | Mine | GSW |
| 21 | 17 | 2 | 5 | 5 | 4 | 68 | 46 (explosives) | | 25 |
| 22 | 21 (combined) | | 5 | – | 3 | 62 | – | – | – |
| 23 | 49 | 5 | 3 | 5 | 4 | 35 | 62 | 35 | 3 |
| 24 | 16 (combined) | | 13 | 4 | 10 | 64 | 63 (fragmentation) | | 37 |
| 25 | 28 | – | 7 (combined) | | | 46 | 78 (explosives) | | 22 |
| 26 | 27 | 3 | 6 | – | 11 | 54 | 38 | 41 | 19 |
| 27 | 13 | 5 | 4 | 6 | 2 | 64 | – | 45 | 24 |

*Explanatory Notes:*
Reference
| 21 | Mechanism: does not add to 100% as included non-penetrating and un-stated categories |
| 22 | Anatomical location: remaining 9% suffered burns and psychological injury |
| 24 | Figures included civilians treated |
| 25 | Anatomical location: 19% unaccounted, burns, combined and undocumented injuries |
| 26 | Mechanism: 2% dues to motor vehicle collision (MVC) |
| 27 | Anatomical location: 6% unknown or multiple injuries |
| | Mechanisms: No IED category and included blunt mechanism |

penetrating wound data in patients who either were killed-in-action (KIA) or wounded-in-action (WIA). Studies which concentrated on a particular organ injury or mechanism were excluded.

Kelly et al.[15] performed an analysis of injury severity and causes of death in Iraq comparing the period 2003–04 and 2006.[15] Explosions (including IEDs) had caused 56% of injuries in 2003–04 rising significantly to 76% in 2006 ($p<0.001$). The biggest cause of death in their study was hemorrhage (87% and 83% in two cohorts, potentially survivable and non-survivable), specifically non-compressible torso hemorrhage. Although EFP-IED as a mechanism was not deliberately mentioned, the authors made the point that IEDs have increased in lethality. Clearly, one should be cautious at ascribing this exclusively to EFP-IED.

Two British studies do specifically include EFP-IED in their analysis of mechanism of injury. [13, 14]

Hodgetts et al.[13] analyzed 76 consecutive trauma related deaths from both Iraq (31 fatalities) and Afghanistan (45 fatalities) between 1 April 2006 to 31 March 2007.[13] Hostile action accounted for 57 of these deaths of which 19 were related to gunshot wounds (GSW) and the remaining 38 to blast and fragmentation. Within the latter group, 17 fatalities were due to "improvised explosive device or explosively formed projectile."

Ramasamy et al.[14] analyzed 100 consecutive British Military trauma patients injured or killed by hostile action between January and October 2006.[14] Fifty-three patients were killed or injured by IEDs and were further analyzed in depth to characterized the injury pattern. The cohort was injured in 23 IED incidents, 21 of which were EFP-IED. There were 2.3 casualties per incident with a range of 1–5. Of the 53 patients, there were 12 fatalities all related to EFP-IED.

Within the fatalities group, the mean new Injury Severity Score (NISS) was 4.67 body areas affected whereas the mean score for the survivors group was 2.61 body areas affected. The precise anatomical distribution is detailed in Table 8.3 (taken from Ramasamy's paper).

**Table 8.3** Anatomical pattern of wounding[13]

| Anatomical locations | IED survivors | IED fatalities |
|---|---|---|
| Lower extremities | 37 (90) | 6 (50) |
| Upper extremities | 37 (90) | 9 (75) |
| Face | 13 (32) | 6 (50) |
| Neck | 8 (20) | 7 (58) |
| Head | 6 (17) | 7 (58) |
| Abdomen | 0 (0) | 5 (42) |
| Pelvis | 0 (0) | 7 (58) |
| Chest/back | 6 (0) | 9 (75) |
| Total anatomical area | 107 | 56 |
| Total patients | 41 | 12 |
| Average anatomical locations per patient | 2.61 | 4.67 |

From Ramasamy.[14] Reprinted with kind permission of Wolters Kluwer Health
Percentage of casualties affected in parentheses ()

This distribution and NISS analysis lead the authors to conclude that injury from EFP-IED was an "all or nothing" phenomenon. Patients caught in the trajectory sustained massive polytrauma which was almost universally fatal or were peripherally related and sustained relatively minor injury.

The mechanism of injury was generally secondary blast injury from metallic fragments. Primary blast injury was only a feature in 3.7% of patients, disagreeing with the suggestion from an earlier paper by Morrison et al. They had postulated this on the basis of a comparison with HEAT injuries.[6]

## 8.5
## Case of an EFP-IED

A male occupant was traveling in a vehicle was subject to an EFP-IED attack. He sustained a single wound to his left shoulder illustrated in Fig. 8.8. Note the discreet wound with a large volume of soft tissue destruction. The plain radiograph in Fig. 8.9 demonstrates the degree of bony injury and retained fragments.

Clinicians managing these injuries need to be aware of the potentially very destructive nature of these wounds. Clearly, prompt surgery to arrest hemorrhage is vital, although often multiple consecutive operations are required in the later reconstructive stages. This is especially the case for limb injuries where there is significant bony and soft tissue loss.

### Summary Points

- Shaped Charges utilize high explosive to collapse a liner material into a high velocity projectile.
- They are utilized in the mining and demolitions industry as they are directional and highly predictable in their behavior.

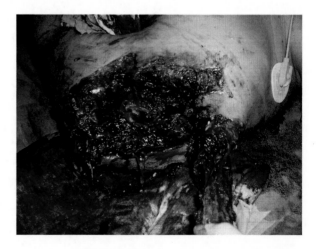

**Fig. 8.8** A view of the *left* shoulder following an EFP-IED injury. Note the significant soft tissue destruction. Orientation: neck at *top right*, *left* arm *top left*

**Fig. 8.9** The plain radiograph of the shoulder in Fig. 8.8 identifying bony destruction and retained fragments

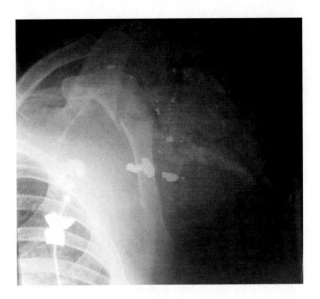

- Militarily, shaped charges are predominantly used as an anti-armor weapon in High Explosive Anti-Tank munitions (HEAT).
- Their mechanism of wound is predominantly by fragmentation and burns.
- Blast and blunt injury are also a feature in armored vehicle crew casualties, although that likely relates to vehicle design.
- Explosively formed projectiles are a sub-set of shaped charges which use a wider, saucer shaped liner to achieve greater standoff performance.
- EFP generates a larger and slower projectile with reduced penetration potential.
- They have emerged militarily in the form of EFP-IED used by irregular forces.
- Despite limited published data, EFP-IEDs appear to inflict catastrophic fragmentation injury to those caught in the trajectory and minor injury to those outwith. Blast injury is a minor component.

**Acknowledgement** An earlier version of this chapter was published as Morrison JJ, Mahoney PF, Hodgetts T. Shaped charges and explosively formed penetrators: background for clinicians. *JR Army Med Corps.* 2007;153(3):184-187 and material is used with permission.

## References

1. Walter WP, Zukas JA. *Fundamentals of Shaped Charges.* 1st ed. Canada: Wiley; 1989.
2. Weickert CA. Demolitions. In: Zukas JA, Walters WP, eds. *Explosive Effects and Applications.* New York: Springer-Verlag; 2003:381-425.
3. Carlucci DE, Jacobson SS. *Ballistics: Theory and Design of Guns and Ammunition.* 1st ed. US: CRC Press; 2008.
4. Walters W. Introduction to Shaped Charges. Defence Technology Information Centre. March 2007. Available at http://handle.dtic.mil/100.2/ADA469696. Accessed June 26, 2008.
5. Bellamy RF. A shaped charge warhead versus a tank. *Mil Med.* 1988;153:246-247.

6. Morrison JJ, Mahoney PF, Hodgetts TJ. Shaped charges and explosively formed penetrators: background for clinicians. *J R Army Med Corps*. 2007;153(3):184-187.

7. Dougherty PJ. Armored vehicle crew casualties. *Mil Med*. 1990;155:417-420.

8. Held M. Warhead hit distribution on main battle tanks in the Gulf war. *J Battlefield Tech*. 2000;3:1-9.

9. Doig A. Some metallurgical aspects of shaped charge liners. *J Battlefield Tech*. 1998;1:1-3.

10. Held M. Liners for shaped charges. *J Battlefield Tech*. 2001;4:1-6.

11. Florence AL, Gefken PR, Kirkpatrick SW. Dynamic plastic buckling of copper cylindrical shells. *Int J Solids Struct*. 1991;27:89-103.

12. Scott B. *Ballistics 2005: 22nd International Symposium on Ballistics*. US: Destech Publications; 2005.

13. Hodgetts T, Davies S, Midwinter M, et al. Operational mortality of UK service personnel in Iraq and Afghanistan: a one year analysis 2006–2007. *J R Army Med Corps*. 2008;153(4): 252-254.

14. Ramasamy A, Harrisson SE, Clasper JC, et al. Injuries from roadside improvised explosive devices. *J Trauma*. 2008;65:910-914.

15. Kelly JF, Ritenour AE, McLaughline DF, et al. Injury severity and causes of death from operation Iraqi freedom and operation enduring freedom: 2003–2004 versus 2006. *J Trauma*. 2008;64:S21-S27.

16. Danon YL, Nili E, Dolev E. Primary treatment of battle casualties in the Lebanon war, 1982. *Isr J Med Sci*. 1984;20:300-302.

17. Shafir R, Nili E, Kedem R. Burn injury and prevention in the Lebanon war, 1982. *Isr J Med Sci*. 1984;20:311-313.

18. Ripple GR, Phillips Y. Military explosions. In: Cooper GJ, Dudley HAF, Gann DS, Little RA, Maynard RL, eds. *Scientific Foundations of Trauma*. Oxford: Butterworth-Heinemann; 1997:247-257.

19. Stankovic Z, Kovacevic V, Karen Z, et al. Morphological characteristics of persons killed in armoured vehicles. *Mil-Med and Pharma Rev*. 1991;48:531-534.

20. Leibovici D, Gofrit ON, Stein M, et al. Blast injuries: bus versus open-air bombings – a comparative study of injuries in survivors of open-air versus confined-space explosions. *J Trauma*. 1996;41:1030-1035.

21. Zouris JM, Walker GJ, Dye J, et al. Wounding patterns for US marines and sailors during Operation Iraqi Freedom, Major Combat Phase. *Mil Med*. 2006;171:246-252.

22. Patel TH, Wenner KA, Price SA. A US army forward surgical team's experience in Operation Iraqi Freedom. *J Trauma*. 2004;57:201-207.

23. Gondusky JS, Reiter MP. Protecting military Cinvoys in Iraq: an examination of battle injuries sustained by a mechanized battalion during Operation Iraqi Freedom II. *Mil Med*. 2005;170:546-549.

24. Hinsley DE, Rosell PAE, Rowlands TK, et al. Penetrating missile injuries during asymmetric warfare in the 2003 Gulf conflict. *Br J Surg*. 2005;92:637-642.

25. Murray CK, Reynolds JC, Schroeder JM, et al. Spectrum of care provided at an Echelon II medical unit during Operation Iraqi Freedom. *Mil Med*. 2005;170(6):516-520.

26. Owens BD, Kragh JF, Wenke JC, et al. Combat wounds in Operation Iraqi Freedom and Operation Enduring Freedom. *J Trauma*. 2008;64:295-299.

27. Galarneau MR, Hancock WC, Konoske P, et al. The navy – marine corps trauma registry. *Mil Med*. 2006;171(8):691-697.

28. Arun N. Shaped bombs magnify Iraq attacks. BBC News, October 10, 2005. Available at http://news.bbc.co.uk/2/hi/middle_east/4320818.stm. Accessed May 6, 2006.

29. Harnden T. Iraqis using "new Hizbollah bombs" to kill British troops. Telegraph Group Limited, April 30, 2006. Available at http://www.telegraph.co.uk/news/main.jhtml?xml=/news/2006/04/30/wiran130.xml. Accessed May 6, 2006.

30. Clay W. Improvised explosive devices in Iraq: effects and countermeasures. *Congressional Research Service*. 2005; **RS22330**: CRS 1-6.

# Suicide Bombs

# 9

Piers R.J. Page and Ian Greaves

## 9.1
## Introduction

It is conventionally accepted that the first suicide bomb was used in the assassination of Tsar Alexander II in 1881. In more recent times, suicide bombing has become an increasingly used technique. Israel has seen regular attacks and most recently Iraq and Afghanistan have seen a large number of incidents. Overall, a recent estimate puts the death toll from this form of attack at 1840 people since 1983. It would appear that the attractions of the suicide bomb to the terrorist are the devastating nature of the injuries which result and the possibility of achieving dramatic religious martyrdom. It is no coincidence that the suicide bomb is a weapon of the religiously motivated terrorist and has played little role in the repertoire of those with secular or purely political aims.

As a tool of paramilitary or terrorist force, suicide bombing has much to offer. With it, very confined spaces and therefore high-density targets can be attacked. There is considerable potential to conceal such a weapon and no complex trigger system is required. Infiltration of the weapon into the location is relatively straightforward. Logistically, teams can be kept very small for launching the attacks as there is no requirement for escape or evasion by the perpetrator after the incident. The kill ratio is enormous; for one life sacrificed, 100 can easily be killed or injured in the right environment. There is also no perpetrator to be questioned and no risk of compromise of the terrorist group. In addition it is difficult to establish effective security measures against suicide bombs.

The technology of suicide bombings can vary significantly. However, the majority of attacks conform to the conventionally recognized model of an explosive package worn as a belt or waistcoat, commonly with fragmentation weapons incorporated in to the design. These primary fragments are easily produced by the incorporation of nails, screws, or nuts on the victim-facing side of the weapon.

P.R.J. Page (✉)
Department of Orthopaedics and Trauma, Frimley Park Hospital, Portsmouth Road, Frimley, Surrey, GU16 7UJ, UK
e-mail: piers.page@gmail.com

A.J. Brooks et al. (eds.), *Ryan's Ballistic Trauma*,
DOI: 10.1007/978-1-84882-124-8_9, © Springer-Verlag London Limited 2011

## 9.2
## Ballistics

As previously mentioned, one of the purposes of suicide weapons is to introduce them into a much higher target density environment than that in which a terrorist may be able to plant a larger IED. As a result, effects may be produced which would require a much larger explosive charge in a different form such as a vehicle borne device. Such an enclosed environment - a bus (sometimes termed an ultra-confined space) or cafe, for example, is a significantly more dangerous place in an explosion than a more open environment, due to the reflection of blast waves within a limited space. Not only will the victims will be struck multiple times by the blast wave, but the peak overpressure of a complex blast wave can be 10 times higher than that from which it originated, as a result of summation of reflected and coincident waves.

Another implication of the close proximity of suicide bombers to their victims is an increased missile energy – although fragments will have a velocity an order of magnitude less than that of a bullet, those striking victims inches or a few feet away will have had minimal chance for their kinetic energy to decay (as opposed to a roadside IED which may be many meters away). The energy decay of such irregularly shaped fragments is rapid and as a result proximity is a key factor in killing potential of these weapons.

The proximity and often centrality of the weapon also means that victims closest are at risk from not only the energy of the fragments but the sheer number of them.

## 9.3
## Primary Injury Patterns

### 9.3.1
### Lung Injury

Blast lung injury (BLI) is a significant cause of morbidity and mortality in these attacks and will lead to a more frequent requirement for ventilatory support amongst the victims. Blast lung injury is associated with very high levels of blast loading and is relatively rare in "conventional" terrorist incidents. It is more common in the victims of suicide bombs as a result of their proximity to the detonation as well as the likelihood of the incident occurring in an enclosed space. It is possible that the requirement for intensive care based ventilatory support will be greater than the capacity of the nearest receiving hospitals. In many areas where suicide bombs are commonly used, such support may not be available at all, significantly increasing the overall mortality. It should be borne in mind when planning the response to these attacks that although BLI patients may not immediately manifest as such, the pressures involved make widespread pulmonary injury likely. This has several implications; a triage system sufficiently sensitive to detect those patients in whom there is a risk of development of lung injury, a clear protocol for their observation and treatment, and an intensive care bed management strategy are among the most important.

### 9.3.2
### Gastrointestinal Injury

It has also been suggested that primary deceleration injuries to abdominal viscera are a significant risk, but there is little consensus here; the Israeli experience in one trauma registry series was that 94.4% of abdominal wounds were secondary and perforating in nature, resulting from fragments (either weapon or environmental). On the other hand, Madrid surgical teams reported a higher rate of primary abdominal injury from the ultra-confined nature of the train explosions on the Madrid train system, and historically another Israeli team reported 2 perforations as primary injuries in a patient group of 29 from a bus bombing. As with the blast lung patients discussed earlier, both patients with abdominal perforation presented late at 3 and 7 days respectively. It is sensible to assume that all patients who have been exposed to a significant blast loading are at risk of gastrointestinal perforation but that the risk is probably relatively small. Clinically, it has proven impossible to identify these patients before there are signs of peritonitis and as a result, careful observation is the appropriate management strategy.

It is worth paying further consideration to the exact mechanism of primary abdominal injury. The blast wave creates a shear force at density interfaces between tissue types. The logical conclusion is that in an attack in a confined space, resulting in a complex wave, there is potential for multiple shear forces to be generated near-simultaneously as the individual impulses of the wave pass through the victim. If each one has different orientation, the overall ballistic effect is of multidirectional shear trauma. It is important that the surgical team are prepared for this before embarking on any surgical procedures.

### 9.4
### Secondary Injury Patterns

The deliberate inclusion of material for its fragmentation effects has become a classical feature of the suicide bomb. Nuts, nails, and ball bearings are all typical of the readily available arsenal of the bomb-maker. The devastating nature of the injuries which result from these fragments should not be underestimated and is a significant factor in the development of psychological problems in survivors and rescue personnel alike.

The injury pattern is much less predictable than seen in conventional munitions using preformed fragments – notched wire in grenades, flechettes, and casing fragments from shells or mines have an a much more uniform shape and size and as a result a more uniform velocity, kinetic energy, and therefore injury pattern.

The implication of this for the surgeon is that there may well be a spectrum of injury from mutilating wounds to multiple superficial flesh wounds. Initially less obvious fragment wounds may be indicative of underlying injury resulting in haemodynamic instability or may act as a focus of infection and source of otherwise inexplicable pyrexia.

Concealed injury is a risk in suicide attacks; those not causing immediate compromise and leaving no obvious external signs. One Israeli case reports a nail with a subtle intra-oral entry wound becoming lodged in a teenage girl's brain. For this reason, the Israeli protocol dictates total body imaging for stable casualties – again, planning must take into account the logistic implications for radiology, should this be considered the adopted standard.

There are some immunological considerations to secondary injury. Firstly, tetanus cover must be established or provided for these casualties; most protocols include automatic boosters regardless of previous vaccination state. Secondly, in addition to intended fragments, suicide attacks show an increased tendency to involve environmental debris (gravel, rubbish, and animal matter, etc.) which will have the expected microbiological implications.

Thirdly, and covered specifically later in the chapter, is the inclusion of allogenic biological material in debris. As suicide bombings have increased in regularity, a growing pattern has emerged of discovery of foreign bone fragments forming part of the secondary injury pattern. The risk of transmission of infection as a result of implantation of body parts is considered below.

## 9.5
## Tertiary Injury Patterns

The most significant form of tertiary injury in these attacks is probably traumatic amputation. Older work from Northern Ireland shows a relationship between extremity of amputation and survival (that is to say that those with more distal amputations had increased survival), and this remains true today.

This knowledge yields two key suggestions. Firstly, pre-hospital care practitioners must be familiar with the use of tourniquets. In the military, the Combat Application Tourniquet (CAT) is universal and has resulted in significant reductions in mortality from traumatic amputation. In the civilian world, however, such devices are more rarely used. Concerns about reperfusion injuries and the risk of adversely affecting the possibility of limb salvage may play a part in this. Current evidence strongly suggests that the risks of both are significantly outweighed by the increased survival rates following early and appropriate tourniquet use.

When planning the response to incidents of this kind, it is important to remember that the immediate response, although immensely challenging, is only one component of the required task. A large caseload of this type of injury will result in a sustained requirement for surgery and intensive care provision over a prolonged period. This will have a significant impact on the normal functioning of the hospital, especially with regard to elective services. Plans may be developed to spread this workload across appropriate centers when the immediate response to the incident is complete.

In less confined bombings, injuries resulting from victims being thrown significant distances may occur. This may be a less significant problem in suicide bombings which are generally detonated in spaces selected for their enclosure.

## 9.6
## Quaternary Injury Profile

Classically, these are burns, inhalational injuries, crush injury, and psychological problems. Flash burns may result from the detonation but significant burns, including inhalational injuries, are relatively unusual unless there is ignition of materials in the immediate vicinity of the explosion. Thermal inhalational injury may further compromise primary blast lung injury, resulting in significant respiratory compromise and exacerbating the need for ventilatory support to victims.

The rise of improvised CBRN devices (both used and intercepted at the planning stage) is another consideration. A detonation insufficiently powerful to shatter glass, for example, should raise extreme suspicion when causing respiratory compromise of a magnitude normally only seen in BLI. The same is true of burns; a scene with little or no fire and yet many burned patients may suggest deployment of a vesicant weapon.

The final aspect is that of psychological damage. Part of the plan for this type of incident should ensure that all patients from the scene are logged to allow follow-up in due course via their primary care provider. Furthermore, these providers should also be prepared for presentation of victims who had no injury warranting medical attention and may have been released from the scene after law enforcement procedures have been followed, or who have self evacuated without coming to the attention of officials at the scene.

## 9.7
## Security and Forensics

Suicide bombings are most commonly employed in the terrorist or insurgent environment, and so the precautions standard to such an incident must be taken. Those dealing with the incident in a pre-hospital environment should consider it a non-permissive environment until the nominated person in charge of scene security informs them otherwise. In most situations this will be the senior police officer at the scene (Police Commander or Police Incident Officer). The potential threats here are manifold – although a secondary device is unlikely it is by no means guaranteed to be absent. The incorporation of CBRN into such an incident potentially renders it both more dangerous and higher profile and so clinicians should be alert to unusual clinical features at the scene suggestive of a toxidrome or non-traumatic manifestation.

Although the responsibility of the incident commander, all responders must be conscious of the risk of admitting an unidentified perpetrator into the casualty chain. Quite apart from any further deliberate acts, a live perpetrator may suggest incomplete or failed detonation of the device and hence substantial risk to the emergency response.

Evidence preservation needs to be incorporated into the medical plan for a suicide bombing – agreement with law enforcement agencies before the event on how clothes, fragments, and biological debris are to be collected will facilitate best care, whilst safeguarding the prospects of any future investigation. It is also important to plan for the scenario where biological material is required for both forensic and clinical purposes.

## 9.8
## Biological Foreign Bodies

Clinicians can expect a significant pattern of secondary injury from a suicide blast. Of particular importance is the risk of casualties sustaining missile wounds from biological material originating from either the bomber or another victim.

The 7th July bombings in London caused numerous casualties; due to the ultra-confined nature of the incidents, the issue of biological material as a missile came to the fore. Wong et al. presented 5 cases some months after, all of whom had sustained secondary injuries involving embedding of allogenic bone. A key outcome was the rapid formulation of a risk and management matrix by the Health Protection Agency; this should now be part of the major incident response planning by healthcare providers. It is also important to note that the response involves primary care and secondary care centers which may be peripheral to the original event and so it is essential that the policy is widely disseminated. The baseline management referred to in the (Table 9.1) below is an accelerated Hepatitis B vaccination program (immediate, 1, 2, and 12 months) and immediate venesection for storage and Hepatitis B and C serology at 3 and 6 months.

Another lesson learned from the London bombings was that all biological debris was surrendered to law enforcement agencies for forensic evidence. This deprived clinicians of any opportunity to test for blood-borne viruses by polymerase chain reaction. Consensus on this between investigators and clinicians is important to ensure neither health care nor due process are compromised.

**Table 9.1** Risk and implementation categories of post-exposure prophylaxis for those sustaining wounds involving biological material

| Category | Wound description | Implementation of treatment |
| --- | --- | --- |
| 1 | Directly injured in explosion with major penetrating injuries leading to damaged skin and admitted to hospital | Post exposure management is feasible for in-patients and recommended as routine with the expectation that most patients will receive vaccination |
| 2 | Directly injured in explosion with penetrating injuries leading to damaged skin and discharged after receiving treatment at A&E | Where there are adequate ED records the patient's GP should be contacted and advised to offer post exposure management. Where GP information has not been retained, individuals contacting their GP or other healthcare provider should be offered post exposure management. |

**Table 9.1**  (continued)

| Category | Wound description | Implementation of treatment |
|---|---|---|
| 3 | Directly injured in explosion with penetrating injuries leading to damaged skin and did not attend A&E | It is unlikely to be possible to systematically contact all people within these categories, but where they present to services (emergency or health care) they should be offered post exposure management. NHS Direct and GPs should be informed of this to be able to respond in the event of victims contacting them. Where public messages and statements are made about health for victims, reference should be made to the need to contact GPs for advice on a number of matters including post traumatic stress, hearing loss as well as BBV risk. This to be distributed locally by HPU to care givers and NHS Direct alerted. |
| 4 | Indirectly injured (leading to damaged skin) as a result of providing assistance to victims of the explosion (for example cut from fragments of glass or metal on bodies of victims) | |
| 5 | Superficial exposure of skin or mucous membranes to blood of victims | Those who contact health care providers should have appropriate risk assessment and post exposure management only if blood exposure to damaged skin or mucous membranes occurred. |

Adapted from Health Protection Agency Guidance

## 9.9
## Conclusion

The suicide bomb is now one of the weapons of choice of the religiously motivated terrorist. It also forms part of the armamentarium of political extremists. It will undoubtedly be a key technique of those who seek to influence politics by the use of terror in the decades to come. Suicide bombs are effective because they inflict devastating injuries in locations which their victims have believed secure.

## Suggested Reading

Aharonson-Daniel L, et al. Suicide bombers form a new injury profile. *Ann Surg.* 2006;244(6): 1018-1023.
Almogy G, et al. Suicide bombing attacks: can external signs predict internal injuries? [see comment]. *Ann Surg.* 2006;243(4):541-546.

Almogy G, et al. Can external signs of trauma guide management?: lessons learned from suicide bombing attacks in Israel. *Arch Surg.* 2005;140(4):390-393.

Almogy G, et al. Suicide bombing attacks: update and modifications to the protocol.[see comment]. *Ann Surg.* 2004;239(3):295-303.

Bala M, et al. Abdominal trauma after terrorist bombing attacks exhibits a unique pattern of injury. *Ann Surg.* 2008;248(2):303-309.

DePalma RG, et al. Blast injuries. [see comment]. *N Engl J Med.* 2005;352(13):1335-1342.

Katz E, et al. Primary blast injury after a bomb explosion in a civilian bus. *Ann Surg.* 1989;209(4): 484-488.

Kluger Y. Bomb explosions in acts of terrorism – detonation, wound ballistics, triage and medical concerns. *Isr Med Assoc J.* 2003;5(4):235-240.

Mellor SG. The relationship of blast loading to death and injury from explosion. *World J Surg.* 1992;16(5):893-898.

Post exposure prophylaxis against hepatitis B for bomb victims and immediate care providers. Consideration of other blood borne viruses (hepatitis C and HIV). 2005 [cited 2009, 26 January 2009]. Available from: http://www.hpa.org.uk/webw/HPAweb&Page&HPAwebAutoListName/ Page/1204542903006?p=1204542903006.

Wong JM-L, et al. Biological foreign body implantation in victims of the London July 7th suicide bombings. *J Trauma-Inj Inf Crit Care.* 2006;60(2):402-404.

# Blast Injury

# 10

Emrys Kirkman, Neal Jacobs, Giles R. Nordmann, Stuart Harrisson, Peter F. Mahoney, and Sarah Watts

## 10.1
## Introduction

Blast injuries are an increasing problem in both military and civilian practice.[1] "Blast injury" refers to the biomechanical and pathophysiological changes and the clinical syndrome resulting from exposure of the living body to detonation of high explosive. Recently published figures from the conflicts in Afghanistan and Iraq indicate that approximately 46% of combat casualties treated initially by Forward Surgical Teams had suffered injuries associated with explosions (blast injury).[2] These data are broadly supported by data published from the Walter Reed Army Medical Center (in Washington) showing that 31% of US combat casualties evacuated back to this specialist hospital in the US had suffered blast injuries[3]. More recent data indicate a higher proportion of casualties (71%) are injured in explosions.[4]

## 10.2
## A Little Physics: Important for Understanding Blast Injuries

To understand the classification and nature of blast injuries we need a brief foray into blast physics. When an explosive detonates it generates an extremely rapid (effectively instantaneous) increase in pressure in the immediate vicinity of the explosion (Fig. 10.1a). This has a "knock on" effect on the surrounding medium (usually air or, in the case of underwater explosion, water), transferring the high pressure as a wave outwards faster than the speed of sound from the site of the explosion. The high pressure (called the peak overpressure) usually lasts only for a very short time (thousandths of a second) at any one point and is followed by a rapid fall in pressure, often to sub-atmospheric levels before returning to approximately normal. This is called the "shock wave." The magnitude of the peak overpressure falls as it travels away from the site of the explosion (Fig. 10.1b), initially by an

E. Kirkman (✉)
Biomedical Sciences, Defence Science and Technology Laboratory,
Porton Down, Salisbury, Wiltshire SP4 0JQ, UK
e-mail: ekirkman@dstl.gov.uk

A.J. Brooks et al. (eds.), *Ryan's Ballistic Trauma*,
DOI: 10.1007/978-1-84882-124-8_10, © Springer-Verlag London Limited 2011

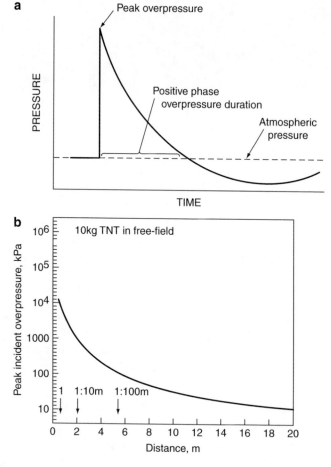

**Fig. 10.1** Schematic representation of a shock wave: (**a**) pressure vs. time at a single point; (**b**) pressure vs. distance from point of detonation

inverse cube relation (doubling the distance reduces the pressure to one-eighth). Because the shock wave is a very brief event with conventional explosives it does not cause the target (object or casualty) to move any great distance (this is not the part of the explosion that "throws things around"). However, the shock wave can cause serious injury (see below). Fragments (of the munition casing and pre-formed fragments contained within the device) and surrounding debris energized by the explosion are propelled outwards and can collide with the target. In addition, the explosion usually gives rise to a very large volume of hot gas. This literally pushes air and debris outwards (more projectile hazard) and acts over a sufficiently long time course to physically throw casualties against other objects. This is called the "blast wind." The shock wave and the blast wind are sometimes collectively called the "blast wave." Finally, for those close to the explosion there is also a large amount of heat which can also cause injury. Armed with this information we are now in a position to classify blast injuries.

## 10.3
## Classification of Blast Injuries

Blast injuries fall into four main categories[5,6]: primary, secondary, and tertiary with miscellaneous additional injuries forming a further (quaternary) group (Table 10.1).

Primary blast injuries result from the interaction of a shock wave with the body. Injury is largely confined to the air-containing organs, such as the lungs, bowel, and ears, often without external signs of injury,[7] although recently there is heightened suspicion that primary blast may also cause brain injury.[8-10]

Secondary blast injury results from the impact of fragments and larger missiles accelerated by the blast. The source of these missiles may be the device itself – its casing or contents such as ball bearings or nails – or from the environment within which the device detonates and may include stones, glass, brick, metal, and wood. Injuries caused by these fragments can be further categorized as penetrating or non-penetrating. This group accounts for the majority of blast injuries, particularly in open spaces.

Tertiary blast injury results from the acceleration of the whole body or parts of the body by the blast wave causing translational impacts of the body with the ground or other fixed objects, and/or traumatic amputation of body parts and stripping of tissue. A further group of miscellaneous injuries includes flash burns, caused by the radiant and convective heat of the explosion, burns caused by the combustion of the environment, crush syndrome, the effects of noxious gaseous products liberated in enclosed spaces, especially carbon monoxide and psychological effects.

The relative frequency of each type of injury is difficult to predict and depends on the quantity and type of explosive, the construction of the explosive device, the proximity of the casualty to the source of the explosion, and the environment within which the charge detonates. The greatest threat to life from the detonation of conventional munitions in an open environment is the penetrating injuries from fragments (secondary blast injury) rather than primary blast injury.[11] This is because the magnitude of the blast overpressure decreases exponentially (see physics, above) with distance away from the site of the blast, so that an individual close enough to the explosion to suffer a primary

**Table 10.1** Classification of blast injuries

| Primary | The effects of the shock wave. The shock wave travels through the body tissues depositing energy (and hence causing damage) especially at gas/liquid interfaces. The lungs are amongst the organs most likely to suffer this form of injury, where it is called "blast lung" |
|---|---|
| Secondary | Fragments and debris energized by the explosion collides with the body causing penetrating injuries |
| Tertiary | The body being thrown against obstacles by the mass movement of air (blast wind) causing blunt injuries |
| Quaternary | Other injuries including burns and crush from collapsed buildings, etc. |

blast injury, e.g., to the lungs, would be very likely to have suffered fatal secondary blast injuries. However, with the use of improved combat body armor, which is very effective in preventing fatal injuries from fragments but has little effect on the shock wave that causes primary blast injury, individuals may avoid immediate life-threatening secondary blast injury only to suffer significant primary blast injury. In addition, modern enhanced blast weapons, which produce few fragments, carry a significantly increased risk of primary blast injury.[11] Furthermore, detonation of an explosive inside structures, e.g., terrorist bombs in buildings, buses, and trains, is also associated with an increased risk of primary blast injury as the shock wave is reflected and amplified by solid structures such as walls.[11,12] This is confirmed by data from civilian terrorist attacks, where bombings occur in confined spaces, which indicate that blast lung is a common feature under this circumstance.[13-15]

## 10.4
## Primary Blast Injuries

Blast lung is the most notable primary blast injury (Fig. 10.2). Blast lung is characterized by contusions of the lungs in which blood contaminates the alveoli (usually without parenchymal laceration). The contusion may range from scattered petechiae to confluent hemorrhages involving the whole lung. The contusions may be bilateral, but they are frequently confined to the lung facing the blast (Fig. 10.2a) and they may continue to spread over the ensuing hours and days.[16] A physiological shunt may be established and the lung compliance will decrease, resulting in stiffer lungs and hypoxia.[17] The injury may progress to acute respiratory distress syndrome (ARDS),[18] often within 24–48 h[19,20] with the worst of the respiratory distress and hypoxemia being seen within the first 72 h.[17,19-24] Blast lung is therefore a condition that evolves (and can worsen) over a period of hours following blast exposure, i.e., a casualty who may not appear "too bad" initially may become critically ill later. Recently a large amount of research has been directed towards understanding the pathology of blast lung, which in time will underpin new treatment strategies.

## 10.5
## Pathophysiology of Blast Lung

The shock wave causes an immediate lung injury which is characterized by rupture of alveolar capillaries, the influx of blood, and extravasation of edema fluid into lung tissue,[25,26] giving rise to hemorrhagic foci which can be substantial depending on the level of blast loading. The intrapulmonary hemorrhage and edema contribute to the initial respiratory compromise in blast lung.[27] The problem is exacerbated because free hemoglobin (Hb) and extravasated blood have been shown to induce free radical reactions which cause

**Fig. 10.2** Photographs showing characteristic "blast lungs" (**a**) from a terminally-anesthetized pig exposed to detonation of a single charge (2.2 kg of EDC1) at a range of 1.5 m from the center of the charge to the outside of the chest wall. The animal was lying supine and exposed to blast from the right side. Note the pulmonary contusions especially on the right side. (**b**) Post mortem lungs from a human blast victim. Note the extensive pulmonary contusions and the characteristic "rib markings" which are now believed to be "intercostal space" markings

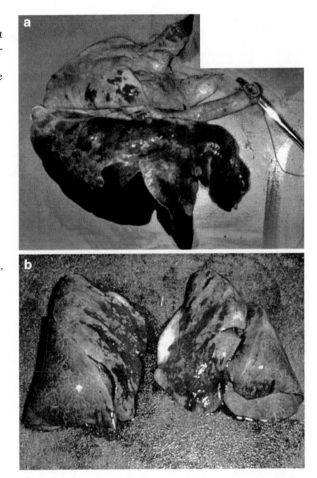

oxidative damage[27] and initiates/augments a pro-inflammatory response.[26] Free Hb also causes an accumulation of inflammatory mediators and chemotactic attractants[28] thereby amplifying the problem.

Within 3 h leucocytes can be demonstrated within the hemorrhagic areas and levels increase for 24 h or more after exposure.[27] This accumulation of leucocytes is associated with increasing levels of myeloperoxidase (MPO) activity, which in turn is indicative of oxidative events and developing inflammation in the affected areas.[27] Histological and electron microscopic examination reveal prominent perivascular edema and extensive alveolar hemorrhages without widespread visible damage to endothelial cells during the first 12 h after exposure.[27] Thereafter (12–24 h after exposure) type 1 epithelial cells show evidence of developing damage followed later (24–56 h after exposure) by secondary damage to endothelial cells which become detached from their basement membrane into the capillary lumen.[27] This process is summarized in Table 10.2.

**Table 10.2** Evolution of blast lung

| Event | Apparent clinical problem | Time (h) |
|---|---|---|
| • Shock wave damage | | 0 |
| • Rupture of alveolar capillaries | | |
| • Blood into interstitium and alveoli | • Reduced gas transfer (esp $O_2$) | |
| • Free Hb and Blood<br>  – Free radicals/oxidative stress<br>  – Augmented inflammatory response<br>  – More edema | • Inflammation<br><br><br>• Reduced gas transfer (esp $O_2$) | |
| • Leucocyte accumulation<br><br>  – More oxidative stress, inflammation<br>  and oedama | • More inflammation and reduced<br>  gas transfer | 3 |
| • Epithelical cell damage evident | • Further impairment | 12–24 |
| • Endothelical cell damage evident | • Lung mechanics | 24–56 |

## 10.6
## Physiological Response to Primary Blast Injury

Primary blast injury results in a characteristic cardiorespiratory response that is mediated in large part by the autonomic nervous system. However, it must also be recognized that other mechanisms such as the release of mediators (e.g., nitric oxide) into the circulation may also play a significant role in the acute response to blast injury.

### 10.6.1
### Cardiorespiratory Response to Primary Blast Injury to the Thorax

A number of experimental studies and clinical reports indicated that primary blast injury to the thorax produces bradycardia,[29-35] prolonged hypotension,[29,30,32,33,35] and apnoea followed by rapid shallow breathing[31,32,34,35] (Fig. 10.3). Initially, it was thought that the bradycardia was a preterminal event, possibly associated with cessation of coronary blood flow.[36] However, more recent studies have demonstrated that the bradycardia is a consistent finding following thoracic blast, even in animals that survive,[35] and that it is an autonomic reflex.

### 10.6.2
### Time Course and Reflex Nature of the Acute Cardiorespiratory Response to Thoracic Blast Injury

A detailed study of the immediate response to primary blast injury to the thorax has shown that the cardiovascular and respiratory responses are not instantaneous; the brady-cardia had a latency of onset of approximately 4 s, while blood pressure began to fall approximately 2 s after blast.[37] This latency is consistent with the response being reflex in

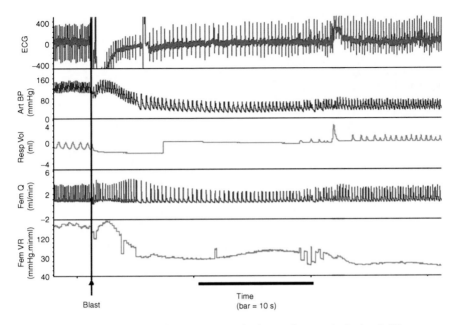

**Fig. 10.3** Typical effects of a single blast exposure to the thorax of an anesthetized male Wistar rat on the electrocardiogram (ECG), systemic arterial blood pressure (Art BP), respiratory tidal volume (Resp Vol, inspiration upwards), femoral arterial blood flow (Fem Q), and femoral vascular resistance (Fem VR). A single blast wave was applied to the ventral thorax at the point indicated (Blast)

nature rather than being the consequence of direct effects, e.g., on the heart or CNS. The initial bradycardia was seen to resolve quickly after blast although some degree of bradycardia persisted for up to 1 h after thoracic blast, while hypotension persisted for at least 2 h (Fig. 10.4). More recent studies have shown that the response also includes a reduction in vascular resistance, at least in skeletal muscle (see Fig. 10.3). Coincident with the cardiopulmonary changes there are early and prolonged falls in arterial oxygen tension following thoracic blast (Fig. 10.5) consistent with the development of pulmonary edema.[38] $PaCO_2$ may fall if pulmonary edema is mild or may rise with more severe pulmonary edema after severe blast injury since pulmonary transfer of carbon dioxide is affected less by edema than the transfer of oxygen. These changes are associated with increases in lung weight indices and lung dry/wet weight ratios, both of which are consistent with the development of pulmonary edema.

## 10.6.3
## Contribution of the Autonomic Nervous System to the Cardiorespiratory Response to Primary Blast Injury

The bradycardia and apnoea seen after blast are both mediated by a vagal reflex.[36,37,39,40] The etiology of the hypotension seen after primary blast injury is complex. The fall in blood pressure appears to be due to a fall in peripheral resistance and cardiac output, the latter because of a myocardial impairment which can last many hours after blast injury[41]

**Fig. 10.4** Cardiovascular effects of exposure to a single blast directed towards the ventral thorax in terminally anesthetized male Wistar rats (alphadolone/alphaxolone 19–12 mg kg$^{-1}$ h$^{-1}$). MBP, mean arterial blood pressure recorded before blast, the peak effect of blast (at time 0 min) and thereafter at the times indicated after blast. Data are mean±s.e.mean

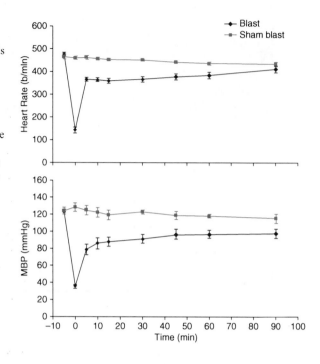

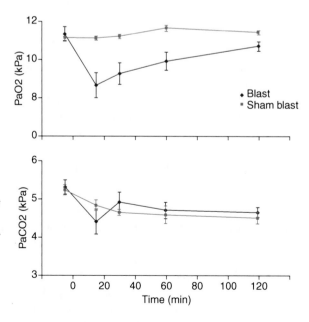

**Fig. 10.5** Blood gas changes after exposure to a single blast directed towards the ventral thorax in terminally anaesthetized male Wistar rats (alphadolone/alphaxolone 19–12 mg kg$^{-1}$ h$^{-1}$). PaO$_2$ and PaCO$_2$, arterial oxygen and carbon dioxide tensions, respectively recorded before blast and thereafter at the times indicated post-blast. Data are mean±s.e.mean

**Fig. 10.6** Effects of primary blast injury due to single blast exposure on myocardial performance *in vivo* in a group of terminally anesthetized Large White pigs. Data were recorded before blast and thereafter at 1.5 and 6 h post blast (B + 1.5 and B + 6 respectively). Data are median (interquartile range). *CI* cardiac output indexed to body weight, *LVSWI* left ventricular stroke work index (Data taken from Harban[41])

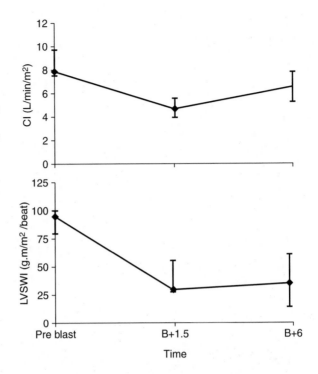

(Fig. 10.6). Although the autonomic nervous system plays some part in the hypotension it is not solely responsible. Recent findings have suggested that primary blast injury causes a rapid release of the potent vasodilator nitric oxide (NO) from the pulmonary circulation.[42-44] It is thought that such a brisk overproduction of NO could lead to a systemic response that includes vasodilatation (J.L. Atkins, WRAIR, personal communication, 2008[45]).

In summary thoracic, but not abdominal,[35] blast produces a triad of bradycardia, hypotension, and apnoea. The bradycardia and apnoea are mediated entirely by a vagal reflex, the most likely candidate being the pulmonary afferent C-fiber reflex. The hypotension appears to be mediated by a reduction in vascular resistance as well as a fall in cardiac output. By 30 min after blast the reduction in vascular resistance is reversed but the myocardial depression seems to persist contributing to long-term hypotension.

## 10.7
### Assessment and Treatment of Casualties with Blast Lung

The broad clinical features associated with blast lung are shown in Table 10.3 and typical chest X-ray (CXR) findings are listed in Table 10.4. It has been argued that CXR however is a poor modality for quantifying the extent of pulmonary contusion (Fig. 10.7a). Computed Tomography (CT, Fig. 10.7b) is better[46,47] but not always available. The presence or absence of tympanic membrane rupture cannot be used as a

**Table 10.3** Clinical features of blast lung

Symptoms
- Dyspnoea
- Cough (dry – frothy sputum)
- Haemoptysis
- Chest pain/discomfort

Signs
- Cyanosis
- Tachypnoea
- Reduced breath sounds
- Coarse crepitations
- Rhonchi
- Dull to percussion
- Features of pneumo/haemopneumothorax
- Haemoptysis
- Subcutaneous emphysema
- Retrosternal crunch (pneumomedistinum)
- Retinal artery air emboli

**Table 10.4** Chest x-ray findings in blast lung

- Pneumothorax
- Haemothorax
- Pneumomediastinum
- Subcutaneous emphysema
- Interstitial emphysema
- Mediastinal emphysema
- Pneumoperitineum – secondary to visceral perforation
- Rib fractures

surrogate marker since it is neither a sensitive nor specific indicator of blast lung. However, although it has been challenged,[48] in the operational environment it remains safe practice to admit patients with a ruptured eardrum for a period of observation whilst other more significant injuries are excluded.[49]

Blast lung has been classified, on clinical grounds, into mild, moderate, and severe categories[50] (Table 10.5). Based on studies of civilian casualties of terrorist bombings mortality was high in those with severe BLI and all of those who survived the first 24 h in this category developed ARDS. All of those who suffered mild and moderate BLI ultimately survived. Thirty-three percent of those with moderate BLI developed ARDS while none of those with mild BLI developed ARDS.[50] Given appropriate intensive care treatment, the prognosis for those with post-blast ARDS is good with complete recovery of lung function within 1 year.[51]

**Fig. 10.7** Investigations from a patient injured by a blast from the patient's left. (**a**) CXR shows bilateral pulmonary infiltrates. (**b**) CT in the same patient shows more clearly the greater extent of the left-sided haemothorax compared to the right

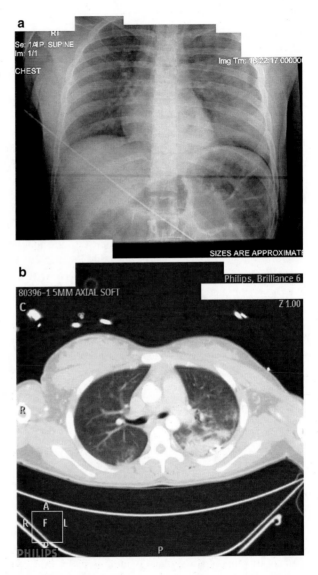

**Table 10.5** Blast lung severity score and proportion of casualties reported to develop ARDS subsequently

| Severity | Mild | Moderate | Severe |
|---|---|---|---|
| PaO$_2$/FiO$_2$ (kPa) | >26.6 | 8.0–26.6 | <8.0 |
| Chest radiograph | Local lung infiltrates | Bilateral or unilateral lung infiltrates | Massive bilateral lung infiltrates |
| Proportion of casualties developing ARDS | 0% | 33% | 100% |

Based on data published by Pizov et al.[50]

### 10.7.1
### Management

Primary blast injury causes the lung to be prone to pneumothorax and significant air emboli can be created.[52] Otherwise, management is similar to that of any other pulmonary contusion with its respective consequences from the pathology with oxygen being the simplest and most effective treatment. Recently there has been increased concern that oxygen is not wholly innocuous and can lead to a range of complications. Consequently guidelines have been published regarding the use of emergency oxygen in adults, which was the subject of a recent editorial in the *British Medical Journal*[53] and recommend the targeting of oxygen to pre-defined arterial saturation levels in a most cases.

Blast lung casualties are susceptible to pulmonary barotrauma (including pneumothorax and air embolism). Unfortunately positive pressure mechanical ventilation with positive end expiratory pressure may be required to maintain adequate oxygenation and the risk of barotrauma may be enhanced by this although more modern ventilation strategies that allow more modest gas exchange targets (permissive hypercapnia) using limited volume excursions and pressure changes have ameliorated these concerns. Prophylactic tube thoracostomies should be considered if air evacuation is planned or close observations are impractical.[54]

Fluid management after blast injury is an area of current research. Conventional wisdom suggested "judicious" fluid resuscitation and allowing the patient to remain hypotensive (e.g., with mean arterial blood pressure no greater than 60 mmHg). However, this approach also has penalties and the significant challenge facing the clinician is the maintenance of adequate tissue oxygenation without overloading the cardiovascular system or exacerbating pulmonary edema.

### 10.8
### Auditory Injuries

The auditory system is very susceptible to blast.[55] Perforation in the anteroinferior part of the pars tensa is the most common manifestation of tympanic injury. Thirty-three percent of injuries are associated with ossicular injury, which does not occur in the absence of tympanic disruption. Cholesteatoma from embedded squamous debris is a long-term complication occurring in up to 12% of blast-perforated ears, dictating long-term follow-up. Associated ossicular injury is a feature of more severe blast injury in as many as a third of reported cases. Sensorineural hearing loss associated with a high-pitched tinnitus frequently occurs immediately following a blast. Hearing loss may resolve in hours or may become permanent in greater than 50% of patients, as has been reported in some series. Although not a priority for treatment, auditory injury should be addressed in 24 h and auditory canal cleaned of all debris. Fifty to 80% of ruptured tympanic membranes will heal spontaneously without further treatment.

## 10.9
## Intestinal Injuries

The injury mechanism includes reflection of the shock wave as it travels across density borders into gas-filled areas of the gut (similar to blast lung injury) causing contusion. In addition displacement and shearing effects can cause tearing of mesenteric and perito-neal attachments with bleeding and devascularizing injury. The characteristic injury seen is a multifocal intramural hematoma beginning in the submucosa, extending with increasing severity to large transmural confluent hematoma and may involve the mesen-tery and vascular supply. Serosal injury should always be considered indicative of trans-mural injury. Cripps[56] identified those lesions at greater risk of perforation in experimental studies in pigs, suggesting that serosal lesions greater than 15 mm in the small intestine and greater than 20 mm in the large bowel are at higher risk of perforation and should be resected. Delayed perforation up to 14 days post injury can occur and most likely is related to progressive ischemia and necrosis with transmural injury or adjacent mesen-teric injury. In the case of immersion blast or in enclosed spaces, primary blast injury to the gut may occur even more frequently than pulmonary injury and at less intense expo-sure to dynamic overpressures.

## 10.10
## Death Following Primary Blast Injury

The immediate cause of death following primary blast injury, in the absence of obvious external injuries, has been the subject of much debate in the literature and a number of theories have been advocated.[32,36,37,57,58] Leaving aside deaths due to the total disruption of the body very close to a charge[36] and secondary changes such as the development of ARDS and unrecognized perforation peritonitis, the chief causes of death will be reviewed. The causes of death can be classified as respiratory and circulatory.

### 10.10.1
### Respiratory Causes

In severe pulmonary blast injury there is massive pulmonary contusion and hemorrhage into the bronchial tree. Bleeding is frequently observed through the mouth and nose[59] and the experimental animals are seen to make a few, terminal, maximally forced respiratory movements for air as they suffocate in extravasated blood.[6,7,32,36] These observations suggest that there is no respiratory center damage[32] as had originally been suggested by earlier workers.[60]

In animals that do not obstruct the airways with blood and froth, early pulmonary pathology is not usually sufficient to account for death.[7,57] The development of pulmonary edema supervening on a physiological shunt through non-aerated contused lung may disturb the pulmonary gas exchange sufficiently to be incompatible with life.[57] Clemedson supported the view of Benzinger[57] that respiratory symptoms are not the cause of death but are the consequence of the circulatory failure.[61,62]

## 10.10.2
## Circulatory Causes

It has been well documented that exposure to blast wave overpressure gives rise to profound changes in the circulatory system. Generally it has been thought that death is secondary to obstruction of the pulmonary capillary bed[32,36,58,61] and a greatly dilated right ventricle is often found at post-mortem.[58] The heart has also been implicated but evidence for *commotio cordis* or sufficient myocardial contusion as the immediate cause of death is scarce.[32,57,58,63,64]

Air embolism in blast injury is the result of air entering the circulation through the damaged alveoli.[57] In animals dying within some minutes of blast injury, air is frequently found intravascularly.[57,58,64] The air bubbles are found, often in large quantities, and always in the arterial side of the circulation. Furthermore, air emboli are only found in animals that die rapidly after exposure and never in those animals that survive to be sacrificed.[58] Air is most commonly found in the coronary arteries, the left side of the heart, and in brain vessels, especially the basilar vessels and in the choroid plexuses. Therefore, in some cases of immediately fatal primary blast injury, air emboli, especially of the coronary arteries, is likely to be the cause of death. Fat embolism as a cause of death has been suggested[65,66] and refuted[32,67] and the time course of hemorrhagic shock from disrupted solid organs is considered too slow to account for immediate death following blast injury.

The majority of the work on death following primary blast injury was performed in the post-war period. Modern authors have concentrated on the cardiorespiratory response in sub-lethal blast exposure and therefore the potential role of the cardiorespiratory response to blast of apnoea, bradycardia, and hypotension in immediate death has not received much attention. There is an interesting correlation between the response to blast injury and that to penetrating brain injury. In both cases the same triad of responses occurs. In 1894, Horsley[68] noted transient apnoea following a side-to-side cerebral injury with a pistol in an animal model. Crockard,[69,70] more recently demonstrated apnoea, bradycardia, and hypotension following a controlled cerebral injury that produced a clean wound away from vital structures and major blood vessels in a primate model. Importantly, the apnoea, without immediate ventilatory support, led to the death of the animal whilst immediate ventilatory support would lead to a recovery of the animal. More recent studies of penetrating brain injury reproduced this cardiorespiratory response[71,72] and have suggested that stress waves, propagating through the brain tissue, damage the cardiorespiratory centers at the base of the fourth ventricle. In support of this concept fissures have been shown in the floor of the fourth ventricle following such penetrating brain injury away from the brain stem that may account for this damage.[73] One conclusion that has been drawn from this parallel is that blast injury may lead to death as a result of the cardiorespiratory response alone, and apnoea in particular.[74] It must be stressed, however, that it is not implied that the response to primary thoracic blast injury is mediated via shock waves transmitted to the brainstem since the apnoea and bradycardia induced by blast can be prevented by vagotomy.[37]

## 10.11
## Secondary Blast Injury

The majority of casualties produced by explosions result from the impact of fragments and debris. In the military environment, the detonation of a high-explosive artillery shell will produce many thousands of metallic fragments of variable mass. Primary fragments, accelerated by the explosive detonation, are classed as either "naturally formed," or "pre-formed." Naturally formed fragments arise from the shattering of a solid casing producing, in general, fragments of variable mass and shape. Pre-formed fragments arise where the case of the device is constructed specifically to control the generation of fragments (such as in grenades and mortars). This results in the production of very small fragments of approximately the same mass and shape, or where the casing contains ball bearings, flechettes, or nails that become primary fragments. In the civilian context the blast-energized debris from explosions, accelerated by the dynamic overpressure, especially in confined spaces will consist of small and large pieces of glass, splintered wood, plaster, gravel, earth, and any other material that is relatively unfixed. These are secondary fragments.

Close to the device the primary and secondary fragments impact the body at many hundreds of meters per second, easily penetrating body cavities, and resulting in a high incidence of serious injuries and death. The wounding power of a missile is dependent on the physical tissue destruction within any given body area or organ and the clinical consequences of the tissue damage within that body area or organ. The anatomical location of the wound is a major factor in the assessment of injury severity.

Amongst fatalities of terrorist bombings in Northern Ireland between 1969 and 1977, 25% had single or multiple penetrating wounds of the thorax, and the abdomen was penetrated in 26%.[75] Penetration of the thorax resulted in a laceration of the major vessels in 18% of fatalities, laceration of the heart in 14%, the lungs in 41%, and the upper respiratory tract in 11%. However, the single most common factors observed in these bomb blast fatalities from penetrating secondary blast injury were penetrating brain injury (66%), skull fracture (51%), and liver laceration (34%).

## 10.12
## Interaction Between the Response to Blast and Hemorrhage

Blast-injured casualties will often sustain hemorrhage as a consequence of their injuries.[75] Hemorrhage initiates a characteristic autonomic response that in turn is modified by the response to injuries such as blast and musculo-skeletal injuries.

The pattern of physiological responses to progressive simple hemorrhage (blood loss in the absence of tissue damage and nociception) is biphasic,[76] with an initial tachycardia (due to vagal inhibition and an activation of sympathetic efferent activity) and maintenance of blood pressure via the arterial baroreceptor reflex (Phase I).[77,78] As haemorrhage progresses, and blood loss exceeds 20–30% of total blood volume, a "depressor" phase (Phase II) becomes apparent. This involves a vagally mediated bradycardia (inhibited by atropine[77]),

**Fig. 10.8** Effects of a progressive "simple" hemorrhage in a male volunteer showing a biphasic response. Blood was withdrawn by venesection until the subject fainted. *TPR* total peripheral resistance, *Syst BP* systolic arterial blood pressure, *CO* cardiac output, *Rt auric p* right atrial pressure (central venous pressure) (From Barcroft.[76] Reprinted with kind permission from Elsevier)

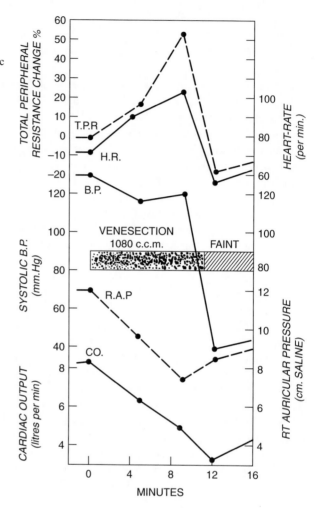

a reduction in peripheral vascular resistance[76,79] and a marked fall in arterial blood pressure (Fig. 10.8). This second phase is not due to a failure of the baroreflex, since the latter's sensitivity is increased at this stage,[80] nor is it a preterminal event,[81,82] but rather it is due to the activation of additional reflex(es). The identity of the afferent limb of the "depressor" reflex is currently uncertain,[83-85] although the cardiac afferent C-fibers may be involved.[86]

Thoracic blast has been shown to augment the bradycardic, hypotensive response to hemorrhage (Fig. 10.9). Furthermore, the effect of blast on the response to hemorrhage can be attenuated by morphine[87] (see Fig. 10.9). However, the mechanism whereby the depressor response to severe hemorrhage is augmented by the response to blast is unknown. In experimental studies enhanced blood loss can be discounted as the underlying cause since there was no post-mortem evidence of additional blood loss into the body cavities. It is therefore possible that the reflex initiated by exposure to blast modifies one of the reflexes mediating the response to hemorrhage.

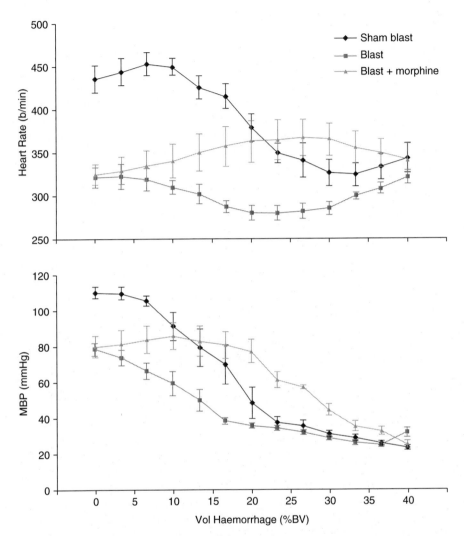

**Fig. 10.9** Effects of a progressive hemorrhage of 40% total estimated blood volume (BV) at a rate of 2% BV min$^{-1}$ on heart rate and mean arterial blood pressure (MBP) in terminally anesthetized rats 10 min after exposure to thoracic blast (or sham blast) and 5 min after administration of morphine (0.5 mg kg$^{-1}$) or vehicle (0.9% saline, 1 mL kg$^{-1}$) i.v. (Based on data from Sawdon.[87] Data are mean±s.e.mean)

Two possibilities are immediately obvious. Either the response to blast inhibits the baroreflex (responsible for the compensatory Phase I of the response to blood loss), or it augments the depressor reflex (responsible for the hypotensive Phase II of the response to hemorrhage). Of these two possibilities the latter appears the most attractive because treatment with morphine (known to block the depressor reflex after simple hemorrhage) also attenuates the bradycardic, hypotensive response to blood loss after blast and uncovers a tachycardic response in its place.[87]

## 10.13
## Effects of Blast Injury on the Response to Fluid Resuscitation After Hemorrhage

The effects of blast injury pose special challenges for the resuscitation of hypovolaemic casualties. The main early management strategies in hemorrhage are the arrest of bleeding and the replacement of circulating volume.[88] During the late twentieth century, aggressive fluid administration was encouraged, but this approach was re-examined within military and civilian medical services. Aggressive fluid resuscitation involves the administration of a relatively large amount of fluid as quickly as possible in an attempt to restore and maintain "normal" arterial blood pressure; the Advanced Trauma Life Support (ATLS) protocol prescribes 2 L of crystalloid solution given intravenously as a bolus, followed by further (variable) aliquots as needed to maintain a normal arterial pressure.[89] In recent years there has been a growing concern that this normalization of blood pressure may lead to clot dislocation and further bleeding,[90-92] consequently military and many civilian medical services now practice hypotensive or limited resuscitation to an end point of a systolic blood pressure of about 80 mmHg (a palpable radial pulse in humans).[93,94] However, this approach is not without penalty since prolonged hypotension can result in poor tissue perfusion and ischemic damage.[95]

In choosing a resuscitation strategy for a hypovolaemic blast casualty two conflicting concerns need to be addressed: poor tissue perfusion and oxygen delivery with hypotensive resuscitation vs. possible fluid overload and re-bleeding with aggressive fluid resuscitation. In casualties who have suffered blast lung, pulmonary oxygen transport will be compromised leading to some degree of hypoxia. The reduced arterial oxygen content will therefore compound the problems of poor tissue perfusion inherent in hypotensive resuscitation strategies. This is likely to be a particular problem when resuscitation needs to be prolonged. Hypotensive strategies have only been validated in the short term (e.g., 75 min reported by Bickell et al.[91] in their clinical trial from the time of the emergency call to operative intervention). However, in military practice much longer times have been reported for the evacuation of a battlefield casualty to a surgical facility for definitive control of the hemorrhage. Recent reports indicate evacuation times of 4–5 h in Afghanistan and 2–20 h in Iraq[96,97] when long distances and operational difficulties are present. In these longer timescales the physiological penalties of poor tissue perfusion arising from hypotensive resuscitation may limit survival.

To address the issue of resuscitation after blast injury and hemorrhage a series of studies were conducted at Dstl Porton Down. The first study was a physiological comparison of early, aggressive, fluid resuscitation (target systolic arterial blood pressure, SBP of 110 mmHg) with the prolonged hypotensive strategy (target SBP of 80 mmHg corresponding to a palpable radial pulse) that represented BATLS at the time (and is currently advocated by NICE[95]). The study was conducted on groups of anesthetized pigs exposed to blast (and no blast) injury and a controlled hemorrhage of 30% total estimated blood volume. The result was that survival time was significantly shorter in the blast-injured hypotensive group[98] (Fig. 10.10) and was associated with overwhelming failure to deliver enough oxygen to tissues, resulting in a profound metabolic acidosis (Fig. 10.11). Two important conclusions can be drawn from this:

**Fig. 10.10** Kaplan-Meier survival plot for two groups of animals subjected to blast (B) before a controlled hemorrhage of 30% total estimated blood volume, 5 min shock phase and fluid resuscitation according to either normotensive (Normot) or hypotensive (Hypot) resuscitation protocols

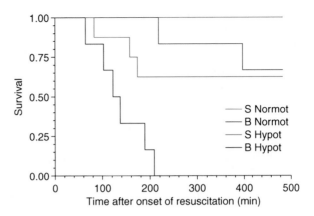

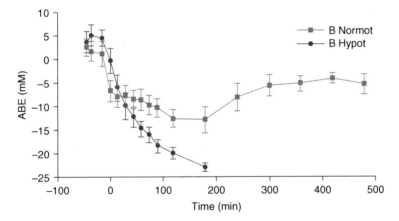

**Fig. 10.11** Arterial actual base excess (ABE) in two groups of animals subjected to blast (B) before a hemorrhage, shock phase, and fluid resuscitation according to either normotensive (Normot) or hypotensive (Hypot) resuscitation protocols. Fluid resuscitation with 0.9% saline in all groups. Time indicates time from onset of resuscitation. First three values represent Baseline 1, Baseline 3, and Blast. Mean values ± SEM

1. Prolonged hypotensive resuscitation is not compatible with survival over extended timelines in casualties with significant blast lung, although shorter periods of hypotension can be tolerated.
2. Aggressive ATLS-style fluid resuscitation did not overload the heart in this experimental study.

However, no inference could be made regarding the likelihood of re-bleeding since the study was specifically designed to assess physiological responses and consequently involved a controlled model of hemorrhage. A more recent study has now been completed to assess the effects of a novel hybrid (initial hypotensive resuscitation followed by later elevation of the target SBP after the first hour) strategy, advocated in current BATLS.[93] The study has shown that novel hybrid resuscitation leads to significantly longer survival times

**Fig. 10.12** (a) Kaplan–Meier survival plot and (**b**) volume of intra-abdominal fluid at post-mortem as a function of survival time in four groups of animals subjected to either sham blast (S) or blast (B) before a controlled hemorrhage of 30% total estimated blood volume and Grade IV liver injury, 5 min shock phase and fluid resuscitation according to either Novel Hybrid (NH) or Hypotensive (Hypot) resuscitation protocols. Fluid resuscitation with 0.9% saline in all groups. Time indicates time from onset of resuscitation

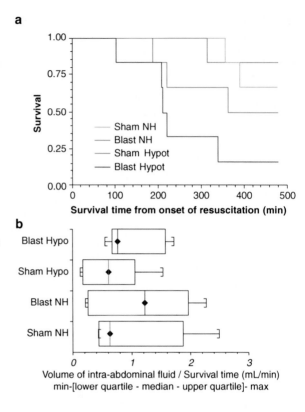

than prolonged hypotensive resuscitation (Fig. 10.12a) in a model of blast injury and hemorrhage. The model incorporated an uncompressed Grade IV liver injury to simulate a survivable battlefield injury which would require resuscitation and is capable of re-bleeding. There was no evidence of increased bleeding in the groups resuscitated with the novel hybrid strategy (Fig. 10.12b).

## 10.14
## Tertiary Blast Injury

The dynamic overpressure following a blast results in the generation of blast winds of high velocity and increased density of air behind the leading edge of the shock wave. This mass movement of air can result in total body disruption, whole body displacement, and collapse of the fabric of a building. Tertiary blast injuries commonly result in blunt injuries often affecting the musculo-skeletal system and/or head. Traumatic amputation of limbs is included in this group by most authors (although a component of this aspect of injury, the initial fracture of long bones, is more likely the consequence of the shock wave). Traumatic amputation generally occurs in very severe cases and is rare in survivors of blast injury at a rate of 1–2%[75,99-103] but common in immediate fatalities.[100,104,105]

## 10.15
## Early Systemic Response to Musculo-Skeletal Injury

The neural nociceptive barrage initiated by musculo-skeletal injury causes profound changes in cardiovascular control resulting in alterations in arterial blood pressure, regional oxygen delivery, and the response to any concomitant hemorrhage, all of which have important implications for morbidity and mortality.

### 10.15.1
### Oxygen Transport

There is an injury-induced diversion of blood supply away from vital organs which has important implications for whole body utilization of the available oxygen delivery ($DO_2$) and a concept known as "critical oxygen delivery." When cardiac output, and hence whole body $DO_2$, is progressively reduced (e.g., because of hemorrhage) the body as a whole responds by extracting more oxygen from the available blood flow to maintain oxygen consumption ($VO_2$). However, this process cannot be extended indefinitely and there comes a point when $VO_2$ starts to fall as $DO_2$ is reduced further. The point at which $VO_2$ becomes dependent on $DO_2$ is called the "critical oxygen delivery" ($DO_{2Crit}$) and represents the point at which organs in the body start to suffer physiological damage because of an inadequate $DO_2$. There is evidence that activation of a neural nociceptive barrage elevates $DO_{2Crit}$ and reduces a patient's ability to extract oxygen from the available blood supply.[106] This increases a patient's susceptibility to problems of reduced oxygen delivery.

The haemodynamic response to muscle ischaemia is mediated by central nervous pathways which involve endogenous opioids.[107,108] It is therefore likely that opioid-ergic drugs may modify this response. One study has shown that mortality after blood loss is increased in animals treated with morphine, despite initial maintenance of a higher blood pressure during and immediately after a controlled hemorrhage in animals treated with morphine compared to placebo.[109]

## 10.16
## Modulation of the Response to Hemorrhage by the Response to Musculo-Skeletal Injury

The biphasic response to "simple" hemorrhage (blood loss in the absence of major tissue damage) is described earlier (see "Interaction Between the Response to Blast and Hemorrhage"). The biphasic response is markedly attenuated by the presence of concomitant tissue injury.[77] The initial increase in heart rate during Phase I of the response to hemorrhage is reduced, and the vagal bradycardia following greater losses

(Phase II) is prevented. The attenuation of the heart rate changes normally associated with blood loss seems to offer some degree of protection against the hypotensive effects of a severe hemorrhage.[77] However this protection may be more apparent than real, as a lower survival rate has been demonstrated in animals subjected to hemorrhage and concomitant electrical stimulation of the sciatic nerve (to simulate injury) compared to animals subjected to hemorrhage alone.[110] It is possible that the better maintenance of blood pressure is achieved at the expense of intense peripheral vasoconstriction leading to ischemic organ damage that will exacerbate the severity of injury. It is tempting to speculate that the splanchnic circulation may be selectively vulnerable to such ischemic damage. There is evidence that when hemorrhage is superimposed on a background of somatic afferent stimulation (to mimic injury) there is a relative redistribution of blood flow from the gut towards skeletal muscle (in contrast to the pattern seen with simple hemorrhage).[111,112] This diversion of blood flow (and oxygen delivery) away from metabolically active organs towards relatively inactive resting skeletal muscle may explain the increase in critical oxygen delivery elicited by somatic afferent nerve stimulation[106] since it effectively "wastes" a proportion of the cardiac output. Ischemic damage to the intestinal mucosa may lead to an increased intestinal permeability and enhanced translocation of endotoxin.[113-115] Therefore the impairment in cardiac function and tissue oxygen delivery associated with blood loss is greater if the hemorrhage is superimposed on nociceptive nerve stimulation compared to hemorrhage alone.[116] If the hemorrhage is superimposed on real rather than simulated tissue injury the tolerance to blood loss is reduced even further[117] (Fig. 10.13).

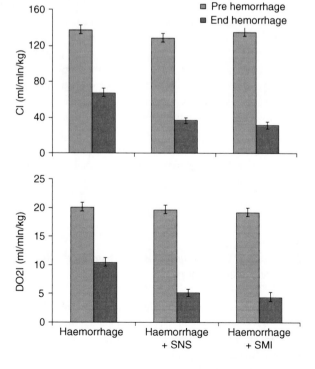

**Fig. 10.13** Effects of somatic afferent nerve stimulation (SNS) and skeletal muscle injury (SMI) on the changes in cardiac output (expressed as cardiac index, CI) and oxygen delivery indexed to body weight (DO2I) produced by a hemorrhage of 40% of the estimated blood volume in anesthetized pigs (Based on data from Rady[116])

## 10.17
## Quaternary Blast Injury: Burns

Burn injuries can be experienced in isolation or as part of multiple injuries. The pattern of burn injury is variable and is dependent on the weapon used. A casualty close enough to a conventional munition to receive burns in an open environment is likely to have suffered severe or fatal secondary (fragment) and primary blast injuries. The incidence of burns in infantry survivors is therefore low; however, this incidence changes when the injuries occur in vehicles, ships, and aircraft. The weapon systems designed to defeat the armor of these vehicles will cause burns due to secondary ignition of fuel and munitions. Casualties injured in these confined environments often have airway burns. In the Falklands campaign a significant numbers of casualties injured in ships suffered burns (34% of those injured). More recent conflicts (e.g., Gulf War 1) have seen casualties injured in armored vehicles. Away from the battlefield, the more recent conflict in Iraq in 2003 saw a large number of civilian casualties with burns secondary to kerosene accidents when local electricity supplies failed.

Burns associated with lung or airway injury can potentially be a significant challenge to a critical care unit deployed with a military field hospital with limited beds and a restricted evacuation policy. Present conflicts have shown that although burn admissions are around 4% of all deployed military hospital admissions,[118] their impact on the critical care department can be significant, generating up to 27% of all critical care admissions.[119]

The mortality of burn injury has decreased over the past 20 years thanks to effective fluid resuscitation, early surgical intervention, infection control, and intensive care organ support. The presence of an inhalational injury in patients with a burn injury can more than double the mortality.[120] Inhalational injury, present in over 25% of burns patients admitted to intensive care[121] causes up to a tenfold increase in the incidence of Acute Respiratory Distress Syndrome (ARDS)[122] and the likelihood of developing pneumonia is doubled.[123]

Inhalational injury can be subdivided[124] into:

- Direct thermal injury above the larynx
- Injury below the larynx
- Local pulmonary and systemic effects of inhaled toxins

## 10.18
## Injuries Above the Larynx

In true supraglottic airway burns the resulting injury is normally thermal. The initial appearance is upper airway edema which develops over a period of hours reaching a maximum between 12 and 36 h post injury. The edema can be severe enough to completely obstruct the airway.

## 10.19
## Injuries Below the Larynx

Sub-laryngeal injury is caused by the inhalation of heated gases and smoke within the bron-chial tree, the injury is predominantly a chemical pneumonitis with bronchial irritation[125] leading to inflammation, mucosal sloughing, and activation of the systemic inflammatory response syndrome. In severe injury this will lead to the development of excess pulmonary secretions, bronchospasm and the acute respiratory distress syndrome (ARDS).[126]

Lung injury is caused by a number of mechanisms. It is not usually due to direct thermal injury except in the case of steam inhalation (where the normal heat-exchanging capability of the upper airway is overwhelmed[127]) but is due to the cytotoxic chemicals and pulmonary irritants within inhaled smoke. Lung injury is heterogeneous because only lung units exposed to the smoke will be injured. Injury mechanisms include inflammation of the lung tissue with loss of cilia resulting in small airway collapse and hypoxaemia. In the airway sloughing of the mucosa occurs causing bronchospasm and the formation of casts may obstruct bronchioles predisposing to atelectasis and pulmo-nary infection. The lung parenchyma surrounding injured airways becomes congested and there is interstitial edema and neutrophil infiltration. The toxic gases present in smoke, e.g., hydrogen cyanide, ammonia, and nitrogen dioxide may cause cellular hypoxia and cause direct lung injury by the activation of inflammatory cascades. It should be noted that this description of lung injury is based on the burns literature. However, when burns combine with blast injury (which can itself cause oxidative stress and inflammation, see "Pathophysiology of Blast Lung") there is a potential, as yet undetermined, of a synergistic interaction and marked worsening of the clinical problems.

## 10.20
## Clinical Assessment and Diagnosis

The diagnosis of inhalational injury is primarily a clinical one based on history and exami-nation of the patient. A history of injury occurring within an enclosed space, an explosion, and (more likely in a civilian setting) decreased sensory awareness due to drugs and alco-hol all make an inhalational injury more likely. The presence of facial burns, singed nasal hair, carbonaceous sputum, and hoarseness of the voice may also point to the presence of an inhalational burn, but have a high false positive rate when taken individually. A tenta-tive diagnosis of inhalation injury can be made using a combination of history, clinical signs (dyspnoea, bronchial irritability, coughing, wheezing, production of copious secre-tions), and pertinent investigations.

As chest x-ray findings are non-specific[128] the present standard for diagnosis confir-mation is fiberoptic bronchoscopy.[129] Typical findings include carbonaceous debris, inflamed and edematous mucosa, and in some cases early mucosal necrosis and sloughing.

## 10.21
## Treatment

Management is primarily supportive and depends on the grade of injury. Initial treatment includes oxygen, bronchodilators, and physiotherapy. The development of airway edema associated with supraglottic burns is a life-threatening complication. In the event of any possibility of airway compromise then early endotracheal intubation is required and the threshold for this should be reduced if patient transfer is anticipated.

### 10.21.1
### Mechanical Ventilation

Low tidal volumes of 6–8 mL/kg of predicted body weight and a plateau pressure of 30 cm $H_2O$ as used in the ARDSnet[130] trial would appear to be the most logical approach. High frequency percussive ventilation (HFPV) is a lung protective strategy that has shown benefit, decreasing both the incidence of pulmonary barotrauma and pneumonia in inhalation injury.[131] Some ovine models have failed to show this[132] but clinical studies have found a significant decrease in both overall morbidity and mortality in a subset of patients with burns injuries treated with HFPV.[133]

### 10.21.2
### Bronchodilators

Inhalational injury to the lower airways can cause wheezing and bronchospasm as a result of the chemical pneumonitis. $\beta$(beta)$_2$ agonists cause relaxation of the bronchial smooth muscle, stimulation of mucociliary clearance, and markedly increase alveolar fluid clearance in the normal lung.[134]

### 10.21.3
### Sodium Bicarbonate

Bronchial lavage with 1.4% bicarbonate has been recommended as beneficial both in neutralizing acidic deposits and assisting in soot decontamination.[125] There are no studies of its use in the management of inhalational injury due to burns, but there is evidence of its ability to improve pulmonary function in the management of inhalational injury due to chlorine gas.[135]

### 10.21.4
### Heparin

Nebulized heparin has been shown to reduce cast formation, decrease lung edema, and improve oxygenation but has not been shown to reduce mortality.[136] Wang et al., found a

100% survival with the use of systemic heparin and HFPV in a smoke induced ovine model of ARDS.[137]

## 10.21.5
### N-Acetylcysteine

Nebulised N-acetylcysteine is a mucolytic agent which acts by rupturing the disulphide bonds which give stability to the mucoprotein network of molecules in the mucus. Its use may improve $PaO_2/FiO_2$ ratios, but has not been shown to reduce mortality in adults.[124] When used in combination with other treatments N-acetylcysteine has been reported to provide beneficial effects. In pediatric patients a combination of nebulised heparin and N-acetylcysteine led to a reduced mortality when compared to a historical control group.[138] In animal models it has been shown to be effective for the treatment of inhalational injury when used with nebulised heparin.[139] However caution should be exercised when using N-acetylcysteine since it is an irritant to the respiratory tract, can cause mucosal changes and may induce bronchospasm.

## 10.21.6
### Therapeutic Bronchoscopy

The use of the fiberoptic bronchoscope has been shown to be of benefit in clearing secretions when all other techniques have failed.[140] Particularly copious or tenacious secretions may require repeated bronchoscopies. There is no evidence to guide the choice or volume of fluid that is best for bronchoalveolar lavage.

## 10.21.7
### Prophylactic Antibiotics and Steroids

There is no evidence to support the use of prophylactic antibiotics in inhalational injuries and their use promotes the growth of drug-resistant organisms.[141] The use of steroids provides no additional improvements in pulmonary function.[142] However, some investigators have found them effective in management of noninfectious pulmonary complications.[143]

## 10.21.8
### Possible Future Treatments for Burns

Thermal injuries have been found to result in diminished plasma arginine levels. Murakami et al.[144] found intravenous L-arginine supplementation improved gas exchange and pulmonary function an in ovine smoke inhalational model at least in part due to its effect on reduction of oxidative stress. A decrease in alpha-tocopherol (vitamin E) plasma levels in burn patients is typically associated with increased mortality and supplementation of Vitamin E prior to injury has been found to increase the $PaO_2/FiO_2$ ratio, ameliorate both peak and pause airway pressure increases, overall ameliorating the acute lung injury caused by burn and smoke inhalation exposure.[145]

## 10.22
## Mild Traumatic Brain Injury Produced by Blast

Until recently attention has focused on the immediately life-threatening effects of blast on a casualty: secondary and tertiary injuries and the effect of blast lung (primary blast injury) with relatively little attention being paid to more subtle effects such as mild traumatic brain injury after blast exposure.[8] Mild traumatic brain injury after blast is presented in this chapter outside of the primary, secondary, and tertiary classification since the predominant mechanism of injury is currently unknown. The traumatic brain injury discussed in this section does not include penetrating brain injury.

A number of authors are concerned that a significant number of casualties surviving the immediate life-threatening effects of blast exhibit the effects of traumatic brain injury. A recent report noted that "As insurgents continue to attack U.S. troops in Iraq, most brain injuries are being caused by IEDs [improvised explosive devices], and closed brain injuries outnumber penetrating ones among patients seen at Walter Reed, where more than 450 patients with traumatic brain injury (TBI) were treated between January 2003 and February 2005. All admitted patients who have been exposed to a blast are routinely evaluated for brain injury; 59% of them have been given a diagnosis of TBI. Of these injuries, 56% are considered moderate or severe, and 44% are mild."[10] There is also anecdotal evidence suggestive of mild TBI after exposure to relatively weak blast.[8] However, a more recent survey of a large cohort (5869) of UK service personnel returning from Iraq indicates that the picture is not as clear-cut as suggested by earlier reports. The UK study used post-concussional syndrome (PCS) as a marker of TBI and concluded that "PCS symptoms are common and some are related to exposures such as blast injury. However, this association is not specific, and the same symptom complex is also related to numerous other risk factors and exposures."[8]

Soldiers with TBI often have symptoms and findings affecting several areas of brain function. Headaches, sleep disturbances, and sensitivity to light and noise are common symptoms. Cognitive changes, diagnosed on mental-status examination or through neuropsychological testing, may include disturbances in attention, memory, or language, as well as delayed reaction time during problem solving. Often, the most troubling symptoms are behavioral ones: mood changes, depression, anxiety, impulsiveness, emotional outbursts, or inappropriate laughter. Some symptoms of TBI overlap with those of post-traumatic stress disorder, and many patients have both conditions.[10] Recent anecdotal and case reports emphasize the occurrence of clinically significant brain injury that is not detected by CT scanning[8] and the difficulty associated with conventional clinical assessment in the multiply-injured blast casualty that can lead to brain injuries not being detected.[146] There is therefore a need for objective markers of TBI after blast injury to allow early identification of those who have suffered brain injury after blast but who do not have overt external signs of this injury.

## 10.23
## Current Animal Models and Evidence of Neuronal Injury After Blast

There is a paucity of experimental studies into the effects of blast on the central nervous system, but there is evidence that blast exposure can lead to demonstrable histological and behavioral changes consistent with brain injury.[147-152] In a recent study on terminally anesthetised rats we have shown that exposure of the head to relatively mild blast leads to the development of edema in the brain.

Anesthetised rats subjected to whole body primary blast injury (without secondary and tertiary injuries) show evidence of neuronal degeneration within 24 h of injury,[147,148,152] caspase-mediated neuronal apoptosis[149] and significant decrement in performance in areas such as rotametric test and forelimb grip strength[152] and active avoidance tasks.[148] The performance changes were shown to persist for at least 5 days.[148] The route of entry of the shock wave into the body is currently the focus of a great deal of speculation. This is very important when designing protective measures. Some workers argue that the shock wave may enter via the thorax and be transmitted to the brain.[153] Local exposure of the thorax to blast has been found to be associated with an early (3 h after blast injury) decrement in behavioral performance, which subsequently recovered by 24 h post injury.[148] The authors of this study attribute the behavioral changes after thoracic exposure to blast to a transmission of the shock wave via the vasculature to the brain,[148] since the head was protected from the blast using a metal plate. Whilst a transmission of the shock wave from the thorax to the brain via the body fluid environment is certainly possible, e.g., neuronal damage has been recorded when explosive charges have been detonated within the body,[154] the shielding used by Cernak et al.[148] to protect the head from direct encroachment of the shock wave may have been inadequate making it impossible to determine the route of entry of the shock wave into the brain. Furthermore, it is not yet certain that it is the shock wave *per se* rather than a secondary consequence of the blast injury that causes the neuronal damage. No blood gas measurements were recorded in these studies so it is impossible to determine whether the effects of blast on the CNS were due to the shock wave or a secondary consequence of another insult e.g., reduction in blood oxygenation due to the thoracic effects of the blast. Such a secondary mechanism is unlikely in the case of Moochhala's study[152] since they reported the absence of blast lung and sustained hypotension. These studies represent an important first step in the field since they clearly demonstrate that blast primary blast injury can be associated with measurable CNS damage, and that the anesthetised rat is a useful model. However, they also leave unanswered a number of important questions regarding the mechanisms of injury, which are vital for the development of protection and treatment strategies.

## 10.24
## Medical Response to Blast Injuries in Terrorist Attacks

Recent reviews have examined broad lessons that have been learned by the medical services responding to explosive attacks.[49] Several major reviews have been written looking at the medical consequences of terrorism over the past 20 years. Frykberg and Tepas[155]

**Table 10.6** Key terms in assessment of medical response to terrorist attack

| Over-triage vs. under-triage | Over triage is the assignment of non- critically injured to higher than appropriate triage groups, resulting in their earlier than necessary evacuation hospitalization. Under-triage is the reverse (i.e., critically injured personnel being given a low priority for treatment and evacuation). Both can result in increased mortality |
|---|---|
| Critical mortality | Mortality rate of critically injured survivors. Critically injured is defined as Injury Severity Score (ISS) >15. As the majority of survivors do not have life threatening injuries, this is considered a better index of care provision |

Modified from Harrisson et al.[49]

published a review article looking at published experience of terrorist bombings between 1969 and 1983. They identified 220 terrorist bombings that had been reported in the medical literature. They demonstrated that although every incident had a unique set of circumstances, there were broad principles in dealing with these situations that could be used. They also established the use of over-triage and critical mortality in assessing these events (Table 10.6), and the relationship between over-triage and deaths among critically injured (the higher the over-triage rate the higher the mortality rate of the critically injured).

De Ceballos et al.[14] discuss the difference created by moving senior staff forward to deal with an incident compared to the situation after the Madrid attacks in 2005. The HEMS service used their helicopter to get staff to the right places but not for the transport of patients.[156] This is thought to have helped reduce the critical mortality rate at their hospital to 15%. In the military context the principle of forward deployment of clinical staff is already being implemented by the DMS with the use of MERT and E-MERT.

## 10.25
## Summary

Detonation of an explosive generates a shock wave, effectively an instantaneous rise in ambient pressure, which travels outwards from the site of the explosion. Fragments and debris are energized both by the explosion and by the mass movement of gas (blast wind) that follows behind the shock wave. Blast injuries are classified according to the biomechanical mechanism of injury. Primary blast injuries are caused by the coupling of the shock wave with the body wall and the generation of stress and to a lesser extent, shear waves within the tissues of the body. The stress wave effects are most pronounced in organs containing interfaces of different densities and therefore the pathology is concentrated in gas containing organ systems such as the lungs. Primary blast injury to the thorax causes a characteristic triad of bradycardia, hypotension, and apnoea. This is a reflex response mediated in large part via the autonomic nervous system with an afferent pathway conducted via the vagus nerve. Nitric oxide is also released from the injured lung and this, together with myocardial depression may make significant contribution to the hypotension. The autonomic response to blast is amenable to pharmacological intervention and can be effected by pre-treatment with drugs such as those used for protection from nerve agents and pain relief.

Secondary blast injuries are mainly ballistic in nature and result from the impact of fragments of the explosive device's casing and other environmental debris with the body causing largely penetrating injuries that may be associated with life-threatening hemorrhage leading to shock. The response to hemorrhage itself is modified by that to blast and pharmacological treatment. The response to blast also modifies that to subsequent fluid resuscitation after hemorrhage. After blast injury metabolic acidosis develops more rapidly during hypotensive resuscitation and survival time is significantly reduced.

Tertiary injuries are the result of displacement of the body or parts of the body by the dynamic overpressure and subsequent collision with the ground or other relatively fixed structures. Most of the pathology will be blunt injury and the head and skeletal system are particularly at risk. The response to blunt injuries to the musculo-skeletal system also modify autonomic outflow, in this case being characterized by elevation in blood pressure and sympathetic activity, vagal inhibition and an attenuation of the hypotensive response to blood loss. These changes may worsen ischaemia-reperfusion injuries and secondary organ damage.

Quaternary injuries include burns. These are more frequent when casualties are injured in vehicles and can include skin and airway/lung injuries which can require prolonged treatment and intensive care. Thermal injury to the upper airway may lead to the development of edema that can occlude the airway. The clinician should be vigilant to this development which can require prompt endotracheal intubation.

Mild traumatic brain injury after blast currently falls outside the classification system since the mechanism (and indeed whether it is specifically associated with blast) is under investigation. However, a number of authorities believe that it is a significant consequence of blast exposure.

**Acknowledgment**   This chapter contains a significant amount of material published in an earlier chapter[45,158] but also addresses additional aspects and important updates. The sections on primary blast injury to the auditory system and intestinal injury are adapted with permission from Baskin & Holcomb.[157]

## References

1. Nelson TJ, Wall DB, Stedje-Larsen ET, Clark RT, Chambers LW, Bohman HR. Predictors of mortality in close proximity blast injuries during Operation Iraqi Freedom. *J Am Coll Surg.* 2006;202:418-422.
2. Rush RM, Stockmaster NR, Stinger HK, et al. Supporting the global war on terror: a tale of two campaigns featuring the 250th Forward Surgical Team (Airborne). *Am J Surg.* 2005; 189:564-570.
3. Montgomery SP, Swiecki CW, Shriver CD. The evaluation of casualties from Operation Iraqi Freedom on return to the continental United States from March to June 2003. *J Am Coll Surg.* 2005;201:7-12.

4. Ritenour AE, Blackbourne LH, Kelly JF, McLaughlin DF, Pearse LA, Holcomb JB, Wade CE. Incidence of primary blast injury in US military overseas contingency operations: a retrospective study. *Ann Surg*. 2010;251(6):1140-1144.
5. Maynard RL, Cooper GJ, Scott R. Mechanism of injury in bomb blasts and explosions. In: Westaby S, ed. *Trauma*. London: Heinemann; 1989.
6. Zuckerman S. Discussion on the problem of blast injuries. *Proc Roy Soc Med*. 1941;34:171-188.
7. Clemedson CJ. Shock wave transmission to the central nervous system. *Acta Physiol Scand*. 1956;37:204-214.
8. Belanger HG, Scott SG, Scholten J, Curtiss G, Vanderploeg RD. Utility of mechanism-of-injury-based assessment and treatment: Blast Injury Program case illustration. *J Rehabil Res Dev*. 2005;42:403-412.
9. Lew HL, Poole JH, Guillory SB, Salerno RM, Leskin G, Sigford B. Persistent problems after traumatic brain injury: the need for long-term follow-up and coordinated care – Guest Editorial. *J Rehabil Res Dev*. 2006;43:VII-VIX.
10. Okie S. Traumatic brain injury in the war zone. *N Engl J Med*. 2005;352:2043-2047.
11. Dearden P. New blast weapons. *J R Army Med Corps*. 2001;147:80-86.
12. Chaloner E. Blast injury in enclosed spaces. *BMJ*. 2005;331:119-120.
13. Avidan V, Hersch M, Armon Y, et al. Blast lung injury: clinical manifestations, treatment, and outcome. *Am J Surg*. 2005;190:927-931.
14. de Ceballos JP, Turegano-Fuentes F, Perez-Diaz D, Sanz-Sanchez M, Martin-Llorente C, Guerrero-Sanz JE. 11 March 2004: the terrorist bomb explosions in Madrid, Spain – an analysis of the logistics, injuries sustained and clinical management of casualties treated at the closest hospital. *Crit Care*. 2005;9:104-111.
15. Marti M, Parron M, Baudraxler F, Royo A, Gomez LN, Varez-Sala R. Blast injuries from Madrid terrorist bombing attacks on March 11, 2004. *Emerg Radiol*. 2006;13:113-122.
16. Cooper GJ. Protection of the lung from blast overpressure by thoracic stress wave decouplers. *J Trauma*. 1996;40:S105-S110.
17. Cohn SM. Pulmonary contusion: review of the clinical entity. *J Trauma*. 1997;42:973-979.
18. Cooper GJ, Townend DJ, Cater SR, Pearce BP. The role of stress waves in thoracic visceral injury from blast loading: modification of stress transmission by foams and high-density materials. *J Biomech*. 1991;24:273-285.
19. Gans L, Kennedy T. Management of unique clinical entities in disaster medicine. *Emerg Med Clin North Am*. 1996;14:301-326.
20. Mellor SG. The pathogenesis of blast injury and its management. *Br J Hosp Med*. 1988;39:536-539.
21. Argyros GJ. Management of primary blast injury. *Toxicology*. 1997;121:105-115.
22. Frykberg ER, Tepas JJ III, Alexander RH. The 1983 Beirut Airport terrorist bombing. Injury patterns and implications for disaster management. *Am Surg*. 1989;55:134-141.
23. Katz E, Ofek B, Adler J, Abramowitz HB, Krausz MM. Primary blast injury after a bomb explosion in a civilian bus. *Ann Surg*. 1989;209:484-488.
24. Leibovici D, Gofrit ON, Stein M, et al. Blast injuries: bus versus open-air bombings – a comparative study of injuries in survivors of open-air versus confined-space explosions. *J Trauma*. 1996;41:1030-1035.
25. Brown RF, Cooper GJ, Maynard RL. The ultrastructure of rat lung following acute primary blast injury. *Int J Exp Pathol*. 1993;74:151-162.
26. Gorbunov NV, Elsayed NM, Kisin ER, Kozlov AV, Kagan VE. Air blast-induced pulmonary oxidative stress: interplay among hemoglobin, antioxidants, and lipid peroxidation. *Am J Physiol*. 1997;272:L320-L334.
27. Gorbunov NV, Asher LV, Ayyagari V, Atkins JL. Inflammatory leukocytes and iron turnover in experimental hemorrhagic lung trauma. *Exp Mol Pathol*. 2006;80:11-25.
28. Gorbunov NV, Mcfaul SJ, Januszkiewicz A, Atkins JL. Pro-inflammatory alterations and status of blood plasma iron in a model of blast-induced lung trauma. *Int J Immunopathol Pharmacol*. 2005;18:547-556.

29. Barrow DW, Rhodes HT. Blast concussion injury. *JAMA*. 1944;125:900-902.
30. Cernak I, Savic J, Malicevic Z, et al. Involvement of the central nervous system in the general response to pulmonary blast injury. *J Trauma*. 1996;40:S100-S104.
31. Clark SL, Ward JW. The effects of rapid compression waves on animals submerged in water. *Surg Gynec Obstet*. 1943;77:403-412.
32. Clemedson CJ. An experimental study of air blast injuries. *Acta Physiol Scand*. 1949;18:1-200.
33. Irwin RJ, Lerner MR, Bealer JF, Brackett DJ, Tuggle DW. Cardiopulmonary physiology of primary blast injury. *J Trauma*. 1997;43:650-655.
34. Jaffin JH, McKinney L, Kinney RC, et al. A laboratory model for studying blast overpressure injury. *J Trauma*. 1987;27:349-356.
35. Guy RJ, Kirkman E, Watkins PE, Cooper GJ. Physiologic responses to primary blast. *J Trauma*. 1998;45:983-987.
36. Krohn PL, Whitteridge D, Zuckerman S. Physiological effects of blast. *Lancet*. 1942;i:252-258.
37. Ohnishi M, Kirkman E, Guy RJ, Watkins PE. Reflex nature of the cardiorespiratory response to primary thoracic blast injury in the anaesthetised rat. *Exp Physiol*. 2001;86:357-364.
38. Damon EG, Yelverton JT, Luft UC, Mitchell K, Jones RK. Acute effects of air blast on pulmonary function in dogs and sheep. *Aerosp Med*. 1971;42:1-9.
39. Irwin RJ, Lerner MR, Bealer JF, Mantor PC, Brackett DJ, Tuggle DW. Shock after blast wave injury is caused by a vagally mediated reflex. *J Trauma*. 1999;47:105-110.
40. Ohnishi M, Kirkman E, Watkins P. Effects of atropine on the bradycardia associated with primary thoracic blast injury in the anaesthetized rat. *Br J Pharmacol*. 1998;123:U60.
41. Harban FMJ, Kirkman E, Kenward CE, Watkins PE. Primary thoracic blast injury causes acute reduction in cardiac function in the anaesthetised pig. *J Physiol London*. 2001;533:81P.
42. Gorbunov NV, Das DK, Goswami SK, Gurusamy N, Atkins JL. Nitric oxide (NO), redox signaling, and pulmonary inflammation in a model of polytrauma. Proceedings of the XIII Congress of the Society for Free Radical Research International Davos, Switzerland; 2006:2-4.
43. Zunic G, Pavlovic R, Malicevic Z, Savic V, Cernak I. Pulmonary blast injury increases nitric oxide production, disturbs arginine metabolism, and alters the plasma free amino acid pool in rabbits during the early posttraumatic period. *Nitric Oxide*. 2000;4:123-128.
44. Zunic G, Romic P, Vueljic M, Jovanikic O. Very early increase in nitric oxide formation and oxidative cell damage associated with the reduction of tissue oxygenation is a trait of blast casualties. *Vojnosanit Pregl*. 2005;62:273-280.
45. Kirkman E, Watts S, Sapsford W, Sawdon M. Effects of blast injury on the autonomic nervous system and the response to resuscitation. In: Elsayed NM, Atkins JL, eds. *Explosion and Blast-Related Injuries*.: Elsevier; 2008:105-142.
46. Schild HH, Strunk H, Weber W, et al. Pulmonary contusion: CT vs plain radiograms. *J Comput Assist Tomogr*. 1989;13:417-420.
47. Wagner RB, Jamieson PM. Pulmonary contusion. Evaluation and classification by computed tomography. *Surg Clin North Am*. 1989;69:31-40.
48. Gofrit ON, Kovalski N, Leibovici D, Shemer J, O'Hana A, Shapira SC. Accurate anatomical location of war injuries: analysis of the Lebanon war fatal casualties and the proposition of new principles for the design of military personal armour system. *Injury*. 1996;27:577-581.
49. Harrisson SE, Kirkman E, Mahoney P. Lessons learnt from explosive attacks. *J R Army Med Corps*. 2007;153:278-282.
50. Pizov R, Oppenheim-Eden A, Matot I, et al. Blast lung injury from an explosion on a civilian bus. *Chest*. 1999;115:165-172.
51. Hirshberg B, Oppenheim-Eden A, Pizov R, et al. Recovery from blast lung injury – one-year follow-up. *Chest*. 1999;116:1683-1688.
52. Keren A, Stessman J, Tzivoni D. Acute myocardial infarction caused by blast injury of the chest. *Br Heart J*. 1981;46:455-457.

53. Leach RM, Davidson AC. Use of emergency oxygen in adults. *Br Med J.* 2009;338:366-367.

54. Sorkine P, Szold O, Kluger Y, et al. Permissive hypercapnia ventilation in patients with severe pulmonary blast injury. *J Trauma.* 1998;45:35-38.

55. Leibovici D, Gofrit ON, Shapira SC. Eardrum perforation in explosion survivors: is it a marker of pulmonary blast injury? *Ann Emerg Med.* 1999;34:168-172.

56. Cripps NP, Cooper GJ. Risk of late perforation in intestinal contusions caused by explosive blast. *Br J Surg.* 1997;84:1298-1303.

57. Benzinger T. Physiological effects of blast in air and water. In *German aviation medicine in World War II.* Washington DC: US Department of the Airforce; 1950.

58. Clemedson CJ, Hultman HI. Air embolism and the cause of death in blast injury. *Mil Surg.* 1954;114:424-437.

59. Zuckerman S. Experimental study of blast injuries to the lungs. *Lancet.* 1940;ii:219-224.

60. Mott FW. The effects of high explosives upon the central nervous system. *Lancet.* 1916;i:331-338.

61. Clemedson CJ, Pettersson H. Genesis of respiratory and circulatory changes in blast injury. *Am J Physiol.* 1953;174:316-320.

62. Clemedson CJ. Respiration and pulmonary gas exchange in blast injury. *J Appl Physiol.* 1953;6:213-220.

63. Desaga H. Blast Injuries. US Department of the Airforce; 1950.

64. Rossle R. Pathology of blast effects. In *German Aviation Medicine in World War II.* Washington DC: US Department of the Airforce; 1950.

65. Hooker DR. Physiological effects of air concussion. *Am J Physiol.* 1924;67:219-273.

66. Robb-Smith AHT. Pulmonary fat embolism. *Lancet.* 1941;1:135.

67. Cohen H, Biskind GR. Pathological aspects of atmospheric blast injuries in man. *Arch Path.* 1946;42:12-34.

68. Horsley V. The destructive effects of projectiles. *Proc R Institution.* 1894;14:228-238.

69. Crockard HA, Brown FD, Johns LM, Mullan S. An experimental cerebral missile injury model in primates. *J Neurosurg.* 1977;46:776-783.

70. Crockard HA, Brown FD, Calica AB. Physiological consequences of experimental missile injury and the use of data analysis to predict survival. *J Neurosurg.* 1977;46:784-794.

71. Carey ME, Sarna GS, Farrell JB, Happel LT. Experimental missile wound to the brain. *J Neurosurg.* 1989;71:754-764.

72. Levett JM, Johns LM, Replogle RL, Mullan S. Cardiovascular effects of experimental cerebral missile injury in primates. *Surg Neurol.* 1980;13:59-64.

73. Sarphie TG, Carey ME, Davidson JF, Soblosky JS. Scanning electron microscopy of the floor of the fourth ventricle in rats subjected to graded impact injury to the sensorimotor cortex. *J Neurosurg.* 1999;90:734-742.

74. Sapsford W. Penetrating brain injury in military conflict: does it merit more research? *J R Army Med Corps.* 2003;149:5-14.

75. Cooper GJ, Maynard RL, Cross NL, Hill JF. Casualties from terrorist bombings. *J Trauma.* 1983;23:955-967.

76. Barcroft H, Edholm OG, McMichael J, Sharpey-Schafer EP. Post-haemorrhage fainting. Study by cardiac output and forearm flow. *Lancet.* 1944;1:489-491.

77. Little RA, Marshall HW, Kirkman E. Attenuation of the acute cardiovascular responses to haemorrhage by tissue injury in the conscious rat. *Q J Exp Physiol.* 1989;74:825-833.

78. Secher NH, Bie P. Bradycardia during reversible haemorrhagic shock – a forgotten observation? *Clin Physiol.* 1985;5:315-323.

79. Evans RG, Ludbrook J. Chemosensitive cardiopulmonary afferents and the haemodynamic response to simulated haemorrhage in conscious rabbits. *Br J Pharmacol.* 1991;102:533-539.

80. Little RA, Randall PE, Redfern WS, Stoner HB, Marshall HW. Components of injury (haemorrhage and tissue ischaemia) affecting cardiovascular reflexes in man and rat. *Q J Exp Physiol.* 1984;69:753-762.

81. Hoffman RL. Rupture of the spleen. A review and report of a case following abdominal hysterectomy. *Am J Obstet Gynecol.* 1972;113:524-530.
82. Sander-Jensen K, Secher NH, Bie P, Warberg J, Schwartz TW. Vagal slowing of the heart during haemorrhage: observations from 20 consecutive hypotensive patients. *Br Med J (Clin Res Ed).* 1986;292:364-366.
83. Kirkman E, Shiozaki T, Little RA. Methiothepin antagonism does not attenuate the bradycardia associated with severe hemorrhage in the anesthetized rat. *Br J Pharmacol.* 1994;112:U58.
84. Scherrer U, Vissing S, Morgan BJ, Hanson P, Victor RG. Vasovagal syncope after infusion of a vasodilator in a heart-transplant recipient. *N Engl J Med.* 1990;322:602-604.
85. Shen YT, Knight DR, Thomas JX Jr, Vatner SF. Relative roles of cardiac receptors and arterial baroreceptors during hemorrhage in conscious dogs. *Circ Res.* 1990;66:397-405.
86. Evans RG, Ventura S, Dampney RA, Ludbrook J. Neural mechanisms in the cardiovascular responses to acute central hypovolaemia. *Clin Exp Pharmacol Physiol.* 2001;28:479-487.
87. Sawdon M, Ohnishi M, Watkins PE, Kirkman E. The effects of primary thoracic blast injury and morphine on the response to haemorrhage in the anaesthetised rat. *Exp Physiol.* 2002; 87:683-689.
88. Hodgetts TJ, Mahoney PF, Russell MQ, Byers M. ABC to<C>ABC: redefining the military trauma paradigm. *Emerg Med J.* 2006;23:745-746.
89. Committee on Trauma ACoS. *Advanced Trauma Life Support (ATLS) Course for Physicians.* Chicago: American College of Surgeons; 2002.
90. Bickell WH, Wall MJ, Pepe PE, et al. Immediate versus delayed fluid resuscitation for hypotensive patients with penetrating torso injuries. *N Engl J Med.* 1994;331:1105-1109.
91. Kowalenko T, Stern S, Dronen S, Xu W. Improved outcome with hypotensive resuscitation of uncontrolled hemorrhagic-shock in a swine model. *J Trauma.* 1992;33:349-353.
92. Stern SA. Low-volume fluid resuscitation for presumed hemorrhagic shock: helpful or harmful? *Curr Opin Crit Care.* 2001;7:422-430.
93. Battlefield Advanced Life Support. UK: Defence Medical Education and Training Agency; 2009.
94. Pre-hospital Initiation of Fluid Replacement Therapy in Trauma. Technology Appraisal 74, UK: NHS National Institute for Clinical Excellence; 2004.
95. Rafie AD, Rath PA, Michell MW, et al. Hypotensive resuscitation of multiple hemorrhages using crystalloid and colloids. *Shock.* 2004;22:262-269.
96. Bilski TR, Baker BC, Grove JR, et al. Battlefield casualties treated at Camp Rhino, Afghanistan: lessons learned. *J Trauma.* 2003;54:814-821.
97. Bohman HR, Stevens RA, Baker BC, Chambers LW. The US Navy's forward resuscitative surgery system during operation Iraqi freedom. *Mil Med.* 2005;170:297-301.
98. Garner J, Watts S, Parry C, Bird J, Cooper G, Kirkman E. Prolonged permissive hypotensive resuscitation is associated with poor outcome in primary blast injury with controlled hemorrhage. *Ann Surg.* 2010;251(6):1131-1139.
99. Brismar B, Bergenwald L. The terrorist bomb explosion in Bologna, Italy, 1980: an analysis of the effects and injuries sustained. *J Trauma.* 1982;22:216-220.
100. Hadden WA, Rutherford WH, Merrett JD. The injuries of terrorist bombing: a study of 1532 consecutive patients. *Br J Surg.* 1978;65:525-531.
101. Hull JB. Traumatic amputation by explosive blast: pattern of injury in survivors. *Br J Surg.* 1992;79:1303-1306.
102. Pyper PC, Graham WJ. Analysis of terrorist injuries treated at Craigavon Area Hospital, Northern Ireland, 1972-1980. *Injury.* 1983;14:332-338.
103. Rignault DP, Deligny MC. The 1986 terrorist bombing experience in Paris. *Ann Surg.* 1989;209:368-373.
104. Hill JF. Blast injuries with particular reference to recent terrorist bombing incidents. *Ann RCS.* 1979;61:4-11.
105. Waterworth TA, Carr MJT. An analysis of the post-mortem findings in the 21 victims of the Birmingham pub bombings. *Injury.* 1975;7:89-95.
106. Kirkman E, Zhang H, Spapen H, Little RA, Vincent JL. Effects of afferent neuralstimulation on critical oxygen delivery: a hemodynamic explanation. Am JPhysiol. 1995;269:R1448-54.

107. Eltrafi A, Kirkman E, Little RA. Reversal of injury induced reduction in baroreflex sensitivity by naloxone in the conscious rat. *Br J Pharmacol.* 1989;96:145.
108. Wyatt J, Kirkman E, Little RA. Reversal of injury induced reductions in baroreflex sensitivity by β-funaltrexamine in the anaesthetized rat. *Physiol Zool.* 1995;68:67.
109. Marshall HW, Prehar S, Kirkman E, Little RA. Morphine increases mortality after haemorrhage in the rat. *J Accid Emerg Med.* 1998;15:133.
110. Overman RR, Wang SC. The contributory role of the afferent nervous factor in experimental shock: sublethal hemorrhage and sciatic nerve stimulation. *Am J Physiol.* 1947;148:289-295.
111. Foex BA, Kirkman E, Little RA. Injury (nociceptive afferent nerve stimulation) modifies the hemodynamic and metabolic responses to hemorrhage in immature swine. *Crit Care Med.* 2004;32:740-746.
112. Mackway-Jones K, Foex BA, Kirkman E, Little RA. Modification of the cardiovascular response to hemorrhage by somatic afferent nerve stimulation with special reference to gut and skeletal muscle blood flow. *J Trauma.* 1999;47:481-485.
113. Deitch EA. Intestinal permeability is increased in burn patients shortly after injury. *Surgery.* 1990;107:411-416.
114. Deitch EA, Adams CA, Lu Q, Xu DZ. Mesenteric lymph from rats subjected to trauma-hemorrhagic shock are injurious to rat pulmonary microvascular endothelial cells as well as human umbilical vein endothelial cells. *Shock.* 2001;16:290-293.
115. Wilmore DW, Smith RJ, O'Dwyer ST, Jacobs DO, Ziegler TR, Wang XD. The gut: a central organ after surgical stress. *Surgery.* 1988;104:917-923.
116. Rady MY, Little RA, Edwards JD, Kirkman E, Faithfull S. The effect of nociceptive stimulation on the changes in hemodynamics and oxygen-transport induced by hemorrhage in anesthetized pigs. *J Trauma.* 1991;31:617-622.
117. Rady MY, Kirkman E, Cranley J, Little RA. A comparison of the effects of skeletal-muscle injury and somatic afferent nerve-stimulation on the response to hemorrhage in anesthetized pigs. *J Trauma.* 1993;35:756-761.
118. Lockey DJ, Nordmann GR, Field JM, Clough D, Henning JD. The deployment of an intensive care facility with a military field hospital to the 2003 conflict in Iraq. *Resuscitation.* 2004;62:261-265.
119. Roberts MJ, Fox MA, Hamilton-Davies C, Dowson S. The experience of the intensive care unit in a British army field hospital during the 2003 Gulf conflict. *J R Army Med Corps.* 2003;149:284-290.
120. Thompson PB, Herndon DN, Traber DL, Abston S. Effect on mortality of inhalation injury. *J Trauma.* 1986;26:163-165.
121. Prior K, Nordmann G, Sim K, Mahoney P, Thomas R. Management of inhalational injuries in UK burns centres – a questionnaire survey. *J Intensive Care Soc.* 2009;10:141-144.
122. Hollingsed TC, Saffle JR, Barton RG, Craft WB, Morris SE. Etiology and consequences of respiratory failure in thermally injured patients. *Am J Surg.* 1993;166:592-596.
123. de La Cal MA, Cerda E, Garcia-Hierro P, et al. Pneumonia in patients with severe burns: a classification according to the concept of the carrier state. *Chest.* 2001;119:1160-1165.
124. Walton JJ, Manara AR. Burns and smoke inhalation. *Anaesth Intens Care Med.* 2005;6:317-321.
125. Hilton PJ, Hepp M. The immediate care of the burned patient. *BJA CEPD Rev.* 2001;1:113-116.
126. Black RG, Kinsella J. Anaesthetic management for burns patients. *BJA CEPD Rev.* 2001; 1:177-180.
127. Einhorn IN. Physiological and toxicological aspects of smoke produced during the combustion of polymeric materials. *Environ Health Perspect.* 1975;11:163-189.
128. Peitzman AB, Shires GT III, Teixidor HS, Curreri PW, Shires GT. Smoke inhalation injury: evaluation of radiographic manifestations and pulmonary dysfunction. *J Trauma.* 1989;29:1232-1238.
129. Kawecki M, Wroblewski P, Sakiel S, Gawel S, Glik J. Fibreoptic bronchoscopy in routine clinical practice in confirming the diagnosis and treatment of inhalation burns. *Burns.* 2007;33:554-560.
130. Oba Y, Salzman GA. Ventilation with lower tidal volumes as compared with traditional tidal volumes for acute lung injury. *N Engl J Med.* 2000;343:813-814.

131. Cioffi WG Jr, Rue LW III, Graves TA, McManus WF, Mason AD Jr, Pruitt BA Jr. Prophylactic use of high-frequency percussive ventilation in patients with inhalation injury. *Ann Surg.* 1991;213:575-580.
132. Schmalstieg FC, Keeney SE, Rudloff HE, et al. Arteriovenous CO2 removal improves survival compared to high frequency percussive and low tidal volume ventilation in a smoke/burn sheep acute respiratory distress syndrome model. *Ann Surg.* 2007;246:512-521.
133. Hall JJ, Hunt JL, Arnoldo BD, Purdue GF. Use of high-frequency percussive ventilation in inhalation injuries. *J Burn Care Res.* 2007;28:396-400.
134. Brower RG, Ware LB, Berthiaume Y, Matthay MA. Treatment of ARDS. *Chest.* 2001; 120:1347-1367.
135. Aslan S, Kandis H, Akgun M, Cakir Z, Inandi T, Gorguner M. The effect of nebulized NaHCO3 treatment on "RADS" due to chlorine gas inhalation. *Inhal Toxicol.* 2006;18:895-900.
136. Murakami K, McGuire R, Cox RA, et al. Heparin nebulization attenuates acute lung injury in sepsis following smoke inhalation in sheep. *Shock.* 2002;18:236-241.
137. Wang D, Zwischenberger JB, Savage C, et al. High-frequency percussive ventilation with systemic heparin improves short-term survival in a LD100 sheep model of acute respiratory distress syndrome. *J Burn Care Res.* 2006;27:463-471.
138. Desai MH, Mlcak R, Richardson J, Nichols R, Herndon DN. Reduction in mortality in pediatric patients with inhalation injury with aerosolized heparin/N-acetylcystine [correction of acetylcystine] therapy. *J Burn Care Rehabil.* 1998;19:210-212.
139. Brown M, Desai M, Traber LD, Herndon DN, Traber DL. Dimethylsulfoxide with heparin in the treatment of smoke inhalation injury. *J Burn Care Rehabil.* 1988;9:22-25.
140. Mlcak RP, Suman OE, Herndon DN. Respiratory management of inhalation injury. *Burns.* 2007;33:2-13.
141. Herndon DN, Thompson PB, Traber DL. Pulmonary injury in burned patients. *Crit Care Clin.* 1985;1:79-96.
142. Cha SI, Kim CH, Lee JH, et al. Isolated smoke inhalation injuries: acute respiratory dysfunction, clinical outcomes, and short-term evolution of pulmonary functions with the effects of steroids. *Burns.* 2007;33:200-208.
143. Irrazabal CL, Capdevila AA, Revich L, et al. Early and late complications among 15 victims exposed to indoor fire and smoke inhalation. *Burns.* 2008;34:533-538.
144. Murakami K, Enkhbaatar P, Yu YM, et al. L-arginine attenuates acute lung injury after smoke inhalation and burn injury in sheep. *Shock.* 2007;28:477-483.
145. Morita N, Shimoda K, Traber MG, et al. Vitamin E attenuates acute lung injury in sheep with burn and smoke inhalation injury. *Redox Rep.* 2006;11:61-70.
146. Lew HL. Rehabilitation needs of an increasing population of patients: traumatic brain injury, polytrauma, and blast-related injuries. *J Rehabil Res Dev.* 2005;42:XIII-XIXV.
147. Cernak I, Wang ZG, Jiang JX, Bian XW, Savic J. Cognitive deficits following blast injury-induced neurotrauma: possible involvement of nitric oxide. *Brain Inj.* 2001;15:593-612.
148. Cernak I, Wang ZG, Jiang JX, Bian XW, Savic J. Ultrastructural and functional characteristics of blast injury-induced neurotrauma. *J Trauma.* 2001;50:695-706.
149. Kato K, Fujimura M, Nakagawa A, et al. Pressure-dependent effect of shock waves on rat brain: induction of neuronal apoptosis mediated by a caspase-dependent pathway. *J Neurosurg.* 2007;106:667-676.
150. Kaur C, Singh J, Lim MK, Ng BL, Yap EPH, Ling EA. The response of neurons and microglia to blast injury in the rat-brain. *Neuropathol Appl Neurobiol.* 1995;21:369-377.
151. Kaur C, Singh J, Lim MK, Ng BL, Yap EP, Ling EA. Ultrastructural changes of macroglial cells in the rat brain following an exposure to a non-penetrative blast. *Ann Acad Med Singapore.* 1997;26:27-29.
152. Moochhala SM, Md S, Lu J, Teng CH, Greengrass C. Neuroprotective role of aminoguanidine in behavioral changes after blast injury. *J Trauma.* 2004;56:393-403.
153. Courtney AC, Courtney MW. A thoracic mechanism of mild traumatic brain injury due to blast pressure waves. *Med Hypotheses.* 2009;72:76-83.

154. Knudsen SK, Oen EO. Blast-induced neurotrauma in whales. *Neurosci Res.* 2003;46: 377-386.
155. Frykberg ER, Tepas JJ III. Terrorist bombings. Lessons learned from Belfast to Beirut. *Ann Surg.* 1988;208:569-576.
156. Lockey DJ, Mackenzie R, Redhead J, et al. London bombings July 2005: the immediate pre-hospital medical response. *Resuscitation.* 2005;66:ix-xii.
157. Baskin TW, Holcomb JB. Bombs, mines, blast, fragmentation and thermobaric mechanisms of injury. In: Mahoney PF, Ryan J, Brookes A, Schwab CW, eds. *Ballistic Trauma: A Practical Guide.* London: Springer-Verlag; 2005:45-66.
158. Kirkman E, Watts S, Cooper G. Blast Injury Research Models. *Phil. Trans. R Soc. B.* 2011; 366:144-159.

# Ballistic Protection

# 11

Alan Hepper, Daniel Longhurst, Graham Cooper, and Philip Gotts

## 11.1
## Introduction

*Personal armor* is the term used to describe items that are worn or carried to provide an individual with protection from energy. In the military and law-enforcement environment, this energy is principally in the form of impact by non-penetrating projectiles or blows, blast waves from explosions, and penetrating missiles.

Energy is the capacity to perform work. The work done on the body may produce contusion and laceration of tissues and fracture of bones. Penetrating missiles deliver energy internally during their passage through tissues. Blast waves and non-penetrating impacts interact with the body wall, and the motion of the body wall resulting from the application of energy couples the external energy into the viscera, where it will do work. Energy may be transferred internally from the motion of the body wall by stress (pressure) waves and shear (the disparate motion of components of tissues and of organs).

Additionally, personal armor is available to offer protection from burns and the acceleration of the body surface resulting from the impact of the moving body against a rigid, unyielding surface – "bump" protection. Many types of personal armor combine protection from penetrating and non-penetrating impacts. For example, military helmets are designed to stop penetrating missiles such as certain classes of bullets or fragments and offer protection against "bump" impacts arising from falls, missiles such as bricks, or obstacles at head height.

This chapter will address principally the retardation of penetrating projectiles. Penetrating projectiles encompass bullets and fragments arising from the detonation of munitions such

A. Hepper (✉)
Biomedical Sciences, Defence Science and Technology Laboratory,
Porton Down, Salisbury, Wiltshire, UK
e-mail: aehepper@dstl.gov.uk

A.J. Brooks et al. (eds.), *Ryan's Ballistic Trauma*,
DOI: 10.1007/978-1-84882-124-8_11, © Springer-Verlag London Limited 2011

as artillery shells, mortars, grenades, and other explosive devices. Knives also may be considered a penetration threat, particularly to law-enforcement officers. Personal armor takes a number of forms that are designed to defeat different ballistic threats:

- Ballistic helmets provide protection from anti-personnel fragments, bump protection or protection from low-energy bullets (fired from revolvers and pistols, for example). In general, ballistic helmets will not stop high-energy bullets from rifles.
- Body armor provides protection from fragments, low- and high-energy bullets, or even slash and stab from knives. The most extensive personal armor systems are Explosive Ordnance Disposal (EOD) suits, popularly known as bomb-disposal suits.
- Hand-held armor consists of ballistic shields, principally designed to protect from bullets.

Apart from EOD suits, there are no modern equivalents to the suit of armor of the Middle Ages. Protection over the whole body against modern ballistic threats would be too heavy for the dismounted soldier or police officer, because the threat is so advanced and the encumbrance would be too great. Therefore modern personal armor covers only the most vulnerable parts of the body – the head and the torso. The helmet covers some proportion of the head, principally the brain (although not completely[1]). The face may be protected with a visor, or the eyes alone may be protected by goggles or other type of eyepiece. Most personal transparent armor components are not usually of a very high ballistic performance. The only exception is the visor used in conjunction with an EOD suit that is a complex, heavy, multilayered item designed to stop high-energy fragments from detonations at very close range. In vehicles, transparent armor is often integrated into the vehicle structure, for example windows and top-cover cupolas, to reduce the burden on the person.

## 11.2
## General Principles of Protection

### 11.2.1
### Mechanics

The technical approaches for stopping penetrating missiles and mitigating non-penetrating impacts are different. The underlying principles of minimizing the effects of energy transfer from a projectile are:

- Absorbing energy in armors by making the projectile do work on materials before it enters the body – breaking materials, stretching them, or compressing them all use energy, or extend the time over which it is applied to the body.
- Redistributing the energy so that other materials or the body wall are more able (due to the reduction in pressure – force per unit area) to withstand the total energy.

The helmet will serve to demonstrate the principles. In simple terms, a helmet comprises a hard shell backed with a foamed material (e.g., a polymer or, historically, rubber).

The helmet will stop a penetrating missile such as an anti-personnel fragment by enabling the fragment to *stretch* armor fibers in the shell, *cutting/breaking* some of them, and *compressing* layers of fibers ahead of it. The foam backing plays little part, except in providing standoff for the deformation and extending the time over which the energy is transferred to the body.

For a non-penetrating missile such as a brick or for the bump of a fall, the hard shell *redistributes* the energy over a larger area of the shell, resulting in a small *deformation*, which is *absorbed* more *slowly* and further *redistributed* by the foamed liner.

The technical approaches are different, but the common themes are:

- Absorb energy
- Redistribute it
- Extend the duration of its application

## 11.2.2
## Coverage

Body armor can be heavy and constrain movement. It is essential that the optimal balance between protection and mobility is maintained. In practice, this dictates that armor must be relevant to the principal ballistic threat and be applied to the most vulnerable areas of the body. Vulnerable in this context may be with respect to saving life or maintaining operational effectiveness (or both) – life saving being the primary aim. For example, the chest plainly is vulnerable to penetrating missiles. For soldiers and law-enforcement officers in static locations who need to be able to return fire, it is essential that the chest has optimal coverage. For a high-energy bullet, this would require a large, rigid plate to defeat the bullet. An infantry soldier who is part of a mobile platoon may find it difficult to carry such a plate and maintain agility and mobility; thus, the armor should be designed to save life, taking account of the medical facilities available. In the context of Northern Ireland, soldiers were issued with small, lightweight plates that covered only the heart and great vessels. Penetrating wounds to the lungs alone have a low mortality with immediate medical care and so the inefficient coverage over the lungs was unlikely to lead to high mortality, but significantly improved the mobility of troops by limiting the bulk and mass of large coverage rigid plates. During deployed operations where clinical and surgical care may be delayed, large ballistic plates are required even for mobile troops to enhance their survivability. Thus, body coverage is an issue dictated by *clinical issues*, in addition to the *ergonomic aspects*.

Knowledge of the clinical consequences and risk to life from low and high-energy penetrating projectiles is necessary to optimize the location of armor. Table 11.1 shows the distribution of wounds in those Killed in Action (KIA), Died of Wounds (DOW), and Wounded for Korea and Vietnam. Also shown in this Table are the presented areas for four regions of the body of a man in a combat posture. It is evident (unsurprisingly) that projectile impacts to the head and thorax are very frequent in the KIA and DOW, and are

**Table 11.1** Percentage distribution of wounds by anatomical areas in Korea and Vietnam conflicts

|                    | Head | Neck | Thorax | Abdomen | Extremities |
|--------------------|------|------|--------|---------|-------------|
| Presented area     | 12   | 16   | 11     | 61      | –           |
| *Korea*            |      |      |        |         |             |
| KIA                | 38   | 10   | 23     | 17      | 11          |
| DOW                | 25   | 7    | 20     | 30      | 15          |
| Wounded who lived  | 7    | 11   | 8      | 7       | 66          |
| *Vietnam*          |      |      |        |         |             |
| KIA                | 34   | 8    | 41     | 10      | 7           |
| DOW                | 46   | 46   | 23     | 21      | 9           |
| Wounded who lived  | 17   | 17   | 9      | 6       | 69          |

*KIA* Killed in Action, *DOW* Died of Wounds
From Carey[2]

out of proportion to their presented areas. The key points emerging from these data from Korea and Vietnam are

- The limbs make up 61% of the presented area, but limb wounds accounted for about 66 and 69% of wounded battle casualties, albeit with a low fatality rate (around 10% of those KIA)
- The head and neck combined are about 12% of the presented area and accounted for 18 and 34% of wounded casualties, but for about 42 and 48% of deaths
- The abdomen and thorax account for 27% of presented area, and for 37 and 51% of battlefield deaths (KIA).

It is also important to recognize that the term "head" encompasses sensory structures, the brain, and other soft/bony tissues, each of which have different vulnerabilities. For example, the eyes make up only 0.27% of the frontal presented area, but are injured in up to 10% of combat casualties.

## 11.2.3
## Wounding Missile

The principal threats to law-enforcement officers are knives and low and high-energy bullets. Military personnel are subjected to a broader range of missiles (in terms of mass, numbers, velocity, direction of attack, and intensity of fire), and the armor systems employed need to reflect this divergence. It also must be recognized that the balance of bullets and fragments in various military conflicts is different. Table 11.2 shows that in general war against other armies (e.g., World War I and World War II), fragments are the principal wounding agent, but in urban or jungle operations against irregular militia or terrorists, bullets predominate. The preferred armor for these different scenarios may be confined to flexible materials such as aramids for anti-personnel fragments, but with a threat

**Table 11.2** Distribution of wounding agents in casualties for wars and campaigns this century (%)

|                   | Bullets | Fragments | Other |
|-------------------|---------|-----------|-------|
| World War I       | 39      | 61        | –     |
| World War II      | 10      | 85        | 5     |
| Korea             | 7       | 92        | 1     |
| Vietnam           | 52      | 44        | 4     |
| Borneo            | 90      | 9         | 1     |
| Northern Ireland  | 55      | 22        | 20    |
| Falkland Islands  | 32      | 56        | 12    |

from high-energy bullets, more substantial armors such as rigid plates are required to counteract the threat. The heads of troops are particularly vulnerable to air-burst munitions and aimed fire of fragmentation weapons at their covert positions and personnel with their upper body exposed (such as vehicle top-covers); thus, helmets are essential to optimize protection. Law-enforcement officers on general patrol duties are not subjected to these threats, so the personal armor should address knife and low-energy bullet attack to the torso, matching the threats the law enforcement officer faces.

## 11.3
## Threats and Testing

When designing or assessing personal armor, it is usual to divide the ballistic threats into three main categories: fragments, low-energy bullets, and high-energy bullets. (Bullets are frequently classed as low and high velocity. For terminal ballistics, it is more appropriate to classify projectiles by their available energy – the capacity to perform work. The kinetic energy of a projectile [Joules] is $0.5 \times$ mass (kg) $\times$ velocity (m/s), i.e., $\frac{1}{2} mv^2$.)

Armors to defeat either low- or high-energy bullets are usually developed to defeat a specific bullet at a specific velocity, often its velocity at the muzzle of the weapon. The wearer would like to be assured that the armor will stop a specific bullet. The test employed is referred to as a *Complete Protection Test*. This is a pass/fail test and therefore sets a threshold that must be exceeded for the armor to pass quality-control tests. It does not provide any information about how far above the stated threshold is the effective performance of the armor.

Fragments have high velocity close to the detonation and generally very low mass; consequently, their available energy is usually low, but with a low presented area giving them a good penetrative capability. Their velocity declines rapidly as range extends. For flexible lightweight armor, it is generally not possible to protect against specific fragmenting munitions at close range. There is a much greater spread of mass, velocity, and shape of fragments from both individual munitions and between different types of munitions. Therefore, a *Complete Protection Test* is not employed. Fragmentation protective armor is specified using a criterion known as the $V_{50}$. The $V_{50}$ is defined as the velocity at which

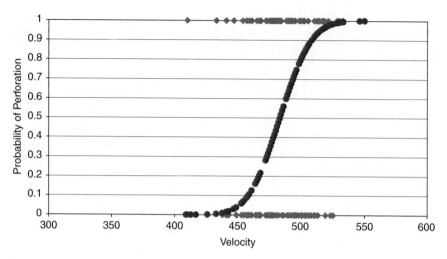

**Fig. 11.1** A $V_{50}$ curve for an armor system

50% of the projectiles are stopped by the armor and 50% perforate. This is a statistical measure and a scientific method that allows the armor designer to rank armor materials and systems. It does not attempt to advise the user of the armor how it will perform in the field, but only how its ballistic performance compares to another armor. Plainly, the 50% of fragments that perforate the armor are capable of producing penetrating trauma. The $V_{50}$ should always be greater than the assessed threat.

For armor, there is no specific velocity above which the projectile will always perforate and below which it is retarded. An example of a relationship between impact velocity and perforation of the armor, from which a $V_{50}$ for armor is determined, is shown in Fig. 11.1. It was obtained by using a series of shots that are penetrating and non-penetrating at known velocities. From these data, an S-shaped curve can be calculated that predicts the probability of penetration with respect to the velocity of the projectile. The velocity at which the probability is predicted to be 50% is the $V_{50}$. Note the considerable overlap in the velocities of nominally identical projectiles that penetrated and those that did not. The $V_{50}$ is not the only measure to assess the performance since the gradient of the S-shaped curve is also a measure of the consistency of the material.

In order to attempt to relate the $V_{50}$ to the effectiveness of the armor in operational use, a Casualty Reduction Analysis model can be used. The operational impact of armor with a particular performance will depend upon a large number of factors that need to be encompassed within a Casualty Reduction Analysis model. This operational impact can be expressed as a function of:

- The coverage of the armor on the body
- The ballistic threat in terms of the number, size, velocity distribution, and trajectory of the projectiles from specific munitions (usually acquired from field trials)
- The presented area of the man and the shielding effects of the ground, structures, and vehicles
- The incapacitation predicted from penetration of fragments through the armor or through other unprotected parts of the body.

These models enable developers to predict the benefits of trade-offs, such as between weight (i.e., coverage), anatomical location of armors, $V_{50}$ performance, and casualty reduction. Additional Operational Analysis tools can also address the effects of a reduction in mobility arising from armor use on the success of the mission and the production of casualties. Placing armor on personnel has many ramifications – some good, some bad; these types of tools are essential to assess the operational consequences. Whether armor stops a particular piece of metal (or not) is not the pinnacle, but a baseline of armor design and deployment, and a thorough understanding of the burden, coverage, and fit is also required. Confidence in the equipment is essential otherwise it will not be worn.

## 11.4
## Materials

The materials used in personal armor depend upon the threat to be defeated and the part of the body to be protected. Similar materials are used for the defeat of fragmentation and low-energy bullets. For the torso, these will be multiple layers of woven, unidirectional, or felted textiles produced from high tensile strength fibers. The most common fibers are ballistic nylon, para-aramids (Kevlar® or Twaron®), and Ultra High Molecular Weight Polyethylenes (UHMWPE) (Dyneema® and Spectra®). The materials can also be encapsulated within a resin matrix and pressed into a rigid composite structure. These rigid composites can be used for helmets.

Composite materials can also be used for protection from high-energy bullets. Composites used for high-energy bullet protection are most usually combined with a ceramic strike face, particularly if the threat projectile contains a steel core rather than only lead. Figure 11.2 shows a ceramic-faced high-energy bullet protective plate that has been struck by a 7.62 mm caliber North Atlantic Treaty Organization (NATO) bullet. The damage to the ceramic strike face is evident over a greater area than the bullet strike location.

The most challenging items of armor are those that are required to be transparent. They require the ballistic resistance, but also good optical quality. The materials used for transparent armor include polycarbonate, polyurethane, acrylic, glass, and glass-ceramics.

## 11.5
## Mechanisms of Projectile Defeat

Some projectiles can be defeated using flexible textile materials and some require a rigid structure. When any projectile of a mass $m$, traveling at a velocity $v$, impacts a target, it possesses kinetic energy ($KE = \frac{1}{2} mv^2$). The energy acts over a very small impact area and enables the projectile to perforate materials. The term often used to describe the ability of a projectile to defeat its target is its *kinetic energy density*, that is, the projectile energy per unit area at the impact site. However, without consideration of projectile material, this term is often used in a misleading way. In the most general terms, an armor system defeats the projectile by preventing perforation, deforming the projectile, absorbing the kinetic energy, and spreading it over a larger area before the projectile has a chance to punch through.

**Fig. 11.2** Alumina ceramic
plate backed by a composite
designed to defeat high-
energy bullets

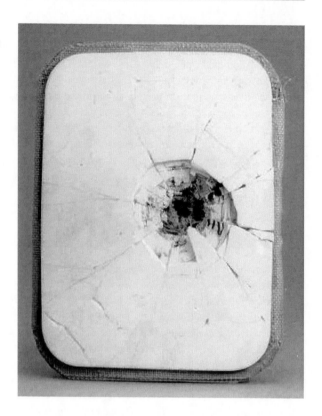

Textile armors, such as those used for fragmentation or low-energy bullet defeat, are usually woven. The yarns used in woven ballistic textiles have a high specific strength and a high
modulus. These properties mean that the fibers are particularly difficult to break. The high
modulus allows the energy to be dissipated as a longitudinal stress wave along the yarn.
Figure 11.3 shows a single cross-over in a woven textile. As the projectile impacts a certain

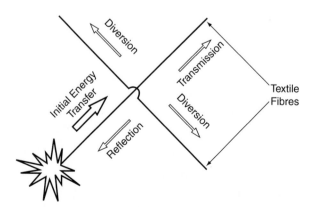

**Fig. 11.3** Distribution of the
bullet's energy in textile
fibers

point on one of the yarns, the energy imparted will travel along the yarn. When it meets the cross-over it divides via a number of possible mechanisms. It can continue along the yarn (transmission), it can be reflected back along the yarn, or it can travel along the crossing yarn (diversion). This is a single cross-over on a single layer. In a one centimeter by one centimeter square there could be well over 100 of these cross-overs. No body armor will consist of a single layer, most will use more than 15 layers, and some more than 40 layers. Not all the energy is dissipated in the first layer and hence the same mechanism continues through the consecutive layers until the projectile does not have sufficient energy to continue. This continual process means that the first layer has been defeated by shearing (cutting) of the yarns. This shearing is a second mechanism of energy absorption and certain materials can absorb more energy using this mechanism than in longitudinal stress wave dissipation.

If a high-velocity bullet is fired from almost any range except the most extreme, it is unlikely to be defeated by textile armor alone. For the defeat of these bullets a hard strike face is often used. In these types of armor the hardness of the strike face is used to break up or distort the projectile before the composite backing spreads the energy over a greater area. Figure 11.4 shows the cross-sectional view of a ceramic-faced, composite-backed armor plate. As the bullet impacts the armor, which usually is harder than the bullet, the nose of the bullet distorts. The shock pressure of the impact also fractures the ceramic. In some ceramics, such as alumina, the fracture pattern takes the form of a conoid (conical fracture), thus imparting the residual energy over a much larger area of the composite backing. Additionally, as the bullet passes through the ceramic, it is initially mushroomed, thus increasing the surface area and reducing the kinetic energy density. It then is broken up by the ceramic as it continues its path to the backing. By the time the remaining parts of the bullet reach the backing it is accompanied by the fragments of ceramic, and these fragments are defeated by the composite backing using a mechanism similar to that of the woven textile described above.

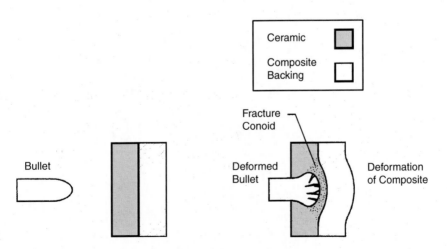

**Fig. 11.4** Defeat of a high-energy projectile by ceramic and composite

## 11.6
## Types of Personal Armor

The ballistic protective tee-shirt does not exist. Materials must be tailored into clothing items that have minimal impact on the performance of the wearer (while still maintaining adequate coverage), and they must be compatible with other equipment the wearer is carrying.

The military ballistic helmet presents the greatest challenges; it needs to be compatible with weapon sights, communications sets, respirators, ocular protection, etc., and still be light and comfortable enough to wear for extended periods.

Body armor on the thorax must enable the wearer to lose heat, aim weapons, sit in a vehicle, crouch, wear load-carrying equipment, etc. If the armor is not comfortable, excessively degrades performance, or the wearer has no confidence in its performance, it will not be worn.

### 11.6.1
### Combat Helmets

Within NATO countries combat helmets are constructed of textile-based composites. The helmet can be constructed of ballistic nylon, para-aramid, or UHMWPE. Figure 11.5 is the UK GS Mk6 Combat Helmet. In this configuration it has the anti-riot (public order) equipment fitted: a polycarbonate visor, with a seal at the top to stop burning fluids pouring down the face, and a blunt impact-resistant and fire-retardant nape protector.

Most combat helmets will be of a similar generic design. The differences that are seen in geometry are due to the requirement for compatibility with other equipment.

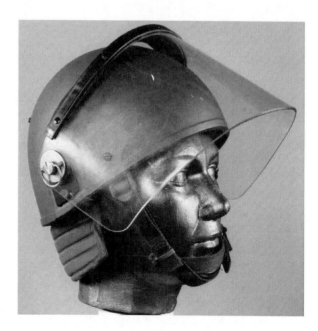

**Fig. 11.5** General combat helmet with antiriot (public order) equipment attached

**Fig. 11.6** Helmet for a crew of armored fighting vehicles

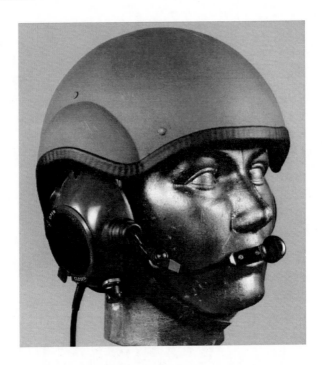

Figure 11.6 is a helmet of crew members of armored fighting vehicles. The shape around the ears is to enable communications equipment to be worn.

Figure 11.7 is a representative low-energy bullet protective helmet, which also has a high level of fragmentation protection.

All UK helmets have a high level of nonballistic impact or "bump" protection. This is achieved using a liner within the helmet shell made of an impact-absorbing material such as closed-cell polymeric foam.

## 11.6.2
### Torso Armor: Ballistic

These items are designed to protect the torso from antipersonnel fragments and low or high-energy bullets. The textile garment alone provides protection from the fragments and/ or low-energy bullets. To increase the level of protection to include that from high-energy bullets a rigid insert plate is added.

Figure 11.8 is the UK's Enhanced Combat Body Armor. The rectangular pocket on the front is the location of the rigid ceramic plate, and Fig. 11.9 is the UK's OSPREY Combat Body Armor (CBA) with larger plates and additional loops to integrate with load carriage equipment.

Figure 11.10 is a police body armor that includes low-energy bullet protection in the garment and larger high-energy bullet protective plates. Most bullet-resistant rigid plates will be of the larger size. The small plate in the UK ECBA (shown in Fig. 11.8) is an

**Fig. 11.7** A ballistic helmet designed to defeat low-energy bullets

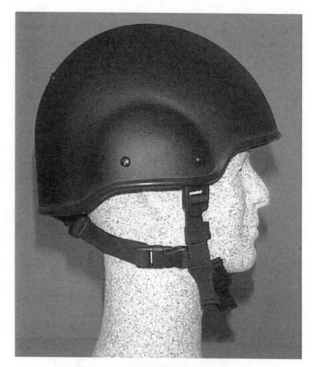

**Fig. 11.8** UK Combat Body Armor principally designed to stop anti-personnel fragments. Note the pocket for inclusion of a plate to defeat high-energy rifle bullets

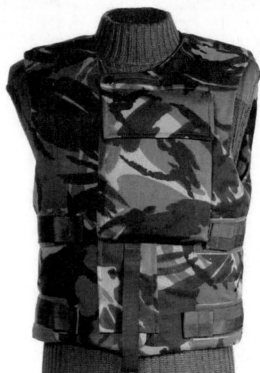

**Fig. 11.9** The UK OSPREY Combat Body Armor

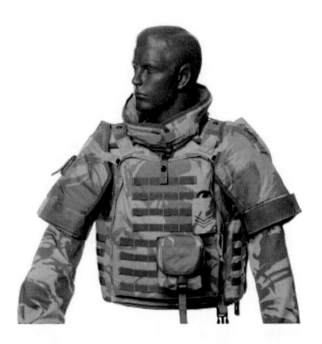

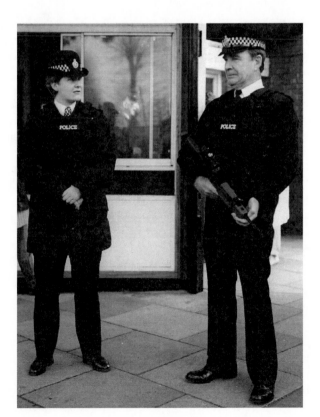

**Fig. 11.10** Police armor – a combination of aramid to defeat low-energy bullets and large plates for high-energy projectiles

**Table 11.3** Comparison of military and police requirements for body armors

| Criteria | Military | Police |
|---|---|---|
| Main threats | Fragmentation<br>High-energy bullets | Stab<br>Low-energy bullets |
| Weight | Low | May be slightly higher when knife protection is included |
| Protection level | Usually a compromise due to other factors | Often has to be complete protection for a specified low-energy bullet threat |
| Specifications | Often designed to meet specific requirements of the user | Usually to a national or international standard |
| Wear time | Could be a very long time or less | Usually for a standard working shift |

exception; it was introduced to keep the weight to an absolute minimum in a theater where rapid medical assistance was available. There are a number of differences between Police and Military Body Armors; these are summarized in Table 11.3.

## 11.6.3
### EOD (Bomb Disposal) Suits

The most extensive ensemble of personal armor is that used by personnel involved in EOD. These operators spend a significant proportion of their time close to large explosive devices that are designed to kill or injure those much further away. Therefore, the requirements for protection are greater than for any other type of user of personal armor. For most users of armor designed to defeat fragment threats, it is assumed that they will not be close enough to the device for any of the associated blast to be an issue (the lethal area for fragments usually considerably exceeds that for blast waves). This is not the case for the EOD operator; he/she is very close to the device and blast overpressure levels will be severe. For this reason an EOD suit should provide protection from both fragmentation and blast. In Figs. 11.11 and 11.12, the area covered by the rigid plate system (on the wearer's front) has blast-protective materials and construction, as well as a very high level of fragmentation protection. The fragmentation protection of the rigid plate may be up to three times that of a CBA. The helmet will be of similar construction to a combat helmet, but of higher performance. The visor should have as high a ballistic performance as the helmet, but it also requires good optical properties.

## 11.6.4
### Torso Armor: Knives

Contrary to expectation, armor that defeats bullets or fragmentation is not necessarily very good at stopping knives or other sharp/edged weapons. Most current knife armors comprise either chain mail backed by ballistic material (Fig. 11.13) or resin impregnated/laminated aramids that combine both knife and ballistic protection.

**Fig. 11.11** 4–9.1. The UK
Mk4 EOD suit (with rigid
plate being removed)

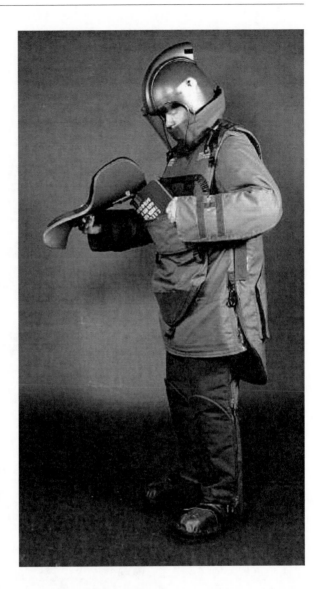

The test standards for knife protection are different to those developed for bullets. Most standards refer to defeating a specific geometry of blade that possesses a specific energy upon impact; in the UK this blade is designed to be representative of the common threat.

In the UK Home Office Standards there are three protection levels, selected dependent upon the risk; an officer on routine patrol will not need the same degree of protection as an officer entering the premises where there is a known knife threat.

Reflecting the various threats, standards refer to energies of 24, 33, and 43 J, with maximum allowable penetrations of 7 mm. Armors are tested to determine compliance by dropping a damped "knife missile" from a drop tower. The damped mass system is designed to replicate a human stab in a repeatable and consistent manner – see Fig. 11.14.

**Fig. 11.12** 4–9.2. The UK
Mk4 (Right) and Mk6 (Left)
EOD suits

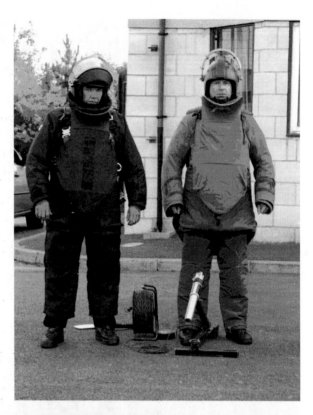

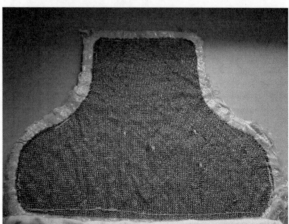

**Fig. 11.13** A representative
knife armor – chain mail
backed with aramid

The UK law-enforcement view on stab armors is that the purpose of the armor is to prevent the officer sustaining "serious or permanent injury"; however, limited knife penetration may occur. Clinicians need to be aware that this penetrating trauma *may* still occur behind knife armors, although the depth of penetration will be reduced significantly

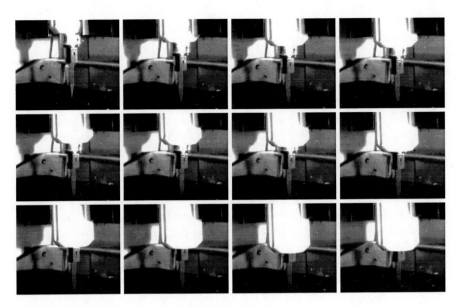

**Fig. 11.14** Knife stab testing using a repeatable dual mass damped drop tube

compared to the unprotected thorax. It is worth noting that, upon post incident inspection of knife-resistant armor (worn by police officers that have been subject to a knife attack), there has been no incidence of knife penetration.

## 11.7
## Medical Issues Associated with Armor Use

### 11.7.1
### Evidence for Reduction in Casualty Numbers

For law-enforcement officers attacked with specific bullets, it is self-evident whether an armor has performed effectively. There is no doubt that thoracic armors save lives.

Gathering evidence that the military use of armor has made a significant benefit in terms of the frequency of KIA; DOW and the Wounded is less clear cut because of confounding factors when comparing casualty rates in different conflicts. The frequency of casualties in these three groups is not determined solely by the threat, the tactical environment and the armor systems deployed. The standard and timeliness of medical care have a significant impact on casualty rates.

In comparing the surgical mortality from thoracic trauma in conflicts in which thoracic armors were not deployed (37% for the US Army in World War I) to those in which they were (10% mortality in Korea), differences can probably be ascribed to developments in cardiovascular trauma management and the use of antibiotics[2] as well as the provision of personal armors. It could also be argued that armors reduce the tempo tactically, and this indirectly may affect the ballistic threat to personnel.

Notwithstanding the caveats raised above, there is evidence that armors make a difference. The percentage wounds (fatal and nonfatal) to the thorax for the US Army in World War II were 13% where thoracic armor was not commonly worn. In Korea, where thoracic armor was worn reasonably routinely, the incidence of thoracic wounds was less – eight percent had fatal or nonfatal thoracic wounds. Carey ascribed the lower-than-predicted incidence of brain wounds sustained by soldiers in a Corps Hospital in Desert Storm to the effectiveness of modern aramid-based helmets and troop discipline in wearing armor.[3] He also noted that brain-injured Iraqi casualties who either wore no helmets or helmets of inferior design and coverage were usually injured over the superior aspect of the cranial vault. For the two US casualties who suffered wounds to the inferior aspect, the projectiles entered the head below the helmet.

In their retrospective review of 125 combat casualties from an urban battle in Somalia, Mabry et al. commented that an important contribution to medical management was the prevention of small fragment wounds to the abdomen. Evidence of penetrating injury invokes the assumption that a perforation of the abdominal wall has occurred and viscera are involved.[1] The armor reduced the requirement for diagnostic procedures and surgical exploration, thereby reducing the medical workload. The battle was dominated by use of AK47 rifles and Rocket Propelled Grenades (RPGs). There was a relatively low rate of penetrating chest wounds, compared to the incidence in Vietnam. Two of the KIA had chest wounds and two had abdominal wounds. In these casualties, the projectiles entered the torso through the soft aramid armor (that is not designed to stop high-energy bullets/fragments). Ceramic plates were not perforated. There were also a number of anecdotal accounts of personnel escaping injury following impact of bullets and fragments on their torso armor.

Burkle et al.[4] undertook a prospective analysis of trauma record data in two military field trauma centers in the Persian Gulf War (1991). The 402 cases were a mixture of US personnel, allies and prisoners of war. Penetrating "shrapnel" (sic) wounds to the chest were observed in 2% of coalition forces but in 15% of "enemy" forces. The disparity in the provision and use of thoracic armor undoubtedly contributed in part to this difference.

## 11.7.2
### Behind Armor Blunt Trauma

Behind-armor blunt trauma (BABT) is the spectrum of non-penetrating injuries to the torso resulting from the impact of projectiles on personal armors. Although the armor may stop the actual penetration of the projectile through the armor, the energy deposited in the armor by the retarded projectile may be transferred through the armor backing and body wall. It may produce serious injury to the thoracic and abdominal contents behind the plate. With very high-energy bullet impacts (such as a 12.7 mm bullet striking a boron carbide plate), the non-penetrating thoracic injuries may result in death.

The existence of BABT as a clinical entity was reported first in the late 1970s amongst police officers wearing flexible body armor struck with handgun bullets. Behind-armor blunt trauma may occur behind flexible textile-based armors and also behind rigid armors principally constructed from ceramic materials.

Behind-armor blunt trauma has been identified as an emerging problem that has implications for the designers of personal armor systems, the operational performance of soldiers and law-enforcement officers, and for the medical management of casualties. There are two principal reasons for its growing prominence:

1. An increase in the caliber and available energy of bullets that may be used in peace-keeping, urban-violence, and other operational scenarios.
2. The desire of the designers of personal armor systems to reduce the weight and thickness of soft armors and armor plates – a strategy that plainly will buy benefit in terms of the burden on personnel, but will exacerbate the problem of dissipating the energy in the armor system. Armors are designed to absorb energy, but the rapid deformations of the armors may result in a greater proportion of the energy of the retarded projectile being propagated into the body.

The earliest case report of the lethal indirect effect of a high-energy round was described in 1969 – the case of a US Army sergeant shot accidentally with an M-16 bullet at close range during the Vietnam War. There was no description of "rigid" body armor or other retardation, but the round did not penetrate the pleural cavity. After a short period of respiratory and haemodynamic stability, the soldier rapidly deteriorated and died within 45 min of admission. Massive pulmonary contusions were seen at post-mortem.

In a civilian setting, Carroll and Soderstrom[5] described five cases of BABT in police officers wearing Kevlar soft-body armor struck by handgun bullets. All survived with no significant cardio-respiratory sequelae.

One of the few accurately documented examples of severe but survivable BABT was presented as recently as 1995[6]. A humanitarian aid worker in Sarajevo was struck by a Soviet 14.5 mm bullet (at unknown range) while wearing "complete" body armor. Apart from skin and muscle damage, his cardio-respiratory status was stable. A chest radiograph revealed no rib fractures and a small haemothorax, which was managed with a chest drain. A subsequent radiograph on the same day revealed a developing pulmonary contusion corresponding to the site of impact. The patient made an uneventful recovery.

The important issue with BABT is that historically it has been associated largely with the defeat of low-energy bullets (such as from handguns) by flexible textile armor systems, however the designs have now matured to reduce the significance of this problem. BABT is now emerging as a significant military problem, particularly behind rigid armor plates designed to defeat high-energy bullets. As a result, many military armor manufacturers offer "trauma attenuating backings" (TABs) to reduce these injuries behind hard armors. It is also plain that the higher-energy threats used in modern times in urban law enforcement render it a problem in the civilian medical scenario.

Behind-armor blunt trauma is caused by the deformation of the rear surface of the armor (plate or textile) occurring as a result of the dissipation of the energy of the retarded bullet. This deformation has a number of biophysical sequelae that are dependent upon its rate (peak velocity) and gross dynamic deformation

- The strike of a bullet on the armor plate generates a short duration stress (pressure) wave that is coupled into the body.
- The rear of the plate then deforms locally at high velocity towards the body and accelerates the body wall – this also generates a stress wave.

- The deflection of the body wall under the armor applies local shear to the wall (e.g., rib) and shear is transferred to underlying tissues—thoracic and abdominal viscera.
- The plate as a whole moves and results in a distributed load to the body, leading to additional torso wall displacement.

Thus, the pathology observed is a combination of stress-wave–induced trauma and shear resulting in local damage to the body wall and viscera. The incidence and severity is dependent upon the energy of the impact and the characteristics of the armor (and TAB, if present). These factors determine the peak velocity and maximum gross deflection of the body wall. The pathology is the commonly observed pattern of non-penetrating trauma from high-energy localized impacts: rib fracture, pulmonary contusion, pulmonary laceration, cardiac contusion, hepatic trauma, and bowel contusion.

Trauma is generally localized to the contact area and underlying tissues (see Fig. 11.15), but the generation of stress waves in the retardation process of high-energy bullets against plates may lead to more widespread pulmonary trauma, similar to that observed in casualties exposed to blast waves – "blast lung."

Law-enforcement agencies publish standards for body armor that are designed to limit the severity of BABT. Manufacturers of armor systems have to demonstrate compliance of their products with these standards. Test procedures are a compromise between fidelity to the biophysical processes of BABT and a test regimen that does not require enormous investment and specialized knowledge from manufacturers. Current standards in the UK are based on the maximum back-face deformation of armor, determined by indentation of Roma Plastilina®. Police armor is assigned to five threat groups ranging from lightweight flexible armor intended for use by unarmed officers in very low-risk patrolling duties (HG1/A – this armor may be used covertly or overtly), to armor designed to stop rifle ammunition and shotguns at close range. The maximum deformation permitted in the Plastilina backing material is 44 mm for the HG1/A group and 25 mm for the more severe threat groups. Similar standards are used in the US.

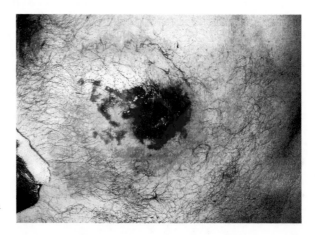

**Fig. 11.15** Typical 9 mm Behind Armor Blunt Trauma through a soft textile armor

NATO has reviewed the threat from BABT in military operations and concluded from the available knowledge that for military rifle bullets:

- The BABT injury potential of defeated very high-energy bullets (i.e., 12.7 mm caliber) is significant.
- That of 7.62 mm bullets is largely dependent on the rigid plate armor design.
- There is no evidence of significant BABT injury from 5.56 mm military bullets.

The energy transferred from armor may be absorbed, dissipated, or redistributed using the TABs placed between the armor system and the body. These TABs vary in design depending on the threat to be countered – in the most extreme example of attenuating the energy transfer of a retarded 12.7 mm bullet, the TABs are constructed from a stiff-foamed polymer of substantial thickness. On the basis of the NATO assessment, the focus for attenuating BABT has been for the 12.7 mm and more severe 7.62 mm threats. For low-energy handgun bullets striking textile armors and 5.56 mm bullets striking rigid plates, the risk of life-threatening injury is very low. Nevertheless, BABT may be present and the physician is advised to recognize the potential for pulmonary, cardiac, and hepatic trauma (dependent upon impact site), even in the absence of a defect on the skin.

## 11.7.3
### Removal of Armor

The removal of clothing for the survey of a casualty is compounded by the presence of body armor and the supine posture. Aramids such as Kevlar cannot be cut with the type of implements normally found in medical facilities. Most thoracic armors open at the front, side, or over the shoulder (or a combination of these) and are sleeveless (although some modular systems provide shoulder and upper arm protection but these are usually detatchable). The armors must be designed to be removed with relative ease.

Medical teams should develop drills to remove armor systems. The particular pattern of armor worn by the law-enforcement or military population they serve will be defined and teams need to familiarize themselves with the nature of the protective equipment issued operationally.[6]

Removal of EOD suits is very problematic as there may be no frontal and side openings (to maintain integrity of the suit when subjected to severe blast, the opening may be at the rear) and the legs and arms will be heavily armored with aramid. The lower-limb armor may be in the form of a salopette, which can be removed relatively easily, but the presence of bulky, relatively tight-fitting sleeves on the upper jacket will make removal with spinal immobilization very difficult. Some suits, such as the UK Mk4 and Mk6, have the aramid seams marked to facilitate emergency removal.

It is difficult to offer specific advice on removal because the designs of suits vary, but the general principles are

- It is futile to try and cut the aramid (unless cutters specifically designed to cut multi-layer aramid are available).
- There is little point in searching for *covert* seams – the designers try to ensure that there are none – so utilize marked seams (if any).

- If time permits, the manufacturers should be able to advise on the removal.
- Undertake a rapid survey of the design of the armor (seeking "Velcro" straps and zips that most likely are to be out of sight for EOD suits) and develop a strategy for its removal. Rolling of the casualty during the primary survey may be inevitable in order to gain access to initiate resuscitation and to effect removal of the arms from sleeves for the secondary survey.

There may be either clinical or tactical requirements in the military to assess casualties who are still wearing body armor. Harcke et al.[7] used plain film and computed tomography of simulated casualties clothed with aramid helmet, torso armor (plate and aramid textile), and demining suit sleeve. Helmets may contain metal components. They concluded that if conditions so dictate, patients wearing military-pattern personal armor can be satisfactorily examined radiographically through the armor systems. This conclusion also is undoubtedly applicable to civilian medical staff dealing with armor systems used by law-enforcement officers.

## 11.7.4
## Perforation of Armor by Bullets

Textile armors will not stop high-energy bullets. If the textile armor is defeated by a bullet, will the presence of the armor exacerbate the trauma? The ballistic basis for this potential problem is that as a result of its passage through the textile, the bullet may be influenced thus:

- Deformation or break-up.
- Induction of yaw (the deviation of the axis of the body of the bullet from its line of flight).
- Instability arising from a reduction in the balance of angular velocity (spin) and longitudinal velocity.

Each of these factors could lead to an increase in the total energy transferred to a target and changes in the distribution of energy along the track.

The scientific evidence is limited and equivocal. The characteristics of the bullet range, strike angle, armor construction, and thickness will all influence the effect that the armor has on the bullet during its passage and it is inappropriate to offer generalized statements. Knudsen[8] demonstrated instability of 7.62 mm AK-47 bullets after passage through soft aramid comprising 28 plies. The yaw induction was also dependent upon strike angle. The consequences of the yaw induction upon a tissue-simulant target behind the armor were not investigated, but intuitively the temporary cavity in tissue would be more proximal and energy transfer would be greater. It is difficult to judge the overall clinical consequences. More recently, experiments in the UK have indicated *increased* stability of 5.45 mm and 5.56 mm bullets after passage through aramid. The temporary cavity volumes were reduced in soap behind the armor when compared to shots into soap with no armor.[9]

This issue requires more research to determine clinical impact, but it is unlikely that torso wounds will be unequivocally significantly increased in *clinical* severity by the passage of a high-energy bullet through textile armor.

If a high-energy bullet defeats ceramic armor, the effects on a soft target behind the plate will be dependent upon how overmatched the bullet is to the armor. If only just over-matched, the steel core of the bullet may emerge from the back face of the armor and enter the body with relatively low energy – the jacket and lead components may be captured in the plate. At the other extreme, multiple bullet fragments arising from erosion of the bullet by the ceramic and pieces of the ceramic armor may perforate the composite backing of the plate to result in gross, but relatively superficial high-energy transfer wounds.

**Acknowledgments**   Graham Smith and John Croft of the Police Scientific Development Branch, Sandridge, UK provided information on knife armors.

## References

1. Mabry RL, Holcomb JB, Baker AM, et al. United States Army rangers in Somalia: an analysis of combat casualties on an urban battlefield. *J Trauma*. 2000;49:515-528.
2. Carey ME. An analysis of US Army combat mortality and morbidity data. *J Trauma*. 1988;28(suppl):S515-S528.
3. Carey ME. Analysis of wounds incurred by US Army Seventh Corps personnel treated in corps hospitals during operation desert Storm, February 20 to March 10, 1991. *J Trauma*. 1996;40(suppl):S165-S169.
4. Burkle FM, Newland C, Meister SJ, Blood CG. Emergency medicine in the Persian Gulf War – Part 3: Battlefield casualties. *Ann Emerg Med*. 1994;23:755-760.
5. Carroll AW, Soderstrom CA. A new non-penetrating ballistic injury. *Ann Surg*. 1978;188: 735-737.
6. Ryan JM, Bailie R, Diack G, Kierle J, Williams T. Safe removal of combat body armor light-weight following battlefield wounding – a timely reminder. *J R Army Med Corps*. 1994;140: 26-28.
7. Harcke T, Schauer DA, Harris RM, Campman SC, Lonergan G. Imaging body armor. *Mil Med*. 2002;167:267-271.
8. Knudsen PJT, Sorensen OH. The destabilising effect of body armour on military rifle bullets. *Int J Legal Med*. 1997;110:82-87.
9. Lanthier J-M. *The Effects of Soft Textile Body Armour on the Wound Ballistics of High Velocity Military Bullets* [MSc Thesis]. Shrivenham, Wiltshire, UK: Cranfield University College of Defence Technology; 2003.

## Further Reading

Abbott TA, Shephard RG. Protection against penetrating injury. In: Cooper GJ, Dudley HAF, Gann S, Gann DS, Little RA, Maynard RL, eds. *Scientific Foundations of Trauma*. Oxford: Butterworth Heinemann; 1997:83-100.
Cannon L. Behind armour blunt trauma – an emerging problem. *J R Army Med Corps*. 2001;147: 87-96.

# Forensic Aspects of Ballistic Injury

# 12

Jeanine Vellema and Hendrik Scholtz

Clinical forensic medicine is best defined as the application of forensic medical knowledge and techniques to the solution of law in the investigation of trauma involving living victims.[1-5] In the setting of emergency departments, these techniques include the correct forensic evaluation, documentation, and photography of traumatic injuries, as well as the recognition and proper handling of evidentiary material for future use in legal proceedings.[1-8]

While the tasks of documenting, gathering, and preserving evidence traditionally have been considered to be the responsibility of the forensic pathologist or the police, the roles of the trauma physician and forensic investigators actually have several areas of complementary interest. These arise from the dual purposes of providing immediate care for the individual victim or patient and the longer-term reduction and prevention of injury and violence in the community as a whole.[6,9]

Appropriate documentation and handling of evidence by trauma personnel assist the forensic pathologist in evaluating cases of initially non-fatal traumatic deaths and assist the police and legal authorities responsible for investigating both civil and criminal cases in deceased and surviving injured patients.[6]

In addition, emergency physicians could play an important role in informing police about patients presenting to them with non-fatal forensic-related problems such as gunshot wounds. In these instances, consent to report must be obtained from the patient so as not to breach physician–patient confidentiality. Patients should be advised that it is in their interest, as well as the interest of the wider community, to report offenses, but it remains the patients' decision whether such offenses are reported.[9,10]

In September 2003, the General Medical Council (GMC) in the UK published "Reporting Gun Shot Wounds. Guidance for Doctors in Accident and Emergency Departments." The guidelines were developed with the Association of Chief Police

J. Vellema (✉)
Division of Forensic Medicine, School of Pathology, University of the Witwatersrand, Johannesburg, South Africa
e-mail: vellema@telkomsa.net

A.J. Brooks et al. (eds.), *Ryan's Ballistic Trauma*,
DOI: 10.1007/978-1-84882-124-8_12, © Springer-Verlag London Limited 2011

Officers and supported by the College of Emergency Medicine. In essence, the guidance is that the police should be informed whenever a person has arrived at a hospital with a gunshot wound, but initially identifying details such as the patient's name and address usually should not be disclosed. The treatment and care of the patient remains the doctor's first concern. If the patient's treatment and condition allow them to speak to the police, then they should be asked if they are willing to do so. If they refuse or cannot consent, then information still may be disclosed if it is believed this is in the public interest or is required by law. The patient should be informed of the disclosure and an appropriate record made in their notes. Copies of the guidelines can be obtained from the GMC.

Thus, while the main priority of trauma physicians always will be to provide timely and optimal care for the individual living patient, they also could serve society in general by applying some forensic principles in their approach to patients who are victims of violence.[5-8]

## 12.1
## The Forensic Evaluation

In a firearm-related injury, the direction that a bullet travels through a body may have little relevance in a patient's clinical management, but it usually has profound medico-legal implications. The appearance of a gunshot wound may not only indicate the bullet's direction and trajectory, but also the type of ammunition and weapon used and the range of gunfire. Additionally, it may assist with the manner of gunshot injury or death with respect to it being accidental, homicidal, or suicidal in nature.[2,11]

Proper forensic evaluation of patients in the clinical environment is often neglected in the hurried setting of a resuscitation.[6-12] Such an evaluation should be documented comprehensively and should include a history and physical examination with accurate descriptions of wound characteristics supplemented by diagrams or line drawings.[3-8,13] Use of a proforma, which includes a simple diagram, has been shown to improve the quality of documentation.[14-17]

Ideally, photographs should be taken whenever possible. However, consent must be obtained first from patients for photography, unless they are unconscious. The consent form must become a permanent part of the patient's medical records. In unconscious patients, "implied consent" is the legal construct used to secure consent when the photographs may aid in the subsequent conviction of those individuals who perpetrated a crime. If implied consent was used, the physician later must obtain consent from either the patient or next of kin.[3]

In addition to the above documentation, recognizing, collecting, and preserving physical evidence while maintaining a "chain of custody" is another important responsibility of trauma personnel; this will be dealt with comprehensively later in this chapter.[1-8,12-16]

## 12.2
## Documentation of Gunshot Wounds

Emergency physicians are ideally positioned to describe and document gunshot-wound appearances before such wounds are altered by surgical intervention or the healing process.[3,17]

The interpretation of gunshot wounds with respect to "entrance and exit," direction of fire, or type of firearm or ammunition used need not be commented on. Clinicians should confine themselves to recording accurately the location, size, and shape of all wounds, as well as any unusual marks or coloration associated with these wounds. Surgical procedures such as drain sites must also be recorded to prevent subsequent interpretive difficulties for the forensic pathologist, should the patient die.[17-21]

Differentiation between entrance and exit wounds can be difficult, and information from patients or witnesses may be false or inaccurate. In a study of 271 gunshot-wound fatalities, it was found that trauma specialists had misclassified 37% of single exiting gunshot wounds with respect to entrance or exit wounds and 73.6% of multiple gunshot wounds had been misinterpreted with respect to total number of wounds, as well as erroneous identification of entrance or exit wounds.[17]

If descriptive documentation is accurate, acknowledged experts in forensic wound ballistics can use these descriptions to make the necessary forensic interpretations pertaining to direction and range of gunfire, as well as type of weapon and ammunition used.[17-22]

An emergency physician may be called upon by the courts to give evidence regarding injuries sustained by a gunshot victim and, in nonfatal gunshot victims, may be the only person who can testify as a witness of fact to the original appearances of the gunshot wounds.

An expert witness is someone who, because of training and depth of experience, may be asked to give an opinion based on the observation of others, as opposed to merely testifying as to the facts of the case.[12]

Thus, a trauma surgeon may be called as a "factual" witness regarding the wound(s) appearances, but may also be called as an expert witness regarding the severity or lethality of a wound. The expert forensic ballistics witnesses may be asked to interpret the documented factual findings in a gunshot-wound victim and define the wound descriptions as entrance or exit, as well as give an expert opinion as to range and direction of fire, type of firearm, and ammunition used.[12]

The quality of both factual and expert testimony will depend on the accuracy of the original clinical documentation, which in turn may influence the outcome of the court case.[1-8,15-22]

## 12.3
## Forensic Concepts

Accurate descriptions of gunshot wounds require a basic understanding of firearms, ammunition, and wound ballistics, as well as the relevant forensic terminology.[2,3] Ballistics is defined as the science of motion of projectiles and can be divided into interior ballistics, the study of the projectile in the gun; external ballistics, the study of the projectile moving through the air; and terminal ballistics, the study of the effects the projectile causes when hitting a target, as well as the counter effects produced on the projectile.

Wound ballistics is considered a subdivision of terminal ballistics, which concerns itself with the motions and effects of a projectile in tissue.[23-25]

Chapters 4 and 5 dealt with firearms and ammunition. Only a brief summary of some pertinent forensic issues pertaining to the above will be given here.

### 12.3.1
### Forensic Aspects of Firearms and Ammunition

When a firearm is discharged, the primer is crushed and ignited by the firing pin producing an intense flame, which ignites the propellant gunpowder in the cartridge case. The rapidly burning gunpowder results in the formation of relatively large volumes of very hot gas within the cartridge case, and the pressure of these gases on the base of the projectile result in the projectile being forced out of the cartridge and propelled through the barrel of the firearm.

As a consequence of these events, the ejected projectile is accompanied by a jet of flame, hot compressed carbon monoxide-rich gases, soot, propellant particles, primer residue, metallic particles stripped from the projectile, and vaporized metal from the projectile and cartridge case.[23-32]

In revolvers, similar substances may emerge from the cylinder-barrel gap, the amount of which will depend on the manufacture, quality, and age of the weapon.[23] These residues are most commonly referred to as gunshot residue (GSR), but the terms cartridge-discharge residue (CDR) or firearm-discharge residue (FDR) also are used.[32]

Additional components that may be expelled and deposited on a bullet when a firearm is discharged are the elements fouling the barrel of a firearm. These could include rust particles, lubricating oil, dirt, and even biological material resulting from blowback of blood and tissue into the barrel of the weapon, as sometimes happens in hard-contact entrance wounds.[23,24,27-31]

This has forensic relevance in that:

1. in addition to the ejected bullet, the residual materials resulting from the discharge of a firearm may impart specific characteristics to the appearances of gunshot entrance wounds depending on the range and angle of discharge of a firearm, the type of firearm, and type of ammunition used;[23-31]
2. the description, detection, and identification of expelled residual materials may provide valuable investigative information, allowing for scientific range estimates, identification of the ammunition or firearm(s) used, and thus identification of the assailant(s).[23,24,32]

It is of major clinico-forensic importance for trauma personnel to recognize that in addition to the bullet and its cartridge case, all of the above barrel emissions constitute potential evidentiary material that may be deposited in and on the clothing, hair, body, and wounds of a gunshot-wound victim, or even an assailant. By being aware of the presence and value of gunshot-related evidence, such evidence may be identified, collected, and preserved rather than inadvertently being destroyed.[1-8,13-16]

### 12.3.2
### Forensic Aspects of Wound Ballistics

Penetrating projectiles can be classified broadly into two major groups, namely fragments and bullets. Fragments from military munitions are the most common wounding agents in war, although fragmentation injuries also may occur following civilian terrorist bombings. Bullets are the predominant penetrating missiles in civilian clinical practice.[33]

Weapons originally designed for military use are also used frequently in civilian settings, leading to blurring of the distinction between military wounds arising from high-velocity rifles and fragments and civilian wounds arising from handguns with lower muzzle velocities.[34]

There are three mechanisms whereby a projectile can cause tissue injury:

1. In a low-energy transfer wound, the projectile crushes and lacerates tissue along the track of the projectile, causing a *permanent cavity*. In addition, bullet and bone fragments can act as secondary missiles, increasing the volume of tissue crushed.[15,23-42]
2. In a high-energy transfer wound, the projectile may impel the walls of the wound track radially outwards, causing a *temporary cavity* lasting 5–10 ms before its collapse, in addition to the permanent mechanical disruption directly produced in (1) (Fig. 12.1).[23-31,33,34,38-42]
3. In wounds where the firearm's muzzle is in contact with the skin at the time of firing, tissues are forced aside by the gases expelled from the barrel of the firearm, causing a localized *blast injury* (Fig. 12.2).[15,38]

Several misconceptions exist about the wounding effects of high-velocity projectiles, particularly when their kinetic energy (as determined by muzzle or impact velocity alone) is presumed to be the sole determinant in size of temporary cavity formation.[33,34,38-43]

The severity and size of a gunshot wound is related directly to the total amount of *kinetic energy transfer* to the tissues, not merely the total amount of kinetic energy possessed by

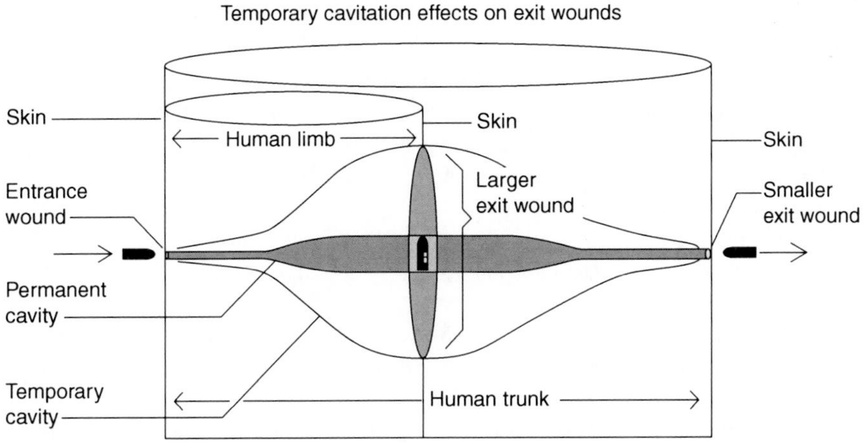

**Fig. 12.1** Schematic profile of the variable sizes of exit wounds caused by the same projectile, as influenced by the diameter of the temporary cavity at the point of exit. The narrow column represents the diameter of a limb and the wider column, the diameter of a trunk

**Fig. 12.2** Contact gunshot wound of the head showing compressed gases expanding between the scalp and the outer table of the skull, with soot deposition in the subcutaneous tissues and on the bone

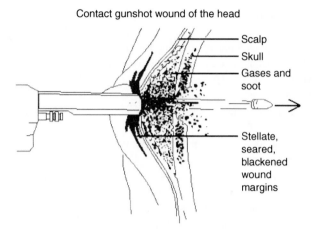

Contact gunshot wound of the head

- Scalp
- Skull
- Gases and soot
- Stellate, seared, blackened wound margins

the projectile. Kinetic energy transfer is proportional to the degree of retardation of the projectile in the tissue, which in turn is determined by four main factors[23,33,34,38-43]:

1. The amount of kinetic energy (KE) possessed by the bullet at the time of the impact, which is dependent on the velocity and mass of the bullet ($KE = \frac{1}{2}mv^2$).[23-25,33]
2. The angle of yaw of a bullet at the time of impact, which in turn is dependent on the physical characteristics of the bullet (its length, diameter, and density), the rate of twist imparted by the barrel, and the density of the air. The greater the angle of yaw when a bullet strikes a body, the greater the retardation of the bullet and consequently the greater the amount of kinetic energy transfer. This explains why unstable projectiles in flight cause larger entrance wounds on impact with the body. Once the bullet enters the denser medium of tissue, its yaw angle increases progressively until the bullet becomes completely unstable, tumbles and rotates by 180°, and ends up traveling base forward. Tumbling of the bullet in tissue increases the presented cross-sectional area of the bullet, resulting in more direct tissue destruction and increased retarding (drag) forces, with consequently greater kinetic energy transfer and larger temporary cavity formation. The sudden increase of the drag force also puts strain on the bullet, which may lead to the break up of the bullet and more tissue destruction.[23]
3. The caliber, construction, and configuration of a bullet also influence the amount of kinetic energy transfer to tissue[23]:
   - Blunt-nose bullets and expanding bullets designed to mushroom in tissues are retarded more than streamlined bullets, resulting in more kinetic energy transfer to the tissue.
   - The caliber and shape (bluntness of the nose) of a bullet determine the initial presented cross-sectional area of the bullet and thus the drag of the bullet, but are of less importance when bullet deformity occurs.
   - Deformation of a bullet depends on both the construction of the bullet and the bullet velocity.
   - Construction of a bullet refers to the jacket, the length, thickness, and hardness of the jacket material, the hardness of the lead in the bullet core, and the presence or absence of special features, such as a hollow point.

- Soft- and hollow-point rifle bullets expand and may shed lead fragments from the core, irrespective of whether they strike bone, resulting in a lead snowstorm image as visualized on X-ray. This fragmenting phenomenon appears to be related to velocity and does not happen with handgun bullets unless they strike bone. The lead fragments in turn act as secondary missiles increasing the size of the wound cavity.
- A full metal-jacketed rifle bullet also may break up in the body without striking bone because of its velocity and tendency to yaw radically. As stated earlier, the significant yaw results in a sudden increase in the drag force, straining the structure of the bullet and resulting in break up of the bullet.

4. The fourth factor influencing kinetic energy transfer is the density, strength, and elasticity of the tissue penetrated by the bullet and the length of the wound track. The denser the tissue, the greater the angle of yaw and consequently the greater the degree of retardation and kinetic energy transfer.[23]

Thus, while the *capacity* of a projectile to cause tissue damage is defined traditionally by its available kinetic energy, the muzzle velocity of a firearm and the impact velocity of a projectile can be misleading indicators of their potential for injury when the *kinetic energy transfer variables* are ignored.[3,33,43]

Temporary cavitation is merely a transient displacement or stretching of tissue where the size of the cavity is determined by the characteristics of the tissue and the amount of energy transferred. The damage and external wound appearances caused by a temporary cavity can vary greatly depending on its size and anatomic location (see Fig. 12.1). Tissues containing a large amount of elastic fibers, such as lung, muscle, or bowel, can withstand some mechanical displacement without significant damage, but denser tissues with few elastic fibers, such as liver and spleen, and encased tissues, such as the brain, may be lacerated severely.

While considered rare, temporary cavitation may cause vascular disruption and bone fractures distant to the permanent wound track.[33,39,40]

## 12.4
## Forensic Terminology and Gunshot Wound Appearances

Gunshot wounds may be either *penetrating* or *perforating*. The term *penetrating* wound is used when a bullet enters the body or a structure, but does not exit. The term *perforating* wound is used when a bullet passes completely through the body or a structure.[23]

### 12.4.1
### Entrance Wounds

Range of fire is the distance from the muzzle to the victim and can be divided into four broad categories: contact, near-contact or close-range, intermediate-range, and distant-range. Each category has specific identifying features that are imparted both by the bullet and the various emissions accompanying the bullet from the muzzle of a firearm.[3,23,24]

The presence of clothing or hair acting as intermediary barriers may obscure the typical wound characteristics of contact, close-range, and intermediate-range wounds. It is of great forensic importance that the integrity of such intermediary barriers be maintained and such items preserved as evidentiary material.

Other intermediary targets such as doors or windows also may influence the appearances of entrance wounds as discussed under the heading, "Atypical Entrance Wounds."[23,24]

It must be noted that the size of an entrance wound is a poor indicator of the caliber of the wounding bullet because of variations in anatomic anchoring and elasticity of skin.[23]

## 12.5
## Contact Wounds

In contact wounds, the muzzle of the firearm is held in contact with the victim's body or clothing at the time of discharge. Contact wounds may be subdivided further into hard-contact, loose-contact, and incomplete- or angled-contact wounds. In the latter, the complete circumference of the muzzle is not in contact with the body.[3,23,24]

In hard-contact wounds, the muzzle is pressed firmly against the body. All the muzzle emissions accompanying the bullet – the flame, the hot gases, the soot, the propellant particles, the primer residue, and metal particles – are forced into the wound (see Fig. 12.2). The wound appearance can vary from a small perforation with searing and blackening of the wound edges caused by the hot gases and flame, to a large, gaping stellate wound, with soot visible within and around the wound, and searing of the wound edges from hot gases and flame.[23,24]

The large wounds occur over areas where only a thin layer of skin overlies bone, such as the head. On discharge of the firearm, the compressed gases injected between the skin and the skull expand to such an extent that the skin stretches and tears. These tears radiate from the center, resulting in a large stellate or cruciform entrance wound with blackened, seared wound tissues and margins.[3,23](Fig. 12.3a, b). The inner wound tissues may appear cherry pink due to the carbon monoxide in the gases.[23]

Stellate lacerated wound appearances are not only found in hard-contact entrance wounds, but also may be found in tangential, ricochet, or tumbling bullet entrance wounds, as well as some exit wounds. However, in these wounds, soot and propellant will not be present within and around the wound, and the wound margins will not be seared.[3,23,24]

In some hard-contact wounds, the gases expanding in the subcutaneous tissues may slam the stretched skin against the muzzle of the firearm with enough force to leave behind a muzzle-imprint abrasion or contusion on the skin (Fig. 12.4). Patterns like these may be helpful in determining the type of firearm used and should be described, documented, and ideally photographed before wound alteration by debridement, surgery, or healing.[3,23,24]

In both loose-contact and incomplete- or angled-contact wounds, soot and other gunshot residues are present within and around the wound. Soot, which is carbon, is produced

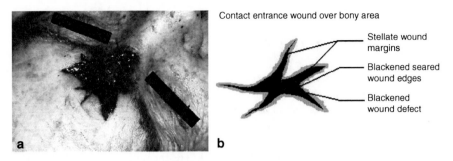

Contact entrance wound over bony area

Stellate wound margins

Blackened seared wound edges

Blackened wound defect

**Fig. 12.3** (**a, b**) Contact gunshot wound of the forehead showing a large, stellate, lacerated wound with soot blackening visible within the wound and on the wound margins

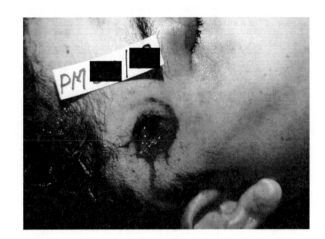

**Fig. 12.4** Hard-contact gunshot wound of the temple, with a partial muzzle-imprint abrasion around the soot-blackened wound

by the combustion of propellant and imparts a black color to the areas where it is deposited. In addition, flame and hot gas emissions result in searing of the skin around the wound. Scattered grains of propellant may accompany the jet of gas and be deposited in the seared and blackened zones of skin. The angle between the muzzle and the skin will determine the soot and searing pattern.[3,23]

In a perpendicular loose- or incomplete-contact wound, the distance between the muzzle and the skin is too small for propellant particles to disperse and mark the skin; the resultant wound appearance is that of a round central defect surrounded by a zone of soot overlying seared skin.[23,24] In an angled loose- or incomplete-contact wound, the zone of searing and soot deposition around the wound is elongated in shape. A fan-shaped pattern of powder tattooing resulting from propellant grains skimming over the seared skin may be observed at the distal end of the entrance wound. This pattern can indicate the direction in which the gun was angled.[23]

## 12.6
## Close-Range or Near-Contact Wounds

There is considerable overlap between the appearance of close-range and loose-contact wounds, making it difficult to differentiate the two. Both have an entrance defect with a surrounding zone of seared, soot-blackened skin. Close-range can be defined as the maximum range at which soot is deposited on the wound or the clothing, usually with a muzzle-to-target distance of up to 30 cm in handguns.

Because some of the soot can be washed away, its presence and configuration should be described accurately and documented, and photographed if possible, prior to cleansing or surgical debridement (Fig. 12.5). Cleaning a wound with a spray of hot water or pouring hydrogen peroxide on wounds caked with clotted blood should wash away or dissolve the blood but preserve the soot pattern. Propellant particles may be deposited in the seared zone surrounding the wound defect, but tattooing from the dispersal of propellant generally is not seen.[23]

## 12.7
## Intermediate Range Wounds

The hallmark of intermediate-range wounds is the phenomenon of so-called powder tattooing. This tattooing consists of numerous reddish-brown punctate abrasions surrounding the entrance wound, caused by unburned and partially burned propellant particles impacting against the skin (Fig. 12.6). Tattooing may be observed in wound-to-muzzle distances between 1 cm and 1 m, but generally is found at distances of less than 60 cm in handguns. The lesions of tattooing are actual small abrasions and thus cannot be washed off.[3,23,24,28,29]

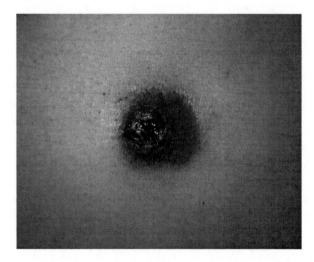

**Fig. 12.5** Slightly angled near-contact wound with the wider zone of soot-blackened skin on the same side as the muzzle of the weapon, i.e., pointing towards the weapon

**Fig. 12.6** Powder tattooing around an intermediate-range gunshot entrance wound

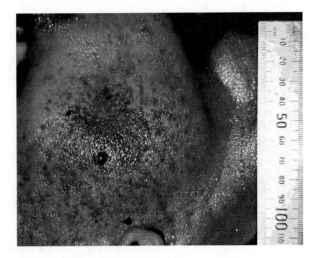

With respect to searing, soot deposition, and powder tattooing, the following must be noted[23]:

- The zone size, concentration, and pattern of both soot deposition and powder tattooing depend on the muzzle-to-target distance and angle, the type of propellant powder and ammunition, the barrel length, and the caliber and type of weapon.
- Accurate documentation and photography of patterns of skin searing, soot deposition, and powder tattooing accompanied by simple line drawings will allow for comparative test-firing studies to give more accurate range-of-fire estimates.
- Test firing is conducted at forensic ballistic laboratories where the offending weapon is fired at a target from different ranges using similar ammunition to that which caused the wound. The target appearances then are compared with those of the wound and the range determined.
- Intermediary barriers such as hair or clothing may obscure or prevent skin searing, soot deposition, or powder tattooing from occurring (Fig. 12.7). At close and intermediate ranges, ball powder may perforate 1–2 layers of cloth to produce powder tattooing, but flake powder usually does not even perforate one layer of cloth. Clothing also may result in redistribution of soot and powder patterns among the layers of clothing or on the skin in a hard-contact wound, altering the wound appearance to that of a loose-contact wound. It also may absorb completely the soot of a close-range wound, altering its appearance to mimic that of a distant-range wound.
- The correct handling of the clothing of gunshot-wound victims as evidentiary material will allow for further forensic investigations pertaining to range, direction, and firearm or ammunition identification to be conducted on such items.
- Microscopic examination and elemental analyses could be performed on excised gunshot wounds to assist with range, as well as entrance versus exit wound determinations.[23,30,37]

**Fig. 12.7** Soot deposition on clothing in a close-range firearm discharge

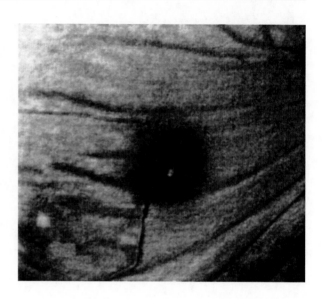

## 12.8
## Distant-Range Wounds

In distant-range entrance wounds, the only marks left on the body are produced by the mechanical action of the bullet perforating the skin. There is no searing, soot deposition, or tattooing associated with the skin defect.[23]

Regardless of range, most entrance wounds have a zone of abraded epidermis surrounding the entrance hole, which is called an "abrasion ring" or "abrasion collar." This abrasion ring traditionally is considered to be caused by friction between the bullet and the epithelium, which occurs as the bullet indents and perforates the skin[23,24,27-31] In a recent study utilizing high-speed photography and the "skin–skull–brain model," it was postulated that the abrasion ring is due to the massive temporary overstretching of the skin adjacent to the bullet perforation.[35] The abrasion ring is due neither to the bullet's rotational movement nor to thermal effects of the bullet on the skin (Fig. 12.8). The width of an abrasion ring varies with the caliber of the firearm, the angle of bullet entry, and the anatomic location. The abrasion ring may be concentric or eccentric, depending on the angle between the bullet and the skin (see Fig. 12.8a).

Distant-range entrance wounds of the palms, soles, and elbows do not have abrasion rings and appear stellate or slit-like due to the thickness and rigidity of the skin in those regions. Some high-velocity distant entrance wounds may have no abrasion ring and may show small "micro-tears" radiating outwards from the edges of the perforation, which may be visualized with a dissecting microscope.[23]

Most distant-range entrance wounds are oval to circular with a punched-out, clean appearance to the margins, totally unlike those of exit wounds.[23] A contusion ring may also be present around the wound defect due to damaged blood vessels in the dermis.[35] However, distant entrance wounds over bony surfaces may have stellate or irregular appearances.[23,24]

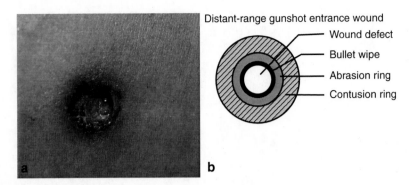

**Fig. 12.8 (a, b)** Slightly angled distant-range gunshot entrance wound with punched-out neat wound margins. A slightly eccentric abrasion ring and narrow contusion ring are present around the wound defect

Distant-range wounds may have a gray coloration to the abrasion ring, which is called bullet wipe. This occurs when powder residue, soot, gun oil, or dirt deposited on the bullet surface as it moves down the barrel is rubbed off the bullet by the skin as the bullet penetrates the body. Bullet wipe is commonly observed in clothing overlying entrance wounds and is also referred to as a grease ring[23,24,27,28,35] (see Fig. 12.8b).

It is not possible to determine an exact range of fire in distant-range entrance wounds. Here, only the ring of bullet wipe may be of value in linking a wound to a weapon because metallic elements from the primer, cartridge case, and bullet may be present in the bullet wipe.[23] However, it must be re-emphasized that soot and propellant from close- and intermediate-range wounds may be deposited on the clothing overlying the wound, resulting in a skin wound that *appears* to be of distant-range.[3,23,24,26-31]

## 12.8.1
### Exit Wounds

Most exit wounds have similar characteristics irrespective of whether they result from contact, intermediate, or distant ranges of firing. An exit wound typically is larger and more irregular than an entrance wound. This is mainly due to two factors[23,24]:

1. increasing projectile instability as it travels through the tissue, resulting in accentuated yaw, eventual tumbling, and the bullet exiting base first if the wound track is long enough;
2. projectile deformation in its passage through the tissues as seen in the mushrooming of a bullet.

Both factors result in a larger area of projectile presented at the exit site, with a resultant larger, more irregular exit wound. Exit wounds result from the stretching force of the bullet overcoming the resistance of the skin. The skin is perforated from the inside out, causing eversion of the wound margins and protrusion of tissue tags through the wound defect[23,24] (Fig. 12.9).

**Fig. 12.9** Irregular exit
wound with eversion of the
wound margins

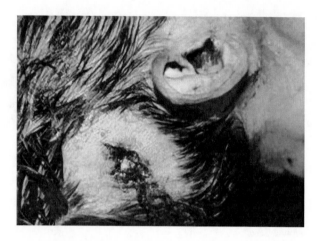

Exit wounds can be difficult to interpret because they vary in size and shape and are not necessarily consistently larger than their preceding entrance wounds. Factors other than projectile deformation and projectile instability affecting the size and appearance of an exit wound include[23,24]:

1. velocity and temporary cavitation effects of a bullet at the point of exit (see Fig. 12.1);
2. fragmentation of the bullet;
3. secondary missile formation, such as bone or jacket fragments accompanying the bullet through the exit wound;
4. bone under the skin in the area of exit;
5. objects pressing against the skin in the area of exit.

## 12.8.2
### Atypical Entrance Wounds

Atypical gunshot entrance wounds occur when bullets become unstable and nonaxial in their flight before striking the body. Unstable nonaxial flight may be caused by intermediary objects, ricochet, inappropriate weapon–ammunition combinations, poor weapon construction, or use of silencers, muzzle brakes, and flash suppressors. Of significance in these instances is that distant-range gunshot entrance wounds may be confused with contact, close-, or intermediate-range entrance wounds, and even exit wounds, particularly when intermediary objects or ricochet bullets are encountered.[23,44]

If a bullet passes through an intermediary object, before penetrating a body, fragments of glass and even bullet fragments may strike the skin, producing stippling around the entrance wound, mimicking an intermediate-range gunshot entrance wound.[23,44–46] Di Maio[23] defines the term "stippling" as multiple punctate abrasions of the skin due to the impact of small fragments of foreign material. If the material is propellant, it is called powder tattooing, but if the stippling is produced by material other than propellant, it is called pseudo-powder tattooing.

**Fig. 12.10** Larger, more irregular stippling or pseudo-powder tattooing due to fragments of glass

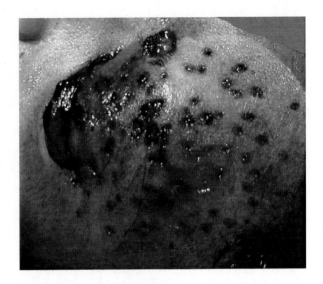

Pseudo-powder tattoo marks generally are larger, more irregular, and more sparse than true powder tattoo marks, and fragments of foreign material from the intermediary object, such as glass, may be found embedded in the marks[23] (Fig. 12.10).

Pseudo-soot blackening effects may occur in ricochet off material such as black asphalt, with deposition of fine black asphalt powder on a victim. Likewise, the lead core of a bullet may disintegrate following ricochet or intermediary object perforation, with powdered or vaporized lead deposition on a victim simulating soot blackening.[23,45-47]

The entrance wound of an unstable or deformed bullet may have a large stellate configuration. In the absence of any stippling or pseudo-soot, it may mimic a contact entrance wound or mimic an exit wound.[23] Bullets recovered from a body following ricochet or intermediate object impaction may be markedly altered in appearance, or even fragmented. If the recovered bullet is handled correctly, forensic scientific examination of such a bullet could reveal the type of material the bullet impacted prior to penetrating the body. This may facilitate the subsequent scene reconstruction and legal proceedings.[13,23,24]

Contact gunshot wounds from firearms fired with silencers, muzzle brakes, or flash suppressors may leave unusual patterns of seared, blackened zones around their entrance wounds (Fig. 12.11). These result from the diversion of muzzle gases by such devices. A silencer may even filter out all the soot and powder emerging from the barrel.[23]

A graze wound resulting from tangential contact with a passing bullet may reveal the direction of fire. Careful hand-lens examination of such a wound may reveal skin tags on the lateral wound margins of the graze-wound trough pointing towards the weapon. The lacerations along the wound-trough margins point in the direction the bullet moved.[23,48] Piling up of tissue may occur at the exit end.[23]

A pseudo-gunshot wound may be defined as an external wound with features resembling those of a gunshot wound, which on further examination is shown to be non-gunshot in origin, such as a stab wound caused by a pointed instrument like a screwdriver (Fig. 12.12).[24,49]

**Fig. 12.11** "Petal" pattern of soot and searing around a contact entrance wound. A flash suppressor was attached to the muzzle of the military rifle used to inflict this wound

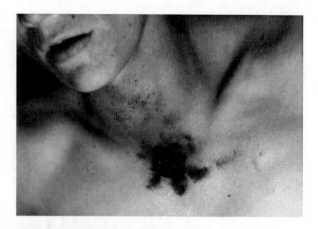

**Fig. 12.12** Oval pseudo-gunshot entrance wound with an "abrasion ring" around the wound defect. This penetrating wound was inflicted with a screwdriver

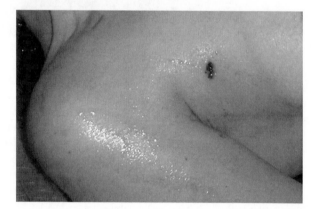

## 12.8.3
### Atypical Exit Wounds

Exit wounds may have abraded margins resembling the abrasion collars of distant entrance wounds. This occurs when the skin is reinforced or supported by a firm object at the instant the bullet exits. The exiting bullet everts the skin, impacting and abrading it against the firm object, such as a floor, a wall, or even tight garments like belts or brassieres. These wounds are called shored exit wounds.[3,23,24] Occasionally, the pattern of the material may be imprinted on the edges of the wound.[23] Elemental analysis of excised shored exit wounds by scanning electron microscope–energy dispersive X-ray spectrometry (SEM-EDX) may reveal the nature of the shoring material.[23,50]

## 12.8.4
### Shotgun Wounds

Shotgun wounds are also classified on the basis of range of fire into contact, close-range, intermediate-range, and distant-range wounds.

The components of a shotgun discharge giving rise to differing wound appearances include the propellant, flame, soot, carbon-monoxide–rich gases, pellets, wads, detonator constituents, and cartridge-case fragments.[23,24,27] The terms used to describe the effects of these shotgun components are the same as for rifled weapons.[24]

The characteristics of shotgun entrance wounds vary with the caliber (gauge) of the weapon, degree of choke, size and number of pellets, as well as the range of fire. Searing, soot deposition, and powder tattooing may be present in close-range and intermediate-range shotgun wounds. The precise range of discharge for a given shotgun can be accurately assessed only by test firing that shotgun with the same brand of ammunition and then comparing the findings with the description of the shotgun wound.[23,24,27]

The wound description should include[23,24,31]:

1. The presence of a wad in the wound and the measurements of the wound defect, as well as the searing, blackening, and powder tattooing patterns around the wound (Close-range: <30 cm).
2. The presence of a wad in the wound and measurements of the wound defect, noting the presence or absence of crenated or scalloped wound edges and surrounding powder tattooing (Intermediate-range: 30–120 cm).
3. Measurement of the diameter of the spread of "satellite" pellet wounds around the measured central defect and the presence or absence of an adjacent wad impact abrasion (Distant-range: >120 cm) (Fig. 12.13).

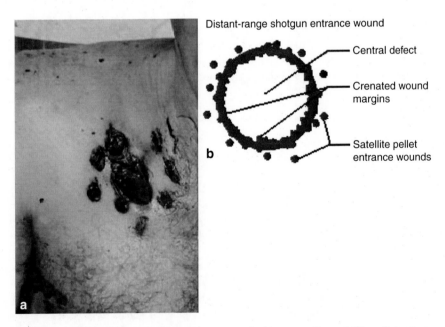

Distant-range shotgun entrance wound

Central defect

Crenated wound margins

Satellite pellet entrance wounds

**Fig. 12.13** (**a, b**) Distant-range shotgun entrance wound with surrounding satellite pellet entrance wounds. Range is estimated at 1.5–2 m

4. The absence of a central wound defect with measurement of the diameter of the spread of pellet wounds (Distant-range: >600–1,000 cm).
5. The presence of a wad or pellets in the clothing.

The range estimates given in brackets above are only a rough guide.

Perforating wounds of the trunk from shotgun pellets are uncommon, but when they do occur, the exit wounds vary from large, irregular, gaping wounds caused by a mass of pellets exiting, to single, slit-like exit wounds produced by single pellets.[23,27]

When found, shotgun pellets and wads should be removed and handled as evidence, as examination of the wad could indicate the gauge of the shotgun and make of the ammunition, whereas the pellets will give the pellet size and shot category.[23]

## 12.9
## Forensic Evidence

The value of forensic evidence in gunshot cases in determining ranges of fire, entrance versus exit wounds, types of ammunition and firearms, manners of injury, and even identification of the assailant cannot be over-emphasized. Therefore the collection, handling, and documentation of evidence during the initial evaluation of a gunshot victim should be standard practice in the emergency setting.[1,3-8] Hospitals should have written protocols that incorporate proper procedures for the collection and retaining of forensic evidence.[6,7,51] A clear understanding of what constitutes evidence is necessary for the successful implementation of such protocols.[4,52]

The term *evidence* is used to describe the nature by which information is presented to the courts; it may be either *informational*, by way of documents and orally, or *physical*, by way of objects such as bullets.[4,52] All physical evidence must be collected carefully, packaged, sealed, and labeled, and it should include the patient's name and hospital number, as well as date and time of specimen collection, specimen type, site of collection, and collector's name and signature.[4,7,13,51,53]

## 12.9.1
## Informational Evidence

In the context of gunshot victims, informational evidence should include a history, examination, and accurate documentation of the gunshot injuries on admission, supplemented with line diagrams, X-rays, and, where possible, photographs. Objective descriptive terminology stating location, size, and shape of wounds, and any unusual marks or coloration should be used to describe the wounds, rather than making potentially inaccurate ballistic interpretations.[1-8,11-22] All iatrogenic interventions must also be recorded to prevent subsequent interpretive difficulties by the forensic pathologist.

X-ray studies indicating the location and the number of bullets in the body must be included. The path and fragmenting nature of a bullet may be revealed, but opinions regarding the type of ammunition used are best left to ballistics experts.[8,11-24] When bone is traversed in the path of a bullet, an X-ray may provide valuable information as to the direction of fire, as the bullet displaces the bone fragments in the direction it travels.[23,24]

## 12.9.2
## Physical Evidence

Physical evidence is real, tangible, or latent matter that can be visualized, measured, or analyzed.[4] Any belongings, body fluids or tissues, or foreign objects found in or on the patient constitute potential evidence. If physical evidence is very small or microscopic, it is referred to as "trace evidence."

In gunshot victims, physical evidence would include:

1. trace evidence such as:
   - gunshot residue (GSR) or blood-spatter on the victim's hands, hair, and clothing[23,32,54-59]
   - hairs, debris, or fibers on the victim's body or clothing[4,7,53,60]
   - blood or tissue under the victim's fingernails[3,23,54]
2. blood, urine, or tissue samples
3. clothing with or without bullet holes
4. bullets and cartridge cases in the victim's body or clothing.[4-7,13,51,53]

## 12.10
## Trace Evidence

The individual collection of trace evidence by "tape lift" or "swabbing" ideally should be performed by trained forensic personnel and falls outside the scope of the trauma surgeon.[4,32] However, by merely collecting and preserving the clothing of a gunshot victim in totality, trace evidence collection and analyses of GSR, fibers, hairs, debris, or blood on the clothing can be performed at forensic laboratories.[4,7,23,32,53-60]

If a physical altercation occurred prior to the shooting incident, fingernail scrapings could be used for comparative DNA analyses. Special crime kits for the collection of such samples are available in most centers, but ideally staff with appropriate forensic training should collect these samples.[1-8,16]

Once the patient is stable, GSR testing on the hands of victims could be performed by forensic investigators, as particles may be detectable for up to 12 h following the shooting incident, using SEM-EDX techniques. A GSR test may determine whether a person has fired a firearm by testing for primer-residue constituents containing barium nitrate, antimony sulfide, and lead peroxide.[23,32-55]

If GSR or DNA testing is to be performed on the patient's hands, the hands should not be cleaned with soap or alcohol. Paper bags should be placed over the hands and secured with elastic bands. Plastic bags should not be used as condensation or moisture in the plastic bags may wash away primer residue or cause fungal degradation of biological evidence.[3,4,7,13,23,53]

## 12.11
## Laboratory Samples

Admission blood samples for alcohol or drug analyses taken prior to dilution by volume expanders or transfusions will yield the most accurate results. Urine specimens also may be used, but they are less valuable for quantification of results.[7] The victim's blood could be used for comparative DNA analysis with blood spatter found at a scene, on a suspect, or on a firearm, as well as with tissue particles found on a spent bullet recovered at a scene.[23,54]

Surgical debridement of a gunshot wound will permanently alter the wound appearance. If not properly documented, photographed, or retained for microscopic evaluation, this may result in misinterpretation by subsequent examiners.[1-8,51] Excised wound margins could allow for microscopic and SEM-EDX evaluation in cases where it is important to[23,30,37,51,55-58]:

- confirm the range of an entrance wound
- establish whether one is dealing with the pseudo-effects of soot blackening or powder tattooing
- establish which of two gunshot wounds is the entrance wound
- ascertain the type of weapon or ammunition used.

For SEM-EDX GSR trace analysis, the excised skin specimen should be placed outer surface upwards on a layer of dry gauze, on top of a piece of cotton wool dampened (not soaked) with formalin, then placed inside a specimen bottle. The skin sample must be secured in this position by placing another piece of dry gauze over it before closing and sealing the bottle. Suspension of the specimen in liquid formalin should be avoided to prevent particles from being washed off prior to analysis (B. A. Kloppers, personal communication).

## 12.12
## Clothing

The clothing of victims often contains valuable clues, including trace evidence and macroscopic bullet holes.[13] Examination of clothing may reveal information as to range and direction of fire, type of ammunition and firearm used, and allow for confirmatory trace evidence analysis. Therefore, all clothing of gunshot victims should be preserved and retained.[3-8,13,23,24,32,54-61]

Emergency personnel should not cut through the convenient starting point of the bullet holes for purposes of removing clothing because disruption of the bullet defect site may destroy evidence. Clothing should be searched for pieces of spent bullets such as bullet jackets.[13,53] It also should be noted whether any garments on the victim were "inside out," as clothing fibers bend in the direction of the path of the bullet, and the true orientation of the fabric may be important to forensic investigators in confirming the circumstances surrounding the incident.[13,23]

Propellant residue and soot will deposit on clothing in contact, close-, and intermediate-range discharges, as they would on skin (see Fig. 12.7). Contact wounds in synthetic material may even cause "burn holes." Bullet-wipe residue also may be observed as a gray to black rim around an entrance hole in clothing. Trace evidence on retained clothing, including fibers, debris, blood spatter, and GSR, may be detected and analyzed to corroborate or complement macroscopic findings with respect to circumstances, range, and direction of fire and type of firearm or ammunition used.[3,23,32,54-60]

Bloody garments should be air dried before being packaged in correctly labeled paper bags to prevent degradation of evidence by fungal or bacterial elements.[4,7,13,23,53]

## 12.13
## Bullets and Cartridge Cases

When bullets or projectile fragments are found or surgically removed from the patient, their integrity must be maintained as much as possible for subsequent ballistic investigations.[23,24,53] A bullet's unique markings are called *class characteristics*, which result from its contact with the rifling in the gun's barrel when the firearm is discharged. They may indicate the make and model of a firearm using comparative analytical techniques.[23,24] Standard metal instruments such as forceps can scratch the jacket or lead of the bullet, producing marks that could hamper or prevent analysis of bullet striations, and thus firearm identification.[23,62] Russel et al.[62] suggested using a "bullet extractor" to accomplish the dual purpose of safe handling (as in the case of bullets with pointed ends, jagged projections, and sharp edges, for example the Black Talon Bullet) and evidence preservation. The bullet extractor is a standard curved Kelly forceps fitted with 2-cm lengths of standard-gauge rubber urinary catheter as protective tips.[62]

The retrieved projectile should be examined for macroscopic trace evidence such as fibers and glass. If none is found, the projectile may be rinsed gently to remove excess blood or body fluids.[62] If the surgeon chooses to mark the bullet with his initials, such marks should be put on the base of the bullet so as not obliterate the rifling marks on the side of the bullet.[23]

Deformed sharp-edged bullets or bullet fragments should be placed in hard plastic containers rather than traditional bullet envelopes to prevent accidental puncture through the envelopes and subsequent loss or injury.[62,63] The bullet container or envelope should be annotated with the date, time, anatomical location of the bullet, the name and hospital number of the gunshot victim, and the collector's name. Tamper-proof seals should be used whenever possible.[23,53,62]

Cartridge cases that may be found in the victim's clothing also have unique microscopic marks on their bottoms or sides, imparted by contact with the firing pin, the breechlock, the magazine of semiautomatic weapons, and extractor and ejector mechanisms. These may be used to identify the type, make, and model of the firearm used. Therefore they should be handled and preserved in the same careful way as described above for bullets.[23]

## 12.13.1
### The Deceased Gunshot Victim

When a gunshot victim dies in the hospital, the clinical documents forwarded to the forensic pathologist must indicate clearly whether any bullets or projectiles were retrieved from the body of the patient. The location of the bullet before retrieval must be noted. The documents must also include a summary history and examination of the victim at the time of admission, accurate admission wound descriptions, and subsequent iatrogenic procedures performed. If the death is delayed for a period of time, a summary of the patient's management, clinical progress, and any complications must also be recorded. If x-rays were taken, the exact location of any remaining projectiles must be documented clearly.[1-8,13,61]

If a gunshot wound victim dies soon after arrival at the hospital, it is recommended that the deceased's hands be encased in paper bags. If the clothing is still on the body, it should not be removed before placing the body in a body bag for transfer to the mortuary.[4] To facilitate the comparison of clothing defects with wounds on the victim's body, all removed clothing still in the custody of the hospital should accompany the body to the mortuary.[53] All intravenous lines, catheters, tubes, sutures, and drains should be left in situ to minimize possible confusion of gunshot wounds with surgical wounds.[4]

## 12.13.2
### The Chain of Custody

The chain of custody is the pathway that physical evidence follows from the time it is collected until it has served its purpose in the legal investigation of an incident. A record of the chain of custody will reflect the number of times a piece of evidence has changed hands or location prior to its final destination.[4] Minimizing the times that evidentiary items change hands will assist in protecting the integrity and credibility of such evidence.[53] Failure to protect the chain of custody may cause evidence to be inadmissible in court, even though it is physically present, as defense attorneys often attempt to cast doubt on the integrity of the evidence by attacking the chain of custody.[4,53]

All potential evidentiary items should be placed in appropriate containers that can be sealed with tape and labeled appropriately.[4,53] A standard chain-of-custody form attached to the container could be used to document all transfers of the evidence, with the dates, details, and signatures of all the individuals who handled the evidence recorded on it. A copy of this chain-of-custody form should be kept in the patient's hospital record. If the chain is properly recorded, hospital personnel may not be required to testify in subsequent court proceedings, especially when testimony is needed simply to establish the chain of custody.[4,51,53]

Written protocols incorporating the proper handling of forensic evidence, together with standard chain-of-custody forms should be implemented at all hospitals.[6,7,51] A hospital "property custodian" should be appointed to safeguard all evidentiary items until their collection by law-enforcement officials.[4,7]

### 12.13.3
### Explosions and Evidence

With the dramatic increase in the incidence of domestic bombings and mass-casualty incidents worldwide, all hospitals must have mass-casualty plans in place in order to optimize medical care for victims.[64,65] In addition, emergency departments must recognize that criminal prosecution or civil litigation against parties responsible for injurious explosions may follow such events. While it may be very difficult in mass-casualty situations, the forensic aspects of documentation and evidence collection must remain in place.[34,65]

A variety of explosive devices exist, including many which are homemade. Emergency health-care workers must protect themselves and their patients from further injury by ensuring that contaminated clothing and potential flammable material is removed from the patient, keeping in mind that all material removed is potential forensic evidence and should be treated as such.[64] Clothing and hair of victims may contain macroscopic and trace evidence that may reflect the type of explosive used, confirm the chemical composition of incendiary devices, indicate the presence or absence of fire or smoke, and may provide clues as to the location of a patient in relation to the blast.[27-29,64]

The patterns of injuries and shrapnel retained in patients may also provide valuable information as to all of the above. Careful descriptions and documentation of all injuries, total-body X-ray investigations, and retrieval of foreign materials during surgery that may include bomb fragments, must be performed.[27,28,34] Small metal objects forming part of the bomb mechanism may be invaluable in allowing experts to recognize the handiwork of a particular bomb maker or terrorist group.[27-29]

### 12.14
### Conclusion

When clinicians are remiss in the adequate forensic evaluation of gunshot patients, it could have far-reaching medico-legal implications in the increasingly litigious construct of society and could result in obstruction of the ends of justice with respect to the forensic and legal needs of individual patients, as well as society in general.[1-8,16,20,52]

Three separate retrospective analyses have shown that clinical records in gunshot cases routinely lack adequate wound descriptions.[14,18-22] In addition, the correct handling of potentially short-lived evidentiary material and the preservation of a chain of custody is frequently neglected in clinical settings.[5-8]

If a gunshot victim is killed outright and examined by a competent forensic pathologist, precise descriptions of the wounds will be obtained and forensic evidence will be handled correctly. However, if the patient initially survives and remains in hospital for a period of time, then wound healing or sepsis and surgical interventions can cause considerable difficulty in interpretation for the forensic pathologist if the documentation of gunshot wounds and iatrogenic procedures and the collection of forensic evidence have been neglected.[13,15,17-20]

In summary, the comprehensive forensic evaluation of a gunshot victim should include the following:

1. recording of the patient's and clinician's names, date and time of admission, full history and examination, and date and time of death (when applicable)
2. recording of anatomical location, size, shape, and characteristics of the gunshot wound(s), including associated marks or coloration
3. recording of surgical resuscitative procedures, as these may obscure or alter gunshot wound appearances, or result in "additional wounds"
4. augmentation of narrative descriptions with X-rays, diagrams, and photographs where possible
5. use of a proforma, including a simple line drawing, to improve the quality of documentation
6. refraining from "forensic interpretations" of gunshot wound appearances with respect to entrance, exit, direction, or range of fire
7. recording of the patient's clinical management, progress, or complications, as well as special investigations and further surgical interventions
8. recording and correct handling of all evidence collected and proper maintenance of the chain of custody.

Lastly, a succinct observation by William S. Smock[3] that reflects the merits of clinical forensic training and the consequent appreciation of the value of forensic evidence in the emergency department, bears iteration:

"What was once considered confounding clutter that gets in the way of patient care (such as clothing and surface dirt) takes on a whole new significance when recognized for what it really is - evidence."[3]

**Acknowledgments**   With special thanks to Fiona Bester, the Deputy Librarian of the University of the Witwatersrand Health Sciences Library, and her members of staff, Senior Superintendent B.A. Kloppers, the Operational Commander of the Ballistics Unit at the Forensic Science Laboratory in Pretoria, and Raymond Cherry, our Departmental Research Assistant, for their invaluable assistance in the preparation of this chapter.

## References

1. Eckert WG, Bell JS, Stein RJ, Tabakman MB, Taff ML, Tedeschi LG. Clinical forensic medicine. *Am J Forensic Med Pathol.* 1986;7:182-185.
2. Smock WS. Forensic emergency medicine. In: Marx JA, ed. *Rosen's Emergency Medicine.* 5th ed. St Louis: Mosby; 2002:828-841.
3. Olshaker JS, Jackson CM, Smock WS. *Forensic Emergency Medicine.* Philadelphia: Lippincott Williams and Wilkins; 2001.
4. Muro GA, Easter CR. Clinical forensics for perioperative nurses. *AORN J.* 1994;60: 585-591. 593.
5. Smock WS, Nichols GR, Fuller PM. Development and implementation of the first clinical forensic medicine training program. *J Forensic Sci.* 1993;38:835-839.

6. Carmona R, Prince K. Trauma and forensic medicine. *J Trauma*. 1989;29:1222-1225.
7. Mittleman RE, Goldberg HS, Waksman DM. Preserving evidence in the emergency department. *Am J Nurs*. 1983;83:1652-1654.
8. Smialek JE. Forensic medicine in the emergency department. *Emerg Med Clin North Am*. 1983;1:693-704.
9. Hargarten SW, Waeckerle JF. Docs and cops: a collaborating or colliding partnership? *Ann Emerg Med*. 2001;38:438-440.
10. Shepherd JP. Emergency medicine and police collaboration to prevent community violence. *Ann Emerg Med*. 2001;38:430-437.
11. Randall T. Clinicians' forensic interpretations of fatal gunshot wounds often miss the mark. *JAMA*. 1993;269:2058. 2061.
12. Apfelbaum JD, Shockley LW, Wahe JW, Moore EE. Entrance and exit gunshot wounds: incorrect terms for the emergency department? *J Emerg Med*. 1998;16:741-745.
13. Godley DR, Smith TK. Some medicolegal aspects of gunshot wounds. *J Trauma*. 1977;17:866-871.
14. Ross RT, Hammen PF, Frantz EI, Pare LE, Boyd CR. Gunshot wounds: evaluating the adequacy of documentation at a Level I trauma center. *J Trauma*. 1998;45:151-152.
15. Bowley DM, Vellema J. Wound ballistics – an update. *Care of the Critically Ill*. 2002;18:133-138.
16. Ryan MT. Clinical forensic medicine. *Ann Emerg Med*. 2000;36:271-273.
17. Collins KA, Lantz PE. Interpretation of fatal, multiple, and exiting gunshot wounds by trauma specialists. *J Forensic Sci*. 1994;39:94-99.
18. Fackler ML, Mason RT. Gunshot wounds: evaluating the adequacy of documentation at a level I trauma center. *J Trauma*. 1999;46:741-742.
19. Fackler ML. How to describe bullet holes. *Ann Emerg Med*. 1994;23:386-387.
20. Fackler ML, Riddick L. Clinicians' inadequate descriptions of gunshot wounds obstruct justice: Clinical journals refuse to expose the problem. Colordo Springs: *Proceedings of the American Academy of Forensic Sciences*. In: Warren EA, Papke BK, eds. 1996:149.
21. Voelker R. New program targets death investigator training. *JAMA*. 1996;275:826.
22. Shuman M, Wright RK. Evaluation of clinician accuracy in describing gunshot wound injuries. *J Forensic Sci*. 1999;44:339-342.
23. Di Maio VJM. *Gunshot Wounds*. 2nd ed. Boca Raton: CRC Press; 1999.
24. Fatteh A. *Medicolegal Investigation of Gunshot wounds*. Philadelphia: JB Lippincott; 1976.
25. Sellier KG, Kneubuehl BP. *Wound Ballistics and the Scientific Background*. Amsterdam: Elsevier Science; 1994.
26. Gordon I, Shapiro HA, Berson SD. *Forensic Medicine*. 3rd ed. Edinburgh: Churchill Livingstone; 1997.
27. Knight B. *Forensic Pathology*. 2nd ed. New York: Oxford University Press; 1996.
28. Spitz WU, Fischer RS. *Medicolegal Investigation of Death*. Springfield: Charles C Thomas; 1993.
29. Mason JK. *Forensic Medicine*. London: Chapman Hall Medical; 1993.
30. Adelson L. *The Pathology of Homicide*. Springfield: Charles C Thomas; 1974.
31. Knight B. *Simpson's Forensic Medicine*. 10th ed. London: Edward Arnold; 1991.
32. Romolo FS, Margot P. Identification of gunshot residue: a critical review. *Forensic Sci Int*. 2001;119:195-211.
33. Cooper GJ, Ryan JM. Interaction of penetrating missiles with tissues: some common misapprehensions and implications for wound management. *Br J Surg*. 1990;77:606-610.
34. Ryan JM, Rich NM, Dale RF, Morgans BT, Cooper GJ. *Ballistic Trauma*. London: Arnold; 1997.
35. Thali MJ, Kneubuehl BP, Zollinger U, Dirnhofer R. A study of the morphology of gunshot entrance wounds, in connection with their dynamic creation, utilizing the "skin-skull-brain model". *Forensic Sci Int*. 2002;125:190-194.

36. Mason JK, Purdue BN. *The Pathology of Trauma*. 3rd ed. New York: Oxford University Press – Arnold; 2000.
37. Adelson L. A microscopic study of dermal gunshot wounds. *Am J Clin Pathol*. 1961;35: 393-402.
38. Fackler ML. Civilian gunshot wounds and ballistics: dispelling the myths. *Emerg Med Clin North Am*. 1998;16:17-28.
39. Fackler ML. Wound ballistics. A review of common misconceptions. *JAMA*. 1988;259: 2730-2736.
40. Fackler ML. Gunshot wound review. *Ann Emerg Med*. 1996;28:194-203.
41. Hollerman JJ, Fackler ML, Coldwell DM, Ben-Menachem Y. Gunshot wounds: 1. Bullets, ballistics, and mechanisms of injury. *AJR Am J Roentgenol*. 1990;155:685-690.
42. Mendelson JA. The relationship between mechanisms of wounding and principles of treatment of missile wounds. *J Trauma*. 1991;31:1181-1202.
43. Lindsey D. The idolatry of velocity, or lies, damn lies, and ballistics. *J Trauma*. 1980;20:1068-1069.
44. Donoghue ER, Kalelkar MB, Richmond JM, Teass SS. Atypical gunshot wounds of entrance: an empirical study. *J Forensic Sci*. 1984;29:379-388.
45. Dixon DS. Tempered plate glass as an intermediate target and its effects on gunshot wound characteristics. *J Forensic Sci*. 1982;27:205-208.
46. Stahl CJ, Jones SR, Johnson FB, Luke JL. The effect of glass as an intermediate target on bullets: experimental studies and report of a case. *J Forensic Sci*. 1979;24:6-17.
47. Sellier K. *Forensic Science Progress, Shot Range Determination Vol 6*. Berlin: Springer-Verlag; 1991.
48. Dixon DS. Determination of direction of fire from graze gunshot wounds. *J Forensic Sci*. 1980;25:272-279.
49. Prahlow JA, McClain JL. Lesions that simulate gunshot wounds – further examples II. *J Clin Forensic Med*. 2001;8:206-213.
50. Dixon DS. Characteristics of shored exit wounds. *J Forensic Sci*. 1981;26:691-698.
51. Murphy GK. The study of gunshot wounds in surgical pathology. *Am J Forensic Med Pathol*. 1980;1:123-130.
52. Mc Lay WDS. *Clinical Forensic Medicine*. 2nd ed. London: Greenwich Medical Media; 1996.
53. Schramm CA. Forensic medicine. What the perioperative nurse needs to know. *AORN J*. 1991;53:669-683, 686-692.
54. Karger B, Nüsse R, Bajanowski T. Backspatter on the firearm and hand in experimental close-range gunshots to the head. *Am J Forensic Med Pathol*. 2002;23:211-213.
55. Zeichner A, Levin N. Casework experience of GSR detection in Israel, on samples from hands, hair, and clothing using an autosearch SEM/EDX system. *J Forensic Sci*. 1995;40: 1082-1085.
56. Wolten GM, Nesbitt RS, Calloway AR, Loper GL, Jones PF. Particle analysis for the detection of gunshot residue I: scanning electron microscopy/energy dispersive x-ray characterization of hand deposits from firing. *J Forensic Sci*. 1979;24:409-422.
57. Wolten GM, Nesbitt RS, Calloway AR. Particle analysis for the detection of gunshot residue III: the case record. *J Forensic Sci*. 1979;24:864-869.
58. Tillman WL. Automated gunshot residue particle search and characterization. *J Forensic Sci*. 1987;32:62-71.
59. Fojtás̆ek L, Vacínová J, Kolá P, Kotrlý M. Distribution of GSR particles in the surroundings of shooting pistol. *Forensic Sci Int*. 2003;132:99-105.
60. Laing DK, Hartshorne AW, Cook R, Robinson G. A fiber data collection for forensic scientists: collection and examination methods. *J Forensic Sci*. 1987;32:364-369.

61. Finck PA. Ballistic and forensic pathologic aspects of missile wounds. Conversion between Anglo-American and metric-system units. *Mil Med*. 1965;130:545-563.

62. Russell MA, Atkinson RD, Klatt EC, Noguchi TT. Safety in bullet recovery procedures: a study of the Black Talon bullet. *Am J Forensic Med Pathol*. 1995;16:120-123.

63. McCormick GM, Young DB, Stewart JC. Wounding effects of the Winchester Black Talon bullet. *Am J Forensic Med Pathol*. 1996;17:124-129.

64. Maxson TR. Management of pediatric trauma: blast victims in a mass casualty incident. *Clin Ped Emerg Med*. 2002;3:256-261.

65. Wightman JM, Gladish SL. Explosions and blast injuries. *Ann Emerg Med*. 2001;37: 664-678.

## Further Reading

Olshaker JS, Jackson CM, Smock WS. *Forensic Emergency Medicine*. Philadelphia: Lippincott Williams and Wilkins; 2001.

Di Maio VJM. *Gunshot Wounds*. 2nd ed. Boca Raton: CRC Press; 1999.

Fatteh A. *Medicolegal Investigation of Gunshot Wounds*. Philadelphia: JB Lippincott; 1976.

Knight B. *Forensic Pathology*. 2nd ed. New York: Oxford University Press; 1996.

Sellier K. *Forensic Science Progress, Shot Range Determination*. vol. 6. Berlin: Springer-Verlag; 1991.

# Part III

---

# Trauma Systems

# Civilian Trauma Systems

# 13

Jason Smith

## 13.1
## Introduction

A trauma system can be defined as an organized and co-ordinated provision of care to all trauma patients, involving injury prevention, pre-hospital, in-hospital, and rehabilitative phases of care. Trauma systems are widely recognized to improve patient outcome from trauma. This makes logical sense, in that haphazard medical care is unlikely to achieve targets for resuscitation and definitive treatment of the population with penetrating trauma. Patients fare better when there is a prepared and co-ordinated response to injury.

Civilian trauma systems developed in the USA in the 1960s, as a result of military experience in Korea and Vietnam, but the development of trauma systems elsewhere in the world has been much less organized.

Expertise has been centralized into trauma centers, maximizing limited resources in one place, with specific retrieval systems in place for both primary (from scene) and secondary (from another medical facility) retrievals to the trauma center. Pre-hospital protocols enable crews to bypass smaller centers in favor of direct transfer to a trauma center, where teams and specialities appropriate to the level of care required are based.

The implementation of plans to deal with trauma patients are often hampered by external factors such as cost, lack of political support, lack of perceived need, and the failure to prove the worth of trauma systems in terms of improving mortality.

Trauma centers have standardized care of trauma patients with protocols for the management of common conditions based on the best evidence available. Data is collected on trauma patients to enable analysis of performance against theoretical models and also in direct comparison with other trauma centers to maintain quality and ensure clinical effectiveness.

J. Smith
Academic Department of Military Emergency Medicine, Royal Centre for Defence Medicine
Birmingham Research Park, Vincent Drive, Birmingham, B15 2SQ UK
e-mail: jasonesmith@doctors.org.uk

A.J. Brooks et al. (eds.), *Ryan's Ballistic Trauma*,
DOI: 10.1007/978-1-84882-124-8_13, © Springer-Verlag London Limited 2011

## 13.2
## Injury Prevention

Part of a good trauma system is prevention of injury, and nowhere more so than in civilian ballistic trauma. Carriage of firearms by members of the public in the USA, among several other complex confounders, accounts for the high rate of penetrating trauma in the USA when compared to Europe and Australasia. Licensing laws and police initiatives such as gun amnesties may go some way to reducing use and injury from such weapons.

## 13.3
## Pre-Hospital Care

### 13.3.1
### Dispatch

The majority of pre-hospital care in the UK, USA, and Australasia is delivered by paramedics and ambulance personnel. Paramedic crews are dispatched to the scene of an incident on the basis of an emergency call using a centralized number (999 in the UK, 911 in the USA).

If a physician response is available, a system needs to be in place to ensure this is activated in response to appropriate situations. In London, emergency calls are screened in the ambulance control center by one of the helicopter emergency medical service (HEMS) paramedics who dispatches the helicopter or vehicle response team on the basis of appropriate mechanism of injury or physiological disturbance. Similarly, trained paramedics are not universally available on ambulances, and calls therefore need to be triaged to facilitate an appropriate response with the appropriate skill level for the patient.

### 13.3.2
### Protocols

The priorities in the pre-hospital management of trauma patients are detection and treatment of life-threatening injuries and delivery to the most appropriate provider of definitive medical care in an appropriate time scale. In practice, this often means treating airway and breathing problems on scene, and circulation problems en route to definitive care. In the presence of ballistic torso trauma and haemodynamic compromise, every minute that delays that patient reaching definitive hemorrhage control increases mortality. This has translated into a "scoop and run" policy for the majority of cases of penetrating trauma. However, other cases may warrant more formal stabilization at scene, for example the head injured patient with a reduced conscious level may benefit from rapid sequence induction of anesthesia and intubation to protect the airway and ensure adequate oxygenation throughout transfer.

### 13.3.3
### Bypass

Definitive care usually means a hospital capable of delivering resuscitation and surgery. As cardiothoracic and neurosurgical expertise is centralized, time to definitive care is reduced if smaller centers without the appropriate expertise are bypassed. This is still a contentious issue in the UK, where the nearest hospital is much more likely to be used, but hospital bypass is much more established practice in the USA and Australasia.

### 13.3.4
### Pre-alert

Communication between pre-hospital and in-hospital clinical teams is vital if an appropriate response is to be mounted to the arrival of the seriously injured patient. Communication can be through radio, telephone or direct electronic transfer of vital signs from the scene. Efforts should be made to make direct contact between the crew at scene and the resuscitation room, as information passed via a third party is likely to become corrupted.

### 13.4
### In-Hospital Care

### 13.4.1
### Trauma Teams

The presence of a multi-disciplinary trauma team during the initial phase of management of the multi-trauma patient has been shown to improve outcome. The activation of such a response needs to be pre-prepared and dependant on information passed from pre-hospital providers. Typically a trauma team response will involve clinicians from emergency medicine, anesthesia, intensive care, and surgery, responsible for the primary survey and resuscitation during the initial phase of in-hospital care.

### 13.4.2
### Hospital Response

Once the trauma team has been activated, other protocols need to be in place for the patient to receive the care they need. For example, if pre-hospital notification is received that a hypotensive trauma patient is inbound, the operating theater needs to be warned that they may be receiving a patient, so an operating room can be prepared to rapidly receive the patient. Similarly the blood bank needs to be informed of the imminent requirement of blood and blood products, and ideally a protocol for massive transfusion needs to be in place. The preparation of expertise and equipment in computed tomography and angiography again takes time, and therefore pre-warning needs to take place if the patient is to receive timely intervention.

### 13.4.3
### Trauma Surgery

Although there are a few individual exceptions, the specialty of trauma surgery does not currently exist in its own right in the UK, where trauma patients are dealt with by general surgeons as part of the emergency surgery cover, with other specialties called in as deemed necessary. However, patients who present with an expanding haematoma following a GSW to the neck may not be best treated by an ENT or maxillofacial surgeon who is not resident on call and who has little experience in dealing with trauma. The trauma surgeons who do exist tend to be specialists in other fields with appropriate experience and an interest in dealing with trauma. Ideally every trauma patient will be admitted under a named trauma surgeon skilled and experienced in dealing with the complex needs of the multi-trauma patient.

### 13.4.4
### Intensive Care

The specific needs of the trauma patient should be appreciated and in trauma centers there are often dedicated critical care beds where nurses and clinicians used to dealing with trauma patients are based.

### 13.4.5
### Rehabilitation

Trauma patients often need specific rehabilitation, for example neuro-rehabilitation, prosthetic services, and psychological support. As these resources are scarce, they are often centralized and therefore not always available to those trauma patients who require them.

### 13.4.6
### Pediatric Trauma

Trauma is the leading cause of death in children over the age of 1 year, and approximately 25% of all injured patients are in the pediatric age group (aged less than 16 years). A quarter of these will have major trauma requiring the input of a multidisciplinary trauma team, mostly as a result of motor vehicle collisions, falls, and interpersonal violence or war. Pediatric trauma is often managed by those with expertise in either pediatrics or trauma, but rarely both. In the UK, in cities where there are children's hospitals, trauma patients are scarce. Trauma centers are often not co-located with pediatric surgery and children's intensive care facilities. This is a problem that has also been recognized in the USA, where the debate is still ongoing as to how best to tackle this dilemma. In 2001, there were at least 31 pediatric trauma centers covering 21 states in the USA. One of the main problems with the pediatric center model is that to get enough exposure, be educationally sound and financially viable, there will be fewer pediatric centers making transfer times longer, and necessitating a greater distance from home and family.

Another option is to have a joint adult and pediatric emergency facility on the same site, with some cross-over between the adult and pediatric trauma teams to ensure the smooth running of the systems in place for adult trauma. Whichever of these options is preferred, there is a necessity for resuscitation facilities with appropriate equipment, and staff who are adequately trained to use the equipment.

## 13.5
## Research and Audit in Trauma

We can no longer assume that we are good at dealing with trauma patients without corroborating data to support the assumption. The process by which data is collected varies from country to country, and region to region, but essentially involves scoring of patients according to anatomical and physiological criteria, and examining outcomes to ensure that patients who would be expected to survive an injury are not dying unnecessarily. A trauma system should have internal quality control mechanisms in place to ensure it is functioning to an acceptable standard. This involves collection of data to ensure that the system is working when compared to national and international standards.

The UK Trauma Audit and Research Network (TARN) is a collaboration of hospitals from all over the UK and has now expanded to involve other European countries. The TARN database is the largest trauma database in Europe with more than 200,000 cases including over 22,000 pediatric patients. Its aim is to collect and analyze clinical and epidemiological data, and provide a statistical base to support clinical audit, and to aid the development of trauma services.

## 13.6
## External Validity of Trauma Systems

External assessment of trauma systems is a useful tool to highlight deficiencies, and the latest large report to be performed in the UK was the report of the National Confidential Enquiry into Patient Outcome and Death (NCEPOD, 2007). The NCEPOD report has highlighted several areas of weakness in trauma systems in the UK, including lack of coordination of pre-hospital and in-hospital clinical governance, lack of senior input to the trauma teams and during surgery, and the need for standardization of transfers of trauma patients. Recommendations include the establishment of regional trauma networks, centralisation of services, and more senior medical input to the care of trauma patients.

## Background and Further Reading

Royal College of Surgeons and British Orthopaedic Association. Better Care for the Severely Injured. London: RCS(Eng); 2000. www.rcseng.ac.uk

The Trauma Audit & Research Network. www.tarn.ac.uk

Trauma: Who cares? National Confidential Enquiry into Patient Outcome and Death. London: NCEPOD; 2007. www.ncepod.org.uk

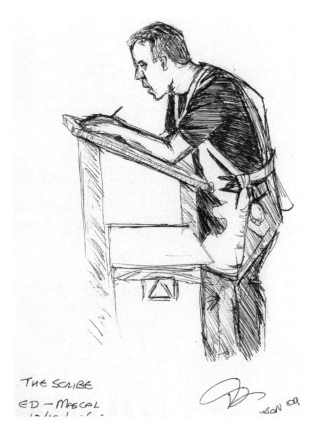

THE SCRIBE
ED — MASCAL

The Scribe
A vital member of the trauma team

# The UK Military Trauma System

# 14

Timothy J. Hodgetts

## 14.1
## Introduction

The UK military trauma system on contemporary operations has evolved substantially in the last decade, drawing on clinical experience from post-conflict peace-enforcing in Kosovo and combat operations in both Iraq and Afghanistan. It has matured so that training, equipment, and clinical guidelines are integrated from point of wounding through to field hospital care, and that clinical practice is rigorously governed from pre-hospital care through to rehabilitation.

This chapter will describe:

- The differences between civilian and military trauma systems.
- The components of the military trauma system.
- Training to support the military trauma system.
- The governance of the military trauma system.

## 14.2
## Military Trauma Is Different

To understand why military and civilian trauma systems are different (including the paradigms of care, and concepts of resuscitation and definitive treatment) requires an understanding of the differences in frequency, severity, and complexity of combat trauma compared to that encountered in the civilian setting.

In a comparison of UK military and civilian contemporary experience, Hodgetts et al.[1] identified that 56.3% of National Health Service (NHS) "major trauma" is related to motor vehicle crashes, whereas it is only 5.1% of major trauma cases treated in British field

T.J. Hodgetts
Academic Department of Military Emergency Medicine, Royal Centre for Defence Medicine, Vincent Drive, Edgbaston, Birmingham Research Park, B15 2SQ, Birmingham, UK
e-mail: prof.admem@rcdm.bham.ac.uk

A.J. Brooks et al. (eds.), *Ryan's Ballistic Trauma*,
DOI: 10.1007/978-1-84882-124-8_14, © Springer-Verlag London Limited 2011

hospitals; furthermore, 83.7% of field hospital major trauma cases related to gunshot, blast, and fragmentation injuries. Banding the Injury Severity Scores demonstrated that the field hospital cohort was significantly more seriously injured than the NHS cohort ($p < 0.0001$), where the NHS cohort was the combined experience of 183 hospitals evaluated in the National Confidential Enquiry into Patient Outcomes and Deaths (2007).[2]

## 14.3
## Comparing Civilian and Military Trauma Systems

Within the military trauma system (Fig. 14.1) there is an expectation that access to professional medical support cannot be immediate: as a result, care is embedded at the point of wounding and individuals are empowered to treat themselves or their "buddies." The standard of individual first aid extends to principles of physiological triage (the *Triage Sieve*, see Chap. 15), basic life support (CPR), use of field dressings, judicious use of a commercial tourniquet, improvised limb splints, administration of intramuscular morphine, and environmental control. One in four combat soldiers receives additional training and equipment to deliver advanced first aid at the point of wounding. In both cases, interventions are focused on simple life-saving treatments, consistently deliverable as casualty treatment "drills" [3,4] that follow the "<C>ABC" paradigm.[5]

Resuscitation priorities have been adjusted from ABC to <C>ABC in response to the observation that *avoidable* battlefield deaths relate predominantly to hemorrhage from limbs. Commercial tourniquets and topical haemostatic agents have been demonstrated to be effective in the treatment of these wounds, with claims of improved survival.[6–8]

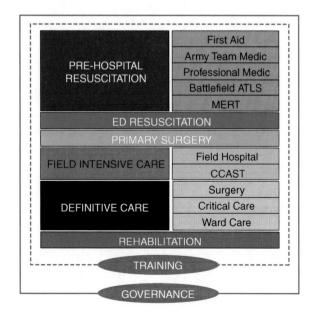

**Fig. 14.1** The UK military trauma system (From: Hodgetts[9] Crown Copyright, reproduced with permission of the editor)

Further amelioration of an anticipated extended pre-hospital timeline in the combat setting has been the introduction of a critical care clinical team (anesthetist or emergency physician; emergency nurse; paramedic) that can fly to the point of wounding and undertake advanced interventions during the flight to hospital: these interventions have included rapid sequence induction of anesthesia, chest drain, surgical airway, thoracotomy, and the administration of blood products (packed red cells and fresh frozen plasma) to the seriously injured. This "Medical Emergency Response Team" (MERT) will follow a "scoop and play" philosophy – it is too dangerous to stay on the ground and attract enemy fire, hence the interventions in flight, day or night, with the regular requirement to treat multiple casualties simultaneously.[10]

Reception at a field hospital involves a consultant-based Trauma Team for every seriously injured casualty: specifically, leadership by a consultant emergency physician and direct involvement of consultants in anesthesia, general surgery, and orthopedic surgery. This compares starkly with UK civilian practice where only 3% of hospitals surveyed had consultant leadership of the Trauma Team out of hours.[2] The principal advantage of clinical seniority is the speed with which critical decisions and decisive action are taken (Fig. 14.2).

This trauma system is developing continuously, incrementally, and by step change. An example has been the implementation of the new concept of *Damage Control Resuscitation*,[11] which incorporates the concept of *Haemostatic Resuscitation* that underpins the early proactive management of the coagulopathy of trauma with packed red cells and plasma in a 1:1 ratio, together with replacement of platelets and fibrinogen and correction of core temperature against pre-determined resuscitation targets.[12]

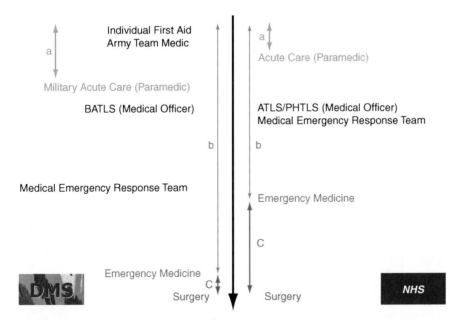

**Fig. 14.2** Emergency medical systems: NHS vs. Defence medical services (From Hodgetts[9] Crown Copyright, reproduced with permission of the editor)

## 14.4
## Systematic Training

There is a single common set of clinical guidelines for acute care from point of wounding through to field hospital care, referred to as Clinical Guidelines for Operations (CGOs).[13] CGOs set the training content for each level of acute care (1st aider; Team Medic; professional medic and paramedic; pre-hospital doctor or nurse; emergency physician or nurse) for all Services and operational areas. There is a single pathway to follow for any medical emergency, whether this is trauma, medical, toxicological (including CBRN), or environmental. This is an unique approach to emergency care and ensures that patients with pathology in more than one domain of the acute care spectrum are managed effectively (a civilian analogy would be a patient who suffers a dysrhythmia and crashes their car in the rain, being trapped in the vehicle and suffering hypothermia: this is a combination of medical, trauma, and environmental problems) (Fig. 14.3a, b).

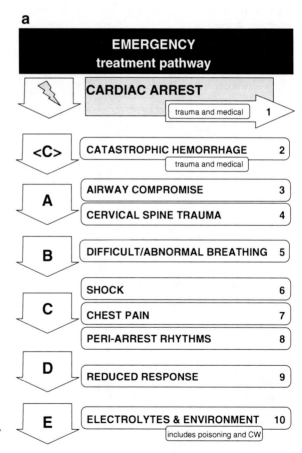

**Fig. 14.3 (a)** Clinical guidelines for operations. The common <C> ABC gateway for all emergencies is shown. **(b)** A pathway for blast injury that is a prompt for the experienced team leader (From ref.[12] Crown Copyright, reproduced with permission)

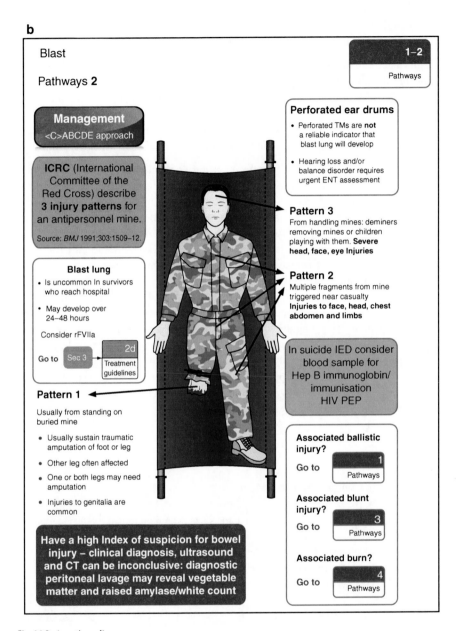

**Fig. 14.3** (continued)

Training in acute care is integrated across the Defence Medical Services with a common standard at each level. Trauma care training for the professional is the 3 day *Battlefield Advanced Trauma Life Support* course.[14] Although it has common roots with the civilian ATLS® course, it has diverged to follow the <C>ABC paradigm and trains doctors, nurses, and paramedics alongside in both individual and team skills. Furthermore, there is recognition that a single approach to resuscitation does not fit each stage of evacuation: there are 4 stages of resuscitation in the combat environment:

- Care Under Fire (drag the patient to safety; simple airway; apply tourniquet for severe limb bleeding; win the fire-fight).
- Tactical Field Care (limited time and equipment; area potentially unsafe; undertake "Tactical Rapid Primary Survey," TRaPS, and associated treatment).
- Field Resuscitation (team based resuscitation by regimental doctor and medics, far forward).
- Advanced Resuscitation (team based resuscitation by experienced Trauma Team).

Advanced Resuscitation takes place on reception at the field hospital – but the boundaries between Field Resuscitation and Advanced Resuscitation are blurred when the experienced MERT is projected forward to the point of wounding.

Common guidelines and systematic training has facilitated a rationalized approach to medical equipment. Each level of care builds on the equipment of the preceding level and for the most part the same equipment is perpetuated within the system once it has been introduced (exceptions exist where lightweight and robust options may be necessary for far forward providers who must carry their treatment equipment when on a dismounted operation).

As preparation for deployment, clinical personnel attend two sophisticated, integrated exercises (separated by several months) where high validity simulated live casualties are treated from point of wounding through a field hospital in real-time.[15] Here there is both microscopic simulation (individual clinical cases) and macroscopic simulation (the whole trauma system is tested continuously for 3 days with all staff functioning as they would in their deployed roles). This gives opportunity after the first exercise for areas of individual and collective performance improvement to be managed, and after the second exercise to validate the hospital for effectiveness to deploy (Fig. 14.4).

## 14.5
## Governance of the Military Trauma System

Trauma management in military operational areas has been highlighted by the Healthcare Commission in 2009 as an example of exemplary practice and one that "the NHS could learn from in the delivery of emergency care."[16]

A framework of governance has been implemented to facilitate best practice, and to ensure that Service personnel who are seriously injured on deployed operations receive exemplary care.[17]

Major Trauma Audit for Clinical Effectiveness (MACE) is a cyclical process of continuous quality improvement through clinical audit. Data on all seriously injured casualties treated by UK Defence Medical Services (UK military, coalition forces, detainees, civilian population) is collected by the deployed Trauma Nurse Coordinator and returned to the Joint Theatre Trauma Registry (JTTR) maintained by the Academic Department of Military Emergency Medicine (ADMEM) at the Royal Centre for Defence Medicine (RCDM) in Birmingham. JTTR holds continuous data on this cohort from 2003, coinciding with the start of hostilities in Iraq. Returns are electronic (where deployed IT systems allow), with

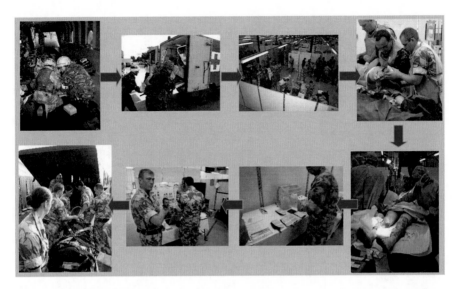

**Fig. 14.4** Integrated training from point of wounding to intensive care or ward treatment within the "HOSPEX" at Army medical services training centre, York (From Hodgetts[9] Crown Copyright, reproduced with permission of the editor)

hard copy accompanying UK military patients evacuated to RCDM for definitive care. Table 14.1 (adapted from Ballistic Trauma 1st Edition) summarizes earlier data collection systems.

The default entry criterion for UK JTTR is a casualty who triggers trauma team activation in a deployed field hospital or Primary Casualty Receiving Facility afloat (Role 2 Enhanced and Role 3). The continuous improvement of care is related to two distinct processes:

(i) A systematic evaluation of outcomes (including a series of performance indicators (PIs) and the analysis of all deaths) that are published as internal reports.
(ii) Near-real time clinical feedback from RCDM through weekly joint theatre clinical case conferences (JTCCC), conducted by telephone.

Performance measurement assesses both the performance in relation to an individual patient and overall system performance. Clinical effectiveness in managing the individual patient is assessed by:

(i) Identification of unexpected survivors and unexpected deaths using internationally accepted mathematical models to predict probability of survival (TRISS Methodology and A Severity Characterisation of Trauma, ASCOT).
(ii) Peer review of all deaths; peer review of all mathematical unexpected outcomes; peer review of all major trauma cases where mathematical models predict expected survival, to determine "clinical unexpected survivors."

Peer review is essential in order to validate the mathematical prediction. Review of all deaths is done jointly with military clinicians, the Home Office pathologist, and experts in

**Table 14.1** Trauma data collection

| Date | Development/event | Significance | Note reference |
|---|---|---|---|
| | Severity of wounds reported vary according to the location of medical facility relative to the conflict and the transport and evacuation available for casualties | May bias the type of injury reported | |
| | e.g., International Committee Red Cross (ICRC) hospitals on the Pakistan/Afghanistan border had traveled a considerable distance to reach the medical facility | Mean delay from wounding to treatment was 4 days thus there were few serious multiple injuries or major injuries involving head, thorax, or abdomen | Rautio and Paavolainen 1988,[18] Coupland and Howell 1988[19] |
| | In contrast Israeli action in Lebanon (1982) | Mean delay seeing a doctor was just 12 min | Rosenblatt et al. 1985 |
| | Problems collecting data during combat | Medical staff are busy and unwilling to record information that is not of immediate benefit to the casualty | Leads to some incomplete or inaccurate records (Hardaway 1978)[20] |
| 1965–1973 | Wound Data and Munitions Effectiveness Team (WDMET) (Vietnam war) | US employed a team specifically to build a database on wounds and wounding munitions | |
| | ICRC wound-scoring and recording system that has been used in their war surgery hospitals in a variety of locations | System is quick and easy to complete and was used in the Gulf conflict | Coupland 1991[21] |
| | | Useful in providing data on the nature and extent of wounds | Bowyer et al. 1993[22] |
| | The British Army's Hostile Action Casualty System (HACS) | Provided information on casualties from the internal security role | Owen-Smith 1981[23] |

Adapted by Kerry Starkey from Ryan[24]

**Fig. 14.5** The joint theatre clinical case conference (Crown Copyright, reproduced with permission)

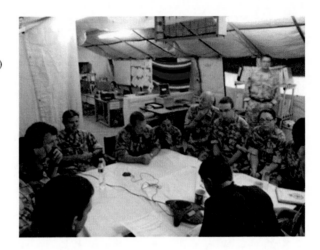

combat body armor development. Unexpected deaths identify system weaknesses, whereas unexpected survivors identify system strengths that require reinforcement. Attendance by ADMEM at each post mortem identifies clinical practice issues, which are actioned in near real-time (within days of occurrence) through the chain of command and the Joint Theatre Clinical Case Conference (Fig. 14.5).

The Joint Theatre Clinical Case Conference (JTCCC, see Fig. 14.5) is held weekly and is coordinated by ADMEM in Birmingham. The telephone conference uses a star phone at each location, with participation from in-theater clinicians in all deployed British field hospitals, RCDM (military and civilian clinicians), the Defence Rehabilitation Centre (Headley Court), and RAF Brize Norton (coordinating all aeromedical movements). Structured feedback is provided on patients admitted during the previous 2 weeks (with written case summaries forwarded the previous day via a secure e-mail system). The conference has repeatedly highlighted issues that are relevant across operational theaters and is the catalyst for rapid policy change, co-ordinated by Surgeon General's Department. Confidentiality is assured by referring to patients only by their Field Hospital admission numbers.

**Acknowledgement**   Original illustrations used in this chapter have been previously published in JR Army Med Corps and are used with permission. Blast pathway Fig. 14.3b originally designed by Col. PF Mahoney.

## References

1. Hodgetts T, Davies S, Russell R, McLeod J. Benchmarking the UK deployed trauma system. *J R Army Med Corps*. 2007;153(4):237-238.
2. National Confidential Enquiry into Patient Outcome and Death, Trauma: Who Cares, November 2007.
3. Battlefield Casualty Drills (5th edition), 2007. Army Code 71638.
4. Team Medic Casualty Drills: Aide Memoire, June 2008. Army Code 64410.

5. Hodgetts TJ, Mahoney PF, Russell MQ, Byers M. ABC to<CABC>: redefining the military trauma paradigm. *Emerg Med J.* 2006;23:745-746.
6. Brodie S, Hodgetts T, Ollerton J, McLeod J, Lambert P, Mahoney PF. Tourniquet use in combat trauma: UK military experience. *J R Army Med Corps.* 2007;153(4):310-313.
7. Beekley AC, Sebesta J, Blackbourne L, Herbert G, Kauvar D, et al. Prehospital tourniquet use in operation Iraqi freedom: effect on hemorrhage control and outcomes. *J Trauma.* 2008;64(2):S28-S37. Supplement.
8. Wedmore I, McManus J, Pusateri A, Holcomb J. A special report on the chitosan-based hemostatic dressing: experience in current combat operations. *J Trauma.* 2006;60(3):655-658.
9. Hodgetts TJ, Mahoney PF. Military pre-hospital care: why is it different? *J R Army Med Corps.* 2009;155(1):4-10.
10. Davis PR, Rickards AC, Ollerton JE. Determining the composition and benefit of the prehospital medical response team in the conflict setting. *J R Army Med Corps.* 2007;153(4): 269-273.
11. Hodgetts T, Mahoney P, Kirkman E. Damage control resuscitation. *J R Army Med Corps.* 2007;153(4):299-300.
12. Kirkman E, Watts S, Hodgetts T, Mahoney P, Rawlinson S, Midwinter M. A proactive approach to the coagulopathy of trauma: the rationale and guidelines for treatment. *J R Army Med Corps.* 2007;153(4):302-306.
13. Development, Concepts & Doctrine Centre (2009). Clinical Guidelines for Operations. Joint Defence Publication 4-03.1.
14. Hodgetts T, Mahoney P, Clasper J, eds. *Battlefield Advanced Trauma Life Support,* 5th edn. Joint Services Publication 570; 2008.
15. Davies TJ, Nadin MN, McArthur DJ, Cox C, Roberts P. Hospex 2008. *J R Army Med Corps.* 2008;154(3):195-197.
16. Healthcare Commission. Defence Medical Services: A review of the clinical governance of the Defence Medical Services in the UK and overseas. Commission for Healthcare Audit and Inspection, March 2009.
17. Smith J, Hodgetts T, Mahoney P, Russell R, Davies S, McLeod J. Trauma governance in the UK DMS. *J R Army Med Corps.* 2007;153(4):239-242.
18. Rautio J, Paavolainen P. Afghan war wounded: experience with 200 cases. *J Trauma.* 1988;28:523-525.
19. Coupland RM, Howell PR. An experience of war surgery and wounds presenting after 3 days on the border of Afghanistan. *Injury.* 1998;19:259-262.
20. Hardaway RM. Viet Nam wound analysis. *J Trauma.* 1978;18:635-643.
21. Coupland RM. *The Red Cross wound classification.* Geneva: International Committee of the Red Cross.
22. Bowyer GW, Stewart MPM, Ryan JM. Gulf war wounds; application of the Red Cross wound classification. *Injury.* 1993;24:597-600.
23. Owen-Smith MS. A computerised data retrieval system for the wounds of war; the Northern Ireland casualties. *J R Army Med Corps.* 1981;127:31-54.
24. Ryan JM, Rich NM, Dale RF, Morgans BT, Cooper GJ (1997). *Ballistic Trauma: Clinical Relevance in Peace and War.* London: Hodder Arnold pp 23-25.
25. Rosenblatt M, Lemer J, Best LA, Peleg H. Thoracic wounds in Israeli battle casualties during the 1982 evacuation of wounded from Lebanon. J Trauma. 1985 Apr;25(4):350-354.

# Part IV

## Prehospital and the Emergency Room

# Triage

# 15

Rob Russell

## 15.1
## Introduction

Incidents involving ballistic trauma are likely to produce more than one casualty. Some incidents (e.g., bombings) may generate large numbers of casualties creating Major Incidents or even Mass Casualties. Once the number of casualties outstrips the medical resources available, a system is required to ensure optimal medical care whilst making the best use of those resources.

Triage is the process of giving patients a priority for treatment and/or evacuation. The term is derived from the French "*trier*" – *to sort or to sieve*, and was originally applied to coffee beans. There are many different Triage systems that operate at different levels, but the overall aim is to enable the right patient to receive the right care at the right time in the right place. In Major Incidents this may also mean "doing the most for the most."

The concept of Triage was developed by Baron Dominique Larrey (1766–1842), Chief Surgeon to the French Armies during the Napoleonic wars.[1] Larrey's first aim was returning fit men to action so minor wounds were treated early. Thereafter, he wanted to identify the sickest for treatment.

Triage systems need to simple and rapid but reliable and reproducible between professionals and casualties. There are many methods in use world-wide. The method used will depend on the situation and the outcome that is needed. Medical and ambulance personnel at the scene of a terrorist bombing require different systems to the surgeon at the hospital deciding the order that the same casualties will go to theater.

Casualties, especially the seriously injured, will get better or worse over time and with medical intervention. The unconscious patient with a moderate isolated head injury will die if their airway is not cleared and supported but once conscious can be simply observed. To take this into account, Triage must be a dynamic process that is repeated regularly.

R. Russell
Academic Department Military Emergency Medicine,
Royal Centre for Defence Medicine and University of Birmingham, Birmingham, UK and
Emergency and Critical Care, Peterborough and Stamford Hospitals NHS Foundation Trust, Peterborough, UK
e-mail: robrussell@doctors.org.uk; rob.russell@pbh-tr.nhs.uk

A.J. Brooks et al. (eds.), *Ryan's Ballistic Trauma*,
DOI: 10.1007/978-1-84882-124-8_15, © Springer-Verlag London Limited 2011

### 15.1.1
### Triage – When?

Triage of one form or another is in day-to-day use in all health systems. Triage of an emergency call at Ambulance Control will determine the type and speed of ambulance response and whether a Doctor is despatched as well. Once the team reaches the patient, Triage is used to decide which hospital the patient goes to, how they get there, and what sort of team meets them on arrival.

Triage takes on even greater significance whenever casualties outnumber the skilled help and other resources available. A two-man ambulance crew attending a two-vehicle motor vehicle crash might be faced with six casualties. The crew must identify those with life-threatening and serious injuries after assessing all the casualties. They must then develop a plan of action for treatment and evacuation until and when assistance arrives.

At the hospital, these same casualties may all arrive in a short period of time. Ideally Ambulance Service Control will have Triaged some to other hospitals, but this may not be possible for geographical reasons. The Emergency Department may not have a resuscitation bay and a trauma team available for each patient. Triage principles will help the Emergency Consultant to determine how to allocate personnel and decide which patients are seen where. Within resuscitation, decisions based on surgical Triage will determine the order that casualties undergo investigations (e.g., X-ray, CT) and are transferred to the operating theater. Some patients may need further Triage for transfer to specialist centers such as neurosurgical or burns units.

### 15.1.2
### Triage – Where?

Triage will start remote from the patient when the first call to the Ambulance Control Center is made and the type of response decided. At the scene, Triage determines the mode of transport to hospital, if there is a choice between road ambulance and helicopter. The destination hospital may also be decided as in some trauma systems (USA, Australia) Triage determines whether the receiving hospital is a trauma center or a general hospital.

At a Major Medical Incident with multiple casualties, Triage will be performed on several occasions. First where the casualties are lying to determine initial priorities for treatment and transport to the Casualty Clearing Station. At the front door of the Casualty Clearing Station casualties will be re-Triaged for treatment within. After treatment, more Triage will decide transport priorities to hospital. Another round of Triage will take place outside the Emergency Department to re-assign treatment priorities. Then after resuscitation and assessment, priorities for surgery, CT scanning, ITU, and possible transfer to a specialist center will be determined.

UK Emergency Departments routinely carry out Triage of all patients on arrival. These circumstances are obviously very different from those pre-hospital, at a major incident or on a military deployment, but the same principles of Triage apply. Immediately life-threatening conditions and injuries are given high priority with minor injuries waiting longer. "Hospital tents" at mass gatherings such as rock festivals and sporting events have also successfully used Triage principles to ensure the best use of limited resources.[2]

## 15.1.3
## Triage – Who?

The identity of the Triage officer(s) will depend on the nature of the incident and where and when Triage is being performed. The Triage Sieve can be performed by anyone, including lay personnel, who has been trained in its use. This is because strict parameters are followed and no clinical judgement is used.

If clinical judgement is allowed at any point in the process, experienced senior staff should be allocated to Triage. Rather than wasting a valuable resource, this will produce accurate Triage, which will ensure optimal use of all resources in delivering the best care for all the casualties. Overtriage – awarding a higher priority to a patient than appropriate diverts personnel and resources away from high-priority patients. Undertriage results in casualties receiving delayed or inadequate care. Baron Larrey understood this and used his best and most experienced surgeons to Triage the wounded for theater.

## 15.2
## Priorities

It is important that a recognized system of Triage categories is used. The NATO "T" is universally recognized. This and the UK pre-hospital system are summarized in Table 15.1.[3] Each Triage priority is also assigned a color for quick recognition of labels. The International Committee of the Red Cross (ICRC) uses its own categories for casualties arriving at its hospitals (Table 15.2).[4]

The T4 or Expectant priority is only used in a "mass casualty" situation, where the number of casualties completely overwhelms the medical resources available and doing "the most for the

**Table 15.1** NATO & UK pre-hospital Triage priorities

| System | | |
|---|---|---|
| Description | T | Color |
| Immediate | 1 | Red |
| Urgent | 2 | Yellow |
| Delayed | 3 | Green |
| Expectant | 4 | Blue |
| Dead | Dead | White |

Immediate priority: Red: casualties requiring immediate procedures to save life.
e.g., airway obstruction, tension pneumothorax
Urgent priority: Yellow: casualties requiring medical treatment within 4–6 h.
e.g., compound fractures
Delayed priority: Green: casualties with injuries that can wait until after 4–6 h.
e.g., small cuts and contusions, minor closed fractures
Expectant priority: Blue: see below
Dead: White: dead casualties must be identified and clearly labeled as such to avoid re-Triage

**Table 15.2** ICRC Triage categories

| | |
|---|---|
| Category I | Patients for whom urgent surgery is required and for whom there is a good chance of reasonable survival. |
| Category II | Patients who do not require surgery. This includes those for whom reasonable survival is unlikely. |
| Category III | Patients who require surgery, but not urgently. |

most" becomes essential. T4 is given to casualties judged to have either non-survivable injuries or whose chances of survival are so small that diverting medical resources to their treatment would compromise the outcome for other casualties. The decision to initiate T4 is taken jointly by the Medical and Ambulance Commanders at the scene or, in the military, by the regional Commander Medical. T4 has not been used in any major incident in the UK to this time.

Using T4 will be against the instincts of all trauma carers but failure to initiate it when appropriate will cost lives. Examples of casualties for whom T4 would be appropriate in a mass casualty situation are severe (>80%) burns or a comatose patient with a penetrating brain injury. Once Triaged T4, casualties should still be given analgesia and comfort. If more resources become available or after other casualties have been treated and evacuated a T4 casualty is still alive, the Triage category should be reviewed.

## 15.3
## Methods

Triage methods may incorporate the mechanism of injury as well as anatomical and/or physiological data from the casualty. Using the mechanism of injury promotes a high index of suspicion for occult injury but can cause over-Triage.[5] Recognition of a mechanism associated with a high chance of serious injury allows the pre-hospital carers to activate a trauma team to receive the casualty. It is not useful when dealing with a large number of casualties. In this situation, the mechanism will have been broadly similar for all, and small variations between individuals, such as positioning in relation to an explosion will not be clear early on. A mechanism-based set of criteria for activation of a trauma team is shown in Table 15.3.

The advantage of using anatomical information is that once the injury has occurred the anatomical data is unlikely to change. However, to collect accurate anatomical information, a full secondary survey of an undressed patient is required so that all injuries are identified. This has to be done by experienced Doctor so that the injuries can be individually and collectively assessed before a priority is given. This requires time and a warm, well-lit environment. Anatomical systems are therefore time-consuming and non-dynamic.

The best indication of the current condition of a casualty is provided by a physiological method. Physiological parameters, such as Respiratory Rate, Pulse, Blood Pressure, and Conscious Level, are easily measured and do not allow for variation in interpretation. One drawback is that physiological systems do not take into account the ability of children and young adults to compensate until in extremis. However, Triage is a dynamic process and should be repeated regularly.

**Table 15.3**  Trauma team activation criteria

| | |
|---|---|
| Anatomical | >1 long-bone fracture – unilateral radius and ulna count as one<br>>1 anatomical area injured<br>Penetrating injury to head, thorax, or abdomen<br>Traumatic amputation or crush injury |
| Mechanism | Fall >6 m<br>Pedestrian or cyclist hit by car<br>Death of other occupant in same vehicle<br>Ejection from vehicle/bicycle<br>Major vehicular deformity or significant intrusion into passenger space<br>Extrication time >20 min<br>Vehicular roll-over |
| Physiological | Respiratory rate >29/min<br>Pulse rate <50 or >130 beats/min<br>Systolic blood pressure <90 mmHg<br>GCS <13 |

A physiological method (Triage Sieve) is best used when a quick snapshot of the casualties' conditions is required, e.g., at the scene of a major incident or at the front door of a Casualty Clearing Station/Emergency Department at times of high patient flow. Anatomical Triage is useful at the hospital in determining the operating priority list. A mixed method (Triage Sort) allows the Triage Officer to employ a physiological system to award a priority but then modify it up or down taking account of the anatomial injuries and is the method of choice if casualty flow allows at the Casualty Clearing Station and Emergency Department.

There are a number of Triage methods in use around the world. Two of the most commonly used methods are described below.

## 15.3.1
### The Triage Sieve[3] (Fig. 15.1)

The Triage Sieve is designed as a fast, snap-shot physiological assessment. It uses mobility, followed by a simple assessment of Airway, Breathing, and Circulation. The Sieve will overtriage patients at both extremes of age, especially those who are normally non-mobile. The pediatric Triage tape has Triage sieves adjusted for length and been validated[6] to address the Triage of young children. The severely injured but mobile patient (e.g., a patient with 40% burns) will be undertriaged by the Sieve. However, Triage is dynamic and these casualties will eventually cease to be mobile and be re-Triaged. In the meantime, they may have been able to self-evacuate to a location where more attention is possible.

The British Military use a modified version of the Triage Sieve use in the field when dealing with single casualties as well as multiple. It employs Catastrophic Hemorrhage and conscious level as well.

**Algorithm Triage Sieve**

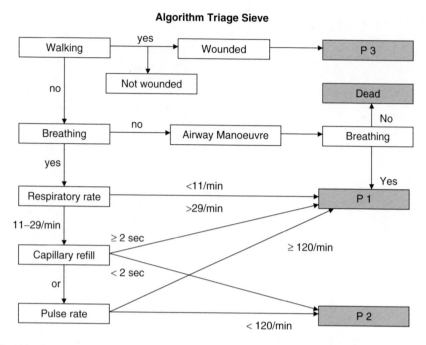

**Fig. 15.1** The algorithm Triage sieve chart (BATLS manual[8]; Advanced Life Support Group[9] with permission)

## 15.3.2
### The Triage Sort

The Triage Sort is a more sophisticated mixed Triage tool but takes longer. The Sort uses the Triage Revised Trauma Score (TRTS) as it's physiological basis but then allows the Triage Officer award a higher or lower priority if anatomical assessment demands it. The TRTS is the unweighted sum of the Revised Trauma Score[7] (RTS) values (Table 15.4).

## 15.4
### Triage Labeling Systems

Once a Triage priority has been assigned, the Triage Officer needs to give each casualty a Triage label. This tells other Triage Officers which casualties have been Triaged and Treatment and Transport teams which patients need treatment and evacuation first.

There are a large number of different labeling systems in use worldwide and there is no accepted national or international standard. As long as everyone who will use a system is familiar with it, this is not a problem. However, confusion can ensue when personnel are operating out of their normal location especially on a multi-national basis.

**Table 15.4** Triage priorities using TRTS

| Respiratory rate (per min) | 0 | 1–5 | 6–9 | 30+ | 10–29 |
|---|---|---|---|---|---|
| Points | 0 | 1 | 2 | 3 | 4 |
| Systolic blood pressure (mmHg) | 0 | 1–49 | 50–75 | 76–89 | 90+ |
| Points | 0 | 1 | 2 | 3 | 4 |
| GCS (total) | 3 | 4–5 | 6–8 | 9–12 | 13–15 |
| Points | 0 | 1 | 2 | 3 | 4 |
| Total score | Priority | | | | |
| | 12 | T3/P3 | Delayed | | |
| | 10–11 | T2/P2 | Urgent | | |
| | 1–9 | T1/P1 | Immediate | | |
| | 0 | | Dead | | |

As Triage is dynamic and reacts to changes in the casualties condition, any labeling system must also be dynamic and react to the patient either getting better and worse. A label must also be easily spotted, simple to use, robust enough to survive in the rain, and easily attached to the casualty. Other useful attributes are having an area of the label for demographic and clinical data to be recorded and updated as the patient moves along the chain of care and each label having a unique identifying number by which the casualty can later be traced through the course of the incident.

A number of labeling systems use a single colored cards for each priority. Information can be written on one side of each card. This type of system is not easily dynamic. When a casualty changes priority, a new card has to be given. Either the old card is removed and any recorded information lost unless copied over, which takes time and risks transposition errors, or it is left with the patient risking confusion as to which of the cards is the current one.

The Mettag label is another common system. It has a plain white main body for casualty information with colored strips at the base. The strips are torn off so that the one left at the bottom denotes the priority. Since the colored strips are small, it can be difficult to see what priority the patient is without going close. Also, this system only allows casualties to get worse, denoted by tearing further strips off. If there is improvement either a new label is required or a discarded strip found and stuck back on.

The best labeling systems available are those that allow all priorities to be shown by the same card. Once information has been recorded, the card is folded so that only one color is visible. If the category changes, more information is recorded and the card refolded with a different color showing, though folding the cards can be tricky if the Triage Officer is unfamiliar with them.

There is no agreed convention on labeling the expectant priority. Blue is commonly used, but both red and green cards annotated "expectant" are alternatives. Some cards allow the Triage officer to fold the corners of the green card back, showing the red behind. Whatever local alternative is in use, all those who may need to know must be informed as part of major incident planning and preparation.

## 15.5
## Summary

Triage sieves and sorts casualties allow optimal care and use of resources. Triage is a dynamic process that operates at many levels, especially with large numbers of casualties and limited resources.

Triage systems must be easy and rapid to use, as well as reliable and reproducible. The information on which Triage decisions are based must be recorded recorded on a Triage label that denotes the priority given.

The aim of Triage at all times is to give the right patient the right care, at the right time, and in the right place.

## References

1. Rignault D, Wherry D. Lessons from the past worth remembering: Larrey and Triage. *Trauma*. 1999;1:86-88.
2. Kerr GW, Parke TRJ. Providing 'T in the Park': pre–hospital care at a major crowd event. *Pre–Hospital Immediate Care*. 1999;3:11-13.
3. Advanced Life Support Group. Major Incident Medical Management and Support – The Practical Approach. London: BMJ Publishing Group; 1995.
4. Coupland RM, Parker PJ, Gray RC. Triage of war wounded: the experience of the International Committee of the Red Cross. *Injury*. 1992;23:507-510.
5. Simon BJ, Legere P, Emhoff T, et al. Vehicular trauma triage by mechanism: avoidance of the unproductive evaluation. *J Trauma*. 1994;37:645-649.
6. Wallis LA, Carley S. Validation of the Paediatric Triage Tape. *Emer Med J*. 2006;23:47-50.
7. Champion HR, Sacco WJ, Copes WS, et al. A revision of the Trauma Score. *J Trauma*. 1989; 29:623-629.
8. BATLS manual (2nd edn) D/AMD/113/23 Army Code No 63726 (2000).
9. Advanced Life Support Group Major Incident Medical Management and Support, 2nd ed. London: BMJ Books; 2002.

# Prehospital Care

# 16

Mark Byers, John-Joe Reilly, and Peter F. Mahoney

## 16.1
## Introduction

Prehospital care of the ballistic casualty should be considered as two intertwined areas:

1. Management of the situation.
2. Management of the casualty.

Managing the situation involves understanding what is happening at the ballistic incident, who is in charge, the medic's role within this situation, and what medical advice and actions are appropriate.

Managing the injured casualty consists of first aid and advanced care *appropriate to the situation.*

## 16.2
## The Situation: Three Environments of Care

Medics who attend ballistic trauma will find themselves providing care in one of three environments: non-permissive, semipermissive, and permissive. This also has been described as Care Under Fire, Tactical Field Care, and Combat Casualty Evacuation Care.[1,2]

### 16.2.1
### The Non-permissive Environment: Care Under Fire

This may occur when a tactically trained medic or medically trained member of an assault team is providing care. A non-permissive environment implies that either the medic or the casualty is under a direct threat. The risks may range from being inside a dangerous structure to being

J.-Joe Reilly (✉)
Academic Department of Military Surgery and Trauma,
Royal Centre for Defence Medicine, University Hospital Birmingham, UK
e-mail: john-joe@doctors.org.uk

A.J. Brooks et al. (eds.), *Ryan's Ballistic Trauma*,
DOI: 10.1007/978-1-84882-124-8_16, © Springer-Verlag London Limited 2011

present during a shooting and under fire. It is not a place in which to deliver medical care. The aim is to extract the casualty in any way practicable without the medic becoming a casualty.

### 16.2.2
### The Semi-Permissive Environment: Tactical Field Care

This environment is not safe, but the direct threat is removed (albeit probably temporarily). Casualty and rescuer might be behind cover, but there is no guarantee the potential assailant or threat will not move and threaten them again.

### 16.2.3
### The Permissive Environment: Combat Casualty Evacuation Care

A permissive environment is a safe environment. In this area the medic should be highly visible and have access to the full range of equipment and resources carried by any prehospital-care practitioner. This does not mean that the medic should delay the casualty's move to hospital.

All three environments will exist around an incident and also can be related to areas of operational control (see Fig. 16.1).

Care in these environments is considered later in the chapter.

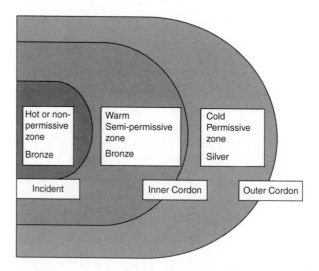

**Fig. 16.1** Zones of care. The non-permissive, semi-permissive, and permissive environments respectively translate to the so called Hot, Warm, and Cold zones around an incident. There is an approximate correlation with the command zones described in the Major Incident Medical Management and Support (MIMMS) course and manual (see ref.[3] and Table 16.3). Bronze describes tactical command at an incident and silver describes operational command. Gold or strategic command is some way distant to the incident. Bronze of MIMMS equates approximately to the Hot (non permissive) and Warm (semi permissive) zones, the areas inside the inner cordon. Silver of MIMMS equates to the Cold (permissive) zone between the inner and outer cordons. The permissive zone beyond the outer cordon is within the Gold area

## 16.3
## The Prehospital Environment

### 16.3.1
### Preparation

Preparing for the prehospital environment begins long before the call out. Prehospital medical practitioners require proper training, the correct clothing and equipment, and an understanding of the environment in which they are working.

### 16.3.2
### Training

The type and level of training required depends on where you are working, for whom you are working, and why you are working there. An individual responding as part of civilian Emergency Medical Service (EMS) has different requirements to the medic working with a military group or police firearms team. A progressive training path is given in Table 16.1.

### 16.3.3
### Clothing

Dress with safety in mind – either to be seen or not to be seen, depending on the setting. Prehospital-care practitioners providing care in a permissive location should wear high-visibility clothing, jackets or tabards, trousers or coveralls, and a helmet that is sufficiently robust and meets the safety specification for the job. The clothing also should conform to the dress codes

**Table 16.1** Training

(a) *Basic first aid*. Basic first aid as taught by British Red Cross, St. John Ambulance, and the Military gives the tools for initial casualty care with minimal resources. Basic first-aid courses can be accessed from local Red Cross and St. John training organizations.

(b) *Specific prehospital training*. Progressive training and qualification in prehospital care is offered and overseen in the UK by the Faculty of Prehospital Care at the Royal College of Surgeons (RCS) of Edinburgh. Training is delivered by organizations such as BASICS Education Ltd. An initial qualification is the RCS's Pre-Hospital Emergency Care Certificate. After this comes the Diploma in Immediate Medical Care (Dip IMC) and the Fellowship in Immediate Medical Care (FIMC). *Contact:* Faculty of Pre-Hospital Care, The Royal College of Surgeons of Edinburgh, Nicolson Street, Edinburgh EH8 9DW; e-mail: fphc@rcsed.ac.uk; BASICS Education Ltd., Turret House, Turret Lane, Ipswich IP4 1DL; e-mail: educ@basics.org.uk.

(c) For Major Incident Management Training: Major Incident Medical Management and Support Course (MIMMS). *Details from:* Advanced Life Support Group, http://www.alsg.org.

(d) *Additional Training*. Additional tactical and field training is needed for individuals providing close medical support to police and military organizations. This needs to be geared around the likely operating environments of these organizations.

of the organization being represented. Clothing should be marked clearly with the name and position/specialty of the practitioner, and at night, they should have reflectors and a torch, preferably a head torch. Guidance for BASICS (British Association for Immediate Care) Doctors on pre-hospital clothing can be found on the BASICS website (http://www.basics.org.uk).

Practitioners in the tactical environment should wear the same protective clothing as the tactical team. This should include, as a minimum, ballistic body armor and a ballistic helmet. This equipment is heavy and unwieldy, and practice is required to operate efficiently in it.

## 16.3.4
### Medical Equipment

This should be adequate for the task, but this needs to be balanced against the necessity to carry it. The practitioner working in a safe area has far more latitude than the practitioner working within a safety cordon. The tactical medic must balance utility with load and should carry as little as possible packed as small as possible. Suggested packing lists can be found in Table 16.2.

**Table 16.2** Suggested packing lists

|  | Tactical field care provider | Civilian pre-hospital care provider |
|---|---|---|
|  | Day Sack / Medical Pouch | Rucksack / Bergen |
| Tactical Clothing | Tactical Medical Vest / Chest webbing | Protective clothing suitable for the operating environment |
| Catastrophic Haemorrhage Control | Combat Application Tourniquet Hemcon$^{Tm}$/Quik Clot$^{Tm}$ (if required) Celox gauze$^{Tm}$ (if required) | Combat Application Tourniquet (if situation dictates) |
| Airway (with C-spine control) | Oro-pharyngeal airway Naso-pharyngeal airway Surgical airway kit | Oro-pharyngeal airway Naso-pharyngeal airway Self inflated Bag/Mask/Valve Set Avanced airway equipment (if trained) Laryngeal Mask Laryngoscope Endotracheal tubes End tidal CO$_2$ monitor Surgical airway kit Cervical collars Spinal stabilisation (blocks, tape etc) |
| Breathing | Asherman$^{Tm}$ chest seals Large bore cannulae | Asherman$^{Tm}$ chest seals Large bore cannulae Chest drain kit |
| Circulation | First field dressings Intravenous cannulae Intravenous fluids (as tactical situation and weight limit allows) Intravenous giving sets FAST-1 Sternal IO Device | Dressings Intravenous cannulae Intravenous fluids Intravenous giving sets Pressure infuser Intraosseous access and infusion kits |

**Table 16.2**  (continued)

|  | Tactical field care provider | Civilian pre-hospital care provider |
|---|---|---|
| Drugs | IM Morphine auto-injector (if required) Antibiotics (dependent upon operating environment) | Opiate analgesic Anti-emetic Benzodiazepine Rapid Sequence Induction drugs (if appropriately trained) Primary care medications |
| Diagnostic Equipment | As dictated by individual training and tactical environment | Stethoscope Sphygmomanometer Torch BM testing kit Opthalmoscope Auroscope |
| Clothing | Tactical clothing as dictated by operational environment | Protective headgear High visibility vest/trousers Protective boots Personal protective equipment (latex gloves/goggles) |
| Paediatric Equipment | Not required | Paediatric aide memories Triage tapes Paediatric trauma pack |
| Packaging and Transport | Folding combat stretcher (if required) Straps Splints Tape | Stretcher (scoop or solid) Straps Splints Extrication kit (if required) |
| Administration | Triage cards Cylume sticks (multiple colours) 9-liner aide memoire Casualty cards Required paperwork Reference books (if required) Permanent markers | Triage cards Casualty cards Aide memoires (as required) Required paperwork |

## 16.4
## The Prehospital Environment

### 16.4.1
### Practice

The ballistic incident may range from an accident at a rural shooting ground to a siege and hostage situation. Each situation presents its own problems. What follows is a generic approach that can be adapted to circumstances.

### 16.4.1.1
### Arriving at the Scene

On receipt of a request to attend an incident involving firearms, it is important to consider:

- *who* has made the request;
- who is in charge of the situation (usually police) If there is no police presence at the scene, it is prudent to confirm they will be attending.
- *where* you are to report [the incident control point (ICP)];
- the *type* of incident;
- routes in and out;
- the numbers of casualties involved;
- who else is attending.

The acronym METHANE (Table 16.3) developed and taught by the Advanced Life Support Group (ALSG) in their Major Incident Medical Management and Support course[3] can be adapted to help remember the information that is required and provides a format for sending a situation report or reporting an incident. Major Incident Medical Management and Support is used by the UK military and is also being taught by a number of North Atlantic Treaty Organization (NATO) armies (T.J. Hodgetts, personal communication, November 2003).

For a simple accident, it may just be a case of being taken to the casualty, ensuring scene safety (such as confirming where the weapon involved is), giving appropriate care, and arranging evacuation to hospital.

A more complex situation may require:

- a clear statement of your tasks;
- the commander's concept of how the operation will progress;
- current intelligence and any information on the numbers and locations of the threat;
- numbers of casualties, locations, and routes to and from them;
- other agencies present, such as police, fire, ambulance, and military;
- clothing and equipment required;
- who is escorting you around the incident;
- the location of support services in the event of a long operation (such as catering);
- signal commands being employed.

Finally, watches should be synchronized to the same time as the commanders (Table 16.4).

**Table 16.3** METHANE report

| |
|---|
| M – My name or name of person requesting assistance |
| E – Exact location of the incident |
| T – Type of incident |
| H – Hazards affecting the incident |
| A – Access routes to the Incident Control Point |
| N – Numbers of casualties and severity |
| E – Emergency services involved or required |

From MIMMS Manual BMJ Books 2002. With permission of BMJ and Prof TJ Hodgetts

**Table 16.4**  Orders process

| |
|---|
| The orders process: Information required by you or those working for you. |
| Ground Brief – a short description of the ground/terrain/environment in which you will be working. |
| Situation Report – Up-to-date information on what is happening, including the threat, casualties, and supporting assets. |
| Task – Your task specifically. |
| Execution of the Task – The commanders' concept of the operation, his intentions and plan, and your role within it. In addition, details of all the tasks delegated to individuals in the team and their place in the overall plan. Finally, coordinating instructions, including timings, movement, and routes to be used. |
| Support Information – Dress and equipment. The location and arrangements of facilities available for feeding, washing, sleeping, and personal hygiene during the task. |
| Signals and Commands – Pre-arranged signals, their meanings, and the command structure. |
| The Time – Synchronize your watch with the commanders. |

## 16.5
## Scene Assessment

The first rule of any prehospital-care incident is safety. This includes safety of the medic, other members of the emergency services, of the public, of the casualty, and of the scene. Every year, prehospital-care providers are injured or killed in both the civilian and military environments because of failing to follow this rule.

Prior to voluntarily entering the scene, the practitioner should understand the level of risk. If a casualty is seen to be lying on the ground, is it safe to approach? If the environment is non-permissive, then a value judgment should be made. The situation will not improve if the rescuer becomes a casualty. A casualty who has suffered a high-velocity head wound is unlikely to survive regardless of the level of care provided, and if the perpetrator were still at large, it would be foolhardy to enter the area. It may be possible to assess the casualty from a safe place, construct a secure approach, and ensure a successful outcome. Do not rush into an incident until a proper assessment of risk has been made and heed advice from the experts.

## 16.6
## Non-permissive Environment

### 16.6.1
### Treatment

This should be rapid and simple:
<C> Catastrophic hemorrhage control by direct pressure, novel haemostatics, or tourniquets.

A. consider turning the casualty to a recovery position or similar to prevent airway obstruction. Cervical spine (C spine) control is not going to be achieved in these circumstances.

Extract the casualty by whatever means is possible. This may mean physically dragging the casualty to cover.

### 16.6.2
### ABC or < C > ABC?

ABC is "airway, breathing, and circulation," the traditional Advanced Trauma Life Support approach to trauma.

<C>ABC stands for "Catastrophic hemorrhage, Airway, Breathing, and Circulation" and is taught on the current UK Battlefield Advanced Trauma Life Support Course – BATLS.[4,5]

Potential survivors of ballistic injury are most at risk from hemorrhage. "Catastrophic hemorrhage, Airway, and Breathing" requires one to deal rapidly with catastrophic or massive hemorrhage by applying pressure to the bleeding point (by kneeling on the wound or the application of a tourniquet) and then move onto airway care. A casualty with non-compressible hemorrhage needs surgical intervention and only the management of *life-threatening* airway and breathing problems should delay their transfer to surgery.

## 16.7
## Semi-Permissive Environment

### 16.7.1
### Treatment

*Within tactical medical care, this is likely to be working within the police cordon.* If the medic has to go forward into this area, an escort should be provided. The medic should be protected at all times while within the cordon by a suitably trained member of the incident team. This is most likely to be a police officer trained in the use of firearms. The officers' role is not to act as a drip stand or extra pair of hands, but to provide security.

The focus remains on getting the medic and casualty to safety, but if time is available, further care can be carried out:

<C>Management of catastrophic bleeding is reassessed along with continuing need for tourniquets

(A) Management of the airway using simple maneuvers and adjuncts such as nasopharyngeal airways. C spine control may be appropriate in a blunt injury, but not in a penetrating injury (see below);

(B) Asherman Chest Seal™ if access to a sucking chest wound is possible; Possibly needle decompression of a tension pneumothorax (very difficult to assess in this location);

(C) Continued hemorrhage control for non catastrophic bleeds.

Extracting the casualty: depends on potential threat. If the situation is volatile, then rapid extraction is needed.

## 16.8
## Cervical Spine Control?

Cervical spine immobilization is employed in the management of the blunt trauma casualty where clinical signs, symptoms, or the mechanism of injury lead one to suspect biomechanical instability in the cervical spine. The concern is that further movement will cause or aggravate a spinal cord injury.

In penetrating trauma, this approach has been reviewed for a number of reasons:

- Ballistic injury to the cervical spine has a very high fatality rate. Much of this is due to adjacent vascular structures being disrupted. Such wounds may or may not involve the spinal cord.[6]
- In the survivor, these wounds generally are accepted to be stable (see Chap. 23) and moving the casualty is unlikely to cause neurological injury.
- Placing collars and other immobilization devices in a non-permissive environment will have minimal benefit, cause evacuation delays, and the delays may endanger both casualty and rescuer.[5,7]
- A cervical collar may obscure developing life-threatening injuries such as a developing hematoma in the neck that can compromise the airway.[8]

In the military environment, cervical spine immobilization for penetrating injury to the neck is not advocated.

Where a penetrating injury has occurred alongside a blunt injury (e.g., casualty shot in the neck and falls off a roof), then immobilization may be carried out for the blunt injury unless to do so would endanger both the casualty and the rescuer.

### 16.8.1
### Permissive Environment

The practitioner can perform the assessments and treatment *appropriate to the casualty's condition*, as will be discussed below. The aim is not to delay definitive hospital treatment.

The decisions that need to be made are how quickly can the patient be transferred safely and by what means can this be achieved?

- *Do nothing at the scene that cannot be carried out safely in transit, and*
- *do nothing in transit that would not be better carried out in a hospital.*

Ballistic trauma is still relatively uncommon in most parts of the UK so it is important to guard against becoming overawed by the injury or the situation.

## 16.9
## Do Not Forget the < C > ABCs

### 16.9.1
### ASSESS

<C>Review management of catastrophic bleeding- including tourniquets.

(A) Is the airway clear? If not, what must be done to secure it? Will a simple adjunct be sufficient, or must the patient have a definitive airway (surgical or endotracheal) to allow transfer?

(B) What is required to improve respiration? Can any defect be closed with an Asherman Chest Seal™? Does the patient now need chest drainage, or will a needle thoracostomy do? How much oxygen is available? Is evacuation by helicopter or other aircraft? Does this influence my decision on chest drainage?

(C) Has all compressible hemorrhage been secured? Is there uncompressible hemorrhage that needs the attention of a surgeon? Does the patient now need intravenous (IV) access, or can it be secured in transit? Does the patient need fluids, and if so, is hypovolemic or normotensive resuscitation appropriate?

(D) What neurological assessment of the patient is required? Does the patient need a Glasgow Coma Score (GCS) or is an AVPU Score sufficient? AVPU means "is the casualty Alert or responding to Voice or only responding Pain or Unresponsive? Is the patient's airway at risk because of neurological trauma and a decreased consciousness level? Assess gross extremity neurology.

(E) Does the patient have any extremity trauma? Does the casualty need limb splintage or pelvic compression straps to improve survival? Can the patient be stabilized on the stretcher and evacuated, or is a traction splint needed first?

A secondary survey rarely is required in pre-hospital care unless time and location dictate it and it usually is achieved better in hospital.

## 16.10
## New Developments

Many of the new developments in the field of pre-hospital care have been driven by combat experience in theaters of operations around the world. The focus of these developments has been wide ranging, however of particular use to pre-hospital practitioners has been the introduction of technologies and equipment that focus on treating the <C> ABC of the injured ballistic casualty.

## 16.11
## Intraosseous Access

The development of devices that enable intraosseous (IO) access to a casualty are particularly noteworthy. IO access has been used since the 1930s, but has gained increasing acceptance over the last 15 years, due to various studies that have shown the efficacy of IO access in emergency situations.[5] Gaining IO access involves using a drill and suitably mounted drill tip catheter to drill into various bony prominences, usually the sternum, tibia, and distal femur. There are also spring-loaded, impact-driven systems that inject catheters to a pre-set depth. The marrow of long bones has a rich network of blood vessels that drain into a central venous canal, emissary veins, and, ultimately, the central circulation. Therefore, the bone marrow functions as a venous access route that cannot collapse when hypovolaemia has occurred. This is particular important when peripheral veins may have collapsed because of vasoconstriction. The intraosseous (IO) route allows medications and fluids to enter the central circulation within seconds. IO access has a high success and low complication rate.[5]

A skilled practitioner can get IO access on a critically injured patient in 10–20 s, which can prove potentially life-saving. There are relatively few absolute contraindications for traditional tibial IO access, however fractures of the tibia and femur at the site of access or above or below is one, for obvious reasons. In this eventuality IO access through the sternum using specialist kits can be attempted.

---

## 16.12
## Novel Haemostatics

Another area of interest to the pre-hospital practitioner is the development of novel agents that promote haemostasis and coagulation with the primary use of arresting potentially catastrophic hemorrhage. The development of these agents has its origins in the second Gulf War. The significantly high casualty rate sustained by United States forces led to an aggressive program of research to try and identify novel topical haemostatic agents that could be used in patients with uncompressible massive external hemorrhage in situations where a tourniquet was either unsuitable (hemorrhage from the major vessels, or junctional wounds in the groin and axilla) or unavailable.[9] There are currently two main products whose usage dominates in the military environment, although there are more in development that will challenge this position in the future. Their use remains controversial.

*Quickclot*© is an inert powder that is derived from volcanic rock. The original version had exothermic properties and was designed to be poured directly into a major wound and stop major hemorrhage. It has been shown to be useful in haemostasis, but does have drawbacks. Its powder nature and exothermic properties (when in contact with liquid) mean that unintentional cutaneous burns – especially when coming into contact with mucous membranes – have been sustained by some when it has been used in a windy environment. New formularies and delivery systems have been introduced to overcome these issues.

*Hemcon*© is a dressing coated in a substance derived from shellfish protein, and is designed to be capable of arresting hemorrhage from high pressure arterial lacerations. It functions by the molecular attraction of red blood cells to form an active clot – and can do this with or without the presence of blood clotting factors. It can also produce a clot in the hypothermic patient, which is a major advantage in the patient that has sustained polytrauma.

This is an area of rapid development and new products are undergoing assessment for pre-hospital use all the time.

## 16.13
## Tourniquets

The use of tourniquets on the battlefield is aimed to control massive compressible external limb hemorrhage. There is a substantial body of evidence to support this assertion.[5] Yet, in the civilian setting the use of tourniquets is still frowned upon in some quarters and positively rejected in others.

Commercially available tourniquets are designed to be applied within a short time frame by the injured soldier – one handed if need be – in order to stop major bleeding from the extremities. Tourniquets have become popular with the military, due the incidence of traumatic amputation associated with ballistic and blast injuries. Tourniquets should always be applied as distally as possible in order to preserve as much viable tissue as is practical.

## 16.14
## Evacuation and the Chain of Care

The prehospital practitioner should not see him or herself as acting in isolation, but as part of a team whose aim is to return the casualty to health. The aim is to do what is appropriate at each level to ensure safe movement onto the next, but not to perform procedures that are better done further down the chain of care.

Within the UK military environment this is described as "roles". Role 1 is care under the direction of a doctor (such as a Regimental Aid Post), Role 3 provides hospital-level care, and Role 4 is definitive care, usually provided away from the conflict, (e.g., the NHS and associated military facilities). Role 2 provides the link between Roles 1 and 3. A Role 2 facility with surgical teams attached is described as "Role 2+".[10]

Monitoring should be employed prior to or during evacuation. The minimal level of monitoring is a fully trained medic looking after the patient and who is capable of dealing with any unexpected emergencies that may occur.

The use of electronic monitors for pulse oximetry, electrocardiogram (ECG), and blood pressure will be dictated by availability and the situation. Prehospital monitoring used by London Helicopter Emergency Medical Service (HEMS) has been described by Morley.[11]

## 16.15
## Packaging and Transfer

The default transport is a properly equipped and crewed emergency ambulance providing a rapid move to a suitable hospital.

At shooting incidents, military, police, and medical helicopters may be in attendance. When used correctly, helicopters can provide a rapid move to hospital, but a number of factors need to be considered.

An Emergency Air Ambulance or a police helicopter with dual police and ambulance tasking should be suitably crewed and equipped to care for and transport casualties. A police helicopter operating only in the police role or military helicopter not configured for casevac is unlikely to have the appropriate crew and equipment. That is not to say they cannot be used effectively if crew and equipment can be carried by them.

Not all hospitals have a helicopter landing site (HLS). Of those that do, few are suitable for night operations in the UK. A significant number are some distance away from the emergency department, and an additional ambulance journey may be required from the HLS to the hospital.

## 16.16
## The Crime Scene

It is nearly always inevitable that, unless at war, a ballistic incident will be a crime scene. This will often apply in peace support and "post conflict" military operations. This has implications for the medic.

If the incident is to be investigated, it is incumbent on all involved to contaminate the scene as little as possible. The practitioner should not interfere with the scene unless it is an unavoidable part of the treatment of a casualty. The dead should not be moved unless it is to gain access to the living. If they are moved, this must be recorded. Artifacts, weapons, and shell casings should not be moved. The death should be confirmed by a doctor in the presence of a police officer. The medical practitioner's movements and role within the incident need to be documented. At the end of the incident, nobody should leave the scene without the permission of the incident commander. Forensics is considered further in Chap. 12.

## 16.17
## Summary

Ballistic trauma produces many problems for the prehospital practitioner. These are not just related to the injuries, but also to the hazards of the situation. Proper training, equipment, and clothing, coupled with an awareness of the dangers encountered and knowledge of how to act and react to the particular circumstances, should lead to the best possible outcome for the casualty and team. Understand the command structure of the incident, the roles and responsibilities of all involved, and the need of the police to investigate the scene. It is not a situation for the amateur, but for a committed and experienced individual who is properly trained. If such an incident is encountered unexpectedly then remember safety, situational awareness, and risk assessment. Clinically do simple procedures well followed by timely transfer of the casualty to an appropriate hospital. Above all else remember individual safety.

## Aide Memoire

Be prepared.

Be familiar with equipment. Keep equipment up to date.

Train regularly with supported service.

Receive METHANE report.

Arrive Safely.

Receive orders.

Non-permissive care: <C>Clear airway.

Semi-permissive care: Minimal care consistent with safety. Transfer as soon as possible.

Permissive care: All you need to, nothing you do not.

Rapid package and transfer by the most appropriate means.

## References

1. Butler FK, Hagmann J, Butler E. Tactical combat casualty care in special operations. *Mil Med.* 1996;161(suppl 3):3-16.
2. De Lorenzo RA, Porter RS. *Tactical Emergency Care: Military and Operational Out of Hospital Medicine.* Upper Saddle River, NJ: Brady Prentice Hall; 1999.
3. Advanced Life Support Group. *Major Incident Medical Management and Support.* 2nd ed. London: BMJ Books; 2005.
4. American College of Surgeons Committee on Trauma. Advanced Trauma Life Support Student Course Manual. 8th ed. Chicago, IL: 2008.
5. Joint Services Publication 570: Battlefield Advanced Trauma Life Support. 4th ed. 2008.
6. Bellamy RF. The nature of combat injuries and the role of ATLS in their management. In: *Combat Casualty Care Guidelines: Operation Desert Storm.* Washington, DC: Office of the Surgeon General, Center of Excellence, Walter Reed Army Medical Center; February 1991.
7. Holcolmb J, Mabry R. Trauma: primary and secondary survey. In: Whitlock WL (chief ed.) *Special Operations Forces Medical Handbook.* Jackson, Wyoming: Teton NewMedia; 2001: 7-1–7-5.
8. Barkana Y, Stein M, Scope A, et al. Prehospital stabilisation of the cervical spine for penetrating injuries of the neck – is it necessary? *Injury.* 2000;31:305-309.
9. Mahoney PF, Russell RJ, Russell MQ, et al. Novel haemostatics in military medicine. *J R Army Med Corps.* 2005;151:139-141.
10. *The Organisation of Medical Support in Army Medical Services Core Doctrine. Principles.* 2000, Crown Copyright.
11. Morley AP. Prehospital monitoring of trauma patients: experience of a helicopter emergency medical service. *Br J Anaesthesia.* 1996;76:726-730.

# Emergency Department Management

**17**

Jason Smith

## 17.1
## Introduction

The Emergency Department management of patients with ballistic trauma should include rapid assessment and life-saving intervention, followed by appropriate investigation and referral for definitive management depending on the haemodynamic status of the patient (Figs. 17.1–17.4).

## 17.2
## Preparation

Prior notification of the imminent arrival of a trauma patient is vital if an adequate and prepared response is to be initiated. Equipment should be prepared, personnel amassed and briefed, and theater and blood bank notified of the imminent arrival of the patient. Penetrating torso trauma should prompt the activation of a multi-disciplinary trauma team, the typical composition of which is described in Fig. 17.5. The team in attendance should be dressed in the appropriate protective equipment (including lead aprons). Equipment preparation should include the means to perform rapid sequence induction of anesthesia and intubation, chest decompression, and vascular access. Radiography should be present and prepared to perform a chest X-ray during the first few minutes of assessment (pre-loading X-ray plates if necessary).

J. Smith
Academic Department of Military Emergency Medicine, Royal Centre for Defence Medicine
Birmingham Research Park, Vincent Drive, Birmingham, B15 2SQ UK
e-mail: jasonesmith@doctors.org.uk

A.J. Brooks et al. (eds.), *Ryan's Ballistic Trauma*,
DOI: 10.1007/978-1-84882-124-8_17, © Springer-Verlag London Limited 2011

**Fig. 17.1** MERT

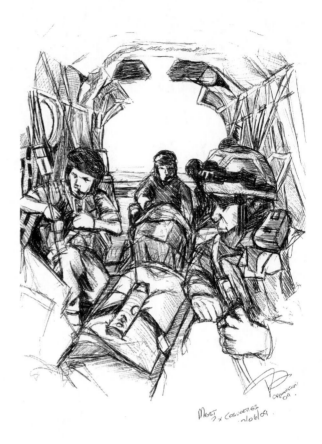

## 17.3
## Arrival

As the patient arrives in the resuscitation room, the trauma team leader should be easily identified. The whole trauma team needs to listen in to a brief handover from the pre-hospital team, prior to transfer from the ambulance stretcher to the resuscitation trolley. This occurs most easily if there is silence other than the person giving the handover. The handover should give a brief summary of events in an easily digestable format, such as the MIST handover (Table 17.1).

The only exception to this is if there is an immediate requirement for definitive airway management, in which case the airway physician and assistant need to address this while the rest of the team take the handover.

The patient then needs to be transferred from stretcher to trolley, followed by a primary survey including assessment and treatment of catastrophic hemorrhage, airway, breathing, circulation, and disability (Table 17.2).

**Fig. 17.2** Work coming in

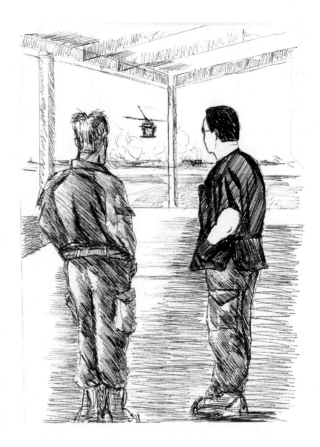

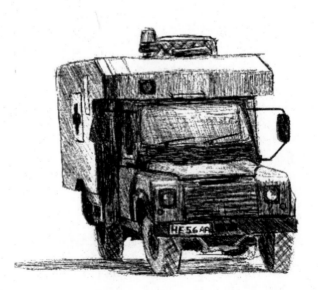

**Fig. 17.3** Ambulance

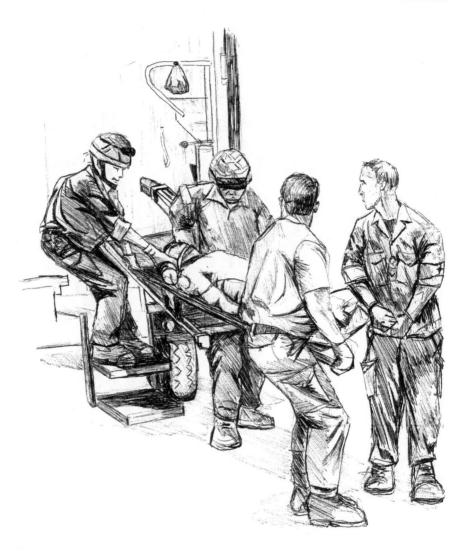

**Fig. 17.4** Offload

## 17.4
### The Primary Survey - < C > ABCDE

Traditional trauma courses teach a vertical and sequential approach to assessing the trauma patient, starting with airway, moving on to breathing and then circulation. In reality, in the presence of a trauma team, this primary survey should happen horizontally or simultaneously, with the airway physician at the head end assessing and managing the airway and administering oxygen, while the primary survey physician assesses breathing, monitoring is attached by an assistant, and intravenous access is gained by the procedures physician.

**Fig. 17.5** A trauma team –
layout of seven personnel
around a resus bay (team
leader, airway plus one,
procedures plus one, survey,
scribe) (Reprinted with
permission from Hodgetts
and Mahoney 2008)

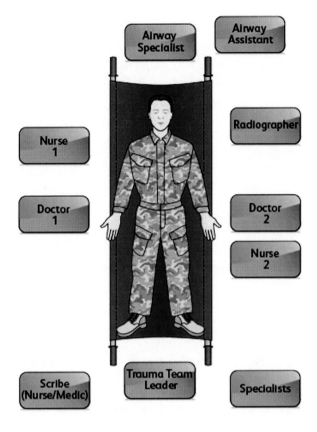

**Table 17.1** MIST handover

| M | Mechanism of injury |
|---|---|
| I | Injuries sustained |
| S | Signs – vital signs including pulse, respiratory rate, blood pressure and Glasgow coma score |
| T | Treatment – pre-hospital treatment administered |

**Table 17.2** Primary survey

| <C> | Catastrophic hemorrhage (control of exsanguinating hemorrhage) |
|---|---|
| A | Airway (and consider cervical spine injury) |
| B | Breathing (give high flow oxygen) |
| C | Circulation (control of hemorrhage and circulatory access) |
| D | Disability |
| E | Exposure and control of environment |

The radiographer should be moving in to perform a chest X-ray, and the team leader and surgeon making an initial assessment of whether or not immediate surgery is indicated. The operating theater staff needs an update at this stage as to whether they need to prepare for the imminent arrival of a trauma patient.

Key questions during the primary survey are:

- Is there uncontrolled external hemorrhage?
- Does the patient require a definitive airway?
- Does the chest need decompression?
- Is the patient cardiovascularly unstable?

## 17.4.1
### Is There Uncontrolled External Hemorrhage?

In the presence of continuing hemorrhage, attention needs to be directed at controlling this by pressure and elevation, use of a tourniquet, sutures, or novel haemostatic agents.

## 17.4.2
### Does the Patient Require a Definitive Airway?

In the presence of airway obstruction, it may be necessary to secure a definitive airway. Indications for this are listed in Table 17.3. This is usually performed by rapid sequence induction of anesthesia and intubation, but in the presence of complicating factors such as an airway burn, or expanding neck haematoma, other methods such as gaseous induction, the use of fibreoptic instruments or a surgical airway may be necessary.

## 17.4.3
### Does the Chest Need Decompression?

When assessing breathing, attention should be paid to symmetry, expansion, air entry, and external evidence of injury. Half of the chest is obscured in the supine trauma patient, so

**Table 17.3** Common indications for tracheal intubation in ballistic trauma

| |
|---|
| Airway obstruction (absolute or impending) <br>   Facial trauma <br>   Expanding neck haematoma |
| Airway burn injury |
| Reduced conscious level including agitation |
| Requirement for anesthesia |
| Requirement for ventilation |

early log roll is essential to detect injury on the back. Physiological parameters including respiratory rate, pulse, blood pressure and oxygen saturation should be measured. In the presence of asymmetrical chest movement, reduced air entry and abnormal physiology, the patient may require urgent chest decompression for treatment of a tension pneumothorax. The classical signs of a tension pneumothorax (deviation of the trachea, engorged neck veins, hyper-resonance) are often not present in the spontaneously ventilating patient.

Decompression could be performed with a needle or cannula, placed into the second intercostal space in the mid-clavicular line, although this method is unreliable and often fails to resolve the problem. Definitive chest decompression by thoracostomy (making the hole through which an intercostal drain is inserted) is often necessary to relieve pressure. This is safe if performed in the fourth or fifth intercostal space, just anterior to the mid-axillary line.

### 17.4.4
### Is the Patient Shocked?

The next question is whether the patient is displaying signs of hemorrhagic shock. In the presence of shock from ballistic injury, the cause is almost always hemorrhage, and control of hemorrhage is therefore the immediate priority. In the meantime, vital organ perfusion should be maintained, although the absolute level of blood pressure (or other physiological target) that should be maintained is still the matter of some debate. A practical solution is to maintain consciousness, although some would advocate titrating intravenous fluid to the maintenance of a radial pulse.

With regard to which fluid to use, there is ongoing debate as to which is the optimal fluid for use in trauma. The role of the newer colloids and hypertonic solutions has yet to be fully established and increasingly there has been a move to the early use of blood and blood products in severely injured ballistic casualties. The reality is that whatever fluid is given, surgical hemorrhage control must be the absolute priority.

### 17.5
### Initial Investigations

In time-critical patients, only those investigations that will immediately alter management should be performed. Typically, for penetrating torso trauma, this will include a chest X-ray, collection of blood for cross-matching, and little else.

At the same time as blood is drawn, however, an initial venous blood gas will give useful information regarding blood pH, serum lactate, and base deficit, and blood should also be sent for a baseline full blood count, clotting profile, and electrolyte screen.

The role of focused assessment with sonography for trauma (FAST) in penetrating torso trauma is less convincing than in blunt trauma. The same principles apply, in that if there is free intra-peritoneal blood, and the patient is shocked, they will require surgery. FAST can be used to triage the body cavities for surgery.

## 17.6
## Secondary Survey

It is particularly important in penetrating trauma that a full and thorough secondary survey is performed to identify wounds that may be entry or exit wounds. This includes a log roll to examine the back, and careful examination of the scalp, axillae, and perineum. Small wounds may be hidden among hair so dried blood needs to be cleaned off and the underlying structures examined.

## 17.7
## Decision Making

Patients with ballistic trauma fall into two groups. They are either physiologically normal or abnormal. The abnormal group can be further subdivided into those in whom critical organ perfusion can be maintained, and those in whom it can not. This final group need urgent surgery to control hemorrhage or they will die. This should not be delayed further and such patients should be transferred to theater within a few minutes of arrival in hospital.

At the other end of the spectrum there is the patient with anatomical evidence of injury but no physiological disturbance. This patient can undergo further investigation in the form of X-rays, contrast-enhanced computed tomography (CT), or angiography as necessary. Somewhere between these lies the group of patients who respond to initial resuscitation, but have had at some time evidence of physiological disturbance. These patients will often require surgery, but there may be time to perform limited investigations such as CT or angiography to better inform the surgeon.

The decision as to the disposal of the patient and the time-critical nature of their condition needs to be made at a senior level, with appropriate senior surgical expertise to support it.

## 17.8
## Handover

Adequate verbal and written handover of the key points are vital for seamless care of the trauma patient. In UK hospitals, the team leader in the resuscitation room will normally be an emergency physician, who will hand over responsibility to in-hospital clinicians as the patient leaves the emergency department. A clear delineation of responsibilities should be in place so there is no confusion. In an ideal world, trauma patients would be admitted under a named trauma surgeon who will oversee care and recruit the expertise of other specialties as necessary. Documentation should be clear and standardized to minimize confusion.

## Further Reading

Hodgetts TJ, Mahoney PF, Russell MQ, Byers M. ABC to<C>ABC: redefining the military trauma paradigm. *Emerg Med J.* 2006a;23:745-746.

Hodgetts T, Mahoney P. Clinical Guidelines for Operations. Joint Defence Publication 4-03.1, Shrivenham, Defence Concepts and Doctrine Centre; 2008.

Hodgetts T, Mahoney P, Evans G, Brooks A. Battlefield Advanced Trauma Life Support. 3rd ed. Joint Service Publication; 2006:570.

# Imaging Triage for Ballistic Trauma

# 18

Jon David Simmons and Tracy R. Bilski

## 18.1
## Introduction

The initial evaluation for ballistic trauma continues to consist of a thorough physical exam followed by evaluation of the physiologic status of the patient. The patient should be fully exposed followed by detailed wound examination to determine projectile trajectory. Based on the suspected path of the missile, determinations can be made as to what structures are likely injured and what interventions may be needed.

All who care for the injured patient agree that there is a limited role for radiological assessment in hemodynamically unstable patients. However, in those patients without physiologic compromise, radiological evaluation can serve as a very useful adjunct in the triage of patients toward more invasive studies, surgical intervention, or non-operative management. The increase of non-operative management has created an expanded role for additional diagnostic modalities including surgeon-performed ultrasound, computed tomography (CT), and angiography. Routine plain film radiographs remain an essential tool in the initial evaluation of all victims of penetrating trauma. With the expansion of these accurate and versatile imaging modalities, many traditional principles in the management of ballistic trauma patients are being redefined.

## 18.2
## Chest, Abdominal, and Pelvic Films

All patients with projectile injuries, irrespective of the area injured, should routinely undergo anteroposterior (AP) radiography of the chest. The use of routine x-ray studies such as the chest and pelvic x-ray may help identify a patient that has a combination of blunt and penetrating trauma that was previously unknown. Additionally, this important and inexpensive

J.D. Simmons (✉)
General Surgery Department, Trauma and Critical Care Surgery Division,
University of Mississippi Medical Center, Jackson, MS, USA
e-mail: drjonsimmons@gmail.com

A.J. Brooks et al. (eds.), *Ryan's Ballistic Trauma*,
DOI: 10.1007/978-1-84882-124-8_18, © Springer-Verlag London Limited 2011

screening tool may quickly exclude many life-threatening conditions. When possible, every effort should be made to perform the chest x-ray with the patient's torso in the upright, seated, or reverse Trendelenberg position. This will allow for an easier diagnosis of free air under the diaphragm from perforated viscus and also may help to better quantify the amount of hemothorax by preventing posterior layering. Other signs such as a wide mediastinum or apical capping could suggest a mediastinal or great vessel injury. Liberal use of the AP and lateral abdominal x-ray and pelvic x-ray should be used when attempting to determine trajectory of one or multiple projectiles. Obtaining x-rays of the chest, abdomen, and pelvis with wound markers (see below) in place can be exceedingly helpful in determining trajectory and can help plan for further diagnostic studies or for operative approaches to the injury.

## 18.3
## Wound Markers

The use of radiopaque markers to identify the entrance and exit wounds may be very useful in determining missile trajectory or as a reference point to a foreign body. This is useful with plain x-ray as well as with CT Scan. We would recommend the use of taped-on metallic paper-clips. Items such as electrocardiogram electrodes should not be used as they can cause confusion when attempting to discern the electrodes placed to monitor the patient from those used to mark the wounds.

## 18.4
## Computed Tomography

Many centers have studied the role of computed tomography (CT) in determining missile trajectory in various anatomic regions, including the neck, chest, and abdomen/pelvis.[1-5] The role of CT has increased significantly due to increasing trend toward non-operative management in all trauma patients. The constant improvement in resolution is allowing surgeons to more accurately determine missile trajectory through tissue planes and determine its adjacency to vital structures. It is important to remember that transporting a patient to the CT scanner can be time consuming and is not indicated in a hemodynamically abnormal patient.

## 18.5
## Magnetic Resonance Imaging (MRI)

Obtaining MRI in ballistic trauma patients is difficult and moreover, its role in the workup of these patients is poorly defined. The ferromagnetic properties of most projectiles preclude its use as the MRI magnet can potentially cause any projectile fragment to move.

Hess[6] and others performed an extensive evaluation of the ferromagnetic properties of 56 different projectiles fired from various air guns, handguns, rifles, and shotguns. They concluded that while not all bullets were ferromagnetic, the only current method of determining if a gunshot victim is suitable for MRI is by pretesting identical missiles before scanning. This limitation therefore prevents MRI from being used as an initial diagnostic tool in ballistic trauma. Furthermore, there are logistical considerations for using MRI as a diagnostic imaging modality - namely its lack of ready availability in many places and the difficulty with MRI compatible monitoring and ventilation equipment.

## 18.6
## Imaging Away from the Emergency Room

The advanced imaging devices are not always in close proximity to the Trauma Bay. Re-warming and initiation of resuscitation is paramount in the early care of the injured trauma patient. It is key that the need for a CT scan or angiography not prevent or delay these treatments. One of the most important roles the trauma team leader plays is to determine the needs of the patient and in what order they are to proceed. A decision to perform imaging outside of the trauma bay (rather than remaining for ongoing resuscitation in one location or proceeding to the operating room) mandates that the risk to the patient from change of location outweigh the risk of diagnostic/therapeutic error from not obtaining the study. This can be a difficult decision at times. It is clear, however, that any severely injured trauma patient transported outside the trauma bay for any reason should be accompanied by a physician member of the trauma team, respiratory therapist, and nurse. This potentially creates an environment amenable to ongoing monitoring, resuscitation, and critical care problem solving, veritably "moving the trauma bay or Intensive Care Unit with the patient." Numerous studies have documented this need; neglecting these principles and allowing patients to be transported to advanced imaging with only a hospital escort is fraught with problems and can lead to adverse patient outcomes.[7,8]

## 18.7
## Imaging of Specific Anatomical Regions

### 18.7.1
### Craniofacial Injury

The initial diagnostic study used to evaluate victims of penetrating injury to the head and/or face is a non-contrast head and/or maxillofacial CT[9,10] (Fig. 18.1). The accuracy of this modality to assess the extent of brain injury and to diagnose or exclude a transcranial trajectory allows rapid triage of patients to surgical intervention, medical management, or expectant observations (Fig. 18.2). Axial, coronal, and/or 3-D reconstructions of a facial CT allows for an assessment of maxillofacial injuries and planning for later

**Fig. 18.1** Mobile Digital X-Ray

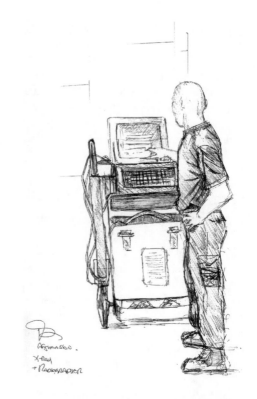

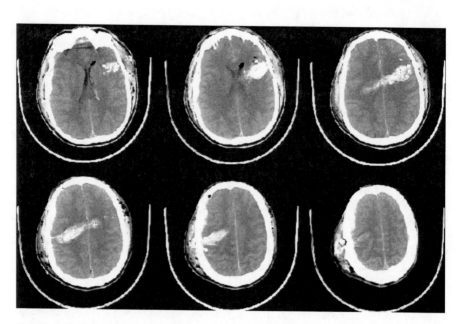

**Fig. 18.2** Self-inflicted gunshot wound to the head with demonstration of transcranial trajectory

surgical intervention. Although most facial fractures do not need repair acutely, certain injuries may require more timely attention and therefore diagnostic studies and appropriate subspecialty consultation should be obtained as soon as possible. Such injuries would include certain ophthalmologic injuries and potential CSF leaks either from a frontal sinus fracture or mastoid fracture. It should be noted that, in cases of severe bullet fragmentation, the scatter effect created by metallic foreign bodies might limit image resolution. Although CT Scan is the mainstay of diagnostic imaging evaluation in these patients, ongoing arterial hemorrhage from gunshot wounds to the face may benefit from early angiographic embolization of bleeding vessels.[11,12]

In patients with penetrating injuries to both the head and torso, hemodynamic stability should guide decision making with regard to diagnostic imaging. In unstable patients, operative interventions aimed at controlling the source of bleeding should take priority over craniofacial imaging, as hypotension significantly increases the mortality associated with traumatic brain injury.[13] In hemodynamically normal patients with combined torso and craniofacial injuries, it is acceptable to obtain a head CT prior to operative intervention provided that the study can be rapidly obtained, patients are adequately monitored, and the team is prepared to urgently transport the patient to the operating room if their condition deteriorates. If CT imaging of at least the head is obtained, neurosurgical intervention directed at the specific injury pattern can ensue simultaneously with laparotomy or thoracotomy, or prior to leaving the operating room. Of note, patients who have sustained isolated craniofacial gunshot wounds do not routinely require immobilization or radiographic evaluation of the cervical spine; however, caution is advised if the complete mechanism of injury is not known (i.e., a blast injury with multiple projectiles and patient having been displaced by the blast wave) or if the patient cannot be fully examined.[14] Often times, these patients require cervical spine films because their mental status exam severely limits the accuracy of bedside assessment of the cervical spine stability.

## 18.7.2
## Neck Injury

The evaluation of hemodynamically normal patients with penetrating neck injuries has changed dramatically over the past 10 years. This change in algorithm is due to general tendencies moving toward non-operative management of trauma patients and the continued advancement in CT resolution and technology. The recent advances in the endovascular field have also changed some of the treatment options for vascular injuries to the neck.

The first step in evaluating penetrating trauma to the neck is to determine hemodynamic stability and rule out "Hard Signs" of injury. "Hard Signs" are physical exam findings that suggest injury to the vascular or aerodigestive tract. These physical exam findings consist of: pulsatile or expanding hematoma, subcutaneous emphysema, wound bubbling, or airway compromise.[15] If the patient is hemodynamically abnormal or presents any hard sign, emergent exploration is warranted regardless of the zone of injury.

By tradition, the management of this complex anatomic region has relied upon classification of the penetration into one of the classic cervical "zones" as described in 1979 by Roon and Christensen[16] (Fig. 18.3). Injuries to zones I and III were largely managed non-operatively by angiography, bronchoscopy, and esophagoscopy to exclude injuries

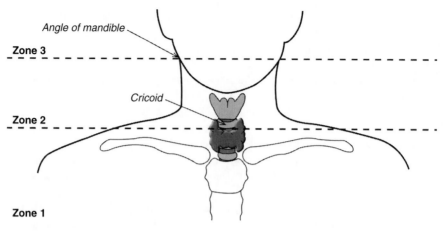

**Fig. 18.3** Zones of the neck for penetrating injury

to the vital arteries or aerodigestive tract.[17,18] Historically, zone II injuries were explored operatively if the injury penetrated the platysma muscle.[19-22] Traditionally the evaluation of penetrating injuries to the neck in the hemodynamically stable patient without "Hard Signs" was the same for all zones of the neck. This consists of arteriography and panendoscopy.[2,23]

The current diagnostic study of choice in hemodynamically normal patients with penetrating neck injuries is a high resolution CT angiogram of the head and neck.[2,24] For zone I injury, this would include CT angiogram of the chest as well. This imaging modality can serve as an excellent diagnostic tool in evaluating the vascular system, esophagus, bronchus, and cervical spine. In those patients in whom trajectory suggests proximity to vital structure or where trajectory is unclear, high resolution, multislice CT and CT angiography serve as a triage tool to select further individualized invasive diagnostic evaluation.

Management of transcervical gunshot wounds deserves special mention as these can lead to major injury in more than one zone.[24] Although there is evidence for both mandatory exploration and for a selective approach to these injuries, Gracias, et al. have shown that if CT demonstrates a trajectory away from vital structures, the need for invasive studies can be eliminated.[2] Hence, these authors recommend high resolution CT angiogram of the head and neck for patients with gunshot wounds as well as the initial diagnostic study.

There is a growing body of literature to support the use of CT angiography in penetrating cervical trauma. Ofer[25] reported a series of patients in whom CT angiography was highly accurate in determining vascular injury with successful non-operative management of patients with negative CT scans. In 2001, a prospective study of Zone II penetrations by Mazolewski[23] demonstrated a 100% sensitivity of trauma-surgeon-evaluated neck CT in identifying injuries requiring operative intervention. That same year, Gracias[2] reported the first series that included patients with gunshots to any of the three neck zones and found that CT was a safe and effective modality "to direct or eliminate further invasive studies in selected stable patients with penetrating neck injury."

In 2002, a prospective study by Munera[26] evaluated 175 patients with penetrating neck injury by CT angiography. They were able to accurately characterize vascular injuries in 27 (15.6%) patients and direct them to appropriate therapy. The other 146 patients were successfully observed without further intervention and without missed injury.

In the evaluation of less-invasive diagnostic techniques, Montalvo found cervical color duplex sonography to be an accurate alternative to angiography in stable patients with Zone II or III injuries who were not actively bleeding.[27] Accurate cervical duplex ultrasound is often not readily available, is operator dependent, and requires specialist expertise in interpretation. In addition, this technology is limited by patient habitus, does not image skull-base injuries, and does not impact the need for evaluation of the aerodigestive tract.

### 18.7.2.1
### Recommendations for the Neck

Any patient with a penetrating injury to the neck who is haemodynamically stable without hard signs of vascular (pulsatile bleeding, expanding hematoma, bruit) or aerodigestive injury (subcutaneous emphysema, wound bubbling, airway compromise) are candidates to undergo a high-resolution CT angiogram of the head and neck (Fig. 18.4). It is a relatively fast screening tool which can accurately identify missile trajectory and injuries to vital

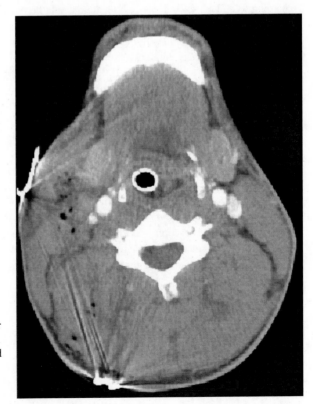

**Fig. 18.4** Computed tomography after gunshot wound to the neck with clear demonstration of trajectory. Injury to the patient's carotid artery, oropharynx, and tracheobronchial tree are excluded

structures. Subsequent esophagoscopy and bronchoscopy can be utilized as necessary after proximity to these structures is determined. If high-resolution CT scanning is unavailable or if CT findings are inconclusive, evaluation should proceed with diagnostic angiography, endoscopy, esophagography, or operative exploration.

### 18.7.3
### Chest Injury

The prevalence of penetrating chest injury is increasing and improved pre-hospital and emergency department protocols have resulted in an increased number of patients with the potential to survive. The triage of penetrating chest injuries have changed dramatically over the past two decades. With the recent popularity of the Focused Assessment with Sonography for Trauma protocols (FAST), evaluation of the heart, lung, and abdomen can be performed within a few minutes.

### 18.7.3.1
### Ultrasound

The FAST exam has dramatically changed the evaluation of penetrating injuries to the chest. According to ATLS protocol, the FAST exam should be performed immediately after the primary survey. Recently, research studies have shown that FAST is equivalent to, or better than, chest radiography for identifying a hemothorax or pneumothorax in trauma patients.

Sonography can detect volumes as small as 20 mL of fluid in the pericardial space, but cannot quantify fluid accumulation.[28,29] Rozycki and colleagues reported a sensitivity of 100% and a specificity of 96.9% for surgeon-performed ultrasonography in diagnosing pericardial effusions.[30] Concomitant hemothorax, epicardial fat pad, and pneumothorax can confound ultrasonographic detection of pericardial effusions. Blaivas and colleagues found that emergency room physicians had trouble distinguishing between epicardial fat pads and pericardial effusions. However, the accuracy increased from 63% to 93% depending on the amount of experience of the ultrasonographer.[31] Meyer and colleagues found significant differences in the sensitivity of echocardiography in identifying serious cardiac injuries in patients with and without hemothoraces (100% vs 56%).[32] In the presence of hemothorax, decompression of pericardial fluid into the pleural space can not be definitively excluded. This was confirmed in a case series of delayed pericardial tamponades that presented without evidence of pericardial fluid on initial echocardiography but all of the patients did have an evident hemothorax on initial exam.[33]

### 18.7.3.2
### Angiography

Angiography is indicated for stable patients sustaining periclavicular injuries who have physical or radiographic findings, such as pulse or neurologic deficit, suggestive or subclavian or axillary vascular injury. Increasingly these injuries may be managed with using endovascular techniques. Patients with no signs of vascular compromise do not require angiography based on proximity alone.[34,35] CTA can be used as an alternative modality for imaging patients with these injury patterns.

### 18.7.4
### Transmedistinal Injury

Hemodynamically stable patients with transmediastinal gunshot wounds, multiple penetrations, or with gunshot wounds of unknown trajectory represent a controversial injury subset in which the appropriate diagnostic pathway continues to evolve. The crucial information that must be obtained from advanced imaging modalities is the status of the mediastinal structures. Patients sustaining transmediastinal trajectories may have injuries to the heart, great vessels, esophagus, or tracheobronchial tree. Each of these injuries is life threatening and delays in diagnosis significantly increase morbidity and mortality.[36]

By following ATLS protocol, any hemodynamically normal patient with penetrating chest injury should get a FAST scan following the primary survey and a chest x-ray following the secondary survey with chest tube placement as needed (Fig. 18.5). Up to 85% of patients with penetrating chest injuries will require a chest tube. The role of a chest tube can be both diagnostic and therapeutic. After chest tube placement on the side of injury, the amount of blood return can be helpful for triage. Output of 1,500 mL initially or 200 mL/h for 2–4 h are indications for thoracotomy.[37] A large air-leak from a tracheobronchial injury can greatly diminish the tidal volume and may also require initial thoracotomy without further imaging. It is the patient without initial need for thoracotomy and who needs additional advanced imaging studies that is controversial.

The traditional workup of transmediastinal gunshot wounds consisted of arteriogram, bronchoscopy, esophagography, and pericardial window.[38,39] Echocardiography would

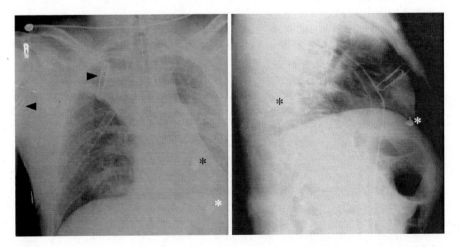

**Fig. 18.5** *Left*: Chest X-ray after multiple gunshot wounds to right chest. *Arrows* demonstrate entrance wounds. Anterior (*white asterisk*) and posterior (*black asterisk*) foreign bodies are seen in the left chest having traversed the mediastinum

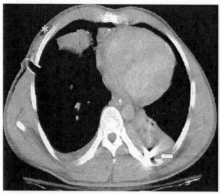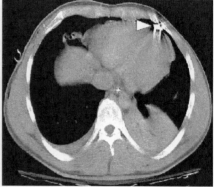

**Fig. 18.6** Chest CT of patient in Fig. 18.5. *Asterisk* demonstrates one entrance wound. Anterior and posterior foreign bodies are seen (*arrow*). The mediastinal structures are clearly at risk for injury and further studies are needed

later provide an accurate alternative to the more invasive pericardial window.[40,41] This approach is very time consuming and requires multiple specialty involvement but has been the standard of care for many years.

The more recent algorithms are replacing the invasive multispecialty approach with contrast enhanced CT scans. The constant improvement in resolution is allowing surgeons to more accurately determine missile trajectory through tissue planes and determine its adjacency to vital structures in the mediastinum.[42] There are multiple small studies that agree with using contrast enhanced CT as a screening tool to identify further necessary studies due to the proximity of the bullet tract which may help avoid unnecessary invasive procedures[4,43,44] (Fig. 18.6).

It is important to emphasize that while contrast-enhanced CT scan has emerged as a useful triage tool in the evaluation of patients with transmediastinal gunshot wounds, positive findings must be followed with traditional studies to guide therapeutic decision-making. Patients with suspected vascular injury based on identified missile trajectory, contrast extravasation, or the presence of mediastinal blood should undergo formal angiography, either as a diagnostic modality to direct operative intervention or as a therapeutic modality for embolization or stent placement at the discretion of the vascular surgeon. This dictum may change as there has already been a shift of practice in blunt aortic injuries. CT angiography with its ability to provide vastly more information and it's ever-improving resolution and 3-D reconstructive ability is surpassing the capability of traditional angiography.[45]

In patients suspected of sustaining esophageal perforation, contrast esophagography, first with water-soluble contrast (Gastrograffin), then with thin barium if needed, is performed to accurately identify injuries. Flexible or rigid endoscopy can also be used as an initial diagnostic modality to exclude or identify thoracic esophageal injuries or to confirm negative esophagography where high clinical suspicion still exists.

Computed tomography findings or missile trajectory that suggests tracheobronchial injury mandates bronchoscopy to identify the level of injury and guide operative intervention.

Formal echocardiography should be used to exclude pericardial violation in patients with questionable findings on surgeon-performed ultrasound or to follow studies limited by emergency department ultrasound equipment, operator inexperience, or patient body habitus.[46]

Finally, after penetrating chest trauma, a subset of hemodynamically normal victims have a normal chest radiograph and no suspected mediastinal involvement. While more common in stab victims, this presentation does occur in gunshot wounds as well. After, initial evaluation, a 3–6 h period of observation in a monitored setting followed by repeat chest radiograph is a safe approach.[47] Patients with normal follow-up chest radiograph can be reliably discharged without further diagnostic studies. While CT can more reliably exclude small pneumothoraces and identify trajectory in these patients, it may not be as cost effective as the above approach.[48]

## 18.7.5
## Abdominal Injury

Traditionally, gunshot wounds to the abdomen have been treated with surgical exploration. Until the last decade, there was no role for advanced imaging for gunshot wounds to the abdomen. Wounds that appeared superficial in the hemodynamically stable patient would then undergo either diagnostic peritoneal lavage or local wound exploration. The recent popularity using diagnostic laparoscopy has also replaced DPL and wound exploration in certain situations. Non-operative treatment of penetrating injuries to the abdomen is still in its infancy. With constant advances in the application of the CT and FAST scans, there is now a select group of patients with penetrating trauma that can be treated non-operatively with close observation.[49-53] Of all the advanced imaging studies used to help with triage of ballistic trauma to the abdomen, the CT scan and FAST have had the most impact. They will be addressed separately below.

## 18.7.5.1
## Ultrasound

As previously described, "FAST" is an acronym for Focused Assessment with Sonography in Trauma. It is routinely used in the triage of all types of traumatic abdominal injuries.[54] According to ATLS protocols, the FAST exam should be performed immediately after the primary survey. This bedside ultrasound is an attractive option for evaluation of the trauma patient. It is portable, quick, and relatively easy to perform. Initially, FAST was used more for blunt trauma but its application in penetrating trauma appears to be equal.[55]

In 2001, Udobi[56] and colleagues prospectively examined 75 stable patients with penetrating trauma to the abdomen, flank, or back with FAST. Their data revealed a sensitivity of 46%, a positive predictive value of 90%, and negative predictive value of 60% for the need for laparotomy based on ultrasound findings. That same year, Boulanger[57] and others reported their experience with FAST in 72 patients. A sensitivity of 67%, a positive predictive value of 92%, and a negative predictive value of 89% were reported for detecting significant intra-abdominal injury with FAST. FAST can also be helpful in the triage of patients with possible thoracoabdominal penetrating injuries.[58] Based on the above, a positive FAST exam is clinically useful in the triage of patients toward laparotomy while a negative study does not reliably exclude injury and warrants further diagnostic imaging.

**Fig. 18.7** Computed tomography of patient with gunshot to the abdomen. Trajectory through adipose tissue without peritoneal violation is demonstrated. Paperclip (*arrow*) marks one skin wound

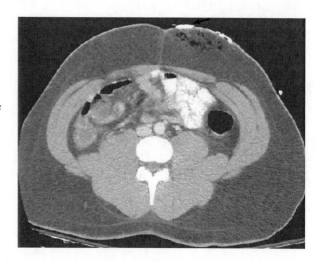

## 18.7.5.2
## CT Scan

The use of CT scan has aided the trauma surgeon in the evaluation of a subset of hemodynamically normal patients with gunshot wounds to the abdomen (Fig. 18.7). Although, it takes an experienced trauma surgeon with a high-resolution CT scan to safely identify these patients. The selective use of non-operative management in ballistic trauma to the abdomen has been shown to be safe and decrease the rates of non-therapeutic laparotomy.[50] These patients usually have one of the following: tangential injuries that do not penetrate the abdominal cavity[3] (see Fig. 18.7), solid organ injury without peritonitis,[59] right upper quadrant thoracoabdominal injuries,[50] and retroperitoneal or renal injuries.[60,61]

In 1998, Grossman and others[3] retrospectively reviewed their experience in evaluating patients with torso gunshot wounds and found that contrast-enhanced abdominal CT is an effective method of determining missile trajectory, and therefore anatomic injury, in selected patients. In 2001, Shanmuganathan and colleagues[61] reported their prospective data on the evaluation of 104 stable patients with penetrating torso trauma with triple-contrast abdominal CT. Computed tomography scans were positive in 35 patients (34%), of which 22 underwent laparotomy and 19 (86%) were therapeutic. Of those patients with negative CT scans, 97% (67/69) were successfully managed non-operatively. They reported a negative predictive value of 100% and 97% accuracy of triple contrast CT scan in selected patients.

In 1999, Demetriades and colleagues[59] published a series of 52 patients with gunshot wounds to the liver as diagnosed by CT scan. Of these patients, 16 remained hemodynamically stable, had no other indication for laparotomy, and were successfully managed non-operatively. Although a diaphragmatic injury may be present in these patients, the presence of the liver abutting the right hemi-diaphragm generally prevents clinically significant complications. In selected patients with isolated liver injuries, angiographic embolization is another option to avoid unnecessary laparotomy and worsening of bleeding in patients with isolated hepatic gunshot wounds.[62-64]

**Fig. 18.8** Computed
tomography of patient with
gunshot to the back. The
missile is seen in the
para-spinous region without
violation of the chest or
spinal canal

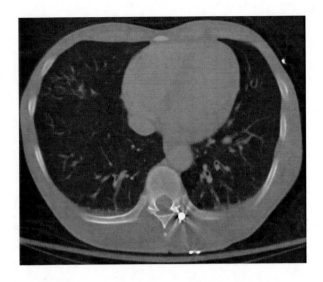

Patients who sustained isolated gunshot wounds to the back or flank are particularly well-suited for evaluation by helical CT scan to identify or exclude significant injury and to avoid unnecessary laparotomy[60,65] with a reported negative predictive value on 100%[66] (Fig. 18.8). In 1987, Hauser reviewed 40 stable patients with posterior penetrating injuries who had been initially evaluated with CT to determine trajectory and identify injuries.[65] Six patients were found to have diagnostic injuries that were confirmed at laparotomy. The other 34 patients were successfully managed non-operatively based on CT exclusion of significant injury. Ginzburg and colleagues[60] reviewed 83 stable patients with abdominal and flank gunshot wounds who were initially evaluated by CT scan. They demonstrated that in 53 patients with no evidence of peritoneal penetration on abdominal CT, non-operative management could safely be pursued.

### 18.7.5.3
### Diaphragm Injuries

The diaphragm is a dome-shaped muscle which separates the chest from the abdomen. The contraction and descent of the diaphragm creates a negative pressure in the chest to facilitate expansion of the lung while the intra-abdominal pressures increase. The negative intrathoracic pressure can range from 7 to 22 cm of water and can reach as much as 100. In the setting of a diaphragm injury or laceration, this large pressure gradient can lead to the herniation of abdominal contents into the chest. The diagnosis of an injury to the diaphragm can be challenging. Most of the literature regarding the diagnosis of diaphragm injuries is in blunt trauma. There is a dearth of literature regarding diagnostic modalities for diaphragm injuries in ballistic trauma. CT scan and plain x-ray of the thoracoabdominal area often cannot reliably rule out a diaphragm laceration.[67,68] The chest x-ray may be diagnostic if a herniation is present but can be normal. Things to suggest herniation on a chest x-ray are: elevation of a hemidiaphragm, mediastinal shift, intrathoracic air bubble, or a coiled nasogastric tube in the left chest.[69] The important principle to remember is that ballistic injury to the diaphragm will likely be associated with other injuries. Right diaphragm injuries are usually butressed by the liver and generally do not need to be repaired. Management of anterior right diaphragm injuries, where the diaphragm is not covered with hepatic parenchyma, is controversial. Left sided injuries need to be repaired to prevent herniation. If herniation is present, reduction of herniated abdominal contents and repair is undertaken to prevent strangulation.

## 18.7.5.4
### Extremity Injury

Ballistic injuries to the extremity are not uncommon in the civilian sector. The immediate task in triage is to determine the presence of bony or arterial injury. In the hemodynamically normal patient, plain radiographs can quickly assess the bony structures in question and additional views can assist in determining needed orthopedic interventions. Determining the presence of a significant vascular injury can be more challenging and is paramount in the management of these patients. The work-up for potential vascular injury in the extremity is well described in the literature.

The diagnosis and management of arterial injuries to the extremity from penetrating trauma was developed from the experience of military surgeons during wartime. Up to 90% of all arterial injuries are in the extremity. In the civilian population, the majority of these are in the upper extremity.[68] The most feared sequelae from extremity arterial trauma is amputation. The outcomes after extremity vascular injury remain variable despite modern diagnostic techniques and surgical therapy.

Patients with "hard signs" of vascular injury require emergent operative attention without the use of diagnostic imaging. Hard signs include: absent or diminished pulse, pulsatile bleeding, expanding hematoma, or signs of distal ischemia. An arteriogram can be performed intraoperatively if deemed necessary by the surgeon.[70] The patients without "hard signs" should then have ankle-brachial indices (ABI) or arterial-pulse indices (API) determined. An ABI or API of greater than 0.9 does not require any further diagnostic testing. Angiographic imaging is reserved for those without hard signs of injury with an ABI less than 0.9. "Soft signs" of vascular injury including: proximity to an artery, nonexpanding hematoma, and neurological deficits, do not require formal angiography as long as the ABI is greater than 0.90. There are currently two options for angiography: standard arteriogram or computed tomographic angiogram (CTA).

The standard arteriogram is performed by an interventional radiologists or vascular surgeon. This is considered the gold standard for diagnosing arterial injuries in the extremity. This has the advantage of the potential to treat an injury with a stent or coil ligation when appropriate.

The CTA is a newer modality which is being used more frequently to diagnose arterial injuries throughout the body. It has the advantage of being less invasive and will also provide more information than the standard arteriogram. One problem is the scatter caused by projectile fragments may hamper your ability to accurately rule out a vascular injury. This is especially true for shotgun injuries.

### 18.7.5.5
### Imaging in Battlefield or Natural Disaster Conditions

While many of the options for the imaging of ballistic trauma victims discussed above are easily accessed in the medical center setting, it is obvious that such technology is often not available in the austere conditions of the battlefield, in military forward surgical units or following a natural disaster. CT scanning and interventional radiology are likely to be options only at higher echelons of care or if main hospitals in the area of question remain functional. Portable digital x-ray and hand-held ultrasound technology are more readily available and are now part of the equipment carried by most military forward surgical units as well as rapid response medical/surgical teams and NGO (non-governmental organization) deployable medical aid teams.

The portable ultrasound machines have also become more capable with the addition of various probes to perform such studies as color Doppler flow, as well as advances aiding diagnosis of pneumothoraces, hemothoraces, ocular injuries, foreign body localization, and others.[71,72]

An additional advance in imaging involves teleradiology. As an evolving technology, this may play a critical role in the evaluation of trauma patients in austere environments. Properly trained medics and healthcare providers could take and transmit images where a radiologist or trauma surgeon can offer experienced interpretation.[73] This technology is not widely used on the battlefield at the time of publishing.

While diagnostic imaging is often useful in the evaluation of ballistic trauma victims, a trauma surgeon is trained to provide operative inspection and direct visualization of trajectories and injuries when clinically appropriate. In mass casualty events and when advanced technologies are unavailable, one must rely on clinical and operative training/judgment. This principle is never more apparent than on the battlefield or on site after a natural disaster.

## 18.8
## Summary

Imaging has become increasingly important in the evaluation of ballistic trauma. Plain x-rays and FAST are valuable in the unstable patient in the emergency room. The role of CT and CT angiography continues to expand in the evaluation of these injuries in the hemodynamically normal patient. Embolization and interventional radiology techniques are increasingly being used to treat a variety of vascular injury especially those where surgical access can be difficult. Continued clinical research is needed to further define the role of advanced imaging in ballistic trauma and to possibly expand its use as technology evolves.

## References

1. Besenski N. Traumatic injuries: imaging of head injuries. *Eur Radiol.* 2002;12(6):1237-1252.
2. Gracias VH, Reilly PM, Philpott J, Klein WP, Singer M, Schwab CW. Computed tomography in the evaluation of penetrating neck trauma: a preliminary study. *Arch Surg.* 2001;136:1231-1235.

3. Grossman MD, May AK, Schwab CW, et al. Determining anatomic injury with computed tomography in selected torso gunshot wounds. *J Trauma*. 1998;45:446-456.

4. Hanpeter DE, Demetriades D, Asensio JA, Berne TV, Velmahos G, Murray J. Helical computed tomographic scan in the evaluation of mediatinal gunshot wounds. *J Trauma*. 2000;49(4):689-695.

5. Demetriades D, Velmahos G. Technology-driven triage of abdominal trauma: The emerging era of nonoperative management. *Annu Rev Med*. 2003;54:1-15.

6. Hess U, Harms J, Schneider A, et al. Assessment of gunshot bullet injuries with the use of magnetic resonance imaging. *J Trauma*. 2000;49(4):704-709.

7. Voigt LP, Pastores SM, Thaler HT, Halpern NA. Review of a large clinical series: intrahospital transport of critically ill patients: outcomes, timing and patterns. *J Intensive Care Med*. 2009;24(2):108-115.

8. Waydhas C. Intrahospital transport of critically ill patients. *Crit Care*. 1999;3(5):R83-R89.

9. Anonymous. Neuroimaging in the management of penetrating brain injury. *J Trauma*. 2001;51(2 Supp):S7-S11.

10. Kim PE, Go JL, Zee CS. Radographic assessment of cranial gunshot wounds. *Neuroimaging Clin N Am*. 2002;12(2):229-248.

11. Demetriades D, Chahwan S, Gomez H, Falabella A, Velmahos G, Yamashita D. Initial evaluation and management of gunshot wounds ot the face. *J Trauma*. 1998;45(1):39-41.

12. Diaz-Daza O, Arraiza FJ, Barkley JM, Whigham CJ. Endovascular therapy of traumatic vascular lesions of the head and neck. *Cardiovasc Intervent Radiol*. 2003;26(3):213-221.

13. Chesnut RM. Avoidance of hypotension: conditio sine qua non of successful severe head injury management. *J Trauma*. 1997;42(5 Suppl):S4-S9.

14. Kaups KL, Davis JW. Patients with gunshot wounds to the head do not require cervical spine immobilization and evaluation. *J Trauma*. 1998;44(5):865-867.

15. Meyer JP, Barrett JA, Schuler JJ, Flanigan DP. Mandatory vs selective exploration for penetrating neck trauma. A prospective assessment. *Arch Surg*. 1987;122(5):592-597.

16. Roon AJ, Christensen N. Evaluation and treatment of penetrating cervical injuries. *J Trauma*. 1979;19(6):391-397.

17. Jurkovich GJ, Zingarelli W, Wallace J, Curreri PW. Penetrating neck trauma: diagnostic studies in the asymptomatic patient. *J Trauma*. 1985;25(9):819-822.

18. Back MR, Baumgartner FJ, Klein SR. Detection and evaluation of aerodigestive tract injuries caused by cervical and transmediastinal gunshot wounds. *J Trauma*. 1997;42(4):680-686.

19. Asensio JA, Valenziano CP, Falcone RE, Grosh JD. Management of penetrating neck injuries. The controversy surrounding zone II injuries. *Surg Clin North Am*. 1991;71(2):267-296.

20. Biffl WL, Moore EE, Rehse DH, Offner PJ, Francoise RJ, Burch JM. Selective management of penetrating neck trauma based on cervical level of injury. *Am J Surg*. 1997;174(6): 678-682.

21. Klyachkin ML, Rohmiller M, Charash WE, Sloan DA, Kearney PA. Penetrating injuries of the neck: selective management evolving. *Am Surg*. 1997;63(2):189-194.

22. Van As AB, van Deurzen DF, Verleisdonk EJ. Gunshots to the neck: selective aniography as part of conservative management. *Injury*. 2002;33(5):453-456.

23. Mazolewski PJ, Curry JD, Browder T, Fildes J. Computed tomographic scan can be used for surgical decision making in zone II penetrating neck injuries. *J Trauma*. 2001;51:315-319.

24. Tisherman SA, Bokhari F, Collier B, et al. Clinical practice guideline: penetrating zone II neck trauma. *J Trauma*. 2008;64(5):1392-1405.

25. Ofer A, Nitecki SS, Braun J, et al. CT angiography of the carotid areteries in trauma to the neck. *Eur J Vasc Endovasc Surg*. 2001;21(5):401-407.

26. Munera F, Soto JA, Palacio D, et al. Penetrating neck injuries: helical CT angiography for initial evaluation. *Radiology*. 2002;370:366-372.

27. Montalvo BM, LeBlang SD, Nunez DB Jr, et al. Color Doppler sonography in penetrating injuries of the neck. *AJNR Am J Neuroradiol*. 1996;17(5):943-951.

28. Thakur RK, Aufderheide TP, Boughner DR. Emergency echocardiographic evaluation of penetrating chest trauma. *Can J Cardiol*. 1994;10:374-376.

29. Rozycki GS, Ochsner MG, Jaffin JH, Champion HR. Prospective evaluation of surgeon's use of ultrasound in the evaluation of trauma patients. *J Trauma*. 1993;34:516-526.

30. Rozycki GS, Feliciano DV, Ochsner MG, et al. The role of ultrasound in patients with possible penetrating cardiac wounds: a prospective multicenter study. *J Trauma*. 1999;46:543-551.

31. Blaivas M, DeBehnke D, Phelan MB. Potential errors in the diagnosis of pericardial effusion on trauma ultrasound for penetrating injuries. *Acad Emerg Med*. 2000;7:1261-1266.

32. Meyer DM, Jessen ME, Grayburn PA. Use of echocardiography to detect occult cardiac injury after penetrating thoracic trauma: a prospective study. *J Trauma*. 1995;39:902-907.

33. Simmons JD, Haraway AN, Schmieg RE Jr, Burgdorf M, Duchesne J. Is there a role for secondary thoracic ultrasound in patients with penetrating injuries to the anterior mediastinum? *Am Surg*. 2008;74(1):11-14.

34. Gasparri MG, Lorelli DR, Kralovich KA, Patton JH Jr. Physical examination plus chest radiography in penetrating periclavicular trauma: the appropriate trigger for angiography. *J Trauma*. 2000;49(6):1029-1033.

35. Gonzalez RP, Falimirski ME. The role of angiography in periclavicular penetrating trauma. *Am Surg*. 1999;65(8):711-714.

36. Asensio JA, Berne J, Demetriades D, et al. Penetrating esophageal injuries: time interval of safety for preoperative evaluation. How long is safe? *J Trauma*. 1997;43(2):319-324.

37. Advanced Trauma Life Support® Student Course Manual (8th ed) 2008; American College of Surgeons.

38. Richardson J.D, Flint LM, Snow NJ, Gray LA Jr, Trinkle JK. Management of transmediastinal gunshot wounds. *Surgery*. 1981;90(4):671-676.

39. Demetriades D. Penetrating injuries to the thoracic great vessels. *J Card Surg*. 1997;12 (2 Suppl):173-180.

40. McIntyre RC Jr, Moore EE, Read RR, Wiebe RL, Grover FL. Transesophageal echocardiography in the evaluation of a transmediastinal gunshot wound: case report. *J Trauma*. 1994;36(1):125127.

41. LiMandri G, Gorenstein LA, Starr JP, Homma S, Avteri J, Gopal AS. Use of transesophageal echocardiography in the detection and consequences of an intracardiac bullet. *Am J Emerg Med*. 1994;12(1):105-106.

42. Demetriades D, Velmahos GC. Penetrating injuries of the chest: indications for operation. *Scand J Surg*. 2002;91(1):41-45.

43. Nagy KK, Gilkey SH, Roberts RR, Fildes JJ, Barrett J. Computed tomography screens stable patients at risk for penetrating cardiac injury. *Acad Emerg Med*. 1996;3(11):1024-1027.

44. Stassen NA, Lukan JK, Spain DA, et al. Reevaluation of diagnostic procedures for transmediastinal gunshot wounds. *J Trauma*. 2002;53:635-638.

45. Demetriades D, Velmahos GC, Scalea TM, et al. Diagnosis and treatment of blunt thoracic aortic injuries: changing perspectives. *J Trauma*. 2008;64(6):1415-1418.

46. Aaland MO, Bryan FC 3rd, Sherman R. Two-dimensional echocardiogram in hemodynamically stable victims of penetrating precordial trauma. *Am Surg*. 1994;60(6):412-415.

47. Kiev J, Kerstein MD. Role of three hour roentgenogram of the chest in pentrating and nonpenetrating injuries of the chest. *Surg Gynecol Obstet*. 1992;175(3):249-253.

48. Shatz DV, de la pedraja J, Erbella J, Hameed M, Vail SJ. Efficacy of follow-up evaluation in penetrating thoracic injuires: 3 vs 6 hour radiographos of the chest. *J Emerg Med*. 2001; 20(3):281-284.

49. Beekley AC, Blackbourne LH, Sebesta JA, et al. Selective nonoperative management of penetrating torso injury from combat fragmentation wounds. *J Trauma*. 2008;64(2 Suppl): S108-S116. Discussion S116-S117.

50. Inaba K, Demetriades D. The nonoperative management of penetrating abdominal trauma. *Adv Surg*. 2007;41:51-62.

51. Isenhour JL, Marx J. Advances in abdominal trauma. *Emerg Med Clin North Am.* 2007; 25(3):713-733. ix.

52. Demetriades D, Hadjizacharia P, Constantinou C, et al. Selective nonoperative management of penetrating abdominal solid organ injuries. *Ann Surg.* 2006;244(4):620-628.

53. Pryor JP, Reilly PM, Dabrowski GP, Grossman MD, Schwab CW. Nonoperative management of abdominal gunshot wounds. *Ann Emerg Med.* 2004;43(3):344-353.

54. Rozycki GS, Ballard RB, Feliciano DV, Schmidt JA, Pennington SD. Surgeon performed ultrasound for the assessment of truncal injuries: lessons learned from 1540 patients. *Ann Surg.* 1998;228(4):557-567.

55. Rozycki GS, Ochsner MG, Jaffin JH, Champion HR. Prospective evaluation of surgeons' use of ultrasound in the evaluation of trauma patients. *J Trauma.* 1993;34:16-527.

56. Udobi KF, Rodriguez A, Chiu WC, Scalea TM. Tole of ultrasonagraphy in penetrating abdominal trauma: a prospective clinical study. *J Trauma.* 2001;51(2):320-325.

57. Boulanger BR, Kearney PA, Tsuei B, Ochoa JB. The routine use of sonography in penetrating torso injury is beneficial. *J Trauma.* 2001;51(2):320-325.

58. Tayal VS, Beatty MA, Marx JA, Tomaszewski CA, Thomason MH. FAST accurate for cardiac and intraperitoneal injury in penetrating anterior chest trauma. *J Ultrasound Med.* 2004;23:467-472.

59. Demetriades D, Gomez H, Chahwan S, et al. Gunshot injuries to the liver: the role of selective nonoperative management. *J Am Coll Surg.* 1999;188(4):343-348.

60. Ginzburg E, Carillo EH, Kopelman T, et al. The role of computed tomography in selective management of gunshot wounds to the amdomen and flank. *J Trauma.* 1998;45:1005-1009.

61. Shanmuganathan K, Mirvis SE, Chiu WC, Killeen KL, Scalea TM. Triple contrast helical CT in penetrating torso trauma: a prospective study to determine peritoneal violation and the need for laparotomy. *AJR Am J Roentgenol.* 2001;177:1247-1256.

62. Carrillo EH, Richardson JD. The current management of hepatic trauma. *Adv Surg.* 2001; 35:39-59.

63. Velmahos GC, Demetriades D, Chahwan S, et al. Angiographic embolization for arrest of bleeding after penetrating trauma to the abdomen. *Am J Surg.* 1999;178(5):367-373.

64. Dondelinger RF, Trotteur G, Ghaye B, Szapiro D. Traumatic injuries: radiological hemostatic intervention at admission. *Eur Radiol.* 2002;12(5):979-993.

65. Hauser CJ, Huprich JE, Bosco P, Gibbons L, Mansour AY, Weiss AR. Triple contrast computed tomography in the evaluation of penetrating posterior abdominal injuires. *Arch Surg.* 1987;122(10):1112-1115.

66. Himmelman RG, Martin M, Gilkey S, Barrett JA. Triple contrast CT scans in penetrating back and flank trauma. *J Trauma.* 1991;31(6):852-855.

67. Nau T, Seitz H, Mousavi M, Vecsei V. The diagnostic dilemma of traumatic rupture of the diaphragm. *Surg Endosc.* 2001;15(9):992-996.

68. Rich NM. Surgeon's response to battlefield vascular trauma. *Am J Surg.* 1993;166:91.

69. Waldschmidt ML, Laws HL. Injuries of the diaphragm. *J Trauma.* 1980;20(7):587-592.

70. Shackleton KL, Stewart ET, Taylor AJ. Traumatic diaphragmatic injuries: spectrum of radiographic findings. *Radiographics.* 1998;18(1):49-59.

71. Ma J, Norvell JG, Subramanian S. Ultrasound applications in mass casualties and extreme environments. *Crit Care Med.* 2007;35(5):S275-S279.

72. Chiao L, Salizhan S, Sargisyan AE, et al. Ocular examination for trauma; clinical ultrasound aboard the International Space Station. *J Trauma.* 2005;58:885-889.

73. Strode CA, Rubal BJ, Gerhardt RT, Bultrin JR, Boyd SY. Wireless and satellite transmission of prehospital focused abdominal sonography for trauma. *Prehosp Emerg Care.* 2003;7(3):375-379.

# Part V

## Advanced Resuscitation and Anaesthesia

Section Editor:
Chester C. Buckenmaier, III

# Damage Control Resuscitation

# 19

Adam J. Brooks and Bryan A. Cotton

## 19.1
## Introduction

The majority of deaths from trauma occur in the first few hours after injury, with hemorrhage accounting for the largest percentage of these deaths within the first hour of arrival at a trauma center.[1-3] Hemorrhagic shock and exsanguination account for more than 80% of deaths in the operating room and nearly 50% of deaths in the first 24 h after injury.[2-4] To address such a lethal model of injury, the concept of Damage Control evolved, based on the tenants of rapid cessation of hemorrhage and expedient control of bowel contamination.[5] The primary aim of Damage Control is to prevent the development of the lethal triad of coagulopathy, hypothermia, and metabolic acidosis (or to abbreviate the procedure once the triad begins to develop).

Since the implementation of Damage Control, institutions have observed dramatic reductions in mortality among the population of patients arriving in extremis after injury.[5,6] Despite these improvements and the tremendous efforts and attention directed at implementation of Damage Control techniques (abbreviated laparotomy, reversal of acidosis, correction of hypothermia), traumatic coagulopathy has been seriously underappreciated.[2,7,8] As such, many patients still succumbed to exsanguination as a result of poorly addressed acute coagulopathy of trauma and shock (ACoTS). Increasing evidence has demonstrated coagulopathy in the severely injured patient is often present in the field or upon arrival to the trauma center.[9-12] More importantly, this early coagulopathy and thrombocytopenia have been correlated with outcome.[12,13]

As a result of this growing body of data from the civilian and military setting, the concept of Damage Control Resuscitation (DCR) has developed.[7,10,11,14-18] DCR is built on the classic Damage Control framework where one attempts to avoid (or minimize) development of the lethal triad and achieve both medical and surgical hemostasis. These efforts are aimed at leaving the operating theater with an alive and physiologically intact patient.

A.J. Brooks (✉)
Emergency Surgery and Major Trauma, Nottingham University NHS Trust,
Nottingham, UK and
Academic Department of Military Surgery and Trauma, Royal Centre for
Defence Medicine, Birmingham, UK
e-mail: adam.brooks@nuh.nhs.uk

A.J. Brooks et al. (eds.), *Ryan's Ballistic Trauma*,
DOI: 10.1007/978-1-84882-124-8_19, © Springer-Verlag London Limited 2011

DCR is composed of three basic components[1]: permissive hypotension - palpable distal pulses in an awake patient,[2] minimizing crystalloid-based resuscitation strategies and[3] the immediate release and administration of pre-defined blood products (packed red blood cells, plasma, and platelets) in ratios similar to that of whole blood.[7,10,19]

## 19.2
## Components of Damage Control Resuscitation

### 19.2.1
### Damage Control Hematology

#### 19.2.1.1
#### Defining the Need

Damage control hematology (DCH) defines the process of delivering large amounts of blood products in an efficient manner in patients who have been identified as having life threatening hemorrhage.[10] Typically, products delivered include packed-red blood cells (PRBC), plasma, and platelets. Adjuncts include cryoprecipitate, recombinant factor VIIa, prothrombin concentrate, intra-operative cell salvage techniques, and fluid warmer/infusion systems. When incorporating this last product, it is critical to ensure that the system is utilized primarily for its product warming properties and not its rapid infusion properties, as these have been associated with increased hemorrhage-related mortality.[20]

Previously, ACoTS was based on laboratory data from the operating room and it was believed that abnormal coagulation laboratory values were not found in the first hours after injury and, when present, were associated with dilution. However, recent studies have shown that greater than 25% of injured patients arrive to the trauma center already coagulopathic and that these patients are at a markedly higher risk of mortality.[12,21,22] Niles et al. evaluated 3,287 combat casualties and found that, of the 391 transfused patients, 38% were coagulopathic on arrival to the combat support hospital.[12] More concerning, mortality among those arriving coagulopathic was 24% (vs 4% among those not coagulopathic on arrival). Civilian centers have found equally concerning data. Cotton et al. demonstrated that among 211 patients receiving massive transfusion (greater than 10 U PRBC in the initial 24 h) the prevalence of coagulopathy was 70%.[10] As with published military data, mortality among patients arriving coagulopathic was markedly greater than for those who were not coagulopathic (67% vs 42%).

#### 19.2.1.2
#### Protocol Development

To address the patient who has significant acute blood loss and arrives at the trauma center already coagulopathic, this aggressive delivery of blood products should begin prior to any laboratory defined anemia or coagulopathy. Therefore, it is critical that strategies are in place to directly (and rapidly) address this coagulopathy. A protocol should be created through the collaborative efforts of a multidisciplinary team. Relevant parties include individuals from emergency medicine, trauma, critical care, transfusion medicine, nursing, pathology, hematology, and anesthesia departments.[10,23,24]

In the absence of a pre-defined massive transfusion protocol, access to the appropriate volume and ratios of blood products may be significantly delayed. The layers of potential delay are too numerous to list here, but include physical ordering of the blood, communication and decision-making between involved parties, and the sending of laboratory samples and timely receipt of their results. Failure to immediately address and treat the evolving coagulopathy so often observed in these patients may lead to a worsening of their coagulopathy, possibly even to exsanguination and death. The transfusion of adequate ratios of blood products not only reduces the chances of developing (or decrease the severity of) traumatic coagulopathy, but also has been shown to improve survival and decrease overall usage of blood.[10,11,17] While few trauma centers had existing protocols in place prior to 2005, an increased number of institutions have implemented pre-defined protocols to address the injured patient requiring rapid release of a massive amount of blood products. One such published protocol is illustrated in Fig. 19.1.

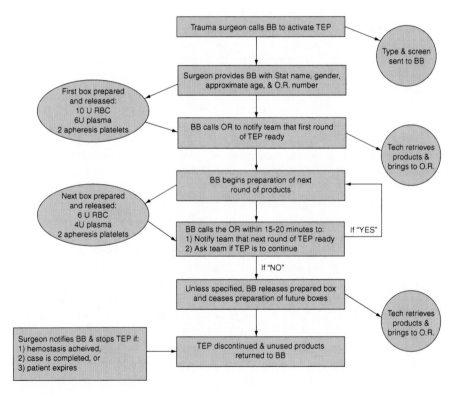

**Fig. 19.1** Massive transfusion protocol activation flowchart (http://www.mc.vanderbilt.edu/surgery/trauma/Protocols/)

### 19.2.1.3
### Identifying Optimal Ratios

To date, there are no prospective data informing clinicians of the optimal ratio of blood products for the MT trauma patient. Given the difficulty associated with performing a randomized controlled trial in this population of patients, several authors have attempted to define the optimal transfusion regimen in the absence of such a study design. Hirshberg et al. created a computer based hemodilution model to simulate the exsanguinating patient.[25] The authors recommended aiming for a ratio of plasma to PRBC of 2:3 and a ratio of platelets to PRBC of 8:10. Ho and colleagues also attempted to define adequate ratios of plasma to RBC through a pharmacokinetic mathematical model simulating the acute coagulopathy seen in trauma patients.[26] This group recommended that the equivalent of whole blood be transfused in order to avoid development or worsening of coagulopathy during the initial resuscitation of an exsanguinating patient; at least 1 unit of plasma and platelets for every red blood cell transfusion (1:1:1).[27]

Civilian and military investigators centers have evaluated their experience to identify the ideal plasma ratios for massive transfusion protocol development. Most civilian data suggests that ratios of at least 2:3 for plasma: PRBC are needed. Cotton and colleagues have demonstrated that patients receiving plasma: RBC at a ratio of 2:3 or greater had lower 30-day mortality when compared to patients receiving less than these ratios.[10,28] Interestingly, ratios of 1:1 did not reduce mortality any further than that observed for 2:3. This was similar to what Kashuk et al. showed in a 5-year retrospective review of 133 patients.[29] However, it is worth noting that only 45 patients in the Cotton data set and 11 patients in the Kashuk study achieved plasma: RBC ratio of 1:1 and their findings may represent a type-II error. Duchesne et al. recently evaluated their 4 year experience of patients who required a massive transfusion and found that those resuscitated with plasma to RBC ratio of 1:1 had a distinct survival advantage over those with a ratio of 1:4.[11] Holcomb et al. recently reported the findings of a retrospective, multi-center study of 466 massively transfused civilian trauma patients.[30] The authors demonstrated that patients receiving higher ratios (<1:2) of plasma to RBC had decreased truncal hemorrhage and increased survival. As well, Sperry et al. recently evaluated 415 blunt trauma patients within a national database and demonstrated that those who achieved a ratio of FFP: RBC < 1:1.5 had a significantly lower mortality rate.[31]

With respect to platelet ratios, there appears to be greater consensus among available data. The large multicenter trial from Holcomb and colleagues noted that patients receiving higher ratios (<1:2) of platelets to RBC had increased survival at 6 h, 24 h, and at 30 days.[30] The authors demonstrated that patients receiving higher ratios (<1:2) of plasma and platelets to RBC had decreased truncal hemorrhage and increased survival at 6 h, 24 h, and at 30 days. Cotton's group has examined the impact of platelet ratios on outcomes. The investigators have found that patients receiving apheresis platelets: RBC at a ratio of 1:5 or greater (1:1 or greater of traditional "packs" of platelets: PRBC) had lower 30-day mortality when compared to massive transfusion patients receiving less than these ratios.[10,28]

## 19.2.1.4
### Protocol Activation and Product Delivery

Typically, activation of a massive transfusion protocol is restricted to attending trauma surgeons and anesthesiologists. This usually occurs through a phone call directly to the blood bank after the faculty member has made the decision based on the clinical data available in the emergency department/trauma resuscitation area. Appropriate demographic data (stat name, approximate age, gender) to which operating room the first "cooler" should go (see Fig. 19.1). The blood bank then releases the pre-defined products in an immediate and sustained fashion.[28] To achieve an appropriate initial response, blood banks usually keep several units of thawed universal donor (AB) plasma and a large number of uncrossed-matched PRBC on hand, ready for immediate release. As each cooler of products is readied, blood banks typically contact the trauma team and notify them that the next cooler is en route and inquire as to whether or not the protocol should continue.

It is inadequate to simply deliver these products and have them transfused as available or in a non-specific time frame and expect to achieve the optimal benefits of a massive transfusion protocol. Failing to timely activate such protocols and deliver the products at the inception of the initial surgery has been associated with significantly worse outcomes.[28] Specifically, failure of the team to immediately transfuse the pre-defined ratios of plasma: PRBC and platelet; PRBC are independently associated with significant increases in 30-day mortality (83% vs 23% and 66% 19%, respectively). The most persistent issue identified by this group (and one that did not improve with provider re-education and academic detailing) was failure to identify the massive transfusion patient early enough and activate the institution's protocol before leaving the emergency department. Activation of the protocol after leaving the emergency department was associated with an almost 3-folds higher risk of death. Because of the lethality of such delays in early protocol activation, this group strongly recommended development and or inclusion of an objective scoring system to augment the clinical acumen of the trauma faculty.

## 19.2.1.5
### Adjuncts

US military experience from the joint theater trauma registry has demonstrated that injured soldiers who underwent massive transfusion and received recombinant factor VIIa early in their course had decreased 30-day mortality.[32] However, this was only retrospective data as is most information about the efficacy of VIIa in trauma. Boffard et al. performed the only randomized study evaluating VIIa in the exsanguinating trauma patient.[33] The authors noted a reduction in the amount of blood transfused (in blunt trauma patients) but did not find a mortality benefit. In light of the data available, many centers have not incorporated VIIa use into their massive transfusion protocols. Another potential adjunct for use in DCR are intra-operative blood salvage techniques (also known as "cell-saver" auto-transfusion devices). Both Timberlake and Ozmen have noted intra-operative blood salvage (IBS) techniques are safe and effective even in patients with intra-abdominal contamination and hemoperitoneum.[34,35] In a randomized controlled trial by Bowley and colleagues, the authors found a reduction in banked blood usage in the IBS group.[36] In addition, they found no difference between the IBS group and controls with respect to post-operative sepsis, survival, coagulopathy, or requirement for clotting factors.

## 19.3
## Permissive Hypotension

While it is recognized that maintaining arterial blood pressure within "normal" ranges may prevent circulatory shock in states of uncontrolled hemorrhage, such an approach in this population of patients may actually worsen bleeding and increase hemorrhage-related deaths. Increasing arterial pressure gradients haven been shown to impair the formation of new clot and dislodge existing clots.[37–39] This concept of clot disruption ("popping the clot") with attempts to "normalize" blood pressure has been well described but has only recently gained momentum in the literature and, more importantly, in clinical practice. Avoiding dislodgment of a hemostatic thrombus, through permissive hypotension, has been demonstrated to reduce bleeding and decrease hemorrhage volume.[2,40–42] The consensus of this literature is to allow the systolic blood pressure to remain at or slightly below 90 mmHg.

The traditional concept of quickly restoring systolic blood pressure to normal ranges is based on out-dated and (for the purpose of patients who are injured prior to arriving to the operating room) flawed hemorrhagic shock models. One such model known as the Wigger's hemorrhage model, was a hemorrhage study in which bleeding was stopped prior to initiating fluid resuscitation.[43] Such "controlled-hemorrhage models" are far from appropriate in studying the pathophysiology of fluid resuscitation with active hemorrhage. Investigators using uncontrolled hemorrhage models have actually demonstrated that resuscitation regimens that produce early increases in blood flow and blood pressure result in greater hemorrhage and mortality.[37,39,41,42,44] These investigators argue that aggressive pursuit of "normal" blood pressure reverses protective vasoconstriction, dislodges early clot formation, and increases hemorrhage occurrence and volume. Unfortunately, there is only one large, randomized human trial that has attempted to extrapolate this data to humans. In that trial, the authors noted a significant improvement in survival among penetrating torso trauma patients in which resuscitation was withheld.[45]

In light of these findings and mounting clinical experience to support it, many experts and consensus groups have published statements and guidelines supporting this concept of permissive (or deliberate) hypotension. These groups were composed of national and international opinion leaders in both the military and civilian trauma arena. In summary, the consensus recommendations are quite similar and are centered upon withholding or minimizing resuscitation prior to achieving surgical control of hemorrhage. Specifically,[1] if the patient is coherent and has a palpable radial pulse, venous access should be placed to "saline lock,"[2] if incoherent or no radial pulse, initiate small boluses of colloid solution (e.g., 500 mL hydroxyethylstarch), and[3] repeat bolus if no response, saline lock access if positive response noted. Importantly, these recommendations reflect that of the groups' evaluations of blunt and penetrating patients, in both military and civilian settings.

## 19.4
## Minimizing Crystalloid-Based Resuscitation

Despite an increased knowledge to the contrary, the advanced trauma life support (ATLS) curriculum recommends resuscitation begin with 2 l of crystalloid in the hypotensive patient, followed by blood products and surgical consultation and/or intervention.[46] Unfortunately, the 2 l fluid boluses are merely a starting point for the aggressive volume replacement that usually follows. Even more concerning is the adoption and application of these guidelines into the pre-hospital environment without any clear benefit. Recent data has shown that performance of pre-hospital procedures (e.g., placement of intra-venous access and subsequent fluid administration) negatively impacts survival in critically injured patients.[40,47,48] While many providers still view the subsequent administration of fluids to be standard of care, neither the animal nor clinical literature would support this approach.

Recent animal data supports the "minimizing" of crystalloid resuscitation until surgical control of hemorrhage has been achieved. Owens and colleagues evaluated the effect of different resuscitation regimens on a group of Yorkshire pigs.[49] In this early, uncontrolled hemorrhage model, peritoneal blood loss and hemoglobin loss were significantly higher in the standard ("euvolemic") crystalloid group. As well, the oxygen delivery was lowest in this group and highest in the low-volume group. Xiao et al. demonstrated that animals whose fluids were titrated to lower mean arterial pressures and smaller volumes had the highest survival when mean arterial blood pressures were in the human equivalent range of 40–60 mmHg.[50] Colloid based agents (e.g., hydroxyethylstarch) and hypertonic saline solutions have been increasingly demonstrated to provide improved perfusion without significant changes in arterial pressure and subsequent hemorrhage volumes.[51–54] Using a murine model of uncontrolled hemorrhage, Krausz et al. compared the administration of lactated Ringer's (LR) and hypertonic saline, combined with splenectomy.[52] The LR solution resulted in significantly more bleeding than infusion of hypertonic saline.

Though they are few, clinical trials performed to date have produced similar findings supporting fluid restriction prior to obtaining control of hemorrhage.[45,55–57] Dalton and colleagues evaluated the effects of pre-hospital fluid administration and noted that 80% patients receive less than 600 mL of fluid in the pre-hospital setting, regardless of mechanism, scene entrapment, or hypotension en route.[58] They were unable to identify benefit from such therapy and recommended withholding fluid administration.

Dutton and colleagues evaluated the concept of "hypotensive resuscitation" and noted that titration of initial fluid therapy to a lower than normal SBP (≥70 mmHg instead of <100 mmHg) during active hemorrhage did not affect mortality.[9] In the early 1990s, Bickell et al. conducted a trial of hypotensive patients with penetrating torso injuries in which individuals were randomized in the field to receive either standard intravenous fluid resuscitation or no fluids. This regimen was continued until the patient reached the operating theater. Despite the lack of fluid resuscitation, the mean blood pressure between the groups was similar while intra-operative blood loss was significantly less in the delayed resuscitation group. More importantly, the mortality rate was significantly lower in the delayed resuscitation group.

As with the pre-hemorrhage control pursuit of "normal" blood pressures, large volume crystalloid-based regimens have been aggressively criticized by several groups and authors.[59-62] Consensus statements from several of these groups were aimed directly at whether to administer fluids prior to hospital arrival (and definitive hemorrhage control). Recommendations included[1] the avoidance of immediate intravenous fluid resuscitation if the patient is coherent and has a palpable radial pulse,[2] the administration of small volume boluses (preferably using colloids) should the patient become incoherent or demonstrate no radial pulse,[3] the titration of fluid boluses until coherence or a palpable radial pulse returns, and[4] the discontinuation of fluids with a positive response to fluid bolus.

## 19.5
## Conclusions

Damage Control Resuscitation continues to develop from its origins on the modern battle-fields of Iraq and Afghanistan. Civilian and military research into all aspects of this approach is ongoing and will likely inform DCR in the future.

## References

1. Acosta JA, Yang JC, Winchell RJ, et al. Lethal injuries and time to death in a level I trauma center. *J Am Coll Surg*. 1998;186:528-533.
2. Kauvar DS, Lefering R, Wade CE. Impact of hemorrhage on trauma outcome: an overview of epidemiology, clinical presentations, and therapeutic considerations. *J Trauma*. 2006;60:S3-S11.
3. Sauaia A, Moore FA, Moore EE, et al. Epidemiology of trauma deaths: a reassessment. *J Trauma*. 1995;38:185-193.
4. Hoyt DB, Bulger EM, Knudson MM, et al. Death in the operating room: an analysis of a multi-center experience. *J Trauma*. 1994;37:426-432.
5. Rotondo MF, Schwab CW, McGonigal MD, et al. Damage control': an approach for improved survival in exsanguinating penetrating abdominal injury. *J Trauma*. 1993;35:375-382. discussion 382-373.
6. Stone HH, Strom PR, Mullins RJ. Management of the major coagulopathy with onset during laparotomy. *Ann Surg*. 1983;197:532-535.
7. Holcomb JB, Jenkins D, Rhee P, et al. Damage control resuscitation: directly addressing the early coagulopathy of trauma. *J Trauma*. 2007;62:307-310.
8. Hutt J, Wallis L. Blood products in trauma resuscitation. *J R Army Med Corps*. 2006; 152:121-127.
9. Brohi K, Singh J, Heron M, et al. Acute traumatic coagulopathy. *J Trauma*. 2003;54:1127-1130.
10. Cotton BA, Gunter OL, Isbell J, et al. Damage control hematology: the impact of a trauma exsanguination protocol on survival and blood product utilization. *J Trauma*. 2008;64: 1177-1182. discussion 1182-1173.

11. Duchesne JC, Hunt JP, Wahl G, et al. Review of current blood transfusions strategies in a mature level I trauma center: were we wrong for the last 60 years? *J Trauma*. 2008;65: 272-276. discussion 276-278.

12. Niles SE, McLaughlin DF, Perkins JG, et al. Increased mortality associated with the early coagulopathy of trauma in combat casualties. *J Trauma*. 2008;64:1459-1463. discussion 1463-1455.

13. Borgman MA, Spinella PC, Perkins JG, et al. The ratio of blood products transfused affects mortality in patients receiving massive transfusions at a combat support hospital 12. *J Trauma*. 2007;63:805-813.

14. Cotton BA, Au BK, Nunez TC, et al. Predefined massive transfusion protocols are associated with a reduction in organ failure and postinjury complications. *J Trauma*. 2009;66:41-48. discussion 48-49.

15. Hess JR, Dutton RB, Holcomb JB, et al. Giving plasma at a 1:1 ratio with red cells in resuscitation: who might benefit? *Transfusion*. 2008;48:1763-1765.

16. Ketchum L, Hess JR, Hiippala S. Indications for early fresh frozen plasma, cryoprecipitate, and platelet transfusion in trauma. *J Trauma*. 2006;60:S51-S58.

17. O'Keeffe T, Refaai M, Tchorz K, et al. A massive transfusion protocol to decrease blood component use and costs. *Arch Surg*. 2008;143:686-690. discussion 690-681.

18. Spinella PC, Perkins JG, Grathwohl KW, et al. Effect of plasma and red blood cell transfusions on survival in patients with combat related traumatic injuries. *J Trauma*. 2008;64: S69-S77. discussion S77-S68.

19. Hess JR, Holcomb JB, Hoyt DB. Damage control resuscitation: the need for specific blood products to treat the coagulopathy of trauma. *Transfusion*. 2006;46:685-686.

20. Hambly PR, Dutton RP. Excess mortality associated with the use of a rapid infusion system at a level 1 trauma center 42. *Resuscitation*. 1996;31:127-133.

21. Brohi K, Singh J, Heron M, et al. Acute traumatic coagulopathy. *J Trauma*. 2003;54:1127-1130.

22. MacLeod JB, Lynn M, McKenney MG, et al. Early coagulopathy predicts mortality in trauma. *J Trauma*. 2003;55:39-44.

23. Bormanis J. Development of a massive transfusion protocol. *Transfus Apher Sci*. 2008;38:57-63.

24. Stainsby D, MacLennan S, Hamilton PJ. Management of massive blood loss: a template guideline. *Br J Anaesth*. 2000;85:487-491.

25. Hirshberg A, Dugas M, Banez EI, et al. Minimizing dilutional coagulopathy in exsanguinating hemorrhage: a computer simulation. *J Trauma*. 2003;54:454-463.

26. Ho AM, Dion PW, Cheng CA, et al. A mathematical model for fresh frozen plasma transfusion strategies during major trauma resuscitation with ongoing hemorrhage. *Can J Surg*. 2005;48:470-478.

27. Ho AM, Karmakar MK, Dion PW. Are we giving enough coagulation factors during major trauma resuscitation? *Am J Surg*. 2005;190:479-484.

28. Cotton BA, Dossett LA, Nunez TC, et al. Room for (performance) improvement: provider-related factors associated with poor outcomes in massive transfusion. *J Trauma*. 2009;67(5): 1004-1012.

29. Kashuk JL, Moore EE, Johnson JL, et al. Postinjury life threatening coagulopathy: is 1:1 fresh frozen plasma:packed red blood cells the answer? *J Trauma*. 2008;65:261-270. discussion 270-261.

30. Holcomb JB, Wade CE, Michalek JE, et al. Increased plasma and platelet to red blood cell ratios improves outcome in 466 massively transfused civilian trauma patients. *Ann Surg*. 2008;248:447-458.

31. Sperry JL, Ochoa JB, Gunn SR, et al. An FFP:PRBC transfusion ratio </=1:1.5 is associated with a lower risk of mortality after massive transfusion. *J Trauma*. 2008;65:986-993.

32. Spinella PC, Perkins JG, McLaughlin DF, et al. The effect of recombinant activated factor VII on mortality in combat-related casualties with severe trauma and massive transfusion. *J Trauma*. 2008;64:286-293. discussion 293-284.

33. Boffard KD, Riou B, Warren B, et al. Recombinant factor VIIa as adjunctive therapy for bleeding control in severely injured trauma patients: two parallel randomized, placebo-controlled, double-blind clinical trials. *J Trauma*. 2005;59:8-15. discussion 15-18.

34. Timberlake GA, McSwain NE Jr. Autotransfusion of blood contaminated by enteric contents: a potentially life-saving measure in the massively hemorrhaging trauma patient? *J Trauma*. 1988;28:855-857.

35. Ozmen V, McSwain NE Jr, Nichols RL, et al. Autotransfusion of potentially culture-positive blood (CPB) in abdominal trauma: preliminary data from a prospective study. *J Trauma*. 1992;32:36-39.

36. Bowley DM, Barker P, Boffard KD. Intraoperative blood salvage in penetrating abdominal trauma: a randomised, controlled trial 6. *World J Surg*. 2006;30:1074-1080.

37. Dries DJ. Hypotensive resuscitation. *Shock*. 1996;6:311-316.

38. Raedler C, Voelckel WG, Wenzel V, et al. Vasopressor response in a porcine model of hypothermic cardiac arrest is improved with active compression-decompression cardiopulmonary resuscitation using the inspiratory impedance threshold valve. *Anesth Analg*. 2002;95:1496-1502. table of contents.

39. Raedler C, Voelckel WG, Wenzel V, et al. Treatment of uncontrolled hemorrhagic shock after liver trauma: fatal effects of fluid resuscitation versus improved outcome after vasopressin. *Anesth Analg*. 2004;98:1759-1766. table of contents.

40. Capone AC, Safar P, Stezoski W, et al. Improved outcome with fluid restriction in treatment of uncontrolled hemorrhagic shock. *J Am Coll Surg*. 1995;180:49-56.

41. Sondeen JL, Coppes VG, Holcomb JB. Blood pressure at which rebleeding occurs after resuscitation in swine with aortic injury 106. *J Trauma*. 2003;54:S110-S117.

42. Sondeen JL, Dubick MA, Holcomb JB, et al. Uncontrolled hemorrhage differs from volume- or pressure-matched controlled hemorrhage in swine 32. *Shock*. 2007;28:426-433.

43. Wiggers CJ. Basic hemodynamic principles essential to interpretation of cardiovascular disorders: the ludwig kast lecture. *Bull N Y Acad Med*. 1942;18:3-17.

44. Stern SA, Dronen SC, Birrer P, et al. Effect of blood pressure on hemorrhage volume and survival in a near-fatal hemorrhage model incorporating a vascular injury. *Ann Emerg Med*. 1993;22:155-163.

45. Bickell WH, Wall MJ Jr, Pepe PE, et al. Immediate versus delayed fluid resuscitation for hypotensive patients with penetrating torso injuries. *N Engl J Med*. 1994;331:1105-1109.

46. Surgeons ACo. *Advanced Trauma Life Support for Doctors*. Chicago, IL: American College of Surgeons; 1997.

47. Cornwell EE 3rd, Belzberg H, Hennigan K, et al. Emergency medical services (EMS) vs non-EMS transport of critically injured patients: a prospective evaluation. *Arch Surg*. 2000;135:315-319.

48. Seamon MJ, Fisher CA, Gaughan J, et al. Prehospital procedures before emergency department thoracotomy: "Scoop and run" saves lives. *J Trauma*. 2007;63:113-120.

49. Owens TM, Watson WC, Prough DS, et al. Limiting initial resuscitation of uncontrolled hemorrhage reduces internal bleeding and subsequent volume requirements. *J Trauma*. 1995;39:200-207. discussion 208-209.

50. Xiao N, Wang XC, Diao YF, et al. Effect of initial fluid resuscitation on subsequent treatment in uncontrolled hemorrhagic shock in rats. *Shock*. 2004;21:276-280.

51. Krausz MM, Bashenko Y, Hirsh M. Crystalloid and colloid resuscitation of uncontrolled hemorrhagic shock following massive splenic injury. *Shock*. 2001;16:383-388.

52. Krausz MM, Hirsh M. Bolus versus continuous fluid resuscitation and splenectomy for treatment of uncontrolled hemorrhagic shock after massive splenic injury. *J Trauma*. 2003;55:62-68.

53. Stern SA, Jwayyed S, Dronen SC, et al. Resuscitation of severe uncontrolled hemorrhage: 7.5% sodium chloride/6% dextran 70 vs 0.9% sodium chloride. *Acad Emerg Med*. 2000;7:847-856.

54. Stern SA, Kowalenko T, Younger J, et al. Comparison of the effects of bolus vs. slow infusion of 7.5% NaCl/6% dextran-70 in a model of near-lethal uncontrolled hemorrhage. *Shock*. 2000;14:616-622.

55. Barak M, Rudin M, Vofsi O, et al. Fluid administration during abdominal surgery influences on coagulation in the postoperative period. *Curr Surg*. 2004;61:459-462.
56. Dutton RP. Low-pressure resuscitation from hemorrhagic shock 39. *Int Anesthesiol Clin*. 2002;40:19-30.
57. Dutton RP, Mackenzie CF, Scalea TM. Hypotensive resuscitation during active hemorrhage: impact on in-hospital mortality 40. *J Trauma*. 2002;52:1141-1146.
58. Dalton AM. Prehospital intravenous fluid replacement in trauma: an outmoded concept? *J R Soc Med*. 1995;88:213-216.
59. Anonymous. Fluid resuscitation in pre-hospital trauma care: a consensus view. *J R Army Med Corps*. 2001;147:147-162.
60. Cotton BA, Jerome R, Collier BR, et al. Eastern Association for the Surgery of Trauma (EAST) practice management guidelines for pre-hospital fluid resuscitaion. *J Trauma*. 2009; 67:389-402.
61. Holcomb JB. Fluid resuscitation in modern combat casualty care: lessons learned from Somalia 107. *J Trauma*. 2003;54:S46-S51.
62. Revell M, Porter K, Greaves I. Fluid resuscitation in prehospital trauma care: a consensus view. *Emerg Med J*. 2002;19:494-498.

# Battlefield Analgesia

# 20

Aaron D. Nelson and Dominic J. Aldington

## 20.1
## Battlefield Pain Management

*It is easier to find men who will volunteer to die, than to find those who are willing to endure pain with patience.*

Julius Caesar

This chapter begins with an overview of pain concepts, pain scoring, and analgesic options. It goes on to review current treatment suggestions for the ballistic casualty at each stage of their care. Finally, a series of appendices offer further information on the drugs, on patient controlled devices, and management of overdoses.

Note: Medication regulatory issues vary around the world and are beyond the scope of this text. Therefore, these issues will not be discussed.

## 20.2
## Introduction

Pain is usually a casualty's primary concern and anecdote suggests analgesia is becoming an increasingly important issue in the medical care of casualties as well.[1] The larger volume of lower intensity casualty generation in most modern conflicts means that medical services are having to worry less about the (overwhelming) quantity of casualties envisaged in a conflict 30 years ago and can now concentrate on the quality of the casualty care[2]; part of this is the consideration of analgesia. Historically in trauma, analgesia was either withheld or severely delayed due to concerns for hemodynamic instability, underestimation of pain with the assumption that a patient's pain correlated with their injury, belief that pain will assist in diagnosis, and excessive concern about addiction. These concerns are

A.D. Nelson (✉)
Department of Anesthesiology and Operative Services, Anesthesiology and Pain Management Division, Brooke Army Medical Center, Fort Sam Houston, TX, USA
e-mail: aaron.d.nelson@us.army.mil

A.J. Brooks et al. (eds.), *Ryan's Ballistic Trauma*,
DOI: 10.1007/978-1-84882-124-8_20, © Springer-Verlag London Limited 2011

compounded by limitations of personnel, equipment, and ability to monitor patients in the military or remote environment.

Secondly, it is also believed that good analgesia can improve casualty outcomes, both physiologically and psychologically.[3] Finally it is true to say that good pain relief is increasingly expected within the wider civilian populations and by extension by our casualty population itself.

## 20.3
## Definitions and Concepts

There are a number of definitions for pain. One of the better recognized is:

"Pain is an unpleasant sensory and emotional experience associated with actual or potential damage or described in terms of such damage."[4] It is imperative that pain be recognized as having both components (sensation and emotional interpretation), as both contribute to not only the understanding of pain, but can be useful therapeutic targets.

Pain can be classified in a number of ways. One is according to its duration. Chronic pain is a pain that last for more than 3 months, while acute pain is the pain that lasts from the time of injury up to this point. Thus, acute pain is the "normal" pain that we experience with an injury and thus is almost a universal experience. These terms, acute and chronic are a temporal distinction and have no relationship to the severity or intensity of the pain. Classification of pain by primary source (i.e. somatic, neuropathic, etc.) can be overlapping or somewhat subjective, but has been used to target certain therapies.

One of the difficulties that exists when treating pain is we tend to believe that we understand pain better than we probably do. Thus the idea that an insult in the periphery activates a receptor, which sends a message of pain along the nervous system up to the brain where we have a "pain" sensation, is a concept that has been taught since the time of Descartes and is still taught today. This pain theory has some practical value. It provides explanations for why we get pain and why some drugs and treatments such as nerve blocks will remove the feeling of pain. However, it does not explain why following amputation some people will experience pain in a limb they no longer have, nor why following a traumatic lower limb amputation from an improvised explosive device blast, a casualty may refuse offers of analgesia because no pain is perceived despite significant tissue damage. It also fails to recognize that pain is an individualized experience that has an interpretive psychological component. Each person will experience pain within their own social context which is influenced by their perceptions on how the injury will impact on current and future functioning.

A more accurate theory likely involves the complex interaction of the sensory and psychological components of pain, together with the dynamic nature of the nervous system. The more traditional view of a "hard wired" system, which we are often taught, is likely too simple a theory for our current understanding of pain. What has become increasingly understood is that pain is not simply an ascending neural transmission, but has significant modulation from descending neural pathways, which can be an important component in treatment.

## 20.4
## Principles of Acute Pain Management

Assessment 0–3; 0–10
Treatment
   Non-medical
      Reassure
      Remove cause
   Medical
      Local anesthetic blocks
      Pain Ladder
         Mild pain – Paracetamol
         Moderate pain – "Weak" Opiate
         Severe pain – "Strong" Opioid
Reassessment of pain and effect of intervention

## 20.5
## Assessment

Subjective measurement of pain is the first step in the management of pain. Historically in severe trauma, this simple step has been the one most frequently absent. A baseline assessment of the patient's perception of pain severity is required to develop an individualized pain treatment plan and then evaluate the effectiveness of the plan. For multiple reasons, the pain experienced by the patient does not always correlate with severity of injury.

There exist a number of validated ways of scoring pain. Commonly people may be asked to score their pain on a scale from 0 to 10, where 0 is no pain and 10 is the worse pain they can imagine. This 0–10 score is derived from the visual analogue score that uses a 100 mm line to evaluate pain. This is of great value in scientific trials but little use in the pre-hospital environment.

In the field environment we need a scale that is quick to use, has a "value" that will guide our decision making and is easily understood by both the casualty and the provider. One such scale runs from 0 to 3. This has the advantage of not only equating to none, mild, moderate, and severe pain, but also of fitting in with the acute pain ladder (see below) thus aiding decision making. It is also easy to understand albeit of less research value.

It is possible to roughly equate these two different verbal numerical scales 0–10 and 0–3 allowing comparisons if necessary.[5] Needless to say care must be taken to ensure that the pain score being used is understood by all; a 3 on a scale up to 10 is not the same as a 3 on a scale up to 3. Both scoring systems should also be accompanied by a patient's perception of the adequacy of their pain control (pain is tolerable, moderately tolerable, or not tolerable for example). There are situations in polytrauma where a patient will complain of 5/10, but state their pain control is very tolerable.

There are problems when gauging pain across different cultures and of course in the case of casualties who cannot communicate- either because they speak different languages or no language- extremes of age or severe injury. In these cases some specialize scores do exist but the fail-safe option is to use clinical judgment and experience to guide therapy.

Pain scores should be recorded prior to any analgesic being given and the scoring of pain is as important as scoring any of the other physiological "vital" signs- heart rate, blood pressure, respiratory rate

## 20.6
## Treatment Options

This section will look at the following options for the treatment of acute pain:

Non Medical
1. Reassurance
2. Remove Cause

Medical
3. Regional Anesthesia
4. Pharmacological options

### 20.6.1
### Reassurance

Simple reassurance can have a significant beneficial effect for both the casualty and those around them.

### 20.6.2
### Cause Removal

If possible the cause of pain should be removed. Fractures should be splinted. Bandages should not be so tight that they function as tourniquets – unless that is their explicit function. Patients should be made as comfortable as possible for transport.

### 20.6.3
### Regional Anesthesia

The aim of regional anesthesia is to reversibly block the transmission of afferent pain signals between the point of injury and the brain. It may take the form of peripheral nerve blocks, distal to the spinal cord, or neuraxial blockade such as epidural and subarachnoid injections. The injections may be performed "blind" using surface anatomy and clinical judgment, or using aids to placement such as stimulating needles and ultrasound. Local anesthetics are usually injected, but may have other agents added to them to enhance their action. They can be administered in the form of single injections or as continuous infusions.

These are not "new" techniques having been described in the military medical literature for the past 60 years[6] when they were the only techniques available. However modern technologies have made their use safer and more reliable leading to an increase in use.[7]

As with any anesthetic technique there are complications associated with regional anesthesia. The two especially devastating consequences may be the development of a compartment syndrome or unintentional intravascular injection. Although a regional anesthetic block does not directly cause compartment syndrome, it may delay its recognition and thus exacerbate the degree of injury, but then this is true of any pain management modality. Because pain management is a vital part of any surgical plan, the best way to minimize the risk of compartment syndrome is a high index of suspicion, and a multimodal pain management plan that minimizes unwanted side effects associated with using any one modality for pain management. For this reason discussion with a surgeon is advisable before a block is performed. Unintentional intravascular injection can result in seizures and cardiovascular collapse. Careful assessment of ability to treat a casualty in the event of local anesthetic toxicity is important to take into consideration prior to utilization of regional techniques. Further detailed information for using regional anesthesia in field conditions can be found in the Military Advanced Regional Anesthesia and Analgesia Handbook (www.bordeninstitute.com).

### 20.6.4
### Pharmacological Options

### 20.6.4.1
### Agent

The pharmacological approach to acute pain treatment can be summed up using the acute pain ladder. The drugs are arranged in a "ladder," with the weakest forming the bottom "rung" and the strongest at the top. There are traditionally three rungs corresponding to mild, moderate, and severe pain.

The bottom rung is traditionally paracetamol (acetaminophen).

The second rung is made of the "weak" opiates such as codeine, tramadol, and pethidine. These may be prepared in combination with paracetamol so care should be given to avoid overdose of the latter. The modern approach is to consider the non-steroidal anti-inflammatory drugs as second line (because of their side effect possibilities).

The final stage is the "strong" opiates such as morphine, oxycodone, hydromorphone, and fentanyl.

The important feature of this ladder system is that under normal situations one would ascend the ladder from the bottom rung up; thus in severe pain all three groups of agent may be necessary and can be combined to improve relief and minimize adverse effects (Table 20.1).

**Table 20.1** Pharmacological options

| Pain score | | | Analgesics used | | |
|---|---|---|---|---|---|
| Numerical | Verbal | | | | |
| 10<br>9<br>8<br>7 | 3 | Severe | | | "Strong" opioid |
| 6<br>5<br>4 | 2 | Moderate | | "Weak" opioid and/or NSAID | "Weak" opioid and/or NSAID |
| 3<br>2<br>1 | 1 | Mild | Paracetamol | Paracetamol | Paracetamol |

## 20.7
## Treatment Phases

The following recommendations are intended only as a guide for therapy. Obviously the patient, clinical situation, and physician experience will greatly influence actual treatment choices. Treatment plans for polytrauma defy protocol driven pain medicine and require individualization for effectiveness. The phrase to keep at the forefront of one's mind is "Primum non nocere."

### 20.7.1
### Prehospital

#### 20.7.1.1
#### Individual

In the ideal situation the casualty will be able to initiate their own analgesic treatment when they feel they need it. In cases of mild or moderate pain it may be that agents from the bottom and middle "rungs" of the pain ladder will be sufficient. Musculoskeletal injuries or minor burns are examples where individual treatment is appropriate.

However, when dealing with severe pain one of the "strong" opiates will be necessary. Clinicians often make the error of going straight to opioid medications, initially ignoring the other "rungs" dictated by the normal approach. Certainly doses of NSAIDs and "weak" opiates provide an analgesic foundation for the successful application of reduced amounts of strong opioid.

**Individual**

Measure and record pain
Morphine 10 mg im 2 hourly

**Unit "Medic"**

Measure and record pain
Morphine 10 mg im
Consider Paracetamol 1 g qds po/pr
   NSAID

**Tactical Transfer**

Measure and record pain
Morphine 10 mg im or 0.1 mg/kg iv
Ketamine 10–20 mg iv 5mins
Consider
   Paracetamol 1 g qds popr/iv
   NSAID
   Local anesthetic peripheral nerve block

**Field Hospital**

Measure and record pain
As above with augmentation according to equipment and experience
Patient controlled analgesia (see below)
Consider Amitriptyline 50 mg po on (see below)

**Strategic Transfer**

Measure and record pain
Continuing what has been started at the field hospital to include PCA, CPNB,
Epidural infusions
Consider transmucosal fentanyl for breakthrough pain

**Base Hospital**

Measure and record pain
Use whatever is necessary

United States special operation forces physicians have had good results with a protocol for a "wound pack" consisting of acetaminophen, rofecoxib (now meloxicam), and a flouro-quinolone.[8,9] Of important note is that this strategy was specifically designed for highly trained military operators who had need to administer medication which would cause little or no effect on mental status and coagulation, and which also conserved limited medical supplies in a situation with a high risk of delayed extraction. This has not been in broad-scale use in regular military units. The wound pack represents a significant step forward in non-opioid based, far-forward, individual pain management and should be evaluated further for a more generalized military use (Fig. 20.1).

Some thought should be given to recording what analgesia has been administered and when, especially if implementing pain management medications that are unit specific (see above), outside the dosing in "common use," or if casualties will be evacuated to different facilities or to multi-national facilities.

**Fig. 20.1** Shock pack

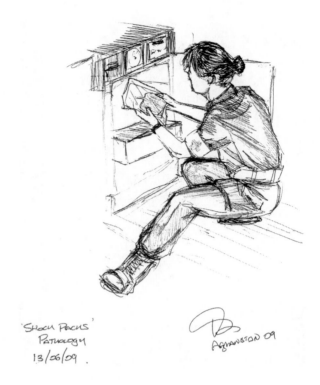

'Shock Packs'
Pathology
13/06/09 .

Aghanistan 09

## 20.7.1.2
## Unit Medic

Analgesia issues should be considered only after providers have ensured adequate airway, breathing, and circulation of the casualty is established.

The team's medical specialist would be expected to provide initial pain assessment of the casualty and provide first line medications as needed. The medic should also be proficient in providing non-pharmacological support particularly reassurance and reduction in the cause of the pain. This is particularly important as judicious use of medical supplies in a forward or austere environment is critical. Furthermore, effort should be made to record f pain scores and the times, doses, and route of analgesics.

Improvements in intravenous and intraosseus access allow intravenous medication administration for appropriately trained forward personnel with the advantage of more predictable pharmacokinetics. Hemodynamically stable casualties may not have intravenous access, leaving oral and IM administration as options.

In 2004, US Army physicians published a study reporting the use of transmucosal fentanyl citrate for analgesia in hemodynamically stable combat casualties with isolated orthopedic injuries.[8,9] The authors identified that transmucosal fentanyl had many characteristics of the "ideal battlefield analgesic," and described its successful use by taping the stick of the fentanyl "pop" to the casualties finger. Important to note, the availability of this strategy was limited to medical officers and senior medics to ensure proper patient evaluation, selection, and monitoring. As this strategy is not commonplace, documentation of timing and dosing of medication becomes vital.

### 20.7.1.3
#### Tactical Transfer

Analgesic provision during the tactical transfer phase is of key importance to the well being of the casualty during evacuation. Clear pain management records should be kept of what occurs and communication if pain treatment plans at patient transfer is vital. Further doses of drugs, or even initial doses of those that have not been given, may be required but again the simple steps of reassurance and reduction of the cause of the pain should not be over looked.

Other agents such as ketamine and simple peripheral nerve blocks may be introduced at this stage. Single injection t peripheral nerve blocks in particular may be especially useful for pain management of extremity trauma during transport and evacuation of casualties to higher levels of care. They offer the advantages of good analgesia with less concern for exacerbation of hemodynamic instability, sedation, nausea, or respiratory depression during the time period when individual monitoring and resources may be limited. Optimally, the duration of the block may match or just exceed the transport duration.

When peripheral blocks are used, it is imperative that there be clear identification of any transport patient who has received a block so that they can be quickly identified and evaluated once they've arrived at the receiving facility. The pre-block extremity evaluation for sensory and motor function should accompany the patient. On arrival, any casualty receiving a block for transport needs to have evaluation of soft tissue compartments in the involved extremity and an assessment of the block to allow oral or intravenous medications to be started/resumed prior to the block wearing off.

What can actually be achieved will depend on the mode of transfer, the duration of transfer, the tactical situation, and skills of providers present.

### 20.7.2
#### Field Hospital

Most deployed field medical establishments should be capable of significant analgesia. Again the most important step is to evaluate the pain whenever the other physiological vital signs are being assessed -Temperature, Pulse, Respirations, Pain; "TPR-Pain."

The Role 3 field hospital should have physicians with advanced pain management skills and the equipment to all allow safer use of stronger analgesics or of more complicated techniques of pain relief.

The first procedures for providing restorative surgery are usually accomplished at the field hospital. A multimodal pain plan using a variety of analgesics can be established with an understanding that the patient will likely soon be evacuated. Agents such as ketamine and sedatives such as benzodiazepines are likely to be used together with more opiates. Patient controlled analgesic (PCA) pumps may also be used allowing the sensate patient to control their own analgesia. A tricyclic antidepressant such as Amitriptyline should also be considered (see "Chronic Pain" below"). Anticonvulsant medications such as Gabapentin, normally thought of as chronic pain medications, have been increasingly recognized as having acute management benefits and can be considered.

> *Regional anaesthetic techniques, particularly PCA, CPNB, and epidural infusions are becoming more common. The use of advanced pain management modalities such as these assumes proper staff training and equipment throughout the evacuation chain.*

## 20.7.3
## Strategic Transfer

A clear understanding of air evacuation policy and procedure is imperative for successful pain care in Role 3 and during strategic transfer. Communication of patient air evacuation pain plans in essential. If specific analgesics are being given the patient should have a good supply of them. If specific personnel (such as doctors) are required to administer the drugs, they should be on the flight; it is assumed that most strategic transfers will be done by air. If specific pieces of equipment such as infusion pumps are required, the transfer personnel need to be happy with their operation and they need to have been "cleared for flight" which can be a lengthy process. Medical staff should also have optional pain plans available in case primary plans fail.

Occasionally unexpected "break-through" pain may occur. If this occurs, an analgesic such as oral transmucosal fentanyl or sublingual fentanyl would be appropriate.

## 20.8
## Chronic Pain

Development of chronic pain following trauma is both common and difficult to treat.[10] It can have a profound effect on both the survivor and their family. There may also be an association with subsequent post-traumatic stress disorder development.

Current evidence and treatments do not support that there is a clear cut treatment that will prevent development of chronic pain. As a result, prevention and treatment have centered on the known risk factors. Intuitively it is felt that good initial analgesia probably helps as will appropriate robust rehabilitation in surroundings appropriate for the individual.

We encourage early use of the drugs used in the management of nerve ("neuropathic") pain in the field hospital prior to return to the level 4 facility. These are started preemptively in an attempt to reduce later problems. Examples of these are tricyclic antidepressants (Amitriptyline 50 mg daily) or some of the anticonvulsants. While the evidence for this approach is weak at present, they do have other more obvious benefits such as enhancing sleep which can be significantly deranged and are thought to be beneficial in the treatment of PTSD as well. Pain and PTSD have overlapping neurologic pathways, and interact in a poorly understood directional relationship. However, the increased rate at which PTSD is seen when chronic pain results directly from a traumatic event indicates a significant interaction in vulnerable individuals.

.The treatment of casualties of traumatic injuries who develop chronic pain absolutely must include consideration and treatment of psychological and social problems that individual will face. From simple interventions from ensuring proper fitting prosthetics for amputees, to large-scale projects such as renovation of living quarters, an aggressive approach to psychosocial problems can have profound effects on a patient's outlook, mood, and interpretation of their level of disability due to pain or injury.

### 20.8.1
### "Addiction" Issues

The use of opioid medication is often stigmatized due to issues of addiction. A clear understanding of this issue and the definitions used is important for pain providerse.

> *Dependence* indicates the potential for withdrawal symptoms associated with dose reduction or cessation. This effect can be seen with many medications and not specifically opioids; one example is slowly reducing steroid doses.
>
> *Tolerance* indicates a reduction in the effect of a specific dose. With opioids this is seen more quickly with nausea and sedation than with analgesia and constipation. Tolerance is a normal physiologic response to chronic administration of many medications, and should be expected.
>
> *Addiction* implies a compulsive use of a substance and the pre-occupation with obtaining it in the face of evidence suggesting further use would lead to harm. Rates of addiction to opioids *in acute pain managment due to traumatic injury* tend to be severely overestimated by health care providers. Although there is a significant range of rates reported in current literature, the rates have nearly universally been cited to be in the low single digits.
>
> *Pseudo-addiction* refers to a healthcare provider's impression that a patient is seeking opioids due to addiction when in fact they are seeking opioids for relief of undertreated pain. This phenomenon can be reduced through use of multimodal pain plans that have less emphasis on opioids.

### 20.9
### The Future

Analgesia will continue to be of increasing importance as our understanding of the impact pain has on morbidity and mortality is further clarified. Pain is now understood to be a disease process itself rather than just a symptom of disease. To aid in this sea change there will be a greater collection of epidemiological data on pain and analgesia and further research to help optimize treatment.

> *Whilst completely novel pain medications are not likely to be available soon, enhancements to delivery technology and improved understanding of use is increasing daily.*

## 20.10
## Summary

Pain is probably the most important aspect of a casualty's injury "experience."
The three point analgesic ladder remains the bedrock of acute pain management.
Pain scores should be recorded as often as other physiological scores.
A host of analgesic agents and routes exist and this is likely to grow further but
intramuscular morphine remains the gold standard for far forward pain care.

## 20.11
## Appendix I: Medication Review

*These are not comprehensive instructions and no responsibility can be taken for doses
suggested.*

Non Steroidal Anti Inflammatory Drugs (NSAIDs)
    Diclofenac
    Ibuprofen
    Specific COX II Inhibitors.
Opioids
    Morphine
    Pethidine
    Fentanyl
    Alfentanil
    Remifentanil
    Methadone
    Hydromorphone
    Weak Opioids
      Codeine
      Tramadol
      Buprenorphine
Other Analgesics
    Ketamine
    Paracetamol
    Methoxyflurane
    Entonox
Peripheral Nerve Blocks

### 20.11.1
### Non Steroidal Anti Inflammatory Drugs (Nsaids)

### 20.11.1.1
### Mechanism

NSAIDs work by inhibiting the action of the enzyme cyclooxygenase. This prevents the production of a number of substances that are thought to produce pain as well as a number of other actions.

### 20.11.1.2
### Effects

In addition to their analgesic and antipyretic actions NSAIDs are associated with a number of other effects.

#### Gastric Irritation

This can result in a spectrum of problems from mild pain to fatal hemorrhage. This side effect is thought to be reduced with the use of COX II inhibitors.

#### Inhibition of Coagulation

This is predominately through inhibition of platelet function although may be less with COX II inhibition.

#### Inhibition of Renal Function

Renal prostaglandin production may be reduced by NSAID administration. This can lead to a critical reduction in renal blood flow which in the presence of hypotension and hypovolaemia can lead to acute renal failure.

#### Inhibition of Bone Repair

This may be significant in long term use delaying fracture repair.

### NSAID Sensitive Asthma

Up to 20% of asthmatics may experience a severe asthma attack on exposure to NSAIDs. Children appear to be relatively protected from this. These are associated with allergic rhinitis, nasal polyps, and middle aged asthma sufferers.

#### 20.11.1.3
#### Agents

### Diclofenac

| Routes | Oral, intravenous and rectal |
|--------|------------------------------|
| Doses  | Adults 150 mg daily.         |

### Ibuprofen

Of the most commonly used NSAIDs ibuprofen has the lowest rate of gastric side effects. This may be in part due to its having the weakest anti inflammatory properties – it does not follow that it necessarily has the weakest analgesic actions.

| Routes | PO. peak analgesia being reached in 1–2 h. |
|--------|---------------------------------------------|
| Doses  | Adult – 1,800 mg daily in 4–6 divided doses. Paeds – 5 mg/kg QDS |

### Ketorolac

Potent NSAID with advantage of having an intravenous formulation. Should be used with great caution in renal compromise. Doses range from 15–30 mg IV.

### Specific COX II Inhibitors

These are thought to reduce the incidence of gastric complications and reductions in platelet function. Their use is also subject to "guidance" from a number of regulatory bodies and it is likely that their use will continue to change with time. Examples include celecoxib and paracoxib.

#### 20.11.1.4
#### Opioids

### Introduction

The term "opiate" refers to naturally occurring substances with morphine like properties whilst "opioid" includes the synthetic analgesics that act via the opioid receptors and are competitively antagonized by naloxone.

An important factor to consider when administering opioids is that individual dose requirements will vary between patients and even for the same patient on different occasions just as pain vaires. For this reason the best approach is to titrate the dose administered according to patient requirement. In this way one can achieve optimum analgesia with the minimum of side effects.

### 20.11.1.5
### Strong Opioids

#### Morphine

The "gold standard" analgesic

#### Effects

1. Cental Nervous System
   Analgesia
   Sedation, followed by euphoria and then dysphoria with increasing dose
   Meiosis, a result of Edinger – Westphal nucleus stimulation
   Nause and Vomiting – the chemoreceptor trigger zone may be indirectly simulated but the vomiting center is not. In fact higher doses may inhibit the system so as to reduce nausea and vomiting.
   Hallucinations in c. 3%

2. *Respiratory System*
   Respiratory depression
   Antitussive effect
   Bronchospasm can occur, usually a result of histamine release.

3. *Cardiovascular System*
   Histamine release is thought to result in a reduction in smooth muscle tone and a mild bradycardia.

4. *Gastrointestinal*
   Gut sphincters contract and motility is reduced leading to constipation and possibly increased vomiting.

5. *Genitourinary*
   Increased tone of the detrusor and sphincter muscles may precipitate urinary retention.

6. *Musculoskeletal*
   Opioids can increase muscle rigidity. This appears to be more common following rapid intravenous administration rather than by other routes.

7. *Skin*
   Puritis, most marked with epidural or intrathecal routes. Antihistamines may help although the role of histamine is uncertain.

8. *Endocrine*
   ADH secretion is increased which may lead to impaired water excretion and hyponatraemia

| Routes | Multiple routes possible, including intranasal. The subcutaneous route is not encouraged because of relatively low lipid solubility. Following intramuscular administration peak analgesia should be reached after c.10–30 min and may last 4 h. In the normal patient this is almost as as fast an onset as the intravenous route. Orally it has a 50% bioavailability. Morphine undergoes extensive biotransformation to active metabolites. Problems can be caused with renal failure causing reduced elimination. |
|---|---|
| Dose | The difficulty is that morphine the dose that can be given will depend upon the pain the patient experiences. There is no clear "upper limit." An initial dose of 0.05–0.1 mg/kg iv or im should be used to start analgesia. In adults 2 mg iv every 5 min to titrate analgesia after an initial bolus. 10 mg im can be repeated every 2 h although under appropriate supervision more than this may be required. |

### Pethidine

It is available as tablets and solution for injection. It is said to produce less biliary tract spasm than morphine although the clinical significance of this is often questioned.

Serious interaction is seen with monoamine oxidase inhibitors including coma, labile circulation, convulsions, and hyperpyrexia.

Anticholinergic effects such as a dry mouth and occasional tachycardia can occur.

It is inactivated in the liver to a number of metabolites including norpethedine which has half the analgesic activity of pethidine, a longer elimination half-life, an association with hallucinations and grand mal seizures, and effects not reversed by naloxone.

| Routes | PO IV, IM |
|---|---|
| Dose | 0.5–1 mg/kg, titrated to effect. |

### Fentanyl

A clear colorless intravenous solution also available in the form of transdermal patches, buccal and sublingual tablets, and a buccal "lollipop."

An iontophoretic "PCA" patch is available.

It has negligible oral bioavailability which means that fentanyl has to be absorbed through the oral mucosa rather than "swallowed."

One vital point to note when using this buccal route is that the lozenge has to "paint" the oral mucosa and not sit statically on one site if the drug is to be optimally absorbed. Tablet forms are now available for sublingual and buccal use that do not require this movement.

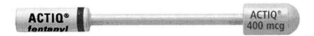

**Fig. 20.2** Actiq® oral transmucosal fentanyl applicator; the "Lollipop"

Fentanyl is said to release less histamine than morphine thus may not reduce blood pressure to the same degree (Fig. 20.2).

| Dose | IV: 1 μ(mu)g/kg. |
|------|------------------|
|      | Oral "lollipop": Approximately 10–1 ratio with intravenous morphine (thus 800 μ(mu)g oral transmucosal fentanyl ≈ 8 mg iv morphine).[10] |

### Alfentanil
This is an opioid that is only really used for sedation and perioperative analgesia.

### Remifentanil

It is a potent analgesic that will only be used perioperatively or for sedation.

### Methadone

This is a synthetic opioid which is used in some parts of the world for the management of acute pain. It is thought to have a wide range of actions and not solely opioid in nature as it may have activity at NMDA receptors. It also has a long half-life.

### Hydromorphone

Thought to have a swifter onset than morphine. Approximately four times more potent orally and eight times more potent via the parenteral route.

### 20.11.1.6
### Weak Opioids

### Codeine

It is approximately one sixth the potency of morphine. It is relatively more effective orally than parenterally.

Intravenous route tends to be avoided because of incidents of hypotension.

It has been suggested codeine is just a prodrug for morphine. However, approximately 9% of the UK population is poor metabolizers of codeine. This may often result in significantly reduced analgesia in this population. Conversely some people may be very good metabolizers and have an excessive response.[11]

| Dose | Adult- 30–60 mg QDS; but more may be necessary. |
|------|------------------------------------------------|

### Tramadol

Tramadol is described as a "weak" opioid and is indicated for the treatment of moderate to severe pain.

The effects are similar to those of morphine. It may make epilepsy more common in those that are susceptible to it.

It should not be given with monoamine oxidase inhibitors.

| Dose | Up to 400 mg daily in divided doses. |
|------|--------------------------------------|

### Buprenorphine

Thought to be 30 times more potent than morphine. There have been suggestions that it is less likely to cause respiratory depression. However even high doses of naloxone have difficulty in antagonizing its actions.

Anecdotal reports suggest nausea and vomiting may be more common with buprenorphine than other opioids.

| Routes | Sublingual, injection (im & iv) |
|--------|--------------------------------|
| Dose   | Sublingual: 200–400 μg QDS |

Intramuscular/slow intravenous: 300–600 μg QDS

### 20.11.1.7
### Other Analgesics

### Ketamine

Ketamine is a relatively unique drug that, like opioids, causes a range of actions from dysphoria and analgesia to death. However it is not an opioid but a phencyclidine derivative.

There is a belief that the stereoselective isomer has a better side effect profile than the racemic mixture but it is the latter that one finds more often.

The traditional use of ketamine was limited to use as an anesthetic agent in the hemodynamically unstable trauma patient. The US Army has been able to frequently utilize subanesthetic doses of ketamine in low rate continuous infusions and PCA combinations in perioperative and acute pain management. Advantages to the use of ketamine in this context have been a reduction in opioids required to reach a given level of pain relief, decreased risk of respiratory depression, reduction of the development of opioid tolerance, prevention of opioid-induced hyperalgesia, and although controversial, reduction of risk of chronic pain.[12]

## 20.11.1.8
## Effects

### CNS

The anesthesia produced is typically described as "dissociative anesthesia."

Limb movement may occur as may groaning. These do not necessarily indicate a light anesthetic.

Sedation occurs in sub-anesthetic doses in common with analgesia.

Dreaming and hallucinations occur especially on emergence and during sedation. These can be vivid and worrying and are more common in adults than children. They may be reduced with concomitant administration of opiates or benzodiazepines.

Consequently the issue of ketamine use in the head injured patient is being reviewed.

There can be preservation of corneal and light reflexes together with slow nystagmic gaze.

### Respiratory System

Respiratory function is relatively well preserved as are airway reflexes. Ketamine is acts as a bronchodilatator.

An increase in salivary and tracheobronchial secretions occurs and this may be problematic.

### Cardiovascular

Ketamine is a potent sympathomimetic. This action tends to mask its myocardial depressant and venodilatation actions, certainly on initial dosage. Myocardial depression is less with ketamine than it is with other intravenous anesthetic agents.

| Routes | Intravenous and intramuscular routes remain the military routes of choice at present. Intranasal route may have some uses. Intramuscular Ketamine has a peak plasma level of about 20 min. |
|---|---|
| Doses | Analgesia and sedation is usually to be found using subanesthetic doses; low infusion rates for analgesia range from 0.5–2mcg/kg/min; infusion for sedation for painful procedures ranging from 5–10mcg/kg/min; PCA mixtures most commonly 1 mg morphine/1 mg ketamine; 10–20 mg bolus aliquots titrated for effect and repeated as required. |

### Paracetamol

In common with many other NSAIDS paracetamol is freely available over the counter either alone or in combination with a number of other drugs. For this reason, as mentioned above, there is a real possibility of overdose, either deliberate or accidental. Commonly described as having "synergy" with other analgesics with approximate 20% opioid-sparing analgesic properties.

### 20.11.1.9
### Effects

#### CNS

The exact site of paracetamol's action is still under debate but as well as being an analgesic it also has good antipyretic properties.

#### GI

Unlike traditional NSAIDs paracetamol is not thought to have an irritant effect on the gastric mucosa.

#### GU

In overdose there is a risk of renal tubular necrosis.

| | |
|---|---|
| Routes | Oral and rectal routes are the most common although intravenous may become more widespread. |
| Dose | The maximum daily dose in adults is quoted as 4 g. In children it is 80 mg/kg. |

### Methoxyflurane

This is an inhaled anesthetic vapor that in low doses gives good pain relief. It is in use with the Australian and New Zealand Defence Forces. However there are side effects and complications associated with it that make its use in British forces unlikely.[13]

### Entonox

This is mixture of oxygen and nitrous oxide. Again it requires a degree of coordination to allow inhalation. It requires a relatively bulky apparatus to provide it. There are also practical issues surrounding its use and storage that make it unattractive for use in the prehospital environment. Below $-6°C$, the pseudocritical temperature of entonox, the mixture undergoes lamination and nitrous oxide enters the liquid phase. Thus initially oxygen alone is delivered and then only nitrous oxide. It should also be avoided in patients with bowel obstruction, pneumothorax, sinus, and middle ear disease.

### Peripheral Nerve Blocks

In depth discussion on the use of peripheral nerve blocks is outside the scope of this chapter.

Limb blocks are the most common blocks used. They can be either as "single shot" injections or as infusions. They may be done "blind" or guided using peripheral nerve stimulators or even ultrasound.

## 20.12
## Appendix II: Patient Controlled Analgesia

### 20.12.1
### Introduction

As the name suggests, this is a technique by which the patient is able to control the administration of their analgesia.

The current British military device is the Baxter "Wristwatch" PCA. US forces have utilized several different PCA pumps (most commonly the Sorenson "Ambit") which have also been utilized for continuous peripheral nerve blockade. There has been effort to switch to a separate, color-coded, standardized pump for each use to avoid confusion.

Typically morphine 2 mg/ml is the solution used with this system. The addition of an antiemetic to this solution is not encouraged.

This system does not provide a one-stop solution to the problems of analgesia for all patients, and it does not transfer all responsibility for analgesia to the patient but it may help reduce nursing workload. However, the patient does need to be monitored by the ward staff to confirm efficacy, and watch for unwanted side effects from the morphine. To aid this it is normal practice for a suitable protocol to be employed on the wards and an example of this is given below.

The fentanyl iontophoretic patch PCA, "Ionsys" does exist but at present there are no plans for its widespread use within the military system.

### 20.12.2
### PCA Protocol

Patient suitability is determined by an anesthetist or the acute pain team in conjunction with ward staff.

The PCA must be prescribed on a suitable drug prescription chart. This does not prevent the prescription of other analgesics although care should be taken with alternative medication that may augment unwanted side effects of the morphine.

Regular recordings of pulse, blood pressure, respiratory rate, pain, and sedation (see below) are required. Typical timings are:

Recovery – 5 min. To include $S_pO_2$ until stable.
Ward – hourly for 4 h and then 4 hourly.

However, if the PCA was started on the ward then as for recovery for the first hour.

### 20.12.3
### Pain and Sedation Score

Tables 20.2 and 20.3.

### 20.13
### Appendix III: Oxygen Administration Protocol

Patients who have one of the following signs should be given supplementary oxygen:

$S_pO_2 < 95\%$ on air
Sedation score of 3 (see pca protocol for scoring scale)
Respiratory rate $< 9$/min

**Table 20.2** Pain score

| Pain score | |
| --- | --- |
| 0 | No pain |
| 1 | Mild pain |
| 2 | Moderate pain |
| 3 | Severe pain |

**Table 20.3** Sedation Ssore

| Sedation score | | |
| --- | --- | --- |
| 0 | No sedation | |
| 1 | Occasionally drowsy | Easy to rouse |
| 2 | Frequently drowsy | Easy to rouse |
| 3 | Severely sedated | Difficult to rouse |

Patients with scores of 3 for either pain or sedation need to be reviewed by the medical staff or the acute pain team

Oxygen should be started at 4l/min via a mask immediately.

Regular recordings of pulse rate, respiratory rate, blood pressure, $S_pO_2$, and sedation should be initiated.

Refer to the Opiate Overdose Protocol if this is thought to be the origin of the respiratory depression.

The medical staff should be informed as soon as possible.

Ensure the location of the resuscitation equipment is confirmed.

## 20.14
## Appendix IV: Protocol Opiate Overdose

Typical signs are:

> Respiratory rate < 9
> Sedation score of 3 (severely sedated, difficult to rouse)
> Reduced $S_pO_2$

Prompt intervention is required to prevent a potentially threatening event occurring.

If opiate overdose is suspected:

> Give oxygen, according to the Oxygen Administration. Protocol
> Give Naloxone 0.4 mg iv bolus. This may need to be repeated after 10–15 min.
> Inform the medical staff as soon as possible.

## 20.15
## Appendix V: Paracetamol Overdose

As little as 5 g of paracetamol taken in a 24 h period may lead to severe hepatic damage. This damage is maximal after 3–4 days but initial symptoms may be sufficiently mild as to not cause undue concern.

Actual plasma paracetamol levels may be difficult to obtain in field conditions. However, if 150 mg/kg has been taken with the last hour administration of activated charcoal is suggested. Antidotes such as acetylcysteine and methionine may protect the liver if given within 12 h of ingestions, although the former may be protective up to 24 h after ingestion.

## 20.16
## Appendix VI: UK : US Drug Names

Often US generic drug names will be different to UK names. Almost always the Brand name will be different and these are used more often in the US than the UK.

This list is not exhaustive (Table 20.4).

**Table 20.4** UK: US drug names

| UK name | US generic name | US brand name |
| --- | --- | --- |
| Paracetamol | Acetaminophen | Tylenol® |
| Paracetamol and oxycodone | Oxycodone and acetaminophen | Percocet® |
| Tramadol | | Ultram® |
| Tramadol + paracetamol | Tramadol and acetaminophen | Ultracet® |
| Hydromorphone | | Dilaudid® Palladone® |
| Fentanyl (oral) | | Actiq® or Fentora® |
| Buprenorphine (sublingual) | | Subutex® |
| Pethidine | Meperidine | Demerol® |

# References

1. Luger TJ, Lederer W, Gassner M, Lockinger A, Ulmer H, Lorenz IH. Acute pain is under-assessed in out-of-hospital emergencies. *Acad Emerg Med.* 2003;10(6):627-632.
2. Bricknell MC, Hanhart N. Stability operations and the implications for military health services support. *J R Army Med Corps.* 2007;153(1):18-21.
3. Joshi GP, Ogunnaike BO. Consequences of inadequate postoperative pain relief and chronic persistent postoperative pain. *Anesthesiol Clin N Am.* 2005;23(1):21-36.
4. Merskey H, Bogduk N. In: Merskey H, Bogduk N, eds. *Classification of Chronic Pain.* 2nd ed. 1994.
5. Collins SL, Moore RA, McQuay HJ. The visual analogue pain intensity scale: what is moderate pain in millimetres? *Pain.* 1997;72(1–2):95-97.
6. Markowitz J. A series of over 100 amputations of the thigh for tropical ulcer. *J R Army Med Corps.* 1947;86:159-170.
7. Baker BC, Buckenmaier C, Narine N, Compeggie ME, Brand GJ, Mongan PD. Battlefield anesthesia: advances in patient care and pain management. *Anesthesiol Clin.* 2007;25(1):131-145. x.
8. Kotwal RS et al. Novel pain management strategy for combat casualty care. *Ann Emerg Med.* 2004;44:121-127.
9. Mabry R, McManus JG. Prehospital advances in the management of severe penetrating trauma. *Crit Care Med.* 2008;36(Suppl):S258-S266.
10. Rivara FM, MacKenzie EJ, Avery B, Nathens M, Jin Wang, Daniel OS. Prevalence of pain in patients 1 year after major trauma. *Arch Surg.* 2008;143(3):282-287.
11. Administration FD. Use of Codeine Products in Nursing Mothers. 2008 [updated 2008; cited 2008, 25 Aug 08]; Available from: http://www.fda.gov/cder/drug/infopage/codeine/default.htm.
12. Malchow RW, Black I. The evolution of pain management in the critically ill trauma patient: emerging concepts from the global war on terrorism. *Crit Care Med.* 2008;36(Suppl):S346-S357.
13. McLennan JV. Is methoxyflurane a suitable battlefield analgesic? *J R Army Med Corps.* 2007;153(2):111-113.

Craig C. McFarland

Pre-hospital Anesthesia

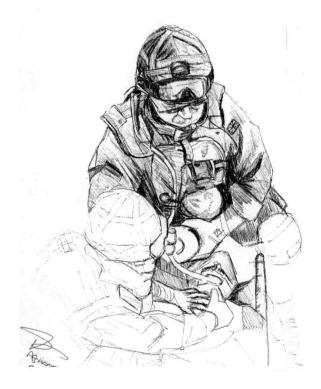

C.C. McFarland
Department of Anesthesia and Operative Services, Brooke Army Medical Center,
Fort Sam Houston, TX, USA and
Uniformed Services University for the Health Sciences, Department of Anesthesiology,
Fort Sam Houston, TX, USA
e-mail: craig.mcfarland@us.army.mil

A.J. Brooks et al. (eds.), *Ryan's Ballistic Trauma*,
DOI: 10.1007/978-1-84882-124-8_21, © Springer-Verlag London Limited 2011

## 21.1
## Introduction

For the ballistic trauma casualty, the intraoperative period is critical. The anesthetic care received in this period can be the difference between life and death – between complication and recovery. This chapter provides practical recommendations to deliver effective anesthesia care to these challenging patients.

Ballistic casualties presenting for anesthesia generally fall into one of two categories:

Late – the stable patient who has been receiving medical care and is returning to the OR for further washing or more definitive treatment. One *may* approach this patient as one would a routine elective case.

Early – the immediate trauma patient who is potentially unstable. One should approach this patient as having a full stomach and shocked physiology. This chapter focuses on this group of ballistic casualties.

## 21.2
## Preparation for Trauma

This is determined by capabilities of the medical team (Level 1 trauma center versus community hospital versus field hospital in an austere environment).

A Level 1 trauma center or robust field hospital has trauma protocols and systems in place. Trauma team nurses and physicians are familiar to each other and ancillary services are plentiful.

Community hospital healthcare providers tend to be less "practiced" in treating trauma. They may lack some ancillary or consultative services.

Austere environment trauma teams may be very practiced in trauma care but their capabilities are limited by scarce medical resources.

- In all cases, effective care is enabled by team members understanding their roles and trauma procedures. In all but the level one trauma center, this requires rehearsal drills before the first casualties arrive.

## 21.3
## Goals of Trauma Anesthesia

The trauma anesthesiologist should focus on the goals of trauma anesthesia. Every clinical decision (choice of induction agents, IV access, monitoring, etc.) can be made confidently when these goals are kept in mind. As in most other anesthesia subspecialties, there may be more than one "right" way to proceed. In these cases, the trauma goals will guide the prudent anesthesiologist. For example, when inducing general anesthesia in a volume depleted victim of multiple gunshot wounds, it is imperative to preserve the patient's tenuous hemodynamics. In this particular scenario, the anesthesiologist may have to choose between ketamine and sodium thiopental. Ketamine's ability to augment blood pressure by increasing sympathetic tone would help to meet the goal of blood pressure preservation. Conversely, sodium thiopental at a dose of 4–5 mg/kg would likely cause a profound decrease in systemic blood pressure, and would therefore be a poor choice for this particular case. However, reduced doses of sodium thiopental have been used effectively for decades in this very situation. To achieve the goal of preserving perfusion, inducing anesthesia with sodium thiopental 1–2 mg/kg would be acceptable. Thus, both techniques, ketamine and reduced-dose sodium thiopental, are methods to induce general anesthesia while preserving vital organ perfusion.

## 21.4
## Goals of Trauma Anesthesia

1. Preserve/improve vital organ perfusion
2. Avoid the triad of hypothermia, coagulopathy, and acidosis
3. Find associated injuries
4. Avoid causing further injury
5. Optimize the patient relative to the entire medical treatment system

### 21.4.1
### Preserve/Improve Vital Organ Perfusion

This involves establishing adequate intravenous access and standard monitoring as well as invasive monitoring when indicated (arterial pressure monitoring or central venous pressure monitoring are examples). The judicious use of fluids (particularly blood and blood products) and vasoactive drugs to support adequate systemic pressures and cardiac output is essential. It may be beneficial to initially accept relatively low blood pressures prior to the operating room theater as part of hypotensive resuscitation. This is discussed elsewhere, in Chapter 19 – Resuscitation.

Adequate, high volume, access and invasive monitoring are imperative. Everyone involved in the case (anesthesiologist, surgeon, nurses, etc.) should understand that priority is initially given to establishing access and monitoring prior to any surgical manipulation. If immediate surgical intervention is required to preserve life, for example to cross-clamp an aorta or pack the abdomen, the anesthesiologist must be provided time following these procedures to "catch up" with needed access and monitoring.

### 21.4.2
### Avoid the Triad of Hypothermia, Coagulopathy, and Acidosis

To a large extent, this is achieved by efforts at improving tissue perfusion. However, correction of hypothermia requires additional measures such as warming all intravenous fluids, warming the ambient temperature, covering any part of the patient not currently being operated on, and using forced air warmers when possible.

Coagulopathy can be assessed by obtaining lab work including platelet count. Thromboelastography can provide a thorough illustration of the patient's coagulation status.[1] But this data is often not timely or unavailable. The anesthesiologist should constantly evaluate the surgical field for blood that is slow to clot and be in frequent communication with the surgeon on this issue.

Acidosis is frequently a result of poor tissue perfusion, but it can also be exacerbated iatrogenically, by acidic crystalloid solutions or inadequate ventilation.

## 21.4.3
### Find Associated (but Less Obvious) Injuries

Ballistic trauma often causes injuries which are quite apparent on presentation. A common pitfall, however, is failing to find other injuries which are not obvious. Trauma teams can easily become fixated on obvious trauma, such as an amputation, while failing to notice a small penetrating chest wound that is a greater medical problem for the patient. Also remember that there may be multiple mechanisms of injury. A victim of a gunshot wound to the chest could sustain a cervical spine injury if he falls to the ground from a height, or overturns his vehicle. Obtaining reports on mechanism of injury from pre-hospital personnel is an important part of trauma resuscitation. Advanced trauma life support (ATLS) protocols advocate primary and secondary surveys with the intent of finding these injuries that otherwise could easily be missed.[2]

## 21.4.4
### Avoid Causing Further Injury

Certain precautions should be considered for every ballistic trauma patient. First, gunshot wounds generally confer a low risk for cervical spine injury.[3] However, if the events surrounding the injury included other mechanisms, the cervical spine may still be at risk, and should be protected during the conduct of the anesthetic. Secondly, victims of trauma are presumed to have full stomachs. Thus, rapid sequence intubation should be performed routinely. In cases where maintaining spontaneous ventilation is desired during intubation, inhaled sevoflurane or boluses of ketamine are options for inducing anesthesia in a controlled manner without inducing apnea.

## 21.4.5
### Optimize the Patient Relative to the Entire Medical Treatment System

This goes beyond maintaining a state of complete relaxation for the surgeon. One must think longitudinally and systemically. Are there other patients waiting who require emergent surgery? If so, should some of the procedures planned for the patient currently in the OR be deferred until later? Is the current patient consuming the hospital's supplies of a scarce resource, such as blood products? If so, should the planned procedure be altered? Can anything be done to decrease postoperative consumption of scarce resources? For example, can multimodal analgesics or regional anesthesia be used to decrease opioid requirements, which may then translate to less supplemental oxygen use, less respiratory depression, and less-intensive nursing care?

### 21.4.6
### Planning Anesthesia

Ballistic trauma casualties are often characterized by full stomachs, hypovolemia, penetration of multiple body regions, and often unstable fractures to include the cervical spine. To avoid missing an injury, the anesthetist should take a standardized approach to casualties, with an understanding of when and how the standard approach should be modified. Additionally, as the patient enters the operating theater, the anesthetist and the surgeon should both agree on the relative urgency of obtaining better intravenous access and invasive monitoring, versus deferring this until after surgery has started. In case of non-compressible, life-threatening hemorrhage, the surgery is begun straight away to staunch catastrophic hemorrhage, with a planned pause after hemorrhage is controlled to allow the anesthetist to complete line placement for continued resuscitation.

When the casualty is ready for anesthesia, a suggested approach is:

### 21.4.6.1
### Induction

The standard induction sequence for trauma anesthesia is preoxygenation and rapid sequence induction with cricoid pressure, followed by endotracheal intubation. As airway management may be made difficult by airway trauma or cervical spine injury, equipment for difficult airways must be available. In addition to a range of endotracheal tubes and laryngeal mask airways, a gum-elastic bougie is desirable. A surgical airway kit is critical, along with a trained provider (surgeon or anesthetist) who is ready to use it (Fig. 21.1).

There are many options for induction agents. No matter which agent is chosen – ketamine, propofol, sodium thiopental, or etomidate – it must be used in a dose consistent with a shocked, hypovolemic patient. Ketamine at a dose of 1 – 2 mg per kilogram (mg/kg) has proved very useful in such patients.[4]

In rapid sequence, a neuromuscular blocker should follow the induction agent. Succinylcholine (1–1.5 mg/kg) is the agent of choice. Exceptions fall in two categories: patients after the acute phase of injury following major burns or multiple trauma, and patients who have extensive denervation of skeletal muscle or upper motor neuron injury, such as paraplegia. These cases can be complicated by succinylcholine-induced severe hyperkalemia.[5] In such instances, rocuronium is desirable due to its rapidity of onset relative to other non-depolarizing neuromuscular blocking drugs,[6] although a systematic review concludes that it is not quite as rapid as succinylcholine.[7]

**Fig. 21.1** "Emergency Airway Management Algorithm" (Emergency airway management algorithm used at the R. Adams Cowley Shock Trauma Center, presented as an example. Individual practitioners and trauma hospitals should determine their own algorithm based on available skills and resources. LMA, laryngeal mask airway (Reproduced from Miller, RD. Miller's Anesthesia. 2005;6:2,455, with kind permission from Elsevier Ltd)

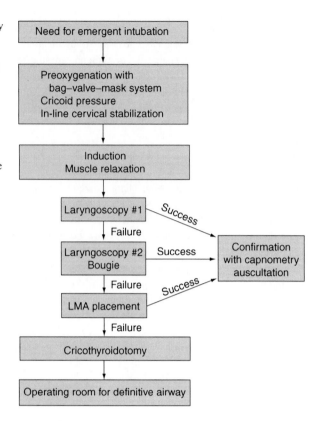

## 21.5
## Maintenance

The maintenance phase of the anesthetic can be carried out with a variety of techniques. In a shocked patient, agents with vasodilatory properties must be given judiciously. An option in this case is to use intermittent boluses of ketamine to maintain anesthesia until hemorrhage is controlled. Once hemodynamics are normalizing, volatile agents can be introduced. Although the use of total intravenous anesthesia for wartime surgery was criticized after World War II,[8] the basis for this criticism was thoroughly debunked after wartime medical records became available to the public.[9] The author of this chapter has found that a mixed solution of ketamine, fentanyl, and dilute propofol can be easily titrated with or without an infusion pump in austere environments where resources are limited (see inset for example). Ketamine has been avoided in head-injured patients, but recent evidence suggests that including ketamine as part of a multi-agent anesthetic does not worsen outcomes in ballistic head injuries.[10] Continued muscle relaxation, if required, can be achieved with any non-depolarizing neuromuscular blocker as the effect of succinylcholine subsides.

As surgery is progressing, the anesthetist must continually assess whether the goals of ballistic trauma anesthesia are being realized. Standard noninvasive monitors of heart rate and rhythm, oxygenation, temperature, and arterial blood pressure are a starting point. Proper assessments of volume status may require central venous pressure in addition to direct arterial pressure measurement. Resuscitation with crystalloids, colloids, and blood products is continued intraoperatively, according to the principles discussed in Chaps. 19 and 23. Aggressive measures may be required to avoid hypothermia, as discussed above. The intraoperative period requires attention to many parallel processes. The anesthetist should establish a method of maintaining anesthesia that confers stable hemodynamics with minimal adjustment. This plan liberates the anesthetist to focus on a variety of patient issues that require attention during the turbulent period of trauma surgery on a shocked patient.

## 21.6
## Multi-Agent TIVA for the Austere Environment

A bag containing 50 mL saline, 40 mL (400 mg) propofol, 5 mL (250 mcg) fentanyl, and 5 mL (250 mg) ketamine is prepared for a final volume of 100 mL. A 20 drop per mL infusion set is used to deliver this preparation.

For an 80 kg patient, adjusting the drip rate to 1 drop per second (1 gtt/s) will result in a propofol rate of 9 mg/kg/h. 1 drop every 2 s equals a rate of 4.5 mg/kg/h. 1 drop every 3 s equals 3 mg/kg/h. In practice, after rapid-sequence induction and intubation of an adult trauma patient, the infusion is begun at 1 gtt/s, then titrated steadily downward as the case progresses. If the patient is not relaxed, spontaneous ventilation may be allowed to return while general anesthesia is maintained.

## 21.7
## Emergence/Post-op

Casualties of ballistic trauma often require ventilator support and continued endotracheal intubation, as well as, intensive care services postoperatively. Much of the intraoperative care continues seamlessly as the patient moves to the ICU setting. Full monitoring and any ongoing resuscitation must not be interrupted.

Upon arrival in the intensive care unit, immediate assessment includes physical examination and laboratory investigations. A well-resuscitated trauma patient ideally would have minimal evidence of the physiological consequences of cellular hypoxia. Some laboratory markers of resuscitation endpoints are presented below, with the caveats that they do not supersede clinical acumen, and that trends are often more significant than isolated numbers. A patient who arrives in the intensive care unit with normal stable vital signs and nominal laboratory values has likely received both effective surgical management and appropriate anesthetic management.

Critical care of the ballistic trauma patient is specifically discussed in Chaps. 19 and 23.

## Endpoints of Resuscitation

pH 7.35–7.45
Base deficit −3.0 or higher with a lactate concentration of 1.0 mmol/L or less
Core temperature >35.5°C
International normalized ratio (INR) <1.5, PT* <16 s, PTT** <42 s
Hemoglobin (Hb) 80 g/L or greater
Platelets >50 × 10⁹/L
Fibrinogen >1 g per liter
*PT = Prothrombin time
**PTT = Partial thromboplastin time

## 21.8
## Problems in the Operating Theater

If the patient's condition unexpectedly deteriorates, the original diagnosis must be reviewed in light of the mechanism of injury and the possible anatomical and physiological consequences. Consider the differential diagnoses listed in Table 21.1. Some of these are fundamental to any general anesthetic, but many are encountered more frequently in trauma settings.

**Table 21.1** Differential diagnoses for the deteriorating patient

| Airway and ventilation | Tension pneumothorax |
| --- | --- |
| | Main stem intubation |
| | Kinked or obstructed endotracheal tube |
| | Undiagnosed chest injury |
| | Malfunctioning chest drain |
| | Developing lung injury (in blast or severe blunt trauma) |
| Circulation | Bleeding from missed injury |
| | Missed high spinal cord lesion |
| | Tension Pneumothorax |
| | Cardiac contusion |
| | Cardiac ischemia |
| | Cardiac tamponade |
| | Anaphylaxis |
| | Dilutional coagulopathy |
| | Disseminated intravascular coagulation (DIC) |

## 21.9
## Conclusion

Anesthesia for ballistic trauma can be challenging and will frequently test both the technical and diagnostic abilities of the anesthetist. Practical management needs to follow a logical sequence of assessment and treatment and should be kept as simple as possible. Frequent discussion between anesthetist and surgeon and reassessment of treatment priorities is vital to maximize the chance of a successful outcome.

## References

1. Kaufmann CR, Dwyer KM, Crews JD, Dols SJ, Trask AL. Usefulness of thromboelastography in assessment of trauma patient coagulation. *J Trauma*. 1997;42:716-720. discussion 720-722.
2. American College of Surgeons. *ATLS advanced trauma life support program for doctors*. 7th ed.
3. Bellamy RF. The nature of combat injuries and the role of ATLS in their management. In: Combat Casualty Care Guidelines: Operation Desert Storm. Washington, DC: Office of the Surgeon General, Center of Excellence, Walter Reed Army Medical Center; February 1991.
4. Wood PR. Ketamine: Pre-hospital and in hospital use. *Trauma*. 2003;5:137-140.
5. Martyn JAJ, Richtsfeld M. Succinylcholine-induced hyperkalemia in acquired pathologic states. *Anesthesiology*. 2006;104:158-169.
6. Magorian T, Flannery KB, Miller RD. Comparison of rocuronium, succinylcholine, and vecuronium for rapid-sequence induction of anesthesia in adult patients. *Anesthesiology*. 1993;79(5):913-918.
7. Perry JJ, Lee JS, Sillberg VAH, Wells GA. Rocuronium versus succinylcholine for rapid sequence induction intubation. *Cochrane Database of Syst. Rev.* 2007; (3), Art. No.: CD002788. doi:10.1002/14651858.CD002788.pub2
8. Halford FJ. A critique of intravenous anesthesia in war surgery. *Anesthesiology*. 1943;4:67-69.
9. Bennetts FE. Thiopentone anaesthesia at Pearl Harbor. *Br J Anaesth*. 1995;75:366-368.
10. Grathwohl KW et al. Total intravenous anesthesia including ketamine versus volatile gas anesthesia for combat-related operative traumatic brain injury. *Anesthesiology*. 2008;109:44-53.

# Regional Anesthesia for the Ballistic Trauma Victim

# 22

Dan Connor

## 22.1
## Introduction

In the last edition of Ballistic Trauma the management of pain following ballistic trauma was mentioned only briefly – the purpose of the book has largely been to act as a practical guide to surgeons, physicians, and anesthetists managing the initial phases of trauma resuscitation. Success of this management saves the casualty's life. Almost invariably however, there will be significant tissue disruption, inflammation, and a systemic stress response that results in the patient experiencing significant pain. The most seriously injured military casualties will be transferred from the conflict zone with sedation and analgesia as a critical care transfer – usually intubated and ventilated. However, the preponderance of casualties will experience isolated limb trauma from gunshot or fragments and will be evacuated thousands of miles in an air evacuation aircraft that is jarring and crowded. Relying on opioid analgesia in this austere environment can be difficult at best and at times deadly. Additionally, these wounded can expect to have one or more visits back to the operating room before or after transfer to the home nation.

This chapter explores the suitability, possibility, and practicalities of using regional anesthesia to provide pain relief for the ballistic casualty after their initial resuscitation.

## 22.2
## Background

Since morphine was first discovered in 1805, it has been used extensively and reliably as first line analgesia for trauma in military and civilian arenas. Ketamine also remains a useful adjunct for the skilled clinician to manage pain as well as induce and maintain anesthesia. However, until recently morphine has been the only reliable option for post-operative pain management

D. Connor
Anaesthetic Department, MDHU Portsmouth, Queen Alexandra Hospital,
Portsmouth, Hampshire, UK
e-mail: danthea@mac.com

A.J. Brooks et al. (eds.), *Ryan's Ballistic Trauma*,
DOI: 10.1007/978-1-84882-124-8_22, © Springer-Verlag London Limited 2011

**Table 22.1** Undesirable effects of morphine

| |
|---|
| Sedation |
| Respiratory depression |
| Euphoria/dysphoria |
| Nausea and vomiting |
| Histamine release |
| Anti-tussive |
| Cardiovascular depression |
| Constipation/ileus |
| Smooth muscle spasm |
| Muscle rigidity |
| Tolerance |
| Dependence |

in the wounded. However, opioids have an extensive list of undesirable side-effects (Table 22.1) which make this class of pain medications less than ideal for this purpose.

During the Vietnam War, Thompson reported the use of single injection peripheral nerve blocks on casualties in an American Army surgical hospital.[1] He performed some of these nerve blocks on soldiers exiting the helicopter to alleviate their pain whilst being transferred and awaiting damage control surgery (personal communication). More recently, injuries sustained by American soldiers in the ongoing wars in Iraq and Afghanistan have hastened the development of the use of regional anesthesia for post-operative analgesia including transfer back through the evacuation chain.[2]

Most anesthetists have a number of regional anesthetic techniques that they regularly employ in their routine clinical practice. However there can be difficulties using these normal strategies to place regional anesthetic blocks and catheters in a casualty who has suffered traumatic amputation of a limb.

Advances in Personal Protective Equipment (PPE) and medical care have resulted in an increased number of survivors. The survival rate for US soldiers is over 90%, but the incidence of severe limb trauma in these survivors has increased.[3]

The challenge to clinicians is to manage these casualties within the constraints of the environment in which they happen to be practising – whether this is military or civilian conflict casualties, or disaster relief such as after a Hurricane or Tsunami.

## 22.3
## Not Managing Pain

As mentioned above, morphine has been the mainstay of pain management, alongside adjunctive oral analgesics such as acetominophen (paracetamol) and non-steroidal anti-inflammatory drugs. However, untreated or inadequately treated acute pain can lead to the development of chronic pain.[4]

The American Pain Foundation surveyed 753 veterans who had returned injured from Operation Iraqi Freedom and Operation Enduring Freedom. Sixty four percent of the veterans reported symptoms of chronic pain, with 70% of those surveyed experiencing severe pain daily. Two thirds of those in chronic pain reported symptoms of depression, one third were experiencing post traumatic stress disorder and 29% had symptoms of both.[5] Ongoing pain is also associated with anxiety, panic attacks, substance abuse, and suicide. Only 6% reported very effective analgesia, with 62% of veterans describing their analgesia as moderately effective.

In a recent survey of UK military personnel returning wounded from Iraq and Afghanistan (Mercer – unpublished), 30% of all those surveyed exhibited signs and symptoms of neuropathic pain as determined by a LANSS score > 12. Of the casualties investigated 100% had been treated with paracetamol, 86% with morphine, 84% with non-steroidal analgesia, 72% with amitriptylline, pregabalin, or gabapentin, but only 4% had received any regional anesthesia.

Predicting which patients will develop chronic pain is not possible. Melzack and Wall's classic paper on the gate theory of pain has provided the framework by which pain specialists approach the management of pain.[6] The concept of central sensitisation and wind-up were introduced. Peripheral sensory neurone activity drives systems that amplify and prolong the incoming sensory message until the experience of this pain becomes dissociated from the peripheral activity. The theory led to the idea that pain could be controlled by modulation – reduce excitation or increase inhibition. Reducing the sensory input with early use of regional anesthesia has been shown to be of benefit,[7] though large case-series and random controlled trials are still lacking.

## 22.4
## Use of Regional Anesthesia in the Civilian Environment

An anesthesiologist's practice in the military environment must be guided by their routine "peacetime" work. There is no benefit to patients in starting to perform regional blocks or place continuous peripheral nerve block (CPNB) catheters for the first time in an acute setting. Equally, the austere battlefield medical environment is not ideal for learning to use ultrasound to locate nerves or even obtain central venous access. These skills are best integrated into practice within a controlled elective environment with full recourse to more experienced colleagues and appropriate learning resources.

The use of regional anesthetic techniques, both single injection and CPNB, are on the increase across the developed world. Todorovic[8] anticipates that by the middle of the twenty-first century more than 75% of surgical interventions will be performed in the outpatient or day-case setting. Examples of major surgery currently being performed in an "ambulatory" environment include hip,[9] knee[10] and shoulder[11] arthroplasties. Regardless of the absolute figure, developments in minimally-invasive techniques, requirement for faster patient discharge, improved ability and success at regional anesthesia will, in turn, promote the general breadth and depth of experience of each individual anesthesiologist with respect to regional anesthesia.

Most anesthesiologists will encounter opportunities in their routine work to develop and improve their regional anesthesia skills with potentially significant benefits for the patient. Ideally, all military anesthesiologists would be skilled practitioners in multiple approaches to block the upper and lower limbs. They should also be accustomed to the placement and management of CPNB catheters and the use of these catheters as part of a multimodal pain care plan.

## 22.5
### Use of Regional Anesthesia in the Military Environment

Since Thompson's narrative about the management of American casualties in Vietnam there had been little reported development in the role or usage of regional anesthesia for military casualties, until the current wars in Iraq and Afghanistan started to produce large numbers of casualties with severely injured extremities.

Working from the Walter Reed Army Medical Center (WRAMC) in Washington, the Army Regional Anesthesia and Pain Management Initiative (ARAPMI) started to prospectively collect data on casualties received from the conflicts that were being managed with any form of regional anesthesia.[12]

Over a 21 month period, battle injury patients who received regional anesthesia procedures following severe extremity trauma were entered into a database. This provided a cohort of 287 patients, the majority of whom were multiply injured, who received a total of 634 operations using advanced regional anesthesia techniques, including 37% who suffered traumatic amputations. Most of the casualties had received damage control surgery along the evacuation chain and so were receiving definitive surgery at WRAMC.

A total of 285 single-injection nerve blocks and 361 indwelling continuous peripheral nerve block (CPNB) catheters amounting to over 1,700 catheter days were placed. The majority of these were primarily used for operations, with only 40 of the total being used purely for pain control. Although pain scoring was not initially a primary outcome of the data collection, pain scores were significantly reduced, and there were few complications in the CPNB group. Though 11.9% experienced some form of complication, the majority of these were minor or technical in nature. Only 1.9% experienced catheter related infection, all of which were minor and treated only with removal of the catheter. The authors pointed out that a contributing factor in this low infection rate was likely the routine use of intravenous antibiotics in this patient population. This compared favorably with other institutions.

However, whilst initiating regional anesthesia in the comfort and sterility of a large institution at the end of the evacuation chain can provide excellent analgesia and facilitate repeat procedures for the wounded, the goal of providing early regional anesthesia soon after wounding to allow pain free procedures and repatriation through the aeromedical evacuation chain – and avoiding the experience of prolonged pain post injury – presents an additional set of challenges.

## 22.5.1
### Use of CPNB in the Field Hospital

Buckenmaier (Chief of ARAPMI at WRAMC) et al.[12] reported the first use of CPNB to evacuate a soldier whose lower limb was damaged enough in Iraq to require amputation. Initial surgery and subsequent transfer back via Germany to the US, including repeat surgical procedures took place using lumbar plexus and sciatic CPNB techniques placed at the twenty-first Combat Support Hospital near Baghdad by Buckenmaier. The casualty's verbal pain scores reduced from 10 to 0 (zero represents no pain, 10 is the worst pain imagined) and surgery was performed without general anesthetic. Buckenmaier accompanied the patient back to Landstuhl in Germany and managed to convince the flight crew to allow the infusion pumps to remain in use in-flight. At the US hospital in Germany concerns about compartment syndrome resulted in the infusions being turned off, but then recommenced as pain scores increased back up to eight out of ten.

This and subsequent cases highlighted the difficulties associated with starting CPNB in this environment. Surgeons are concerned about compartment syndrome. Air Force medical staff has very strict rules about using non-flight tested equipment in their aircraft, and are also not trained in the use of CPNB but are skilled in the use of morphine. This equally applies to receiving hospitals where staff may not be used to managing CPNB.

Despite these important evacuation chain issues, CPNB has become an accepted component in the pain management of American wounded. Currently, the largest impediment to the routine use of regional anesthesia has been the lack of trained personnel in theater who are skilled and/or available to provide acute pain management services. Pain management has traditionally been an assumed or implied duty of the anesthetist, but experience from the current conflicts suggest that appropriately trained personnel must be deployed specifically for pain management if wounded are to receive these important medical interventions routinely. Recently, the British military has tested this concept with the deployment of an acute pain service at Camp Bastion Hospital, Afghanistan. Data from this first experience is pending.

## 22.5.2
### Use of Ultrasound in a Military Environment

Another anticipated difficulty for anesthesiologists using single injection or CPNB regional techniques is how to identify the appropriate anatomy when a traditional stimulator technique may not work because of loss of tissue, or traumatic amputation. Authors have reported stimulating phantom limbs,[13] but this can be unreliable as well as distressing. Plunkett et al.[14] reported the use of ultrasound to place a supraclavicular catheter in a soldier who had experienced multiple injuries including an above elbow amputation and also a tracheostomy, reducing communication to hand signals. Peripheral nerve stimulation would have not been possible in this relatively routine war wound.

Ultrasound guidance for placement of single injection and CPNB catheters has been reported to improve block performance times and/or number of needle passes, improve success rates, speed the onset of the block, increase the duration of block in children and provide a local anesthetic sparing effect.[15,16] These benefits coupled with the common amputations seen in modern war, make a high fidelity ultrasound machine a highly desirable addition to the deployed military anesthesiologists armamentarium. In addition these machines are useful for placement of central venous catheters, FAST (Focused Assessment with Sonography in Trauma)[17] exams, and general imaging purposes.

However, the use of ultrasound requires additional skills, experience, and knowledge and therefore would need to be part of an anesthesiologist's routine practice to enable use of ultrasound-guided techniques in a military environment.

## 22.6
## Risks of Regional Anesthesia

Advocating placement of catheters for CPNB, and also single injection regional techniques for peri-operative analgesia is only appropriate when the clinician is aware of the risks associated with these procedures.

Table 22.2 summarizes the main risks and complications associated with regional anesthesia. Many of these risks can be mitigated and the incidence is reduced by experience at performing the blocks, knowledge of the anatomy, and good attention to detail.

### 22.6.1
### Infection

Of concern has been potential for an increased risk of infection when placing CPNB catheters following blast injury, as many of the solders have extensive debris and tissue damage and have a high incidence of systemic infections following severe trauma. So far there does not appear to be a concomitant increase (versus civilian practice) in catheter

**Table 22.2** Risks associated with regional anaesthesia techniques

| Risk associated with any nerve block | Additional risks for catheter techniques |
|---|---|
| Infection | Increased risk of infection |
| Haematoma/bleeding | Catheter failure |
| Nerve damage (permanent and temporary) | Catheter disconnection |
| Inadvertent intra-vascular injection | Catheter migration |
| Failure | Catheter leak |
| Pneumothorax (upper limb and paravertebral blocks) | Catheter removal with bleeding diathesis |
| Local anesthetic toxicity | Retained catheter |
| Masking of compartment syndrome | |

related infections, though the ARAPMI Regional Anesthesia Tracking System (RATS) is likely to generate more data on this. Also, epidural analgesia is used for some military casualties being repatriated with significant bilateral injuries. The risk of infection in the epidural space is much greater to an individual, than abscess formation alongside a peripheral nerve.

### 22.6.2
### Coagulopathy

The risk of placing or removing CPNB catheters in patients who are anticoagulated or coagulopathic presents a definite risk, particularly in the ballistic trauma population who are likely to receive a massive blood transfusion and then later be given prophylactic low-molecular weight heparins. Recent publications support the use and removal of CPNB catheters against a set of practice parameters for patients receiving LMWH,[18] and also in patients receiving lumbar plexus CPNB for total hip arthroplasty whilst anticoagulated with warfarin.[17,19] Whilst the recommendations are not that this is an inherently safe practice, it allows for experienced clinicians to balance the risks against the benefits.

### 22.6.3
### Compartment Syndrome

A significant concern for clinicians managing patients after ballistic injury is the potential for high quality regional anesthesia masking the development of compartment syndrome. In the author's experience, where the development of compartment syndrome is of immediate concern, the surgeon will generally have performed a prophylactic compartment release.

In a systematic review of nearly 2,000 cases of acute traumatic compartment syndrome (awaiting publication in *Trauma*) Hayakawa found 13 cases in eight case reports where effective analgesia masked the onset of symptoms and therefore delayed diagnosis and treatment. Six of these were related to epidurals, six cases were masked by patients on PCA morphine and one following a femoral nerve block. The authors point out that neither the denominator or numerator are known, and that there is likely to be under-reporting of cases where effective analgesia was in use but compartment syndrome was effectively diagnosed and treated.

The currently available evidence therefore suggests that PCA morphine is as likely to mask, or delay the diagnosis of acute traumatic compartment syndrome, as central neuraxial block. Because this complication is uncommon, large prospective data series will be required to elicit whether effective regional anesthesia does lead to delayed diagnosis and management. It is important to note that most anesthetists differentiate between a surgical level of block (motor, sensory, and sympathetic) where issues of compartment syndrome should be surgically managed and an analgesic level of block (sensory and sympathetic, with motor sparing) which is maintained by CPNB. Ischemic pain is usually not masked by an analgesic level block.

The most effective strategy is one of a high index of suspicion, careful continuous clinical assessment of high risk cases and prompt intervention when appropriate. Analgesic plans that emphasize multimodal therapy (the use of multiple analgesic medications that work by diverse mechanisms but synergistically) tend to reduce unwanted side effects of any single pain medication, to include the masking of compartment syndrome. Analgesia should be provided via whatever modality is appropriate for the patient's condition, though where CPNB is in use, managing local anesthetic dose to provide analgesia with minimum motor blockade may assist in the clinical assessment.

## 22.6.4
### Local Anesthetic Toxicity

The risk of local anesthetic toxicity is increased with increasing doses of local anesthetic, particularly in highly vascular tissues, and especially with intravascular injection. Specific strategies to reduce the risk of this complication include:

- Standard monitoring with audible oxygen saturation tone.
- Oxygen supplementation.
- Slow, incremental injection (5 mL every 10–15 s).
- Gentle aspiration for blood before injection and every 5 mL thereafter.
- Initial injection of local anesthetic test dose containing at least 5–15 µg epinephrine with observation for heart rate change > 10 beats/min, blood pressure changes > 15 mmHg, or lead II T-wave amplitude decrease of 25%.
- Pretreatment with benzodiazepines to increase the seizure threshold to local anesthetic toxicity.
- Patient either awake or sedated, but still able to maintain meaningful communication with the physician.
- Resuscitation equipment and medications readily available at all times.
- If seizures occur, patient care includes airway maintenance, supplemental oxygen, and termination of the seizure with propofol (25–50 mg) or thiopental (50 mg).
- Local anesthetic toxicity that leads to cardiovascular collapse should immediately be managed with prompt institution of advanced cardiac life support (ACLS) protocols.
- Intralipid (KabiVitrum Inc, Alameda, Calif) 20% 1 mL/kg every 3–5 min, up to 3 mL/kg, administered during ACLS for local anesthetic toxicity can be life saving. Follow this bolus with an Intralipid 20% infusion of 0.25 mL/kg/min for 2.5 h (see Appendix A).

Local anesthetic choice for regional anesthesia is also an important consideration when attempting to minimize toxic risk. Generally, the greatest risk to the patient for local anesthetic toxicity occurs during the initial placement of the block which consists of a bolus of local anesthetic. Bupivacaine is a popular long acting local anesthetic used in regional anesthesia. Unfortunately, its use in large volume techniques had been reportedly associated with prolonged resuscitation following accidental intravascular injection. Bupivacaine has the lowest recommended dosages of any of the amide local anesthetics. If patient safety were the only issue (other than cost, convenience, or availability) involved in long-acting local anesthetic selection, less toxic options (ropivacaine) would likely be used for large volume blocks. This issue remains controversial. WRAMC recommendations for local anesthetic dosages for single injection block and CPNB provided in Appendix B.

### 22.6.5
### Ultrasound

Using ultrasound reduces the number of needle passes required to successfully place a regional block[13] and should therefore reduce significant complications, though currently there are no randomized controlled trials of sufficient size (and may never be) to prove this hypothesis. In skilled hands, carefully bolusing local anesthetic under direct vision may reduce the risk of inadvertent intravascular injection of local anesthetic and perhaps inadvertent neural damage. Ultrasound guided block also allows for dynamic injection of local anesthetic around nerve targets as opposed to the static injection typical of nerve stimulation techniques. This typically results in the shorter block onset characteristic of ultrasound guided blocks.

This balance of potentially significant risks must be weighed against the potential benefits – both for the patient and also for the anesthesiologist in a resource and personnel limited combat support or field hospital.

### 22.7
### Benefits of Regional Anesthesia

Compared to morphine, continuous peripheral nerve block analgesia provides superior post-operative analgesia compared to morphine at all time points and also a reduction therefore in opioid related side effects (see Table 22.1).[20]

However, there are other significant benefits in the field hospital environment.

### 22.7.1
### Adaptability

Whilst the aim with all military severely injured casualties is early repatriation, this may not always be possible. The ballistic trauma victim will invariably require repeat visits to the operating theater after their damage control surgery. In both the current conflicts in Iraq and Afghanistan the Allied Forces also look after local nationals who may remain with the hospital for many surgical procedures.

A CPNB catheter facilitates these procedures since re-establishment of a surgical block involves merely dosing the CPNB catheter. This in turn decreases overall time in the operating theater and recovery, allows for safe short notice deferment or rescheduling of patients when unexpected emergency patients arrive, and decreases the level of input required from nursing staff on the ward. CPNB also decreases patient opioid consumption and allows the patient to maintain pain control between procedures when patient bolus capable pumps are used.

## 22.7.2
## Humanity

Many of the patients managed in the deployed military (and humanitarian) environment may be separated by a language barrier. This affects their ability to communicate pain effectively. This issue is particularly pertinent for children who are equally susceptible to ballistic trauma in areas of conflict. Mariano and colleagues reported favourably on the use of ultrasound guided CPNB catheters on medical missions in developing countries.[21] There may therefore be a double benefit in terms of adaptability and improved analgesia in this group of patients with whom communication and cultural differences in attitude to pain may result in inadequately treated pain otherwise.

## 22.7.3
## Critical Care

Malchow and Black summarize the "paradigm shift" that has occurred during the past 5 years with respect to management of pain in the critically injured combat casualty.[22] The complications of pain and side effects of opioids, increased intensive care stay, and subsequent development of chronic pain have decreased with an aggressive opioid sparing acute pain management strategy that includes a variety of oral and intravenous pharmacological strategies, as well as the use of regional anesthesia.

## 22.7.4
## Acute Traumatic Brain Injury (ATBI)

In addition to the critical care data, soldiers and civilians who are involved in blast injury are at high risk of development of mild to severe ATBI. This group of patients are at particular risk of developing chronic pain, which is a finding independent of the occurrence of Post Traumatic Stress Disorder, depression and common in patients with fairly minor ATBI.[23] They are also the group who are more likely to be unable to, or to ineffectively communicate their pain experience. Therefore any strategy to reduce pain from the outset should be considered highly desirable.

## 22.7.5
## Chronic Pain

Current data from non-severely injured soldiers returning from Iraq and Afghanistan, registering for Veterans Affairs care indicate that pain problems will be among the most common complaints.[24] Clark and colleagues[25] suggest a revision in pain classification for combat trauma pain, where other factors such as PTSD, breakthrough pain, and psychosocial factors all impact upon the progression of initially unremitting acute pain to develop in to chronic pain. The ARAPMI RATS data may provide an answer as to whether regional anesthesia has a direct impact upon the development of chronic pain in this group of patients. The data for avoidance of the specific entity of phantom limb pain is also equivocal at present. However, the concept of providing early effective analgesia would intuitively seem to reduce the nociceptive inputs that are required for the "wind-up" phenomenon that leads to chronic pain – not withstanding the earlier advantages of cardiovascular stability and reduced pain during transfer.

## 22.7.6
## Transfer

To repatriate a casualty requires a significant number of patient moves. The author of this chapter placed a femoral CPNB catheter in a British soldier in Afghanistan following fragmentation injury that had disrupted his femur. The patient's pain was rated as severe post insertion of a Denholm pin for traction, and was exacerbated by movement – particularly of the traction weights. Pain had not been controlled with large doses of morphine, but relief was almost immediate after femoral nerve blockade was commenced. Repatriation to the UK and definitive surgery required eleven transfers (Table 22.3) all of which generates unavoidable movement of the "immobilized" leg and therefore the potential for pain. Lack of approved equipment for aeromedical transfer meant that this patient's femoral nerve catheter was bolused as required by an anesthetist, but pain scores remained at mild to none including following definitive surgery in the UK.

The example illustrates the benefit to the individual of being able to utilize catheter based regional anesthesia – notwithstanding putative advantages in reducing risk of developing chronic pain. Additionally, this example illustrates the need for a military pain infusion pump that allows physician infusion program adjustment and patient controlled bolus capability (Table 22.4).

**Table 22.3** Transfers and transport for a military casualty

| From | To | Mode of transport |
| --- | --- | --- |
| Ward, Camp Bastion | Ambulance | Trolley |
| Ambulance | Tactical flight | Stretcher |
| Camp bastion | Kandahar | Air |
| Tactical flight | Ambulance | Stretcher |
| Airfield | Medical facility Kandahar airhead | Ambulance |
| Medical facility | Airfield | Ambulance |
| Ambulance | Aeromed flight | Stretcher |
| Kandahar | UK | Air |
| UK Airport | Birmingham | Ambulance |
| Ambulance | Receiving ward | Trolley |
| Ward | Theater | Trolley |
| Definitive surgery | Ward | Trolley |

**Table 22.4** Desirable characteristics of a military pain infusion pump

| |
|---|
| Easily identifiable by shape and color |
| Used only for pain service infusions |
| Lightweight and compact |
| Reprogrammable for basal rate, bolus amount, lockout interval, and infusion volume |
| Battery operated with long battery life |
| Program lock-out to prevent program tampering |
| Simple and intuitive operation |
| Medication free-flow protection |
| Latex free |
| Visual and audible alarms |
| Stable infusion rate at extremes of temperature and pressure |
| Inexpensive |
| Durable for long service life without needing maintenance |
| Certified for use in US military aircraft |

Buckenmaier 3rd.[34] With kind permission from The Henry M. Jackson Foundation for the Advancement of Military Medicine, Inc.

## 22.8
## Challenges and Obstacles

As has been highlighted, many of the challenges and obstacles that exist in providing safe and effective regional anesthesia in this unique environment for this challenging group of patients exists with the anesthesiologist performing the procedure – skills and knowledge are required that must already be part of an individual clinician's routine clinical practice. To facilitate the placement of CPNB catheters and use them effectively there is a necessary amount of specialist equipment that is required (Fig. 22.1).

### 22.8.1
### Multidisciplinary

The management of acute pain following polytrauma must be a surgical team effort. The theater team need to be trained in the principles and practice of multimodal analgesia and regional anesthesia. The surgeons have to be part of the decision making process and need to be comfortable with the presence of a CPNB catheter. The ward nurses and flight nurses have to be trained to understand the management of acute pain problems with CPNB infusions. The equipment needs to be approved by the aeromedical team to ensure there are no flight safety issues. The receiving hospitals also need to have CPNB catheters as part of their normal lexicon of healthcare.

**Fig. 22.1** Set-up for peripheral nerve block (**A**) Sterile surface.(**B**) Sterile gloves (full aseptic technique including gown is required for CPNB catheter).(**C**) Chlorhexidine in alcohol cleaning solution (or similar).(**D**) Marker pen and ruler (mark site before sedation).(**E**) Sterile drape. (**F**) Sedation available (midazolam, fentanyl, etc). (**G**) 1% lidocaine with 23G needle.(**H**) Local anesthetic.(**I**) Stimulating needle.(**J**) Peripheral nerve stimulator (optional if using M).(**K**) Sterile swabs.(**L**) Opsite spray dressing (or similar).(**M**) Ultrasound machine and gel (optional).(**N**) Sharps disposal bin and clinical waste bag for correct disposal post-procedure

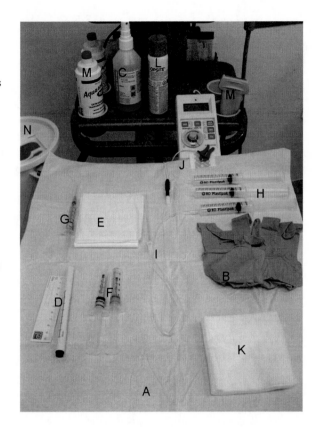

## 22.8.2
## Multimodal

Regional anesthesia has been the focus of this chapter. Specific methods of providing effective and appropriate analgesia for specific wound entities are not within its scope. Neither has an analysis of the most effective drugs or regimens for provision of single injection or CPNB analgesia. What must be highlighted is that regional anesthesia is only part of the answer. Morphine will always have a place in the analgesic pharmacopoeia, but all attempts should be made to reduce the required dose.

- Paracetamol (acetaminophen) has a low side effect profile and excellent morphine sparing capacity.
- Non-steroidal anti-inflammatory drugs should be considered for each patient.
- Alpha2-adrenergic receptor antagonists such as clonidine have an analgesic and sedative effect (and can prolong duration of action of local anesthetic blocks).
- NMDA antagonists – in particular ketamine – can reduce morphine consumption and may reduce wind-up.[26]
- The anticonvulsant gabapentin is also currently used following traumatic amputation, as based upon current best evidence it may reduce the incidence of chronic pain.

## 22.9
## Summary

Regional anesthesia has a place in the management of the ballistic trauma victim as part of a multimodal approach to the management of severe limb trauma. Its use is limited only by the skills and competencies of the multi-disciplinary team, though the aim must always be to provide the patient with the most effective analgesia available for their situation. Further information on the military application of regional anesthesia can be found in the Military Advanced Regional Anesthesia and Analgesia Handbook (Borden Institute, Washington DC, 2009 www.bordeninstitute.army.mil or www.ARAPMI.org).

These patients are young men and women who will have just been involved in a harrowing life changing incident. It behoves all who are involved in their care to ensure that our skills and competencies match their bravery.

## 22.10
## Appendix A

### 22.10.1
### Intralipid

Local anesthetic toxicity is rare, but potentially life threatening as it is associated with cardiac dysrhythmias and cardiac arrest that are refractory to normal management techniques. The development of Intralipid (Pharmacia & Upjohn, Somerset County, New Jersey, US) complements the supportive management of airway maintenance, ventilation and circulatory support in accordance with standard advanced life support protocols.

The mechanism of action of Intralipid is uncertain. It may act as a lipid "sink" that chelates the local anesthetic agent, or may simply protect the myocardium. Initial animal studies[27] have been augmented by a series of case reports in humans.[28-30] In view of the infrequent nature of this complication the evidence base is unlikely to extend beyond case reports. However, the treatment of local anesthetic toxicity has been supported by editorials in peer-reviewed journals[31,32] and the UK National Patient Safety Agency has also reported favorably on its use.[33] Most UK hospitals now stock intralipid in areas where regional anesthesia is conducted. Its availability should be considered as part of any deployed regional anesthesia capability.

## 22.11
## Appendix B

**Table 22.5** Standard adult ropivacaine dosages for single injection and continuous regional anesthesia at Walter Reed Army Medical Center

| Regional anesthesia technique | Adult single injection[a] | Continuous infusion of 0.2% Ropivacaine | Patient-controlled bolus rate of 0.2% Ropivacaine[b] (mL bolus/20 min lockout) | Notes |
|---|---|---|---|---|
| Interscalene | 30–40 mL of 0.5% ropivacaine | 8–10 | 2–3 | Often supplemented with an intercostal brachial nerve block |
| Supraclavicular | 30–40 mL of 0.5% ropivacaine | 8–10 | 2–3 | Shortest latency block of the brachial plexus |
| Infraclavicular | 35–40 mL of 0.5% ropivacaine | 10–12 | 2–3 | Catheter techniques less effective compared to supraclavicular catheters |
| Axillary | 40 mL of 0.5% ropivacaine | 10–12 | 2–3 | Catheter techniques less common |
| Paravertebral | 3–5 mL of 0.5% ropivacaine per level blocked | 8–10 | 2–3 | Catheters effective in thoracic region only |
| Lumbar plexus (posterior approach) | 30–40 mL of 0.5% ropivacaine | 8–10 | 2–3 | Epidural spread is a concern |
| Femoral | 20–30 mL of 0.5% ropivacaine | 8–10 | 2–3 | Catheter techniques may miss the obturator or lateral femoral cutaneous nerves |
| Sciatic (anterior or posterior approach) | 20–30 mL of 0.5% ropivacaine | 8–10 | 2–3 | Proximal approaches to the sciatic nerve preferable for catheters |
| Sciatic (lateral or popliteal approach) | 35–40 mL of 0.5% ropivacaine | 10–12 | 2–3 | Often the only approach available to the sciatic nerve following polytrauma |
| Lumbar plexus or femoral + sciatic | 50–60 mL of 0.5% ropivacaine between both sites | 5–10 for both catheters | 2–3 on one catheter | Infusion rates divided between catheters based on distribution of patient's pain |
| Epidural | 20–25 mL of 0.5% ropivacaine | 6–10 thoracic 10–20 lumbar | 2–3 | Opioids often added to infusions |
| Spinal | 5–15 mg of 1.0% ropivacaine | NA | NA | Opioids often added to injections |

*NA* not applicable

[a] Mepivacaine 1.5% can be used in place of ropivacaine at the volumes noted when a shorter duration block is desirable

[b] Occasionally, a 5 mL bolus per 30 min lockout is used in selected patients. Generally, total infusion (continuous plus bolus) > 20 mL/h are avoided

Buckenmaier 3rd.[34] With kind permission from The Henry M. Jackson Foundation for the Advancement of Military Medicine, Inc.

# References

1. Thompson GE. Narration: Anesthesia for battle casualties in Vietnam. *JAMA*. 1967;201:218-219.
2. Stojadinovic A, Auton A, Peoples GE, McKnight GM, et al. Responding to challenges in modern combat casualty care: Innovative use of advanced regional anesthesia. *Pain Med*. 2006;7(4):330-338.
3. Borden Institute, Walter Reed Army Medical Centre. *Emergency war surgery: Third United States revision*. U.S. government printing office; 2004: 3.1-3.17.
4. Clark ME, Bair MJ, Buckenmaier CC 3rd, Gironda RJ, Walker RL. Pain and combat injuries in OEF/OIF. *J Rehabil Res Dev*. 2007;44(2):179-194.
5. http://www.painfoundation.org/page.asp?file=Newsroom/PainSurveys.htm.
6. Melzack R, Wall PD. Pain mechanisms: A new theory. *Science*. 1965;150(699):971-979.
7. Grant AJ, Wood C. Continuous regional analgesia by intraneural block: Effect on postoperative opioid requirements and phantom limb pain following amputation. *Scott Med J*. 2008; 53(1):4-6.
8. Jevtovic-Todorovic V. Standards of care for ambulatory surgery. Are we up to speed. *Minerva Anestesiol*. 2006;72:13-20.
9. Ilfeld BM, Gearen P, Enneking F, Berry L, et al. Total hip arthroplasty as an overnight-stay procedure using continuous psoas compartment nerve block: A prospective feasibility study. *Reg Anesth Pain Med*. 2006;31:172-176.
10. Ilfeld BM, Gearen P, Enneking F, Berry L. Total knee arthroplasty as an overnight stay procedure using continuous femoral nerve blocks at home. A prospective feasibility study. *Anesth Analg*. 2006;102:87-90.
11. Fredrickson MJ, Ball CM, Dalgleish AJ. Successful continuous interscalene analgesia for ambulatory shoulder surgery in a private practice setting. *Reg Anesth Pain Med*. 2008;33(2):122-128.
12. Buckenmaier CC III, McKnight GM, Winkley JV, Bleckner LL, et al. Continuous peripheral nerve block for battlefield anesthesia and evacuation. *Reg Anesth Pain Med*. 2005;30(2):202-205.
13. Klein SM, Eck J, Nielsen K, Steele SM. Anesthetizing the phantom: Peripheral nerve stimulation of a non-existent extremity. *Anesthesiology*. 2004;102:248-257.
14. Plunkett AR, Brown DS, Rogers JM, Buckenmaier CC. Supraclavicular continuous peripheral nerve block in a wounded soldier: When ultrasound is the only option. *Br J Anaesth*. 2006; 97(5):715-717.
15. de Tran QH, Munoz L, Russo G, Finlayson RJ. Ultrasonography and stimulating perineural catheters for nerve blocks: A review of the evidence. *Can J Anesth*. 2008;55(7):447-457.
16. Koscielniak-Nielsen ZJ. Ultrasound-guided peripheral nerve blocks: What are the benefits? *Acta Anaesthesiol Scand*. 2008;52(6):727-737.
17. Scalea TM, Rodriguez A, Chiu WC, Brenneman FD, et al. Focused Assessment with Sonography for Trauma (FAST): Results from an international consensus conference. *J Trauma*. 1999;46:466-472.
18. Buckenmaier CC 3rd, Bleckner LL. Continuous peripheral nerve block in combat casualties receiving low-molecular weight heparin. *Br J Anaesth*. 2008;97:874-877.
19. Chelly JE, Szczodry DM, Neumann KJ. International normalized ratio and prothrombin time values before the removal of a lumbar plexus catheter in patients receiving warfarin after total hip replacementdagger. *Br J Anaesth*. 2008;101:250-254.
20. Richman JM, Liu SS, Courpas G, Wong R, et al. Does continuous peripheral nerve block provide superior pain control to opioids? A meta-analysis. *Anesth Analg*. 2006;102(1):248-257.
21. Mariano ER, Ilfeld BM, Cheng GS, Nicodemus HF, Suresh S. Feasibility of ultrasound-guided peripheral nerve block catheters for pain control on pediatric medical missions in developing countries. *Pediatr Anaesth*. 2008;18(7):598-601.
22. Malchow RJ, Black IH. The evolution of pain management in the critically ill trauma patient: Emerging concepts from the global war on terrorism. *Crit Care Med*. 2008;36(7 Suppl): S346-S357.

23. Nampiaparampil DE. Prevalance of chronic pain after traumatic brain injury: A systematic review. *JAMA*. 2008;300(6):711-719.

24. Gironda RJ, Clark ME, Massengale JP, Walker RL. Pain among veterans of Operations Enduring Freedom and Iraqi Freedom. *Pain Med*. 2006;7(4):339-343.

25. Clark ME, Bair MJ, Buckenmaier CC, Gironda RJ 3rd, Walker RL. Pain and combat injuries in soldiers returning from Operations Enduring Freedom and Iraqi Freedom: Implications for research and practice. *J Rehabil Res Dev*. 2007;44(2):179-194.

26. Himmelseher S, Durieux ME. Ketamine for perioperative pain management. *Anesthesiol*. 2005;102:211-220.

27. Weinberg G, Ripper R, Feinstein DL, Hoffman W. Lipid emulsion infusion rescues dogs from bupivacaine-induced cardiac toxicity. *Reg Anesth Pain Med*. 2003;28(3):198-202.

28. Rosenblatt MA, Abel M, Fischer GW, Itzkovich CJ, Eisenkraft JB. Successful use of a 20% Lipid emulsion to resuscitate a patient after a presumed bupivacaine related cardiac arrest. *Anaesthesiology*. 2006;105:217-218.

29. Litz RJ, Popp M, Stehr SN, Koch TI. Successful resuscitation of a patient with ropivacaine induced asystole after axillary plexus block using lipid infusion. *Anaesthesia*. 2006;61: 800-801.

30. Foxall G, McCahon R, Lamb J, Hardman JG, Bedforth NM. Levobupivacaine induced seizures and cardiovascular collapse treated with Intralipid. *Anaesthesia*. 2007;62:516-518.

31. Weinberg G. Lipid infusion resuscitation for local anesthetic toxicity: Proof of clinical efficacy. *Anesthesiology*. 2006;105:7-8.

32. Picard J, Meek T. *Anaesthesia*. 2006;61:107-109.

33. Patient safety alert 21 (28 March 2007) – Safer practice with epidural injections and infusions. London: National patient safety agency (www.npsa.nhs.uk).

34. Bleckner L, Buckenmaier C 3rd, eds. *Military Advanced Regional Anesthesia and Analgesia Handbook*. Washington, DC: Borden Institute; 2009.

# Part VI

## Clinical Care

Mark J. Midwinter and Adam J. Brooks

## 23.1
## Introduction

Damage Control Surgery (DCS) is an operative strategy that sacrifices the completeness of the immediate surgical repair in order to address the physiological consequences of the combined trauma of the injury and surgery. In the past this has been very much focussed on abdominal trauma and the idea of performing an "abbreviated laparotomy." However the concepts outlined here are applicable to injury beyond the abdomen.[1-3]

The principles of Damage Control Surgery (DCS) have been well described for over 20 years but have been slow to gain universal acceptance. However, it is now recognized that severely injured trauma patients are more likely to die from the metabolic consequences of the injury rather than the completeness of the immediate surgical repair to damaged organs (Fig. 23.1).

## 23.2
## Pathophysiology

The central observation behind the philosophy of DCS is the adverse effects of the combined triad of hypothermia, acidosis, and coagulopathy in the trauma patient.[1,4,5] Hypothermia leads to $\alpha$(alpha)-adrenergic stimulation with vasoconstriction, exacerbating any organ hypoperfusion that may already be present secondary to hypotension from the injury. This leads to worsening acidosis. Both hypothermia and acidosis may be further exacerbated by aggressive fluid resuscitation, especially with normal saline. Hypothermia and acidosis combined with the consumption, dilution, and failure to replace clotting factors leads to a coagulopathy.[6,7] Even if major surgical bleeding is controlled at this stage the patient will continue to

M.J. Midwinter (✉)
Academic Department of Military Surgery and Trauma, Royal Centre for Defence Medicine,
University Hospital, Birmingham, UK
e-mail: prof.milsurg@rcdm.bham.ac.uk

A.J. Brooks et al. (eds.), *Ryan's Ballistic Trauma*,
DOI: 10.1007/978-1-84882-124-8_23, © Springer-Verlag London Limited 2011

**Fig. 23.1** General and Plastic
Surgeons undertaking a
damage control proceedure
together on deployment

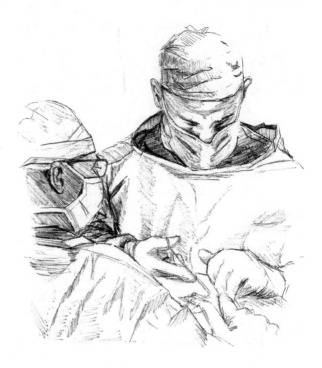

bleed from all cut surfaces prolonging the bloody vicious cycle of hypothermia, acidosis, and coagulopathy. The degree of coagulopathy is under-estimated by standard laboratory tests of coagulation.[8] Coagulopathy has been shown to be a marker of injury severity, rather than just a result of dilution by fluid administration and the effect of hypothermia, the acute coagulopathy of trauma. It has also been shown to be related to mortality[15].

Hypothermia is directly correlated to injury severity and an independent risk factor for mortality, reaching 100% when core temperature is less than 32°C in patients undergoing a laparotomy.[9,10]

## 23.3
## Indications for DCS

The decision to perform a DCS procedure is an active decision that should be reached immediately pre-operatively or within a few minutes of starting the procedure to avoid the vicious cycle being entered rather than employing DCS as a measure of desperation once the consequences outlined above are established. Attempts to define physiological measures when a DCS approach should be adopted have been suggested. An injury severity score of more than 25, systolic blood pressure less than 70 mmHg, core temperature less than 34°C, and pH less than 7.1 have been suggested as indicators for DCS[11] where as others have included lactate or base deficit, blood transfusion requirement, or injury mechanism and complexes.[12] DCS is only applicable to a minority of trauma patients and if used too liberally may be no better or even worse than immediate definitive surgery. However, too strict a definition as to when to adopt the approach particularly based on laboratory indicies, can mean that the adverse physiological consequences are already established. Experience and rapid surgical assessment are key to making a positive, informed decision to adopt a DCS strategy.

## 23.4
## Four Stage Approach to DCS

Classically four stages of DCS are described.[1]

### 23.4.1
### Stage 0

The first stage is the patient selection and decision making described above. This should occur rapidly in the ED or even in the prehospital phase. Alternatively the decision should be made immediately pre-operatively or within minutes of the start of surgery.

### 23.4.2
### Stage 1

The second DCS stage is the intra-operative stage. The priorities are hemorrhage control, limiting contamination, and temporary closure. Hemorrhage control may be achieved by ligation, suture, tamponade (by packing or balloon), or shunting. Definitive vascular repair by grafting or anastomosis is not a DCS procedure. Contamination control is achieved by closure of the ends of the injured hollow viscus. Anastomoses and stomas are not fashioned in DCS. Pre-emptive strategies to prevent compartment syndromes such as fasciotomies and laparostomy are employed. Time in the operating room should be limited and once hemorrhage control and contamination limitation are achieved temporary closure or cover is established to allow the patient to be moved to critical care environment. Time in stage 1 should as short as possible however, taking a patient with active surgical bleeding patient to the ITU is futile.

### 23.4.3
### Stage 2

Once the patient is in the critical care environment continued attempts at correcting the physiological consequences of the injury and metabolic failure are pursued. These will have started in the pre-operative and operative phases. Addressing the physiological consequences of trauma and the coagulopathy in particular as part of a Damage Control

Resuscitation (DCR) strategy from the outset of resuscitation may result in improved physiology intra-operatively but surgery should not be delayed to achieve this goal[13] DCR and DCS should occur concurrently. Active rewarming measures with air-warming devices, fluid warmers, or arteriovenous warming techniques as well as warm ambient environment are employed.[10] Perfusion is restored to the body tissues. By warming and optimizing perfusion the acidosis usually corrects and the oxygen debt from the anaerobic metabolism is repaid. Coagulopathy is corrected by addressing the hypothermia and acidosis and the administration of fresh frozen plasma, cryoprecipitate, and platelets as necessary.[13,14]

Early return to the operating theater can be indicated if there is obvious ongoing surgical bleeding or unaddressed compartment syndromes develop.

## 23.4.4
## Stage 3

Timing of the planned return to the operating theater is dictated by the improvement in the patient's physiological status. It has been suggested that the following indicies are used to guide timing to re-operation; a base deficit greater than −4 mmol/L, lactate of less than 2.5 mmol/L, core temperature greater than 35°C and an international normalization ratio of less than 1.25 normal.

Before the decision to return to the operating theater is made, plans to assemble the appropriate surgical team must be put in place to ensure that the optimum repairs of the injuries are performed. This may require more than one surgical specialty, but with a clearly identified leader to orchestrate the procedures and take a global view of the patient's condition. At this stage anastomoses are fashioned or stomas raised and vascular repairs performed.

Formal closure may not be possible at stage 3 as there may still be significant edema or clinical risk of developing a compartment syndrome (abdominal or extremity). Therefore a planned further operative phase for closing or covering the laparotomy may need to be made.

## References

1. Johnson JW, Gracias VH, Schwab CW, Reilly PM, et al. Evolution in damage control for exsanguinating penetrating abdominal injury. *J Trauma.* 2001;51(2):261-269. discussion 269-71.
2. Rezende-Neto J, Marques A, Guedes LJ, Teixeira LC. Damage control principles applied to penetrating neck and mandibular injuries. *J Trauma Injury Infection Crit Care.* 2008;64: 1142-1143.
3. Wall MJ, Soltero E. Damage control for thoracic injuries. *Surg Clin North Am.* 1977;77(4): 863-877.
4. Rotondo M, Schwab CW, McGonigal MD, Phillips GR, et al. 'Damage Control': An approach for improved survival in exsanguinating penetrating abdominal injury. *J Trauma Injury Infection Crit Care.* 1993;35(3):375-383.

5. Burch JM, Oritz VB, Richardson RJ. Abbreviated laparotomy and planned reoperation for critically injured patients. *Ann Surg*. 1992;215:476-484.

6. Gregory JS, Flancbaum L, Townsend MC, Clouther CT, Jonasson O. Incidence and timing of hypothermia in trauma patients undergoing operations. *J Trauma Injury Infection Crit Care*. 1991;31(6):795-800.

7. Steinemann S, Shackford SR, Davis JW. Implications of admission hypothermia in trauma patients. *J Trauma Injury Infection Crit Care*. 1990;30(2):200-202.

8. Kheirabadi B, Crissey J, Deguzman R, Holcomb J. In vivo bleeding time and in vitro thromboelastography measurements are better indicators of dilutional hypothermic coagulopathy than prothrombin time. *J Trauma Injury Infection Crit Care*. 2007;62(6):1352-1361.

9. Jurkovich GJ WBG, Luterman A, Curerri P. Hypothermia in trauma victims: An ominous predictor of survival. *J Trauma Injury Infection Crit Care*. 1987;27:1019-1024.

10. Morris J Jr, Eddy V, Blinman T, Rutherford E, Sharp K. The staged celiotomy for trauma: Issues in packing and reconstruction. *Ann Surg*. 1993;217:576-586.

11. Moore EE, Burch JM, Franciose R, Offner P, Biffl W. Staged physiologic restoration and damage control surgery. *World J Surg*. 1998;22(12):1184-1190.

12. Talbert S, Trooskin S, Scalea T, Vieux E, et al. Packing and re-exploration for patients with non-hepatic injuries. *J Trauma Injury Infection Crit Care*. 1992;33:121-125.

13. Holcomb J, Jenkins D, Rhee P, Johannigman J, et al. Damage control resuscitation: Directly addressing the early coagulopathy of trauma. *J Trauma Injury Infection Crit Care*. 2007;62:307-310.

14. Kirkman E, Watts S, Hodgetts T, Mahoney P, Rawlinson S, Midwinter M. A proactive approach to the coagulopathy of trauma: The rational and guidelines for treatment. *J Royal Army Medical Corps*. 2008;153(4):302-306.

15. Brohi K, Singh J, Heron M, Coats T. Acute traumatic coagulopathy. *J Trauma Injury Infection Crit Care*. 2003;54(6):1127-1130.

# Management of Ballistic Trauma to the Head

# 24

Geoffrey S.F. Ling, Chris J. Neal, and James M. Ecklund

## 24.1
## Introduction

Historically, the vast majority of penetrating head injuries (PHI) resulted from military combat operations; however, during the latter part of the twentieth century, these injuries have increased in incidence in civilian trauma centers. The difference in military and civilian PHI is often the nature of the penetrating projectile. In a combat situation, a majority of penetrating missile wounds are from either explosive munitions producing low-velocity fragmentation injuries or high-velocity bullets fired from various ranges.[1]

Civilian gunshot wounds primarily result from low-velocity bullets fired at close range, typically from handguns.[2] This accounts for a significant proportion of civilian injuries in the form of homicides, suicides, and accidents, with an estimated 2.4 deaths per 100,000 each year in the United States.[3,4] With the recent increased threat of terrorist attacks, the penetrating and blast injuries traditionally seen during military conflicts may become more frequently seen in some civilian centers. As a consequence of the large number of patients with PHI treated during wartime, a number of the advances and refinements in the care of these patients have emerged from the military experience.

Prior to 1900, PHIs generally were considered fatal. MacCleod reported a 100% mortality in 86 cases of penetrating or perforating head injury during the Crimean War. During the American Civil War, the death rate from pyemia of wounds to the head was as high as 95% in some series. Few surgical interventions were performed because of the high rate of infectious complications. The introduction of Lister's antiseptic technique in 1867, more sophisticated understanding of cerebral localization during the late 1800s, advances in surgical technique during World War I (WWI), and antibiotics during World War II (WWII) gradually led to new optimism regarding the care of these patients.[5,6]

Major Harvey Cushing encouraged the systematic evaluation and treatment of patients with PHI during WWI. He emphasized the importance of early meticulous debridement of all devitalized tissue and removal of all visualized fragments of bone and/or metal.

G.S.F. Ling (✉)
Medical Corps, US Army, University of the Health Sciences, MD, Bethesda, USA
e-mail: gling@usuhs.mil

A.J. Brooks et al. (eds.), *Ryan's Ballistic Trauma*,
DOI: 10.1007/978-1-84882-124-8_24, © Springer-Verlag London Limited 2011

The application of his techniques reduced the operative mortality from 56% to 28% within 3 months at Base Camp 5.[5-9]

World War II brought with it the broad application of antibiotics and the importance of dural repair. Operative mortality was reduced to 14.5% during this conflict.[10,11] During the Korean War, an improved medical evacuation system and the eventual placement of neurosurgeons in combat zones resulted in more immediate surgical interventions. This early intervention proved especially efficacious in the treatment of intracranial hematomas and resulted in fewer infectious complications. Surgical mortality was reduced to as low as 10% in some series during this conflict.[12]

As a result of anecdotal reports describing delayed abscess development in PHI from WWII and Korea, the practice of aggressively removing all bone and metallic fragments in an attempt to reduce postoperative infection was mandated in the US Army during Vietnam. This approach sometimes subjected a patient to multiple operations and occasional increased operative morbidity for what was felt to be an "adequate" debridement.[13]

Critical review of the results of patients at five and 14 years in the Vietnam Head Injury Study (VHIS) ultimately showed no difference in rates of infection or seizures in those patients with retained bone or metallic fragments as seen on computed tomography (CT). This data was applied during the Israeli–Lebanese conflict where Branvold and colleagues[14] described a debridement strategy in 113 patients based on preservation of viable tissue with limited debridement. Fragments were removed with gentle irrigation and fragments that were not easily obtainable were left.

Of the 43 patients with long-term follow up, there was a 51% incidence of retained fragments and no relationship to the development of intracranial abscess formation. Additionally, there was not an increased incidence of posttraumatic epilepsy with retained bone fragments.[14] These important experiences were instrumental in the evolution of the modern surgical management of PHI.

## 24.2
## Ballistics

To understand penetrating trauma, it is important to have a basic understanding of ballistics. Wound ballistics is the study of the projectile's action in human tissue. The ballistic properties of a projectile are dependent primarily on its velocity, size, and shape. The primary injury to the brain is related directly to these properties. Secondary projectiles such as skull fragments may cause further damage.

Penetrating head injury can result from both low- and high-velocity projectiles. Lower-velocity sharp projectiles such as arrows (120 – 250 ft/s) create a tract of primary tissue damage without significant bruising or blunt tearing of surrounding tissue. Higher-velocity projectiles are preceded by a brief (2 ms) sonic shock wave, followed by the penetration of the projectile. In addition to the destruction of tissue in the projectile's path, there is a transmission of kinetic energy resulting in a temporary cavitation effect. In brain tissue, which is relatively inelastic, the cavity is often 10 – 20 times the size of the projectile. After expansion, the cavity collapses under negative pressure that may draw in external debris. The size of the cavity is dependent on the kinetic energy of the projectile.

Kinetic energy (KE) can be expressed in the equation $KE = 1/2 \, mv^2$. While mass is directly proportional to the kinetic energy, it is the velocity that is its key determinant.[15,16] The shape of the projectile determines the ballistic coefficient, which is its ability to overcome air resistance and maintain velocity. The shape also influences the yaw, which is the projectile's rotation around its long axis. While small amounts of circular motion (precession and nutation) occur during flight, projectiles often will tumble when striking tissue. Yaw is maximized when the projectile is rotated at 90° to its long axis.[15,16] This imparts more kinetic energy to the tissue, increases the size of the temporary cavity, and increases tissue destruction. For example, a 0.45 automatic pistol (muzzle velocity of 869 ft per second and a short round-nosed projectile with little yaw) will create a very small temporary cavity; conversely, a 7.62 mm North Atlantic Treaty Organization (NATO) rifle (muzzle velocity 2,830 ft/s and a long sharp nose with maximum yaw) will create a very large temporary cavity.

Projectiles also can deform or fragment upon striking tissue. Copper jacketing lead bullets, as mandated for military rounds by The Hague Peace Conference (1899), helps limit the fragmentation potential. Irregularities made by scoring the surface of the bullet (dum dums) lead to increased fragmentation, creating multiple injury tracts as each fragment becomes a new projectile. The Glaser round is filled with small pellets that disperse on impact. Hollow-point rounds, often seen in civilian shootings, expand their diameter in the direction of flight upon impact, thus creating a larger primary wound tract and more destructive temporary cavitation effects. Explosive bullets such as the Devastator round are designed to detonate on impact and thus will produce extensive tissue injury with additional kinetic energy transfer.[17]

## 24.3
## Injury Classification

Since WWI, PHIs have been classified in an attempt to correlate the type of injury with prognosis. Cushing's original classification of nine different injury patterns was refined by Matson in WWII to four categories, which are explained in Table 24.1. Currently, a PHI is described as a tangential wound, a penetrating wound, or a perforating wound.[15]

### 24.3.1
### Tangential Wound

A tangential wound (Fig. 24.1) occurs when a projectile strikes the head at an oblique angle and may produce scalp lacerations, skull fractures, and cerebral contusions. The projectile may traverse the subgaleal space and exit or remain lodged in the scalp. The presence of a hematoma, depressed skull fracture, or cerebrospinal fluid (CSF) leak may necessitate surgical intervention. Otherwise, local wound care may be applied. These

**Table 24.1** Cushing and Matson's classification of craniocerebral injuries

| Grade | Cushing (WWI) description | Grade | Matson (WWII) description |
|---|---|---|---|
| I | Scalp lacerations, skull intact | I | Scalp wound |
| II | Skull fractures, dura intact | II | Skull fracture, dura intact |
| III | Depressed skull fracture and dural laceration | III | Skull fracture with dural/brain penetration<br>(a) Gutter-type (grazing) – in-driven bone with no missile fragments<br>(b) Penetrating – missile fragments in brain<br>(c) Perforating – through and through |
| IV | In-driven bone fragments | IV | Complicating factors:<br>(a) Ventricular penetration<br>(b) Fractures of orbit or sinus<br>(c) Injury of dural sinus |
| V | Penetrating wound with projective lodged | | |
| VI | Wounds penetrating ventricles with:<br><br>(A) Bone fragments<br>(B) Projectile | | |
| VII | Wounds involving:<br><br>(A) Orbitonasal region<br>(B) Auropetrosal region | | |
| VIII | Perforating wounds | | |
| IX | Bursting skull fracture, extensive cerebral contusion | | |

injuries generally carry a better prognosis with less severe neurological deficits, but they may present with seizures or focal deficit depending on location and extent of injury.

### 24.3.2
### Penetrating Wound

The velocity of the projectile is the main determinant of its energy. If the projectile has enough energy to only penetrate the brain parenchyma, the injury is referred to as

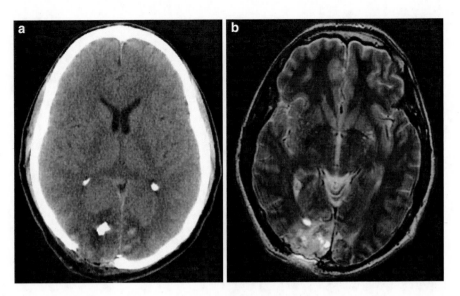

**Fig. 24.1** (**a**) CT of tangential wound to right occipital region from AK47 while wearing military helmet. Wound was emergently debrided at nearby field hospital. Note the in-driven bone fragments. (**b**) MRI of same patient revealing underlying contusion after CT confirmation of no residual metal fragments

penetrating. Energy absorbed by the skull often results in fragments of bone that act as secondary projectiles within the brain. Contusions, lacerations, or hematomas may be caused by these injuries (Fig. 24.2).

Depending on the amount of energy, the projectile may produce unusual tracts within the calvaria that may be detected on CT, but missed on plain films. The projectile may ricochet after hitting the inner table opposite of its entry, creating a new tract within the parenchyma. It also may change directions when it hits dura after penetrating the outer and inner tables of the skull. This unusual occurrence is called *careening*. The projectile then travels along the inner table of the skull, with the potential to damage the venous sinuses.

### 24.3.3
### Perforating Wound

The most destructive pattern of injury is the perforating wound (Fig. 24.3), which is defined by an entry and exit wound with a tract through brain parenchyma. This injury requires a higher-velocity projectile than with a penetrating injury, and thus imparts a higher amount of kinetic energy to the tissue. Local and distant structures are damaged from the cavitation effect the projectile imparts, resulting in multiple fractures, contusions, and hematomas.

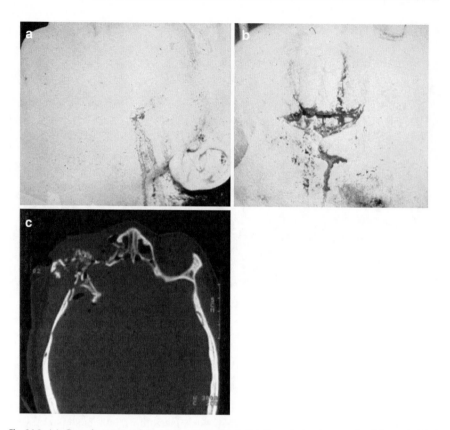

**Fig. 24.2** (**a**) Gun shot entrance wound in left cheek (**b**) Gun shot exit wounds right periorbital region. Note the increased size of the exit wound compared to the entrance wound. (**c**) CT demonstrating intracranial involvement

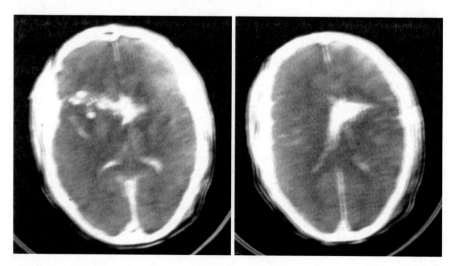

**Fig. 24.3** CT of a perforating GSW with a transventricular tract

## 24.4
## Initial Resuscitation and Management

In civilian trauma, activation of the local emergency medical service (EMS) system allows initial resuscitation efforts to be made in the field to include intravenous (IV) access and intubation when warranted. The use of a helicopter allows for faster transport from the scene or outlying hospital to a neurosurgical center for early intervention.[18,19]

A combat situation provides a different operating environment for PHIs. Initial care is provided by a medic carrying limited supplies and diagnostic equipment. In contrast to civilian systems, combat injuries are triaged in the field and at every level of care. Due to limited capabilities, the goal of combat medicine is to do the greatest good for the most people, thus maintaining the fighting force. If a patient is triaged as expectant, they are not prioritized for rapid evacuation, allowing those resources to be shifted to other, salvageable patients. Military neurosurgeons are viewed as assets, deployed where most beneficial.[20] Depending on the theater of operations, neurosurgical support may be located at a variety of locations or echelons.

A military neurosurgeon may be located in an austere field hospital. Alternatively, he or she may be in a more sophisticated environment further along the evacuation chain. In urban conflict this may be an urban hospital. Head injuries will need to be triaged and initially managed by medics, general surgeons, or general medical officers at more forward locations. Medical evacuation for these patients, either by ground or air, can be delayed as a result of equipment challenges, the terrain, the weather, or the tactical situation. Proactive training and neurosurgical exposure to farforward providers and utilization of telemedicine for neurosurgical consultation can greatly facilitate the care of these patients.

In either a civilian or combat environment, patients with a PHI often experience a period of apnea and hypotension. Early intubation and appropriate fluid resuscitation may reduce the secondary complications from these events.[18,19] A challenge to early intubation in the field can be cervical immobilization. Kennedy and colleagues[21] reviewed the incidence of spine injury in patients with isolated gunshot wounds (GSWs) to the head. They found no spine injuries in 105 patients, suggesting that immobilization may not be necessary, facilitating intubation (see also Chaps. 16 and 25).

As in any trauma, Advanced Trauma Life Support/Battlefield Advanced Trauma Life Support (ATLS/BATLS) guidelines are followed, with a focus on preventing hypoxia and hypotension. Both of these events significantly worsen the outcome of patients with head injury. Once IV access is obtained, laboratory evaluation to include electrolytes, complete blood count (CBC), prothrombin time/partial thromboplastin time (PT/PTT), type and screen/cross, urinalysis, and toxicology panel should be sent. A brief history from medics, family members, or paramedics is taken to include the mechanism of injury, neurological examination at the scene, periods of hypoxia or hypotension, and known past medical history or allergies. During the primary and secondary survey, the patient is inspected thoroughly for entry and exit wounds, which should also include the oral cavity. A temporary clean, bulky dressing is applied to the wounds.

A brief neurological exam is performed, remembering that the patient should be fully resuscitated before determining a prognosis. The patient's Glascow Coma Scale (GCS) score, the presence of hypotension or hypoxia, and any use of pharmacological agents should be noted.[22] If the patient has a GCS score of less than 8 or cannot otherwise protect their airway, intubation for adequate airway protection, oxygenation, and ventilation should be considered. Brainstem reflexes and pupillary exam, to include size, symmetry, and reactivity, are noted. Evaluation for CSF leak is performed at this point, including inspection of the tympanic membranes and nares. Antiepileptic agents and broad-spectrum antibiotics are administered.

## 24.5
## Neuroimaging

Plain radiographic studies of the skull can provide a quick impression on the nature of the injury and evaluate for the presence of intracranial fragments and air, especially in circumstances where a CT scan is unavailable. The true trajectory of the fragment may be misleading in the presence of ricochet or careening fragments (Figs. 24.4 and 24.5).[23] If rapid access to a CT scanner is possible, plain films are not required. Noncontrast CT with bone windows allow for precise localization of bone and projectile fragments, identification of the trajectory, and characterization of brain injury (Fig. 24.5). The presence of mass effect and classification of hematomas, either epidural, subdural, parechymal, or intraventricular, can be performed.[23]

Angiography is recommended when there is a high suspicion for vascular injury. From Aarabi's experience in the Iran–Iraq war, there was a four to ten time increased risk of traumatic aneurysm development in patients with facio-orbito or pterional entry, intracranial hematoma, or projectile trajectories that cross dural compartments.[24] Haddad and colleagues documented 15 cases of traumatic aneurysms from the Lebanese conflict: 14 from fragmentation injuries and one from a bullet. From their experience, they recommended an

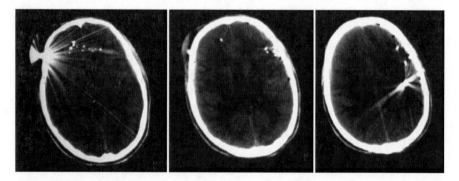

**Fig. 24.4** CT of GSW from close range demonstrating ricochet of fragment posteriorly off contralateral skull. Plain film correlation alone with right frontotemporal entrance wound would lead to an incorrect assumption of true wound tract

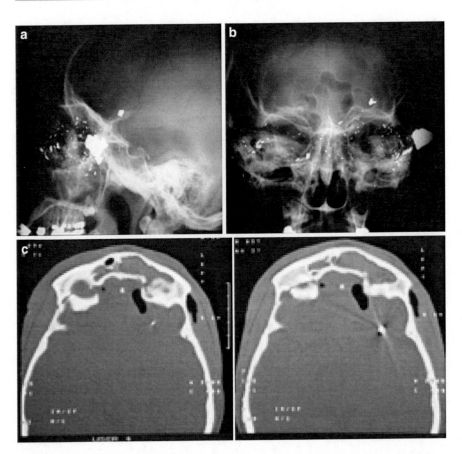

**Fig. 24.5** Lat (**a**) and AP (**b**) skull X-rays of GSW provides some information on retained fragments, presumed tract of injury, and involved structures. (**c**) CT scan gives much better anatomic delineation injury

angiogram for patients with retained fragments, no associated exit wound, and an intracranial hematoma in the distal portion of the trajectory.[25] Other high-risk injuries include a projectile trajectory through or near the Sylvian fissure, supraclinoid carotid artery, basilar cisterns, or major venous sinuses. After stabilization, any PHI patient who develops a new or unexplained subarachnoid hemorrhage or delayed hematoma should also undergo angiography (Fig. 24.6).[23,26]

Magnetic resonance imaging (MRI) currently is not recommended in the acute management of PHI.[23] Retained ferromagnetic fragments produce artifact, distortion, and also can rotate from the magnetic torque.[27-29]

Magnetic resonance imaging may be beneficial in certain cases where the projectile is not retained or is known to contain no metallic elements.

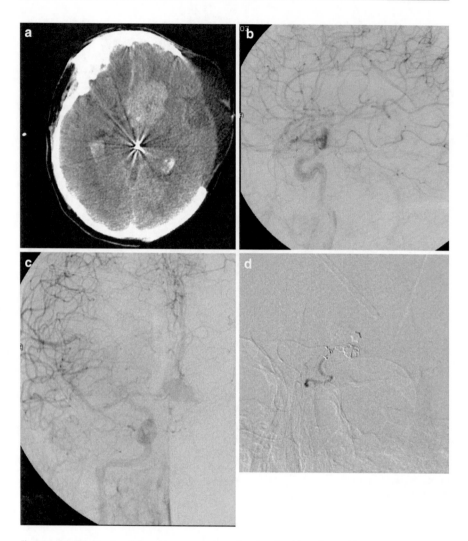

**Fig. 24.6** (**a**) CT showing delayed hematoma in patient involved in a shrapnel injury to base of skull and orbit. (**b**) Lateral and (**c**) AP angiogram revealing pseudoaneurysm of anterior cerebral artery. (**d**) Psuedoaneurysm was treated by endovascular coiling. The patient's initial angiogram after injury was negative

## 24.6
## Preoperative Treatment

Increased intracranial pressure (ICP) is common after PHI.[30–33] The exact pathophysiology behind this elevation is not completely understood. The available data suggests that maintenance of an ICP less than 20 mmHg has a more favorable prognosis than those with uncontrolled intracranial hypertension.[34] Increased intracranial pressure monitoring should be initiated when the clinician is unable to assess a patient's neurological exam, commonly at a GCS score of less than or equal to 8. There are various means to monitor ICP, the most common being intraventricular catheters and intraparenchymal monitors. Intraventricular catheters offer the therapeutic advantage of CSF drainage for treatment of elevated ICP.

Even if ICP monitoring has not been initiated, treatment should be started if the patient demonstrates clinical evidence of herniation or progressive neurological decline. General treatment measures include elevation of the head of bed to 30–45°, keeping the head midline to avoid venous outflow constriction, light sedation, and avoiding hypotension, hypoxemia, or hypercarbia.[35] Cerebral perfusion pressure (CPP) should be kept >60 mmHg.36 Elevated ICP affects the CPP through the relationship: CPP = MAP − ICP. More aggressive treatment measures include increased sedation, CSF drainage, and administration of osmotic agents such as mannitol (0.25–1.00 g/kg).[35]

Hyperventilation reduces ICP through cerebral vasoconstriction, and therefore carries the risk of hypoperfusion from decreased cerebral blood flow. Because of this risk, hyperventilation should be employed sparingly, and only for brief periods while other treatment modalities are instituted.

Projectiles can impart various forces on the cerebral vasculature resulting in arterial wall transection. Depending on the location, the patient may develop a subarachnoid hemorrhage, an intracerebral hematoma, and/or intraventricular hematoma (Fig. 24.7). Subarachnoid hemorrhage is seen in 31 – 78% of PHI cases on CT scan.[36] Both Aldrich and colleagues and Levy and colleagues have shown that the presence of subarachnoid hemorrhage correlates significantly with patient mortality.[37,38]

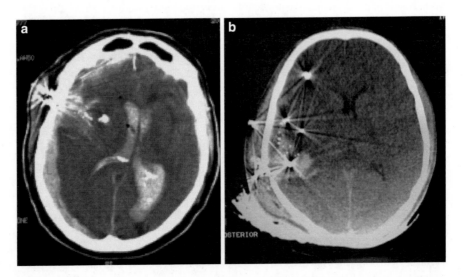

**Fig. 24.7** (**a**) CT of GSW revealing small intraparenchymal hematoma, intraventricular hemorrhage, and a large subdural hematoma with marked mass effect. (**b**) CT of shrapnel wound with small intraparenchymal hematoma

Ten percent of combat-related PHIs are associated with dural sinus involvement.[39] This can lead to massive intraoperative hemorrhage. When the trajectory of the projectile raises the potential of dural sinus injury, preoperative planning should include appropriate hemodynamic support, including blood products and air embolism monitoring, availability of proper equipment, and personnel familiar with surgical techniques for managing venous sinus injury.

Traumatically induced pseudoaneurysms or traumatic intracranial aneurysms (TICA) may occur, with 0.4 – 0.7% of all intracranial aneurysms caused by trauma, 20% of these from PHI.[24,36] The incidence of TICAs is reported between 3% and 33.3% in PHI patients.[24,26,40,41] Angiography is the standard in detection of vascular injuries, but a single angiogram does not rule out the possibility of a TICA.[24,26,40] Since TICAs are not usually true aneurysms, clipping may not be effective. Endovascular techniques or trapping of the lesion are alternative treatment options.

Seizures are common after PHI. They typically are divided into early and late; early defined loosely in the literature as within the first 7 days. Between 30 and 50% of PHI patients develop seizures. Four to 10% of these are early seizures while 80% occur within the first 2 years.[42,43] Data from the VHIS indicated that after 15 years of follow up, nearly 50% of PHI patients with epilepsy stopped having seizures.[43] If PHI patients do not have seizures within the first 3 years, 95% will remain seizure free.[44] Few studies exist that examine only PHI patients and the use of prophylactic antiepileptic drugs. The current guidelines extrapolated from those patients with nonpenetrating traumatic brain injury recommend antiepileptic drugs during the first week to prevent early posttraumatic seizures. No data supports the use of these medications prophylatically beyond the first 7 days in the PHI population to prevent late posttraumatic seizures.[45]

Penetrating head injury wounds are considered contaminated, both superficially and deep. Negative pressure from the projectile's cavitary effect can draw superficial contaminant and debris deep into the wound. The primary projectile, either bullet or fragment, that remains intracranial is not sterile; insufficient heat is generated from the firing mechanism and high velocity for adequate sterilization.[46,47] Broad-spectrum antibiotics are initiated as soon as possible. In civilian PHI, coverage for Staphylococcus and Streptococcus should be of primary concern. With military combat injuries, coverage should also include Acinetobacter, and may be further broadened depending on the area of operations.[48,49]

## 24.7
## Surgical Management

The foundation for surgical management of PHI is found in the work performed by Cushing during WWI: craniectomy, thorough debridement of devitalized scalp, bone, brain, metal and bony fragments, and meticulous closure. This approach remained relatively unchanged through Vietnam. Data from the VHIS and modern military conflicts do not support vigorous removal of all bone and metallic fragments or repeat craniotomies solely for removal of additional fragments. Debridement should be confined to nonviable brain, with removal of readily accessible fragments of bone and metal.[50]

Taha and colleagues reported on a subset of PHI patients that were treated with simple wound closure and a 3-day course of IV antibiotics.[51] Patients met the following criteria: initial GCS score greater than 10, presented within 6 h of injury, entry wound less than 2 cm, no exit wound, trajectory not through the proximal Sylvain fissure, and no significant intracranial hematoma. These criteria attempted to eliminate patients whose injury would produce a significant amount of devitalized tissue. Out of 32 patients, they reported no deaths and one brain abscess that ultimately was treated without complication. Local wound care and closure is a treatment option recognized by the *Guidelines of Penetrating Brain Injury* for similarly selected patients.

The early identification and evacuation of hematomas is important in effecting the outcome of PBI. Some authors have stated that the only indication for surgery, outside of wound care, is the reduction of mass effect, and thus intracranial pressure, from a hematoma.[33,52] The rapid evacuation of hematomas creating significant mass effect is the standard practice. If a hematoma is not removed in a salvageable patient, ICP monitoring should be considered to confirm the decision and to guide further therapy.

All PHI patients should be evaluated vigorously and monitored continuously for the presence of a CSF leak. In a report based on the VHIS, only 50% of CSF leaks were located at the wound site. The remaining were assumed to be caused by injury from the projectile's concussive effect.[32] Mortality for these patients was 22.8% versus 5.1% for those without a CSF leak. The presence of a CSF leak is the variable most highly correlated with intracranial infection in PHI patients. In the VHIS, 44% of the fistulas closed spontaneously.[53] However, if the leak is persistent or delayed in onset, treatment with either CSF diversion or direct surgical repair should be instituted. During any primary surgical treatment of PHI a meticulous, watertight closure of the dura, including the use of temporalis fascia, fascia lata, or graft material, is essential.

Air sinus injuries present an increased risk for CSF leak, especially with an orbital-facial wound. Analysis of a 2-year period during the Korean War revealed a 15% incidence of air sinus injury with combat PHI[54] Delay.

In repair of this injury increases the risk of infection.[7,8,10,54] Management may include craniotomy and anterior fossa reconstruction, exoneration of the frontal sinus, and watertight dural closure. For temporal bone injuries, a mastoidectomy or middle ear exploration with Eustachian tube packing may be required.

## 24.8
## Postoperative Care

Postoperatively, the patient is monitored in an intensive-care setting. As mentioned, ICP is monitored and treated for a goal ICP of less than 20 and CPP of greater than 60.[55] Any persistent, unexplained elevation in ICP or deterioration in neurologic status warrants an emergent CT scan of the head to identify a new mass lesion, most typically a delayed hematoma. A new hemorrhage after surgery should raise the suspicion of an underlying vascular injury or coagulopathy. In certain cases, typically young patients with nondominant hemisphere lesions, a decompressive craniectomy, and duroplasty may be considered in refractory increased intracranial pressure.

The development of hydrocephalus is another potential complication. In a patient with a ventriculostomy, the inability to wean over 7–14 days with persistent high CSF outflow at normal pressure is a good indication the patient will need CSF diversion. Hydrocephalus also may develop in a delayed fashion with a slowly deteriorating neurological exam. If the CT reveals ventriculomegaly, including an enlarged fourth ventricle with no focal mass effect, a lumbar puncture may be performed to record an opening pressure. The final timing for definitive CSF diversion is determined by the presence of other injuries, nutritional status, and infectious complications.

The presence of fever, elevated white cell count, and meningeal signs are concerns for postoperative meningitis. If a ventriculostomy is in place, CSF may be sent for laboratory inquiry. In addition to evaluating the ICP monitoring system, a thorough examination for a CSF fistula should be performed. Not all CSF leaks are present on admission. In review of the VHIS, 72% of CSF leaks appear within the first 2 weeks of injury.[53]

In the initial evaluation and postoperative period, a coagulation panel should be evaluated, as PHI is a known etiology for coagulopathy. The brain parenchyma contains thromboplastin that can activate the extrinsic coagulation cascade. If high levels are released, the patient may develop a disseminated intravascular coagulopathy (DIC). Because the degree of the coagulopathy is related to the amount of thromboplastin released from injured tissue, the presence of DIC represents a large area of parenchymal injury and portends a worse prognosis.[19,56]

As discussed above, the patient should remain on antiepileptic medication for 7 days post injury for the prevention of early seizures. Antibiotics generally are used for a 7–14 day course for isolated PHI. A longer duration may be required based on systemic infection or other complicating factors.

## 24.9
## Prognosis

In comparing outcomes with PHI patients and those with nonpenetrating traumatic brain injuries, PHI patients fare worse. They have an overall mortality of 88%, compared to 32.5% in nonpenetrating traumatic brain injury.[37,57] Typically, death occurs soon after the injury, with 70% occurring within the first 24 h.[57] An accurate assessment of prognosis for each patient is essential to determine the appropriateness of treatment, especially in a military or other resource-constrained environment.

The *Guidelines to Penetrating Brain Injuries* evaluated the literature on five prognostic variables: age, epidemiology, systemic measures, neurological measures, and neuroimaging measures. An understanding of these variables and their outcome can help provide direction in the treatment of the patient and counseling family members on what can be expected.

In general, the older a patient is the higher mortality they typically have. In the limited studies that evaluated age and prognosis, age greater than 50 years was associated with increased mortality. However, a majority of PHI patients are in their second to third decade.[57]

In the civilian population, gunshot wounds are the most common type of PHI, with a majority of these being suicide attempts. Suicide PHIs are associated with a higher mortality.[57] The question has been raised whether suicide outcomes are based on the injury pattern or the degree of resuscitation based on the belief of a worse outcome.[58] This pattern is different in military PHI, where fragmentation injuries instead of gunshot wounds, are found in those patients who survive transport to higher echelons of care. The high velocity associated with military bullet wounds typically causes a devastating intracranial wound. One series reported a mortality with this wound to be 82% higher than with fragmentation wounds.[14]

Given the velocity, and hence the amount of energy imparted by a projectile to achieve a perforating wound, it is not surprising that these injuries are associated with the highest mortality. While no statistically significant data exists, penetrating wounds tend to have a higher mortality than tangential.[57] Surprisingly, there does not tend to be a correlation between outcome and caliber of weapon. This is likely because the energy imparted to the tissue also is related to the velocity, which can be quite variable.[57]

From the patient's presentation and neurological status, several poor prognostic indicators can be determined. Systemic insults after a PHI can worsen the patient's outcome. Periods of hypotension, respiratory distress, and the presence of a coagulopathy all are associated with increased mortality.[57] From a neurologic perspective, the patient's GCS is one of the strongest predictors of mortality and outcome.[57] In civilian settings, most patients present with a GCS of 3 – 5. These patients have the highest rate of mortality and poor outcome. In military series, more patients present with GCS of 13 – 15, and thus have a better outcome. This reflects more fragment injuries, a more rigid field triage system, and a slower evacuation system. An abnormal pupillary exam is common after PHI and can result from orbital trauma, medications, cerebral herniation, or brainstem injury. Patient who present with unequal or fixed and dilated pupils have an increased mortality.[57] There is little data that exists on the prognostic value of ICP in PHI. What is available suggests that elevated ICP within the first 72 h predicts higher mortality.[57]

As previously discussed, a CT scan is the diagnostic modality of choice. Three prognostic indicators can be determined from the patient's initial scan: projectile track, evidence of increased ICP, and the presence of hemorrhage or mass lesion. Projectile trajectories associated with increased mortality include bihemispheric lesions, multilobar lesions, and those that involve the ventricular system. One exception may be a bifrontal injury. Basilar cistern effacement on CT, indicative of elevated ICP, is associated with increased mortality. Midline shift alone, however, is not. The presence of large contusions and/or subarachnoid hemorrhage is associated with increased mortality. A stronger correlation, however, exists between increased mortality and the presence of intraventricular hemorrhage.[57]

Given these prognostic indicators, the provider must decide on who would benefit from surgery and aggressive management. Grahm and colleagues reported on 100 consecutive cases of gunshot wounds to the head in an attempt to answer this question.[18] No patient with a postresuscitation GCS of 3 – 5 and only 20% of those with GCS of 6 – 8 had a satisfactory outcome, defined as either good or moderately impaired on the Glasgow Outcome Scale. From their experience, they recommend that all patients with gunshot wounds to the head be resuscitated aggressively and transferred to a trauma center. Patients with a large, extraaxial hematoma, despite their GCS, should undergo surgical therapy. In those patients without a hematoma and a GCS of 3 – 5, no further treatment should be offered. In patients with a GCS score of 6 – 8 and transventricular or dominant hemisphere multilobar injuries in the absence of an extraaxial hematoma, further treatment should not be offered. A patient with a GCS of 6 – 8 without these findings on CT and all those with GCS of 9 – 15 should be offered aggressive therapy, as this is the population with the best chance at a satisfactory outcome.[18]

The management of the patient with ballistic trauma to the head requires aggressive resuscitation and accurate triage based on clinical and CT findings. When surgical intervention is required, strict attention must be paid to the principles of watertight dural closure and wound coverage after an adequate debridement of devitalized tissue and easily accessible fragments is completed. Aggressive intensive care unit management includes avoidance of hypotension, hypoxia, control of ICP and CPP, use of antibiotics and anticonvulsants, and vigilant monitoring for CSF fistulas and pseudoaneurysms. Unfortunately, this current era of terrorist threats mandates that all physicians should have a basic understanding ballistic trauma to the head.

## References

1. Berman JM, Butterworth JF, Prough DS. Neurological injuries. In: Zajtchuk R, Bellamy RF, eds. *Textbook of Military Medicine*, vol. 1. Washington: Office of the Surgeon General; 1995:375-424.
2. Shaffrey ME, Polin RS, Phillips CD, Germanson T, Shaffrey CI, Jane JA. Classification of civilian craniocerebral gunshot wounds: A multivariate analysis predictive of mortality. *J Neurotrauma*. 1992;9(Suppl 1):S279-S285.
3. Cooper P. Gunshot wounds of the brain. In: Cooper P, ed. *Head Injury*. 2nd ed. Baltimore, MD: Williams and Wilkins; 1987:313-326.
4. Sosin D, Sacks J, Smith S. Head injury associated deaths in the United States from 1979–1986. *JAMA*. 1989;262L:2251-2255.
5. West CGH. A short history of the management of penetrating missile injuries of the head. *Surg Neurol*. 1981;16:145-149.
6. Schmidek S. Operative neurosurgical techniques. Section 2, Chapter 7: Penetrating Brain Injuries.. Orlando, FL. Grune & Stratton 1988.
7. Cushing H. Notes on penetrating wounds of the brain. *Brit Med J*. 1918;221–226
8. Cushing H. A study of a series of wounds involving the brain and its enveloping structures. *Br J Surg*. 1918;5:558-684.
9. Tilney NL. The marrow of tragedy. *Surg Gynecol Obstet*. 1983;157:380-388.
10. Matson DD. *The Treatment of Acute Craniocerebral Injuries Due to Missiles*. Springfield, IL: Charles C Thomas; 1948.
11. War Surgery Supplement. *Br J Surg*. 1947;34(137).
12. Lewin W, Gibson MR. Missile head wounds in the Korean campaign: A survey of British casualties. *Br J Surg*. 1956;43:628-632.
13. Carey ME, Young HF, Mathis JL. The neurosurgical treatment of craniocerebra missile wounds in Vietnam. *Surg Gynecol Obstet*. 1972;135:386-390.
14. Brandvold B, Levi L, Feinsod M, George E. Penetrating craniocerebral injuries in the Israeli involvement in the Lebanese conflict, 1982–1985. *J Neurosurg*. 1990;72:15-21.
15. Ordog GJ. Wound ballistics: Theory and practice. *Ann Emerg Med*. 1984;13(12): 1113-1122.

16. Barach E, Tomlanovich M, Nowak R. Ballistics: A pathophysiologic examination of the wounding mechanisms of firearm: part 1. *J Trauma.* 1986;26(3):225-235.
17. Sykes LN, Champion HR, Fouty WJ. Dum-dums, hollow-points, and devastors: Techniques designed to increase wounding potential of bullets. *J Trauma.* 1988;28(5):618-623.
18. Grahm T, Williams F Jr, Harrington T, Spetzler R. Civilian gunshot wounds to the head: A prospective study. *Neurosurgery.* 1990;27:696-700.
19. Kauffman HH, Makela ME, Lee KF, Haid RW Jr, Gildenberg PL. Gunshot wounds to the head: A perspective. *Neurosurgery.* 1986;18:689-695.
20. Knightly JJ, Pullliam MW. Military head injuries. In: Narayan RK, Willberger JE, Povlishock JT, eds. *Neurotrauma.* New York: McGraw-Hill; 1996:891-902.
21. Kennedy FR, Gonzalez P, Beitler A, Sterling-Scott R, Fleming AW. Incidence of cervical spine injury in patients with gunshot wounds to the head. *South Med J.* 1994;87:621-623.
22. Trask T, Narayan RK. Civilian penetrating head injury. In: Narayan RK, Wilberger JE, Povlishock JT, eds. *Neurotrauma.* New York: McGraw-Hill; 1996:869-889.
23. Neuroimaging in the management of penetrating brain injury. *J Trauma.* 2001;51:S7-S11.
24. Aarabi B. Management of traumatic aneurysms caused by high-velocity missile head wounds. *Neurosurg Clin North Am.* 1995;6:775-797.
25. Haddad FS, Haddad GF, Taha J. Traumatic intracranial aneurysms caused by missiles: Their presentation and management. *Neurosurgery.* 1991;28:1-7.
26. Amirjamshidi A, Rahmat H, Abbassioun K. Traumatic aneurysms and arteriovenous fistulas of intracranial vessels associated with penetrating head injuries occuring during war: Principles and pitfalls in diagnosis and management. *J Neurosurg.* 1996;84:769-780.
27. Oliver C, Kabala J. Air gun pellet injury: The safety of MR imaging. *Clin Radiol.* 1997;52:299-300.
28. Smith AS, Hurst GC, Durek JL, Diaz PJ. MR of ballistic materials: Imaging artifacts and potential hazards. *Am J Neruoradiol.* 1991;12:567-572.
29. Teitelbaum GP, Yee CA, Van Horn DD, Kim HS, Colletti PM. Metallic ballistic fragments: MR imaging safety and artifacts. *Radiology.* 1990;175:855-859.
30. Crockard HA. Early intracranial pressure studies in gunshot wounds of the brain. *J Trauma.* 1975;15:339-347.
31. Lillard PL. Five year experience with penetrating craniocerebral gunshot wounds. *Surg Neurol.* 1978;9:79-83.
32. Nagib MG, Rockswold GL, Sherman RS, Lagaard MW. Civilian gunshot wounds to the brain: Prognosis and management. *Neurosurgery.* 1986;18:533-537.
33. Sarnaik AP, Kopec J, Moylan P, Alvarez D, Canady A. Role of aggressive intracranial pressure in management of pediatric craniocerebral gunshot wounds with unfavorable features. *J Trauma.* 1989;29:1424-1437.
34. Intracranial pressure monitoring in the management of penetrating brain injury. *J Trauma.* 2001;51:S12-S15.
35. Bullock R, Chesnut RM, Clifton G, et al. Guidelines for the management of severe head injury. *Eur J Ernerg Med.* 1996;3:109-127.
36. Vascular complications of penetrating brain injury. *J Trauma.* 2001;51:S26-S28.
37. Aldrich EF, Eisnberg HM, Saydjari C, et al. Predictors of mortality in severely head-injured patients with civilian gunshot wound: A report from the NIH Traumatic Coma Data Bank. *Surg Neurol.* 1992;38:418-423.
38. Levy ML, Rezai A, Masri LS, et al. The significance of subarachnoid hemorrhage after penetrating craniocerebral injury: Correlations with angiography and outcome in civilian population. *Neurosurgery.* 1993;32:532-540.
39. Kapp JP, Gielchinsky I. Management of combat wounds of the dural venous sinuses. *Surgery.* 1972;71:913-917.
40. Aarabi B. Traumatic aneurysms of brain due to high velocity missile head wounds. *Neurosurgery.* 1988;22:1056-1063.

41. Jinkins JR, Dadsetan MR, Sener RN, Desai S, Williams RG. Value of acutephase angiography in the detection of vascular injuries caused by gunshot wounds to the head: Analysis of 12 cases. *AJR Am J Roentgenol*. 1992;159:365-368.
42. Caverness WF, Meirowsky AM, Rish BL, et al. The nature of posttraumatic epilepsy. *J Neurosurg*. 1979;50:545-553.
43. Salazar AM, Jabbari B, Vance SC, Grafman J, Amin D, Dillon JD. Epilepsy after penetrating head injury, I: Clinical correlates—a report of the Vietnam Head Injury Study. *Neurology*. 1985;35:1406-1414.
44. Weiss GH, Salazar AM, Vance SC, Grafman JH, Jabbian B. Predicting posttraumatic epilepsy in penetrating head injury patients. *Arch Neurol*. 1986;43:771-773.
45. Antiseizure prophylaxis for penetrating brain injury. *J Trauma*. 2001;51:241-243.
46. Thoreby FP, Darlow HM. The mechanism of primary infection of bullet wounds. *Br J Surg*. 1967;54:359.
47. Wolf AW. Autosterilization in low-velocity bullets. *J Trauma*. 1978;18:63.
48. Taha JM, Saba MI, Brown JA. Missile injuries to the brain treated by simple wound closure: Results of a protocol during the Lebanese conflict. *Neurosurgery*. 1991;29:380-383.
49. Taha JM, Haddad FS, Brown JA. Intracranial infection after missile injuries to the brain: Report of 30 cases from the Lebanon conflict. *Neurosurgery*. 1991;29:864-868.
50. Surgical management of penetrating brain injury. *J Trauma*. 2001;51:S16-S25.
51. Suddaby L, Weir B, Forsyth C. The management of.22 caliber gunshot wounds of the brain: A review of 49 cases. *Can J Neurol Sci*. 1987;14:268-272.
52. Arendall REH, Meirowsky AM. Air sinus wounds: an analysis of 163 consecutive cases incurred in the Korean War, 1950–1952. *Neurosurgery*. 1983;13:377-380.
53. Kearney TJ, Bentt L, Grode M, Lee S, Hiatt JR, Shabot MM. Coagulopathy and catecholamines in severe head injury. *J Trauma*. 1992;32:608-612.
54. Part 2: Prognosis in penetrating brain injury [review]. *J Trauma*. 2001;51(suppl 2):S44-S86.
55. BTF Website https://www.braintrauma.org/coma-guidelines.
56. Marshall LF, Maas AI, Marshall SB, Bricolo A, et al. A mutlicenter trial on the efficacy of using tirilazad mesylatein cases of head injury. *J Neurosurg*. 1998;89:519-525.
57. Kaufman HH, Schwab K, Salazar AM. A national survery of neurosurgical care for penetrating head injury. *Surg Neurol*. 1991:36(5):370-377.
58. Shoung HM, Sichez JP, Pertuiset B. The early prognosis of craniocerebral gunshot wounds in civilian practice as an aid to the choice of treatment. *Acta Neurochir (Wien)*. 1985;74:27-30.

# Spinal Injury

# 25

Neil Buxton

## 25.1
## Introduction

A spinal cord injury can be devastating to the victim. The management of spinal cord injury secondary to gunshot wounds or other ballistic injuries is still controversial. In the United States of America, a gunshot wound is the second most common cause of spinal cord injury. In one civilian series, up to 25% of all spinal cord injuries were secondary to gunshot wounds. This is a condition affecting mainly young people under 30 years of age, more than 90% of whom are males. Over a third will be under the influence of alcohol or drugs, and nearly half will be shot from behind. Over half of such injuries will present with complete paraplegia. By the nature of the inflicting injury, more than one quarter will have associated injuries. The majority of the gunshot wounds affect the thoracic spine, with the lumbar spine being second most common.

## 25.2
## History

In World War I, only patients with incomplete injuries survived. Overall mortality rate was 71.8%, with urinary sepsis being the main cause of death. At this time there was also a 62.2% operative mortality rate. Complete injuries were only treated with wound debridement. Laminectomy was reserved for incomplete injuries that were experiencing further neurological deterioration.

In World War II, surgery was offered to all, but the mortality rate had been reduced to 11.4%. In the Korean War, operative mortality was only 1%. Improved casualty evacuation times seen in the Vietnam War did nothing to further improve neurological recovery.

Civilian series have been even less encouraging. Stabbings have been found no less devastating than gunshot wounds to the spine.

N. Buxton
Neurosurgery Department, Walton Centre Liverpool, Liverpool, UK
e-mail: neilbuxton@doctors.org.uk

A.J. Brooks et al. (eds.), *Ryan's Ballistic Trauma*,
DOI: 10.1007/978-1-84882-124-8_25, © Springer-Verlag London Limited 2011

## 25.3
## Pathophysiology

A complete spinal cord injury is one whereby there is no function below the level of the injury. Some spinal cord reflexes may return. A physiologically complete injury does not require complete transection of the spinal cord.

With modern high-velocity weapons, it is not necessary to hit the spinal cord directly to cause a spinal cord injury; hitting the bony components of the spine can cause microscopically detectable spinal cord injury up to 15 cm from the level of the primary injury. There is usually intramedullary hemorrhage and more rarely extradural or subdural hemorrhage, even with a direct cord injury.

## 25.4
## Initial Management and Assessment

Each victim of such an injury should undergo a full normal resuscitation protocol with appropriate management of life-threatening injuries along Advanced Trauma Life Support/ Battlefield Advanced Trauma Life Support (ATLS/BATLS) guidelines. In such an injury, it is important to remember that, until proven otherwise, hypotension is due to blood loss and not spinal cord shock.

Having resuscitated the patient, stabilized them, and treated the other life-threatening injuries, the patient is then ready to be assessed by the neurosurgeon, and, in times of conflict, this may take many hours to days to achieve. However, it generally is agreed that early assessment of the neurological status is deemed vital and ideally should be carried out within 24 h of the injury, always after the resuscitation. This is important because the presenting neurological and autonomic status have considerable implications for the prognosis. Therefore, the first medical attendant who sees the casualty after resuscitation needs to fully examine them from a neurological point of view, and, of course, this should be recorded with care. This is of paramount importance for prognostication, as 90% of presenting neurological deficits are permanent.

The neurological examination needs to record the sensory status, strength of muscle groups, tone in the limbs, reflexes, and sphincter status.

Simple measures such as nasogastric tube, bladder catheterization, and nursing management to prevent decubitus ulcers and deep venous thrombosis are vital for the overall care of such an injured patient. For the medical attendant, the neurological examination should be repeated periodically in order to document recovery and/or deterioration.

## 25.5
## Spinal Shock

This results in flaccid paralysis distal to the injury. The reflexes and tone return to become hyperactive by 6–12 weeks. The more rapid the return of the reflexes, the poorer the prognosis for neurological recovery in patients with complete injuries.

Neurogenic shock with bradycardia, hypotension, and hypothermia is due to autonomic paralysis and is managed with fluid replacement and active warming. Atropine may even be required, especially if the pulse rate drops below 40 beats/min.

## 25.6
## Investigations

### 25.6.1
### Plain X-Ray

This will demonstrate the bony anatomy and the presence and position of any retained foreign bodies.

### 25.6.2
### Computed Tomography (CT)

Computed tomography provides good bony detail, but in the presence of metal fragments will have significant artifact. Computed tomography is excellent for three-dimensional reconstruction of the bony anatomy, but in the face of a fragment injury, the radiological artifact may be too great to make the pictures meaningful.

### 25.6.3
### Magnetic Resonance Imaging (MRI)

Magnetic resonance imaging is extremely useful for the soft tissues, in particular spinal cord anatomy. This is a particularly important modality, as early realization that complete transection of the cord has occurred is extremely useful for prognostication. The problem with MRI scanning is that there is a theoretical risk of the magnetic field causing foreign body movement, as well as artifact, even though there are records of the MRI being used safely in patients with fragmentation injuries. Magnetic resonance imaging is essential to investigate delayed deterioration.

### 25.6.4
### Myelography

This may be necessary where metal fragments and metal artifact prevent the use of CT or MRI.

## 25.7
## Instability

Battlefield gunshot wounds to the neck causing neurological deficit have a high fatality rate. In those surviving, it generally is accepted that the neck injury is not unstable.

It is important that the mechanism of injury be elicited during the history as, especially during the transition to war phase, there are many motor-vehicle accidents and those injured in them would be expected to have potentially unstable spinal injuries. It is essential to treat any person so injured who has reduced or impaired levels of consciousness due to intoxication or the injury as having a spinal injury until positively proven otherwise. In such an instance, where practical, full ATLS-type management should be initiated. In a mass casualty situation, or where the tactical situation is unsafe, the expediency of life-saving treatment may necessitate reduced diligence with respect to spinal immobilization.

It is important to remember that some penetrating injuries, if treated as unstable, may actually be to the detriment of the casualty as, for example, putting on a cervical collar for a penetrating neck injury has in some instances been found to mask significant deterioration. Indeed, in these casualties, subsequent investigations have found that the spinal injury was, in fact, not unstable after all. Quite clearly, if an unstable injury is missed, the consequences for the casualty are potentially devastating; this is why the mechanism of injury is important in the history. In fact, in a purely penetrating injury of the neck, it is recommended that a supportive collar not be used at all.

## 25.8
## Operation?

There is considerable controversy regarding whether or not to decompress the spinal cord or theca. The initial neurological status remains the most important factor for overall expected outcomes. Initial military experience from the major wars of the twentieth century suggested that highly aggressive surgical therapy should be the approach; however, in recent years, with increasing civilian experience, a more conservative approach has been adopted. With regard to incomplete spinal cord injuries alone, it has been found that removal of the penetrating fragment, if impinging upon the spinal cord, does improve overall motor function in some reported series. In some published studies where surgery was undertaken in nearly all cases, there have been some instances where the neurological status has actually been made worse by surgery.

For foreign bodies present in or around the cauda equina, many studies have supported the removal of the foreign body, but this can be a technical challenge at operation because the foreign bodies can move. Having the patient positioned slightly head up and using fluoroscopy to aid identification of the foreign body position is recommended.

There is considerable agreement that where there is cerebrospinal fluid leakage, progressive neurological deficit, or spinal instability, surgery should be undertaken, although surgery for instability may be controversial to some authorities. In war, if casualty evacuation is needed, the spinal injury casualty will need to be made stable by surgical fixation so transfer can be made more easily and safely. The removal of the foreign body to prevent later sepsis remains controversial, as many studies have indicated that foreign body retention does not actually increase the risks. In cases were the penetrating fragment traverses the abdominal cavity, and therefore possibly the bowels, prior to entering the spinal canal, the life-threatening injuries are recommended to be dealt with first, followed by thorough wash out from anteriorly with a prolonged high-dose usage of antibiotics. It is hardly surprising that penetration of the colon is associated with the highest risks of infection, although some studies have suggested that transoral is higher still. Retained foreign bodies can cause problems in other areas, in particularly plumbism (lead poisoning), but this is an infrequent complication of lead fragments. It has been recognized that lead fragments in joint spaces or disk spaces should be removed, as toxicity is likely. Of more concern are copper-jacketed projectiles, as these are particularly toxic and it is recommended that, whatever the situation, any copper-jacketed projectile be removed at surgery as soon as possible.

## 25.9
## Role of Antibiotics and Other Drugs

It is recommended that high-dose broad-spectrum antibiotics be administered intravenously for 7–10 days, especially if there is a retained foreign body or if the projectile has traversed a hollow viscous.

Antacids are recommended to minimize the risk of stress ulceration.

Methylprednisolone has been advocated in the management of blunt spinal cord injury, but a number of studies have not found methylprednisolone to be of any clinical benefit in gunshot-wound–induced spinal cord injury. Indeed, in one series, increased rate of complications was found and attributed to the use of steroids. There is currently ongoing controversy regarding the use of steroids, even in the previously advocated blunt spinal cord injury; therefore, at this moment in time, the use of steroids in penetrating spinal cord injury cannot be recommended.

## 25.10
## General Nursing Care/Postoperative Care

The management of a spinally injured patient, whether it be due to penetrating injury or blunt, are virtually identical from the nursing and postoperative management aspects. The casualty needs a nasogastric tube, bladder management, aseptic management of catheters, careful pressure area care, and early physiotherapy and rehabilitation. Careful fluid management and catheter management needs to be maintained with avoidance of urinary tract infections and catheter blockage in the long-term care. With increasing sophistication in the management, these patients are living significant lengths of time and represent a considerable nursing challenge.

Care of such a casualty needs to be addressed at identifying missed injuries, such as peripheral fractures, but with emphasis on ruling out a second spinal injury. Other severe injuries, such as abdominal trauma and head injury, should have been recognized in the primary or secondary survey and dealt with accordingly. A low threshold for investigating for other injuries should be maintained throughout the care of such a patient.

Other important considerations include hypovolemia; ruling out active bleeding may be difficult, but is vital. Once a sinister cause is excluded, then fluid resuscitation to maintain a blood pressure between 80 and 100 mmHg systolic is appropriate. Adequate urine output is the best marker.

Hypothermia due to sympathetic failure causing peripheral vasodilatation should be actively managed.

Bradycardia due to decreased sympathetic drive can be so severe as to lead to asystolic arrest. Atropine may be necessary. Hypoxia and tracheal toilet can be enough to exacerbate the bradycardia to produce arrest.

Autonomic dysreflexia (mass reflex) can occur in over 50% of those with injuries higher than T6. There is an uncontrolled sympathetic reflex to usually only mildly noxious stimuli such as a full bladder or bowel. There is flushing, headache, sweating, anxiety, and hypertension with bradycardia. Removal of the stimulus and elevation of the head of the bed are needed. Failure to resolve the hypertension may require drug therapy such as hydralazine. Untreated, this hypertension can be fatal. Therefore, prevention by nursing diligence is necessary.

Prophylaxis for DVT and PE is essential. Care to prevent chest problems due to reduced chest excursions, poor cough reflex, etc., is important. Chest infections are common. Breathing control is impaired.

There may be ileus, constipation, gastric reflux, and gastric stress ulcers. All need appropriate management and, in the case of bowel motility and ulcer prophylaxis. Nutritional advice and support is required early to minimize the effects of posttraumatic catabolism.

Improved urological care has reduced the long-term death rate. Improved catheter technology and the introduction of intermittent self-catheterization have brought about significant improvements. There should be a low threshold for treating urinary tract infections and periodic renal tract ultrasound to assess bladder capacity and any ureteric reflux.

Pressure area care and prevention of ulcers can make the difference between a relatively normal life and a prolonged hospital stay. The worst cases end up with osteomyelitis and major plastic and reconstructive surgery.

Pain can be a long-term problem. It may be due to spasm, or it can be neurogenic or analogous to phantom limb pain. Multidisciplinary pain team management is recommended.

Delayed deterioration should always prompt urgent investigation for posttraumatic syringomyelia, arachnoid adhesions, etc. Appropriate therapy is indicated to preserve function above the original level of injury. Therefore, any complaint of neurological change no matter how bizarre or minor must be taken seriously, and ideally, periodic complete physical examination of the patient is needed.

Early physiotherapy and transfer to a dedicated spinal injury facility is essential for their optimal rehabilitation. This will include psychosocial, sexual, vocational, educational, and recreational rehabilitation in a multidisciplinary setting.

## 25.11
## Evacuation/Transfer

The patients having such an injury in an austere military environment will need careful and well-managed nursing care in order to facilitate their safe evacuation and transfer. As previously mentioned, they should be transferred to a dedicated spinal unit at the earliest opportunity for appropriate rehabilitation and management. It is reasonable to suggest that in the presence of a spinal fracture that an operative fixation will facilitate the early and easier transfer of such an injured patient, as less emphasis would need to be placed on prevention of further injury in the presence of an unstable spine.

## 25.12
## Summary

The management of penetrating spinal cord injuries due to gunshot wounds or fragment injuries is, in the initial phase, as for any ATLS/BATLS protocol. In the battlefield, the chance of the injury being unstable in survivors due to a penetrating injury is very small. It is important to recognize the mechanism of injury and manage the patient accordingly. For example, a casualty involved in a motor-vehicle accident will be at higher risk of an unstable spinal injury than one who has just been shot by a 5.56-mm round. Surviving casualties who have such penetrating neck injuries are extremely unlikely to have an unstable neck, and therefore the application of a stabilizing collar may in fact be detrimental to their care. As with the majority of spinal cord injuries and spinal injuries in general, other life-threatening injuries always take priority. North Atlantic Treaty Organization (NATO) guidelines are specific regarding the management of spinal injuries; they state that complete injuries do not require surgery, surgery being indicated for progressive neurological deficit and spinal instability. To this recommendation should be added that surgery should be applied in the presence of CSF leaks, delayed infections or foreign body reactions, and/or the presence of copper-jacketed rounds or lead foreign bodies in a joint or disk space. In addition, if there is radicular pain where the foreign body can clearly be demonstrated to be compromising a root on appropriate imaging, then this also should be removed. Decompressive laminectomy and foreign body removal for the sake of it is no longer justified. The use of steroids is not recommended at this time. High-dose antibiotics for at least 7–10 days are indicated.

Overall, the most important factor for a prognosis is the presenting neurological status. In 90% of casualties, the presenting neurological deficit is permanent. However, the mortality from a spinal cord injury alone is low, and with the best long-term care available, life expectancy can be virtually normal and that life can be fruitful and useful to society.

## Further Reading

Tator CH, Benzel EC, eds. *Contemporary Management of Spinal Cord Injury: From Impact to Rehabilitation*. Park Ridge, IL: AANS; 2000.

# Eyes

# 26

Robert A.H. Scott

## 26.1
## Introduction

The eyes occupy 0.1% of the total and 0.27% of the anterior surface of the body; vision is the most important sense which magnifies the significance of an ocular injury. Visual loss is likely to lead to loss of career, major lifestyle changes, and disfigurement. Unlike in peacetime where unilateral injuries are the rule, ocular war injuries are bilateral in 15–25% of cases.[1,2]

The use of body armor issued to soldiers in theaters of war makes explosions more survivable but leave the face and eyes relatively exposed. Before the twentieth century, the eye casualty rate was less than four times its expected percentage based on body surface area alone. This has increased to over 50 times the expected percentage in the late twentieth and early twenty-first centuries. Injured personnel, who once would have died of thoracic and abdominal wounds, now present with non-fatal injuries to their eyes and extremities.

The development of more efficient weapons with higher explosive and fragmentation power has led to a continuous increase in the proportion of eye injuries over the years (Table 26.1). In the nineteenth century wars, less than 2% of the battle casualties had documented eye injuries. Until the Korean War, the documented eye injuries were between 2% and 3%. There has been a large increase in such injuries encountered over the past 40 years to between 5% and 7% in the three Arab-Israeli conflicts, attributed to the predominantly urban and tank warfare experienced.[3,4] Subsequent urbanization of warfare, increased explosive power of weapons combined with relatively poor uptake of ocular protection in relation to protection of the rest of the body contributed to a further increase

R.A.H. Scott
Vitreoretinal Surgery Service, Ophthalmology, Royal Centre for Defence Medicine,
Birmingham Research Park, Birmingham, UK
e-mail: rahscott@btinternet.com

A.J. Brooks et al. (eds.), *Ryan's Ballistic Trauma*,
DOI: 10.1007/978-1-84882-124-8_26, © Springer-Verlag London Limited 2011

**Table 26.1** Incidence of war-related eye injuries from the nineteenth to twenty-first century

| War | Year | Population | % Non-fatal injuries |
| --- | --- | --- | --- |
| Crimean | 1854–56 | British | 0.65 |
| Crimean | 1854–56 | French | 1.75 |
| American Civil | 1861–65 | American | 0.5 |
| Franco- Prussian | 1870–71 | German | 0.86 |
| Franco-Prussian | 1870–71 | French | 0.81 |
| Russo- Turkish | 1877–78 | Russian | 2.5 |
| Sino-Japanese | 1894 | Unknown | 1.2 |
| Russo-Japanese | 1904–05 | Japanese | 2.22 |
| Russo-Japanese | 1904–05 | Russian | 2 |

in the proportion of eye injuries; increasing to 13% in Operation Desert Storm 1991.[5] Prioritization of combat eye protection may have contributed to the reduction of the proportion of eye injuries to 6% in Operations Iraqi Freedom and Enduring Freedom (2001–2005).[6]

The largest study of combat-related eye trauma, 5,320 cases from the Iran-Iraq War, between 1980 and 1988, revealed two large groups of eye injuries where modern diagnostic and treatment modalities could be used to improve the prognosis. These were retained foreign bodies (17%) and posterior segment injuries (59%).[7]

Ocular injuries from terrorist bombings have a similar incidence to those of modern warfare ranging from 3% in the Manchester bomb to 10% in the Okalhoma City and Dharan blasts. The pattern of injury in these incidents are from missile fragments and small fragments of glass, cement, mortar, and other debris associated with the blast that cause minimal damage if they impact on the clothes or skin, but significant morbidity if they hit the eye.[8-10]

Adequate eye protection would reduce the number of eye injuries in warfare, particularly secondary blast injuries. Cotter and La Piana analyzed the data from the Vietnam War and, using a theoretical model, proposed that had the standard current US Army 2 mm thick defense goggle been worn, 52% of eye injuries would have been prevented.[8] Applying this figure to the Vietnam War overall, 5,000 eye injuries from US and allied forces could have been prevented by the use of eye protection.[9]

Eye protection is provided to US and UK service personnel. Its uptake is variable as combatants will often complain that eye protection degrades their vision due to misting, a poor field of view from the frames and it will scratches easily. Enforced use of eye protection in US military convoys in Iraq in 2004 reduced the incidence of eye injuries to 0.5% from a conflict wide incidence of 6%; back to the levels experienced in the Crimean War.[10] (Fig. 26.1).

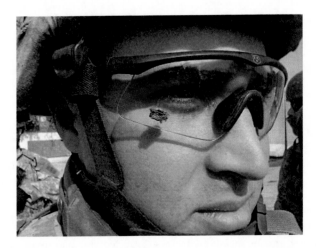

**Fig. 26.1** US infantryman with "Sawfly" combat eye protection with an embedded fragment and an abridged version of his recollection of the incident.[59] "I am an Infantry Platoon Leader, currently deployed to Mosul, Iraq in Support of OIF. Our patrol was struck by a massive IED, launching shrapnel and debris at high velocities toward the vehicle. I was thrown into the hull of the Stryker and later discovered that my eye-pro, the "Sawfly" *yellow* tinted lenses, prevented a shard of shrapnel from contacting my face, saving my eyesight and preventing serious injury. The shrapnel punctured the lens, but did not penetrate. The shrapnel was large enough to dislodge the eyewear from my face and force me into the vehicle. I wore the glasses the rest of the patrol, confident they could still do the job." (Photograph courtesy of Revision Eyewear, London, UK)

## 26.2
## Assessment of the Injured Eye

### 26.2.1
### History

Meticulous note-keeping is essential as eye injuries will often require preparation of legal and insurance reports or police statements. The time and date of the injury as well as the attendance in eye casualty should be recorded. The mechanism of injury should be described in detail including the circumstances of the injury. An accurate list of all injuries to the eye, its adnexae, and other injuries to the body should be made; this is especially important with multitrauma cases. Foreign bodies should be examined and the patient asked about their likely composition and type. Any eye protection or eyewear used at the time of injury should be noted. This information is particularly important for medicolegal reasons.

Previous first-aid treatment given should be detailed. The past ocular history should be recorded, as it may affect ophthalmic management and prognosis. It should be established if the eye was a seeing eye before the injury and any history of amblyopia in either eye.

The general medical history may be important for patient management and should include the tetanus immune status, as with any casualty patient. Known allergies are important as systemic antibiotics are often prescribed.

## 26.2.2
## Examination

Ocular trauma patients are often particularly stressed as they are worried about losing their vision and should be made as comfortable and relaxed as possible. It is important to assess if two eyes are present and if they are grossly intact, this can be difficult to assess with extensive ocular adnexal swelling and an examination under anesthetic may be required. Associated cranial trauma should be considered especially if there are associated facial injuries; or penetrating orbital and ocular trauma.

*Visual assessment* is by measuring the best-corrected visual acuity of each eye separately with a Snellen chart using normal visual correction. The acuity is measured as a fraction of the distance from the chart (6 m) divided by the size of letter a normal observer should see at that distance. The fraction 6/6 represents what a normal person can see at 6 m; a vision of 6/12 is what the patient sees at 6 m and a normal patient sees at 12 m, half the acuity. A reduced chart using smaller letters at a closer distance can be used in the examination room.

Spectacles are often lost or broken in ocular trauma; if the vision is measured while looking through a pin-hole the effects of uncorrected refractive error or mild media opacity are counteracted. If no letters can be read, the ability to count fingers, to see hand movements, and to perceive light are recorded in that order as CF, HM, PL, and NPL (nil perception of light) respectively. If the vision is PL, the ability to project which quadrant the light is shining from is recorded.

Pupil examination is performed; shape, symmetry, the red reflex, and pupil reactions to light stimulation are recorded. A distorted pupil suggests anterior segment trauma, iris plugging of a penetrating injury or prolapse of vitreous or lens into the anterior segment. Transillumination defects of the iris may be due to iris root tears or the passage of an intraocular foreign body. Iris sphincter rupture causes notching of the pupil margin and indicates significant ocular trauma.

The pupillary red reflex is visualized using a direct ophthalmoscope at 50 cm. It is absent if there is opacity of the ocular media such as cataract, vitreous hemorrhage, or total retinal detachment. Afferent pupillary reactions must be tested and recorded using the Marcus Gunn swinging flashlight test. A bright pen torch can be used even when one eye is closed. In an *afferent pupillary defect* there is a decreased direct response caused by decreased visual function in one eye; due to optic nerve or retinal damage. In the *swinging flashlight test* a light is rapidly moved back and forth between the eyes every 2 to 3 s. The afferent pupillary defect becomes obvious when the flashlight is moved from the normal to the affected eye, and the affected pupil *dilates* in response to light. Under normal conditions, the pupil remains constricted when the light is shone at it.

*Facial structures* are assessed for cheek swelling, flattening, or asymmetry from a malar fracture. The horizontal and vertical alignment of the pupils and canthi from the bridge of the nose is measured with a ruler. An increase (telecanthus) indicates a mid-facial fracture. An inferiorly displaced lateral canthus indicates a zygomatic fracture.

Enophthalmos, where the eye is sunken, suggests a blow-out fracture, usually involving the maxillary floor. Proptosis, a bulging eye, suggests an orbital haematoma; if combined with loss of vision and a tense orbit a retrobulbar hemorrhage should be diagnosed. This is an ocular emergency requiring immediate surgical decompression with a lateral canthotomy. The orbital rim is palpated for steps indicating a fracture; or crepitus indicating surgical emphysema from a fracture in an air sinus. Infraorbital hypoaesthesia indicates infraorbital nerve involvement in an orbital floor fracture.

*Eyelid examination* is initially of the lid contours; asymmetry may be from ruptured canthal tendons that attach the ends of the lid to the orbit. A flattened upper lid may indicate a globe rupture. Lid foreign bodies are detected by lid eversion. Here the conjunctiva is anesthetised with Benoxinate Hydrochloride 0.4% drops; the upper lid everted by placing a cotton-wool bud stick over the lid crease; pinching the eyelashes and folding the lid tarsal plate over the stick. If a foreign body is seen on the tarsal surface, it can be wiped off using the cotton wool bud. If a foreign body is suspected in the upper fornix, such as a lost contact lens, a Desmarres retractor is used to double evert the eyelid. If globe rupture is suspected the lid must not be everted in case it puts pressure on the globe and causes extrusion of ocular contents.

Lid wound assessment includes an estimation of the depth to assess if it is partial or full-thickness; any tissue loss that might increase the risk of corneal exposure; if there is any lacrimal cannalicular involvement causing persistent epiphora; wound contamination that would require prophylactic antibiotic cover and the presence of ptosis indicating lid levator muscle damage.

*Extraocular muscle assessment* is initially with the cover/uncover test and alternate cover test performed with the eyes in the primary position (looking straight ahead). The eyes are then tested for diplopia in all 9 positions of gaze while following a pen torch or target and the alternate cover test is performed to check the ocular balance in each position of gaze (Fig. 26.2).

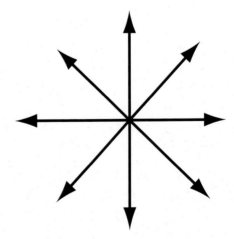

**Fig. 26.2** The nine positions of gaze (includes straight ahead)

*Globe examination is initially* performed using a pen torch to examine the anterior segment, pupil reactions, lids, and adnexae. An estimation of the anterior chamber depth can be made by holding the torch side on to the limbus.

*Direct ophthalmoscopy* is a readily available and portable examination technique. The patient is asked to look straight ahead at a distant point. The same eye is used by the observer to look through the ophthalmoscope as is examined. Positive lenses are dialed to visualize the anterior segment and will detect corneal lacerations, hyphaema, the red reflex, and pupil abnormalities. The lens power is typically reduced to examine the posterior segment. The view is limited to the disk and macula, a more peripheral view is possible if the patient moves their eyes.

*Slit lamp biomicroscopy* is the best examination technique for the anterior segment and allows an excellent view of the posterior segment. Basic proficiency with the technique is recommended, even if just for anterior segment examination. Foreign bodies are easily visualized and removed from the cornea and conjunctiva. Anterior segment inflammation of the can be assessed as inflammatory cells and flare from aqueous protein can be seen in the slit beam.

*Indirect ophthalmoscopy* is used to diagnose retinal tears and detachments using a head mounted light and a hand-held lens, if combined with scleral indentation, a view of the retina up to the ora can be achieved. This technique is difficult to master and is usually performed by ophthalmologists.

If it is impossible to examine the injured eye, examination under anesthetic is indicated (EUA). An EUA is usually used if the patient is a child, unable to tolerate an examination, if there is too much swelling around the eye or if there is a suspected occult globe rupture.

Pupil dilation (mydriasis) is useful for posterior segment examination, but must only be performed after the pupil reactions have been assessed, an anterior penetrating injury or globe rupture has been excluded and the anterior chamber is judged not to be shallow. Common topical mydriatics used are Tropicamide 1% that gives 2–3 h dilation and Cyclopentolate 1% that gives 12–24 h dilation. Mydriatic drops paralyze the ciliary muscles (accommodation) and the sphincter pupillae muscle (dilation) by reversible muscarinic inhibition. The patient is warned that their vision will be blurred and driving is not advised while the drops are working.

## 26.2.3
### Special Investigations

A plain skull x-ray is performed to exclude cranial and facial fractures and will visualize radio-opaque foreign bodies. If an intraocular foreign body (IOFB) is suspected. The request should be for views in up and down gaze. An IOFB will move with the eye whereas an orbital FB will remain still (Fig. 26.3).

CT scans are the test of choice for orbital and IOFB localization. A consultation with the CT technician is helpful in selecting the optimal section so as to reduce the risk of a false-negative result. Helical CT scans have a very high identification rate.[11] A CT scan will often diagnose other unsuspected cranial and facial injuries (Fig. 26.4).

**Fig. 26.3** Plain skull x-ray of Palestinian protestor demonstrating orbital foreign body. It was a rubber bullet fired by the Israeli Defence Force embedded in the orbit that had destroyed his globe, which required primary enucleation

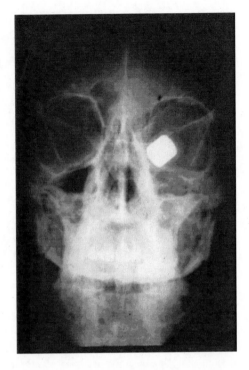

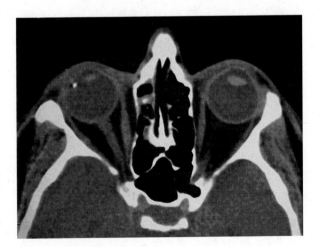

**Fig. 26.4** CT scan of eye demonstrating IOFB in blast injury patient

Ultrasound is useful for IOFB localization and can be used even in the presence of a ruptured globe. It can detect non radio-opaque or very small IOFB that are not detected by x-ray or CT scan. It can often localize orbital FB and help with surgical removal (Fig. 26.5).

**Fig. 26.5** An ultrasound biomicroscopic image showing metallic foreign body (*arrow*) and its shadowing effect (*asterisk*) in the ciliary body.[60] (Reprinted from Özdal[16]. With kind permission from Nature Publishing Group)

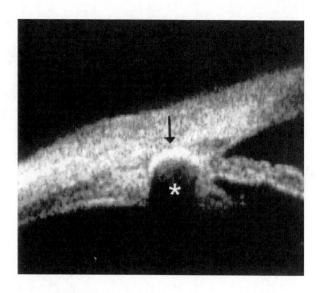

Magnetic resonance imaging (MRI) is contraindicated for metallic IOFB. The magnetic flux may cause them to move within the eye and cause further intraocular damage.

Ancillary tests of ocular function include electrodiagnostic tests of optic nerve and retinal function. These can be useful in severe trauma to help decide if visual function has been lost. Electroretinography (ERG) is useful in the diagnosis of siderosis or chalchosis. A visual field test is performed if optic nerve or tract damage is suspected. If an eye is lost a visual field test is performed of the good eye to confirm that it is normal.

Microscopy and microbiological culture of aqueous/vitreous samples is requested if endophthalmitis suspected. A positive result does not guarantee infection and a negative result does not exclude it.

## 26.3
## Primary Blast Injuries

A primary blast injury (PBI) occurs from the interaction of an explosive shockwave and the body. Short duration shock waves with a high peak dynamic overpressure are thought to damage the body through a form of body-stress coupling causing pressure differentials across the different tissues with shearing and, at a particular limit, pathological damage.

The eye consists of several coats that interface with each other. These vary considerably in their elasticity and density. The mechanism of primary ocular blast injury is from the shock wave rupturing or disinserting these layers from each other. It has been postulated that reflection of the shock wave by the orbit amplifies the effect.[12]

The eyes are less susceptible to a PBI than the air filled organs. At a level of blast sufficient to cause an eye injury accompanying injuries other organs especially the lungs and the bowel are likely. These other injuries are more life threatening and the patient will have to survive them before the eye injury becomes important. The eye only sustains a primary blast injury when the rest of the body is protected either by positioning or by special clothing. Improved eye protection from secondary injury and improved survivability from blast injuries have made pure PBI more common.[13] Factors that influence the effect of blast upon the eye include the peak overpressure achieved and the duration of the pressure at the eye. These two factors are related to the distance that the eye is from the explosion. The eye is more susceptible to a PBI if it points towards the explosion. Usually the wounding effect of an ocular blast injury will be a combination of primary and secondary processes.

### 26.3.1
### Experience

Cases of PBI occur in the subgroup of patients with intraocular lesions who did not sustain a penetrating or perforating ocular blast injury. That group of patients has remained roughly constant in proportion since the Second World War, at an average of 19.3% of all eye injuries (see Table 26.3). In the 21 cases of PBI reported in the literature the pattern of injury is summarized in Fig. 26.1.[14,15] The posterior segment is predominantly affected in approximately 57% of cases, even though the blast wave had to traverse the anterior segment to reach it. The anatomy of this area is made up of several fragile coats with markedly differing physical characteristics making the posterior ocular structures more susceptible to the blast wave.

The prognosis from ocular blast injuries is generally recorded as poor, in papers ranging from 1942 to 1987 the incidence of PBI ranged from 3.3% to 4.5% of ocular blast injury cases. A final visual acuity of 6/12 or better was achieved in 16–32% of these. Injuries to the optic nerve, choroid, and retina carried a worse prognosis than those to the anterior segment, adnexae, or intraocular hemorrhage.[15-17]

### 26.3.2
### Injury Pattern

Different theaters of war produce a similar spectrum of ocular PBI. The proportion of each particular injury varies as to the type of explosive used and the surrounding conditions. The injuries can be divided anatomically.

### 26.3.3
### Anterior Segment

Conjunctival lacerations and subconjunctival hemorrhages are common after explosions. The hemorrhage may be direct or indirect. The direct type is the effect of the blast wave acting upon the blood vessels themselves. The blast may indirectly cause a venous hemorrhage if it is sudden and to the abdomen by raising the venous pressure.[18]

**Fig. 26.6** Traumatic lens
dislocation

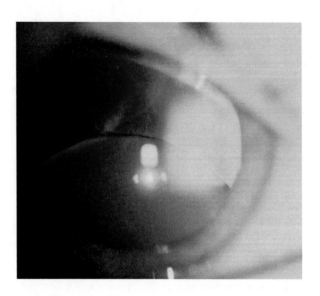

   Iris and ciliary body involvement is the most frequently reported blast injury in the
form of hyphaema due to avulsion of an iris blood vessel. The peripheral vessels are most
susceptible to this injury. Iris sphincter rupture and spiral tears are also well documented.[16]
The ciliary body cleaves at the junction between circular and radial fibers leading to angle
recession, this predisposes to secondary glaucoma.[19] Ciliary muscle atrophy will commonly cause reduced accommodation making reading difficult with associated eyestrain.
   Lens dislocation and subluxation are recorded in many clinical reports of ocular blast
injuries (Fig. 26.6). There is a myopic shift in refraction as the lens assumes a more spherical shape due to loss of zonular attachments. Traumatic cataracts are also recorded,
predominantly of the flocculate type. Lenticular injuries predispose to secondary glaucoma through phacomorphic or phacoanaphylactic mechanisms. Lenticular damage may
not be due to the primary blast injury alone as there is often a concomitant intralenticular
foreign body.[20]

## 26.3.4
## Posterior Segment

Posterior vitreous detachment from the retina may occur from a blast wave exerting a
shearing force at the vitreoretinal interface. At areas of special attachment this force dis-
rupts the underlying tissue.[21] Avulsed blood vessels cause a vitreous hemorrhage and
peripheral retinal tears lead to detachments. Traction over the macular causes tears and
holes with loss of central vision.
   Retinal vasoconstriction from the blast wave may be persistent leading to retinal ischaemia and necrosis.[22] Berlin's edema occurs when locally produced metabolites stimulate
vasodilatation leading to retinal swelling and hemorrhage. This resorbs over a few days
leaving a variable pattern of retinal atrophy. Vision is markedly reduced during the edematous phase though recovery of some or all the visual function is the rule after a few
weeks.[23]

Retinal hemorrhages may be interstitial, preretinal, or subhyaloid. The hemorrhage often breaks forward into the vitreous. Interstitial hemorrhages take weeks to absorb, preretinal and subhyaloid hemorrhages take somewhat longer. Vitreous hemorrhages take months to resorb and may require a vitrectomy.[24]

Tears and disinsertions of the retina have been reported and are usually inferior.[25] Such giant retinal tears and dialyses are particularly associated with ocular contusion and not with primary blast injuries.

Macular lesions are common after blast injuries. The area has a rich choroidal capillary bed, a thick retinal Henle's fiber layer and a poor retinal circulation. Fluid is readily absorbed from the choroid to Henle's layer and retained due to the relatively poor blood supply. If the edema is persistent macular cysts may form leading to lamellar and full thickness holes. Macular holes are usually a late effect after the injury often with a tractional component from an incompletely detached vitreous predisposing to the accumulation of sub retinal fluid with subsequent enlargement.[26]

Macular pigmentation is common and due to retinal pigment epithelial disturbance. This is often the only macular change. This pigmentation is usually asymptomatic, atrophic changes are rare but lead to a profound loss of visual acuity.[27]

Suprachoroidal or intrachoroidal hemorrhage from rupture of the short ciliary vessels may pass through the retina into the vitreous cavity, especially if these layers have already been damaged. Choroidal hemorrhages are typically localized and resolve to leave a patch of chorioretinal atrophy with a corresponding visual field defect.

Choroidal rupture at the level of the relatively inelastic Bruch's membrane is a common ocular PBI. The appearance is characteristically of a crescentic yellow brown streak sprinkled with blood which absorbs to leave a sharply defined scar with pigmented margins. The scar is usually concentric with and temporal to the optic disk (Fig. 26.7). Usually there are single tears which often involve the macula.[28]

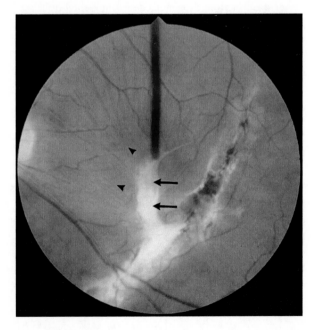

**Fig. 26.7** Photograph of left eye with a choroidal rupture extending to the macula, with secondary epiretinal membrane formation (*arrow*) and a striated appearance of adjacent neuroretina secondary to traction (*arrowheads*)

### 26.3.5
### Optic Nerve

Optic neuropathy is a well recorded if uncommon PBI associated with large blast forces.[29] There are several possible mechanisms of injury which cause optic neuropathy. Optic atrophy can follow massive retinal atrophy with axonal loss following widespread retinal edema. Blast wave induced vasoconstriction of the optic nerve blood supply causes traumatic optic neuropathy. The shearing force at the level of the lamina cribrosa can mechanically disrupt optic nerve axons as they enter the eye. A retrobulbar hemorrhage from rupture of the vortex veins as they leave the globe compressing the optic nerve blood supply to induce necrosis of the nervous tissue.[30]

### 26.3.6
### Orbit

The interface between the air of the maxillary sinus and the orbital floor is thought to promote an atypical blowout fracture at this site as a primary blast effect. This rare blast injury is associated with high intensity blast waves which usually also damage the eye.[31]

## 26.4
## Secondary Blast Injuries

Secondary blast injuries (SBI) are due to the impact of fragment from the explosive device itself or from exogenous debris propelled by the explosion.[32] They are the most common form of high explosive ocular injuries. The projectiles cause penetrating and perforating injuries to the globe and ocular adnexae. Until recently, it was rare to find a case of PBI without any evidence of contusion or any secondary injury to the eye or adnexae.[33,34]

## 26.5
## Birmingham Eye Trauma Terminology System

The Birmingham eye trauma terminology system (BETTS) is a standardized system used to describe and share eye injury information. The eyewall is composed of the Sclera and cornea, though the eye has three coats posterior to the limbus, for clinical and practical purposes ocular wounds are graded according to damage to the most external layer. This common method of describing eye injuries is particularly useful in the management of battlefield trauma cases where the patient will have been transferred to multiple care teams, often from different countries with different languages (Table 26.2).[35]

**Table 26.2** Birmingham eye trauma terminology system (BETTS)

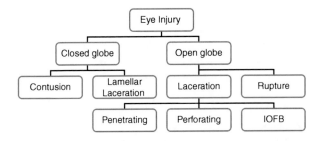

## 26.6
## Closed Globe Injuries

These are common to both primary and secondary blast injuries, but secondary blast injuries are caused by the impact of an object. When a blunt object strikes the eye it causes shortening anteroposteriorly and elongation equatorially. The lens-iris diaphragm is displaced posteriorly centrally while the peripheral structures are expanding outwards. This causes tearing of the ocular tissues, particularly in the iridocorneal angle. When the compressing object is larger than the orbit it pushes the globe posteriorly to suddenly increase the orbital pressure. The pressure is relieved by a blow-out fracture of the orbit, typically inferiorly into the maxillary sinus. This phenomenon often protects the globe from injury though there is up to a 30% incidence of ruptured globe reported in conjunction with orbital fracture.[36]

## 26.7
## Corneal Contusion Injuries

Corneal abrasions are very common after blast injuries. The cornea is very resilient to blunt trauma, which in the absence of previous surgical wounds will often only cause corneal abrasions. Diagnosis is on slit lamp examination of the cornea with flourescein staining after an anesthetic drop is instilled to allow examination of the eye. The underlying corneal stroma is clear in corneal abrasion; a stromal infiltrate may indicate bacterial or fungal keratitis.

Treatment is with topical antibiotic ointment to lubricate the eye surface and reduce the chance of a secondary infection. If the eye is painful, topical cycloplegic or non-steroidal anti-inflammatory drops can be prescribed.[37] There is no evidence that application of an occlusive eye patch improves healing, comfort, or visual outcome and this should not be performed.[38] If the abrasion is persistent a switch to a non-preserved antibiotic along with topical ocular lubricants is made, until healing occurs.

Recurrent erosions occasionally occur after an initial abrasion. They occur classically in the morning as the corneal epithelium sticks to the upper lid conjunctiva while the lids are closed at night and is torn off on waking. Treatment is with frequent topical lubricant drops during the day and ointment at night.

Corneal foreign bodies (FB) are intensely painful, especially if superficial. Radiographic investigation is mandatory to exclude an intraocular foreign body. Diagnosis is on slit lamp examination of the cornea with flourescein staining after an anesthetic drop is instilled to allow examination of the eye. There is often a sterile infiltrate surrounding the FB, especially if it has been present for more than 24 h. There may be superficial punctuate staining of the cornea and mild anterior chamber inflammation. The eyelids are everted and if necessary double everted to exclude the presence of multiple FB. After blast injuries, particularly mine blast injuries there are often multiple deep stromal foreign bodies. After an initial period of inflammation these characteristically become quiescent and the FB inert in the stroma even years after the injury. Apart from problems of glare from light reflecting off the stromal FB, they are often symptomless. Caspar's rings of the cornea are endothelial contusion injuries, without stromal or Descemet's membrane tears. They are multiple, disciform lesions 0.5–1.1 mm in diameter and lie under corneal foreign bodies. As a rule, they spontaneously resolve within 4–5 days with no harmful effects.[39]

Superficial foreign bodies are removed under topical anesthesia at the slit lamp using a hypodermic needle. Occasionally a rust ring forms around a corneal foreign body that can be difficult to remove with a needle. These are removed with a rotating Alger brush. Stromal foreign bodies are more difficult to remove and the corneal entry track must be opened to remove them; often irrigation is the best method of dislodging them from their cavity.

Multiple conjunctival FB are largely removed with saline irrigation. Retained FB are easily removed under topical anesthesia with a cotton wool bud or forceps. The history must exclude a scleral laceration or IOFB and if there is a chance of an IOFB then radiographic investigation is mandatory. Eversion and double eversion of the eyelid should be performed if a subtarsal or forniceal FB is suspected.

## 26.8
## Iris and Ciliary Body Contusion Injuries

Traumatic iritis is similar to uveitic iritis, but with a history of trauma. There is reduced vision, ocular pain, and photophobia. Examination shows perilimbal injection with anterior chamber cells and flare. Management is with a topical cycloplegic agent to relieve pain. Topical steroids are of limited value unless the iritis is prolonged. Retinal examination should be performed to exclude traumatic retinal tears.

Iridocorneal angle recession is where the ciliary body is torn in a manner such that the longitudinal muscle remains attached to its insertion at the scleral spur, while the circular muscle, with the pars plicata and the iris root, is displaced posteriorly. It is common after blunt trauma and diagnosed on slit lamp gonioscopy and is associated with damage to the trabecular meshwork. This impedes aqueous flow from the eye and can cause a rise in the intraocular pressure with secondary glaucoma in 7–9% of cases.[40,41]

In less than 20% of cases of angle recession there is progression to glaucoma. If less than one quadrant of the angle is recessed the chance of secondary glaucoma is minimal if more than two quadrants are affected there is a 10% risk of glaucoma if more than three quadrants are affected the risk of glaucoma is very high.[42,43] Patients with angle recession without glaucoma need to be followed annually for the development of glaucoma; patient education is important as the risk is lifelong. Treatment of glaucoma is initially with topical aqueous suppressant drops and drainage surgery if medical treatments fail. Pilocarpine drops may increase the intraocular pressure in traumatic glaucoma by decreasing uveoscleral outflow.[44]

Iridodialysis is a detachment of the iris root from the ciliary body and can produce corectopia (displaced pupil) and pseudopolycoria (more than one pupil). Glare and diplopia are common symptoms as light enters the eye from through two areas. Patients require lifelong glaucoma monitoring as the iridocorneal angle damage predisposes towards a raised intraocular pressure. If there is diplopia, a contact lens with an artificial iris can be considered. The best treatment is with direct surgical closure of the defect.[45]

Cyclodialysis clefts are from traumatic separation of the ciliary body from the sclera, this allows aqueous to exit directly to the subchoroidal space and causes ocular hypotony. Diagnosis is by gonioscopy or an anterior segment ultrasound scan. Management is with topical atropine for 6–8 weeks as spontaeneous resolution is usual. If it is persistent transcleral diode laser to the cleft is applied. Direct surgical closure is required if medical treatments fail.[46]

Hyphaema is caused by bleeding in the anterior chamber and describes layering of RBC in the inferior anterior chamber (see Fig. 26.2). The height from the inferior limbus is measured to guide management and chart progress (Table 26.3).

Microhyphaema is a small hyphaema in which there are only suspended red blood cells (RBCs) in the anterior chamber with no layered clot. The main complications are raised intraocular pressure and rebleeds. Approximately 10% of patients with traumatic hyphaema have traumatic retinal tears. Retinal tears or detachments must be excluded by posterior segment examination or ultrasound scan if there is no view. Gonioscopy must be performed at some stage to exclude iridocorneal angle recession that may cause late secondary glaucoma. Corneal blood-staining may occur if there is prolonged hyphaema with a high intraocular pressure (Fig. 26.8).

Management of hyphaema is by bed rest with 30° head elevation for 4 days to reduce episcleral venous pressure and promote settling of red blood cells. Sickle cell anemia in susceptible groups is excluded. Elective anticoagulants are discontinued and patients put on light activity for 2 weeks. Atropine 1% drops and topical steroids are prescribed for 2 weeks.

A raised intraocular pressure occurs in 30% of cases and is treated with oral or topical ocular antihypertensives. Diamox is contraindicated if there is sickle cell trait or disease.

**Table 26.3** Hyphaema grading by proportion of anterior chamber filled with blood

| Grade | Proportion of anterior chamber filled with blood |
| --- | --- |
| + | < 1/3 |
| ++ | 1/3–1/2 |
| +++ | > 1/2 but subtotal |
| ++++ | Total hyphaema "8 ball" |

**Fig. 26.8** Traumatic hyphaema with inferior level of blood in anterior chamber

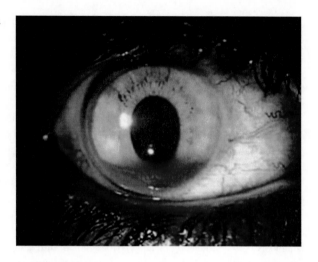

Rebleeding occurs in 4–40% of cases, usually 2–5 days post-injury. Surgical wash-out of the anterior chamber is required for 5% of cases. Iridocorneal angle recession or iridodialysis occurs in 75% of cases, but only 5% go on to develop secondary glaucoma.[47]

## 26.9
## Lens Contusion

Contusion rosette cataracts are classic of blunt trauma and may not appear for years after the injury; causing glare and loss of vision. Anterior and posterior subcapsular cataracts are also common after trauma. A Vossius' ring, a circular deposit of iris pigment epithelium, may be seen on the anterior lens capsule. It is a sign of previous blunt trauma and is asymptomatic, it fades with time. It should be differentiated from old posterior synechia from anterior uveitis.

Lens subluxation is a partially dislocated crystalline lens caused by incomplete zonular dehiscence from trauma. The lens equator is visible through the pupil and the lens (phakodonesis) and overlying iris (iridodonesis) is mobile. If the zonular dehiscence is complete lens dislocation can occur into the anterior chamber or posterior segment. Lens dislocation and subluxation cause sudden loss of visual acuity depending on the position of the lens. If it occurs after relatively minor trauma exclude Marfan's disease, homocystinuria, Weill-Marchesani syndrome, Ehlers-Danlos syndrome, and syphilis. Dislocation of the lens into the subconjunctival or subtenons space can occur through a scleral rupture. The lens is removed and the eyewall defect repaired. Anterior and posterior capsular rupture may occur after contusion injuries. Once any associated injuries and inflammation is managed cataract extraction is performed.

In anterior chamber dislocation, the lens should be repositioned after pupil dilation and supine positioning with corneal indentation with a gonioprism at a slit lamp. Posterior segment dislocation, if there is an intact lens capsule it can be managed conservatively. If there is a chance of capsular damage pars plans vitreolensectomy with intraocular lens implantation is performed. Leakage of lens protein in the vitreous causes severe inflammation and secondary glaucoma.

Surgical removal of traumatic cataracts is by phacoemulsification and lens implantation is performed is there is a visually significant cataract. Traumatic cataracts can be complex cases due to lens zonular dehiscence.

## 26.10
## Posterior Segment Contusion Injuries

*Commotio retinae* (Berlin's edema) describes the transient gray-white opacification at the level of the deep sensory retina after blunt trauma. It settles over 4–6 weeks leaving retinal pigment epithelial disturbance, retinal atrophy, optic atrophy, and on occasion a traumatic macular hole. Visual loss may be transient or permanent according to the extent of macular involvement.

*Choroidal ruptures* are typically crescent-shaped and sited at the posterior pole. They occur when the eye is deformed by a blunt injury. Bruch's membrane of the choroid is relatively non-elastic and ruptures while the more elastic retina and sclera remain intact. They are associated with subretinal hemorrhages that clear to reveal the rupture. Visual recovery is the rule, but can be reduced if the rupture involves the fovea, if there is choroidal subretinal neovascularisation or massive intraocular scarring.

*Sclopetaria*, traumatic chorioretinal rupture is from a concussion injury where an object strikes the eye at high velocity but does not penetrate the eye. The choroid and retina are locally disrupted by the transmitted energy (coup) and at the opposite side of the eye (contracoup) to give an acute traumatic degeneration of the choroid and retina. There are often dramatic retinal tears with associated shallow retinal detachment. These characteristically do not require active treatment as scarring from the surrounding tissue seals the retinal break.

*Optic nerve avulsion* occurs when an object intrudes between the globe and orbital wall to disinsert the optic nerve. There is sudden visual loss that is irreversible. Diagnosis is by ophthalmoscopy where there is loss of the optic disk and confirmed by ultrasound or CT scan.

*Traumatic optic neuropathy* occurs when the concussive wave causes profound vasoconstriction of the pial vessels that supply the optic nerve. The ensuing neural deficit reduces the visual acuity, brightness sense, and color vision. It is typically associated with a relative afferent pupillary defect. Management options for traumatic optic neuropathy management include observation, high dose systemic steroids, and surgical decompression of the optic canal. There is no evidence of superiority of medical and surgical treatment over observation and the interventional treatments carry a high risk of side-effects and complications.

## 26.11
## Traumatic Retinal Tears and Detachments

Retinal dialyses describe a peripheral retinal disinsertion between the edge of the retina and the ora serrata from sudden expansion of the ocular equator from blunt injury. They are responsible for up to 84% trauma related retinal detachments. Myopic patients are more susceptible and the commonest areas for post-traumatic dialyses are the superonasal and inferotemporal retinal quadrants. The detachment evolves slowly, often years after the trauma, as the vitreous body is formed in young people and keeps the dialysis closed. Diagnosis is when vision is lost due to macular involvement or as an incidental finding during routine ophthalmic examination.

Irregular retinal breaks can form as a result of direct contusion. The retina is separated from the vitreous base and the retinal edge typically has a rolled edge. The vitreous base can be disinserted over the edge of the retinal tear, like a bucket handle. If the tear is greater than 3 clock hours it is termed a traumatic giant retinal tear. If left untreated, a retinal detachment occurs with a high chance of proliferative retinopathy (retinal scarring) and a poor visual prognosis, so early diagnosis and treatment are indicated.

Eyes sustaining penetrating or open globe trauma have a high risk of retinal detachment, occurring in 10–45% of cases. Proliferative vitreoretinopathy (PVR) is the commonest cause of recurrent retinal detachment. PVR can be considered a wound healing response in a specialized tissue, leading to the formation of fibrocellular membranes on both the surfaces of the detached retina and the posterior hyaloid face. Contraction of these membranes results in retinal detachment.[48,49]

The incidence of PVR is highest in perforating (through and through) injuries at 46% of eyes and lowest in intraocular foreign body injuries at 11%; if intraocular foreign bodies are excluded the mean incidence is 27% for all open globe trauma.[5]

Traumatic macular holes form as a result of acute changes in vitreoretinal traction over the macular area from ocular contusion, they are typically 300–500 microns in diameter but if there is an element of retinal necrosis they can be much larger. Only 1% progress to retinal detachment and there is a good visual prognosis with successful macular hole surgery.

Other retinal breaks can form as a result of an induced posterior vitreous detachment from the injury. If there is an area of increased vitreoretinal traction, typically over blood vessels a retinal tear forms often with a vitreous hemorrhage. The tears will often be associated with a rhegmatogenous retinal detachment.

Retinal tears and detachments are managed surgically with retinopexy for retinal tears and vitrectomy and internal tamponade or cryopexy and buckling procedures for retinal detachment. If an intraocular gas is used, the patient cannot travel by air until it has resorbed, in case of sudden gas expansion at altitude. Retinal detachments associated with penetrating trauma is particularly susceptible to postoperative retinal scarring (proliferative vitreoretinopathy). This reduces the anatomical and visual outcomes of surgery and the patient should be warned of the guarded prognosis.

## 26.12
## Lamellar Lacerations

*Corneoscleral non-penetrating lacerations* are diagnosed by careful ophthalmoscopy. Siedel's sign indicates a penetrating injury of the anterior segment. Here, a drop of Sodium Flourescein dye is applied to the cornea and is observed with a slit lamp's cobalt blue light. Any fluid leaking out of the eye dilutes the yellow Flourescein and can be observed as a lighter green fluorescent wave.

If leaking, a corneal laceration requires direct suturing using 10/0 nylon sutures under an operating microscope. Deep multiple perpendicular symmetrical short sutures using 10/0 nylon on a half circle needle are used near the central cornea to avoid the visual axis where possible. Longer sutures can be used in the periphery. The first bite is to the central part of the laceration to the peripheral cornea; so called "ship to shore."

Occasionally corneal lacerations can be managed with a bandage contact lens if the laceration is small and self-sealing (Fig. 26.9). *Conjunctival lacerations* heal rapidly and rarely need suturing. A 7/0 vicryl (absorbable) tacking suture is used if required. Topical antibiotic drops are given for 1 week. A contact lens will protect the eye until referral can be made to an ophthalmologist as it stops the flap from dislodging. Topical antibiotics must be given for 1–2 weeks after the laceration.

## 26.13
## Open Globe Injuries

### 26.13.1
### Penetrating and Perforating Injuries

Penetrating eye injuries are sharp eye injuries that have a single entrance wound from the injury (Fig. 26.10). If more than one wound is present, each must have been caused by a

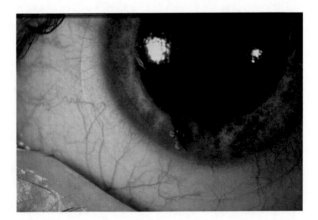

**Fig. 26.9** Corneal perforation covered by bandage contact lens

**Fig. 26.10** Penetrating injury to eye from screw

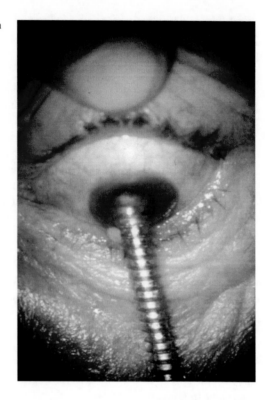

different agent. Perforating eye injuries have an entrance and exit wound; both wounds are caused by the same agent.

The signs are often obvious with an entry/exit site and extrusion of ocular tissue. If there has been an occult penetration there may be early ocular hypotony that recovers after a few hours; anterior segment disruption; vitreous hemorrhage and retinal breaks. Vision can be lost if there is a suprachoroidal hemorrhage as the ocular contents are extruded through the wound.

The eye is protected by a Cartella shield and the patient admitted for bed rest and made nil by mouth preoperatively. Prophylactic systemic antibiotics are prescribed and Tetanus toxoid is given if required. A CT scan is performed to rule out intraorbital, intracranial, or intraocular foreign bodies or penetration. An ultrasound scan is used to localize a posterior rupture/exit site.

Management is by urgent primary surgical repair, this can be followed by a definitive secondary procedure at during the same procedure or at a later date depending on the experience of the surgeon.

## 26.13.2
## Globe Rupture

Globe rupture is a full-thickness wound of the eyewall from a blunt injury. The eye is filled with incompressible liquid and the impact causes sufficient pressure to rupture the eye at its weakest point, by an inside-out mechanism. Rupture is commonly at the impact site, or an area of corneal or scleral weakness such as an old cataract wound.

Clinical signs of scleral rupture include: periocular hemorrhage with hemorrhagic chemosis, a visual acuity of PL or less, afferent pupillary defect, ocular hypotony, an abnormally deep or shallow anterior chamber, an irregular pupil. There is often extrusion of the ocular contents. Globe rupture must be excluded by ultrasound scan in all cases of hyphaema or post-traumatic media opacity that prevents indirect ophthalmoscopy of the fundus.

The eye should not be manipulated in case of extrusion of its contents and a protective Cartella eye shield is fitted. Surgical exploration and primary repair is performed if globe rupture is suspected. The conjunctiva is reflected back and the sclera is systematically examined with particular reference to the thinnest area of sclera that lies under the rectus muscles. Secondary procedures for intraocular hemorrhage are delayed for up to 14 days to allow the blood clot to liquefy, when it can be surgically drained as part of a vitrectomy procedure.

Associated retinal detachments and tears are managed by vitrectomy, retinopexy, and internal tamponade. Suxamethonium should be avoided during the anesthetic as it may cause increased venous pressure and an intraocular hemorrhage. Enucleation as a primary procedure should be avoided unless the patient has been properly counseled and consented. It is better to perform a primary repair and obtain a staff opinion, before the eye is enucleated or eviscerated with an orbital implant as a secondary procedure.

## 26.14
## Intraocular Foreign Bodies

Intraocular foreign bodies (IOFB) cause 14–17% of all ocular war injuries[50,51]; they are a very important subset of eye injuries as they have a modifiable outcome using modern diagnostic, therapeutic, and surgical techniques. They must be excluded in all cases of ocular blast injury. The final resting place of and damage caused by an IOFB depends on the size, the shape, and the momentum of the object at the time of impact, and the site of ocular penetration. In modern warfare a large proportion of IOFB are from grit and stones thrown up by explosions, they are frequently multiple. Appropriate eye protection would significantly reduce the incidence of IOFB injuries.[52]

Increasing IOFB mass is associated with posterior segment injury, retinal impact, and poor vision. The frequency of globe penetration by an IOFB is determined by its shape; blade-shaped > disk-shaped > cylindrical > spherical.[53] Secondary complications from IOFB occur in half of patients; including endophthalmitis, corneal scarring, elevated intraocular pressure, cataract, retinal detachment, and metallosis (e.g., chalcosis, siderosis). There is another type of foreign body particularly associated with explosive injuries where a thin jet of molten metal is injected into the eye through a tiny entry wound. This type of injury may be associated with retinal burns.

Siderosis occurs if a ferrous IOFB is left in-situ, iron dispersion throughout the globe causes retinal toxicity; IOFB removal is usually followed by visual and ERG recovery.[54] Chalcosis occurs from IOFB that contain more than 85% Copper, which is retinotoxic can cause profound visual loss associated with a greenish hue to the affected cornea. Diagnosis can be confirmed by copper assay of an aqueous fluid sample, though the ERG is also reduced.

Systemic and topical antibiotic therapy should be started prior to surgical intervention to prevent endophthalmitis. Topical corticosteroids are used to minimize inflammation and a tetanus booster may be appropriate. Surgical removal of a posterior segment IOFB is by pars plana vitrectomy and is as an emergency if the risk of endophthalmitis is high. In other cases the surgeon has the option of deferring intervention as long as a combination of systemic and topical antibiotic coverage is given and can achieve a good visual outcome without an increased risk of endophthalmitis or other deleterious side effects. The recommended systemic and topical antibiotic are 3rd-generation fluoroquinolones such as Laevofloxacin as they have a wide spectrum of antimicrobial effect including against Pseudomonas Auruginosa and therapeutic penetration into the eye.

The aim of surgery is initially to obtain a view of the posterior segment, performing a lensectomy if required; then perform a pars plana vitrectomy. The posterior hyaloid is removed, and retinal impact sites are treated with prophylactic retinopexy. The IOFB is identified and withdrawn through the sclerotomy using forceps or an internal magnet; if the IOFB is very large it can be delivered via the anterior chamber through a corneal incision that can be sutured. Occasionally an external electromagnet is used to remove IOFB especially if it is buried in the ciliary body.

Anterior chamber IOFBs are not removed through the original wound, but through a paracentesis at 90–180° to it. Viscoelastics reduce the risk of iatrogenic damage to the lens and corneal endothelium. Intralenticular IOFBs occasionally can be left in-situ unless there is a risk of metallosis. The prognosis from an IOFB injury is relatively good with over 50% of eyes achieving useful vision.

In warfare related IOFB injuries poor visual outcomes and postoperative complications were also related to extensive intraocular injury. In 79 of 70 US soldiers deployed in support of operations Iraqi Freedom and Enduring Freedom sustaining IOFB injuries 53.4% achieved visual acuity of 20/40 or better, whereas 77.5% achieved visual acuity of better than 20/200. There were no cases of endophthalmitis (0/79 eyes; 95% confidence interval, 0%–3.1%), siderosis bulbi, or sympathetic ophthalmia despite a mean time to IOFB removal of 38 days post-inury. Among the eyes, 10.3% had nil light perception or had been enucleated by the 6-month follow-up visit.[55]

## 26.15
## Ocular Adnexal Injuries

The eyelids should be carefully examined, asymmetry may be from ruptured canthal tendons that attach the ends of the lid to the orbit. A flattened upper lid may indicate a globe rupture. Lid wound assessment includes the depth (partial/full-thickness); tissue loss (corneal exposure); lacrimal/cannalicular involvement (epiphora); wound contamination and ptosis (levator damage).

The eyelids can be left unrepaired for several days as long as the cornea is protected from exposure by a Cartella shield and ocular lubricants. They have an excellent blood supply and debridement of tissue should be avoided. Superficial lacerations that do not involve the lid margins can be repaired with 6/0 vicryl sutures. Bleeding should be stopped using tacking sutures if necessary. Pressure on the globe should be avoided in case of rupture. If there is lid avulsion a cartella shield is placed over the eye for protection and topical lubricants applied to prevent corneal exposure.

Where the lid margins have been involved, if the cannaliculi have been involved or the levator muscle has been damaged, referral to an ophthalmologist for an oculoplastic repair is recommended. Complex reconstruction of the lid with cannalicular repair as a first procedure can prevent future complications from inappropriate interventions. If there has been tissue loss normal plastic surgery repair may not be appropriate and referral to an oculoplastic surgeon is indicated so that tissue sparing techniques can be used to give the best possible cosmetic result.

Orbital blowout fractures are usually of the orbital floor with herniation of orbital contents into the maxillary sinus, followed by the medial wall with herniation into the ethmoidal sinus. The rectus muscles, usually the inferior rectus, can be trapped as they herniate into the sinuses causing restriction of eye movement.

Patients present after facial trauma with blurred vision, a sunken eye, diplopia, and restriction of eye movements, especially on upgaze. Epistaxis and eyelid swelling following nose blowing due to air being blown into the orbit through the maxillary sinus (surgical emphysema). Initially there is tender periorbital ecchymosis and edema. Enophthalmos can be obscured by tissue swelling and the eye may be proptotic due to orbital hemorrhage. This swelling also may restrict extraocular muscle motility, mimicking entrapment.

Palpation of the orbital rim may reveal a bony step and point tenderness due to a fracture. Inferior periorbital hypoaesthesia indicates trauma to the infraorbital nerve, this usually recovers over a few weeks. Examination of the globe is essential to check ocular function and to exclude a rupture. Ocular misalignment, hypotropia or hypertropia, and limitation of eye movements indicate an orbital fracture. Forced duction tests differentiate entrapment or traumatic dysfunction of the rectus muscles. Orbital x-ray and CT scanning will diagnose an orbital floor blow out fracture with characteristic herniation of orbital contents into the maxillary sinus and often a sinus hemorrhage.

Orbital fractures including blowout fractures are not urgent cases. Prophylactic systemic antibiotics are prescribed and a CT scan or x-ray is performed to exclude an orbital foreign. The patient is instructed not to blow their nose and force air and mucus out of the sinuses and into the orbital cavity. Management of orbital blow out fractures is conservative if there is no enophthalmos or rectus muscle tethering. Adult patients are observed for 1–2 weeks in case of spontaneous resolution. If there is more than 2 mm enophthalmos or significant restriction of eye movement with a positive forced duction test, orbital floor reconstruction with an implant is performed.

*Retrobulbar hemorrhage* is an ocular emergency where bleeding into the orbital space can result in compression of the optic nerve, leading to ischaemia and blindness. It is particularly associated with infraorbital, le Fort, and Zygomatic orbital/facial fractures. Rapid diagnosis and treatment within 100 min, may avoid permanent vision loss.

It is characterized by severe ocular PAIN, rapid tense PROPTOSIS, The PUPIL REACTIONS to light are lost, ocular PARALYSIS where ocular movements are lost and VISUAL LOSS where the vision is reduced like a falling curtain. Lateral canthotomy and inferior cantholysis is performed immediately to decompress the orbit and intravenous acetazolamide and intravenous mannitol is given to lower the intraocular pressure.

*Orbital foreign bodies* (FB) are common ballistic injuries and are commonly associated with significant ocular and orbital injuries. Management of these cases is dependent on the composition and the location of the FB. Ancillary radiographic studies including plain X-ray and CT scans of the orbits can be helpful in localizing the FB. Surgery to remove the FB should be considered in each case, but FB that are not readily accessible can usually be left safely in place.[56]

## 26.16
## Recovery from Primary and Secondary Ocular Blast Injuries

Quere recorded the progress of 132 cases of ocular injury, between 1957 and 1961 during the Franco-Algerian war.[19] These cases were virtually all due to land mine explosions. The nature of the munitions predisposed to a mixture of primary and secondary blast injuries from the explosion and from debris and dirt. Patients sustaining an ocular blast injury were very likely to have multiple injuries to the rest of the body of equal or higher priority. He divided recovery of vision into three stages.

The first stage of active general treatment and healing lasted for 3 weeks. Poor vision at this time did not preclude a satisfactory outcome. The second stage was from 4 to 12 weeks. Here the cases assumed individual clinical patterns requiring specific treatments. An accurate prediction of the final acuity could be made at this time. This depended largely on the state of the macula and other chorioretinal damage. The intraocular pressure recovered at this stage. The third, delayed, stage allowed very few late changes in visual acuity. Late improvements outnumbered late complications which tended to be from retinal disease. These stages are summarized in Table 26.4. After 3 years 25% of the primarily affected eyes achieved a visual acuity equivalent to 6/12 or better. The same criteria for recovery applied to all the injuries whether the injury was predominantly due to primary or secondary blast effects.

The results of these studies provide a guide to the effects of explosive blast injuries to the eye, including PBI and SBI. The anterior segment appears to be more affected than the posterior segment. The impacting fragments preferentially disrupt the anterior segment causing a SBI. The blast wave itself predominantly damages the posterior segment.

**Table 26.4** Stages of recovery from primary and secondary ocular blast injuries

| Stage of recovery post-injury | Time | Phase of recovery | Prognosis |
|---|---|---|---|
| 1 | 0–3 Weeks | Rapid recovery | Poor V A does not preclude good recovery |
| 2 | 4–12 Weeks | Specific syndromes | Final V A can be predicted at this time |
| 3 | 3 Months – 3 Years | Late changes (rare) | Unpredictable but late recovery > exacerbation |

The visual outcome is largely determined by the extent of retinal and especially macular involvement from the original injury. None of the studies mentions if ocular protection was used or if it had any effect upon the injury.

The treatment of the ocular injuries varied between the studies according to the technology and facilities available to the ophthalmologists. For the most part, ocular PBI is initially treated expectantly as the integrity of the eye is virtually always preserved. After 4–12 weeks when specific ocular syndromes become manifest the eye may become amenable to treatment. It is at this stage, for example, that glaucoma becomes manifest or that a vitrectomy might be considered for persistent vitreous hemorrhage.

## 26.17
## Tertiary Blast Injuries

Tertiary ocular blast injuries are from the effects of being thrown into fixed objects or structural collapse and fragmentation of buildings and vehicles by an explosion. Any body part may be affected and the injury pattern includes: fractures, traumatic amputations, and open and closed head injuries, crush injuries as well as extensive blunt and penetrating trauma. As well as direct contusion penetrating and perforating injuries tertiary blast can cause indirect ocular effects.

*Purtscher's retinopathy* is a sudden onset multifocal, vaso-occlusive event that is associated with head and chest trauma. It causes a sudden loss of vision that slowly recovers over weeks and months. The appearance is of multiple patches of superficial retinal whitening with retinal hemorrhages surrounding a hyperaemic optic nerve head.

*Fat embolism syndrome* is a potentially fatal complication from long bone fractures that can affect the respiratory and central nervous systems. Reduced vision is found in 50% of cases and it will commonly cause. The retinal appearance is identical to Purtcher's retinopathy; multiple patches of superficial retinal whitening with retinal hemorrhages surrounding a hyperaemic optic nerve head. Visual recovery is usually good though permanent patchy visual field loss will occasionally occur.

*Terson's syndrome* is a vitreous hemorrhage that occurs after an intracranial hemorrhage. It is commonest (3–8%) after a subarachnoid hemorrhage and is often bilateral. It is thought to be related to an acute rise in intracranial pressure that is transmitted to the retina to cause rupture of the papillary and retinal capillaries. The hemorrhage is thought to form initially between the retina and internal limiting membrane disperses into the vitreous hemorrhage. It is often diagnosed when a patient recovers from the subarachnoid hemorrhage and is found to be profoundly blind. They are associated with the development of significant epiretinal membranes and the visual prognosis is often poor.

*Water-shed infarcts* of the parieto-occipital lobes of the cerebral cortex, are associated with severe blood loss and profound hypotension. The infarct occurs at the borders of cerebral circulation that are sensitive to ischaemic insults. These classically cause bilateral visual pathway damage with cortical blindness.[57]

*Non-arteritic ischaemic optic neuropathy* (NAION) where there is visual loss in one or both eyes with associated optic atrophy due to optic nerve ischaemia will follow severe blood loss and profound hypotension occurs only if there is co-existing vascular disease such as ischaemic heart disease, hypercholesterolaemia, hypertension, and diabetes mellitus, with a higher risk in older patients. Pre-injury ocular risk factors include hypermetropia, a raised intraocular pressure, and a "crowded" optic disk with a low cup to disk ratio of the optic nerve head.

*Valsalva retinopathy* is a sudden loss of vision from a preretinal hemorrhage that occurs when there is a sudden increase in intrathoracic pressure. It typically occurs after heavy lifting or straining at stool coughing or vomiting, but is also common after explosions. Spontaeneous recovery is the rule.[58]

## 26.18
## Quaternary Blast Injury

These are explosion related injuries or illnesses not due to primary, secondary, or tertiary injuries. There may be exacerbations of pre-existing conditions, such as glaucoma or cataracts. Chemical and thermal burns are common around the eye and adnexae in association with ballistic injuries.

*Thermal burns* are often from contact with hot liquids, hot gases, or molten metals. Tissue damage is usually limited to the superficial epithelium, but thermal necrosis and ocular penetration can occur. Topical antibiotics are prescribed for epithelial defects and conjunctivitis. Initially the lid swelling may protect the corneal surface, but sloughing and contracture can lead to corneal exposure, requiring topical ocular lubricants.

*Chemical burns* are blinding emergencies. Alkaline agents such as lye or cement penetrate cell membranes and cause more damage than Acidic agents Acid burns are usually from battery acid explosions which precipitate on reaction with ocular proteins. Corneal epithelial defects range from superficial epitheliopathy to total epithelial loss. Limbal ischaemia is a whitened area without blood flow around the eye. The whiter the eye is the worse the burn. Other signs include focal areas of conjunctival chemosis, hyperaemia, conjunctival hemorrhages, eyelid edema, mild iritis, and periocular burns. The Roper-Hall classification of ocular chemical burns relates the visual prognosis to the amount of corneal damage and limbal ischaemia (Table 26.5).

**Table 26.5** Roper-hall classification of ocular chemical burns

| Grade | Prognosis | Limbal ischemia | Corneal involvement |
| --- | --- | --- | --- |
| I | Good | None | Epithelial Damage |
| II | Good | Less than 1/3 | Haze but the iris details are visible |
| III | Guarded | 1/3 to 1/2 | Total epithelial loss, haze obscures iris details |
| IV | Poor | Greater than 1/2 | Cornea opaque, iris and pupil obscured |

Management of chemical burns is with immediate copious irrigation with Ringer's lactated solution for 30 min or an amphoteric solution such as Diphoterine (normal saline or even tap water are crude alternatives). The pH should be measured after 5 min on ceasing irrigation and if it is not neutral (pH7.0) then irrigation continued until neutral.

The conjunctival fornices are swept with a glass rod to remove retained debris and break conjunctival adhesions. Topical antibiotic ointment and cycloplegic drops are prescribed along with oral Ascorbic acid (vitamin C) to promote fibroblast activity. Oral analgesia is used if required. Topical steroids are used cautiously within the first week as they may cause corneoscleral melting. Raised intraocular pressure is treated with topical or systemic ocular antihypertensives. Amniotic membrane grafts promote corneal surface healing and are especially useful in the management of severe burns.

*Sympathetic ophthalmia* is a bilateral panuveitis that causes a painful red eye with visual loss, in a patient with a history of uveal tissue prolapse from an eye injury. It occurs in approximately 1:500 cases of open globe injury. The injured eye is termed the exciting eye and the fellow eye is the sympathizing eye. Exposure of retinal specific proteins to the immune system during the injury of one eye causes an autoimmune reaction to both eyes at a later date. It can occur as early as 5 days and as late as 60 years after the injury, though 90% of cases occur within the first year. The typical appearance is of granulomatous panuveitis with mutton-fat keratoprecipitates, usually with multiple yellow Dalen-Fuchs subretinal nodules apparent on fundoscopy.

It is commonly thought that prevention of sympathetic ophthalmia is by enucleation of blind traumatized eyes within 7–14 days of the injury. There is little immunological evidence to support this management or time limit, though it provides a convenient time to make definitive decisions about the management of the globe. Evisceration of the globe contents with an orbital implant will usually give a better cosmetic result. Topical and systemic steroids are the mainstay of sympathetic ophthalmia treatment, with further immunosuppression as required.

*Endophthalmitis* after ocular trauma is an exogenous intraocular infection from foreign bodies, and/or blunt or penetrating ocular trauma. The ocular tissues are disrupted by direct invasion by the organism or from the inflammatory mediators of the immune response. Delay in the repair of a penetrating globe injury is correlated with increased risk of developing endophthalmitis.

Symptoms include visual loss, headache, photophobia, and intense ocular and periocular inflammation with a painful injected eye and ocular discharge. Signs of eyelid swelling and erythema with an injected conjunctiva and sclera and a hypopyon (layering of inflammatory cells in the anterior chamber) associated with a reduced or absent red reflex due to vitritis. The casualty may have a fever. The absence of pain and hypopyon do not rule out endophthalmitis.

In traumatic endophthalmitis, bacteria or fungi are introduced at the time of injury. It is common after penetrating ocular trauma in the civilian setting particularly in rural settings. The incidence is rare after battlefield ocular injuries, probably as a result of early treatment with systemic antibiotics. Staphylococcal, streptococcal, and Bacillus species are the most common in traumatic endophthalmitis.

Diagnosis is usually clinically, the presence of an intraocular foreign body must be ruled out. Systemic broad spectrum antibiotics are given as well as intensive topical fortified antibiotics; cycloplegic drops are given to reduce pain. The globe perforation is repaired and intravitreal antibiotics are injected. If the visual acuity is less than hand movements a pars plana vitrectomy is performed. If a fungal endophthalmitis is suspected intravitreal amphotericin B is given with systemic fluconazole.

The prognosis is generally poor but can be extremely variable because of the variety of organisms involved. The visual acuity at the time of the diagnosis and the causative agent are most predictive of outcome. The prognosis appears to also be related to the patient's underlying health and fitness.

## References

1. Belkin M. Ocular war injuries in the Yom Kippur war. *J Ocul Ther Surg*. 1983;2:40-9.
2. Gombos GM. Ocular war injuries in Jerusalem. *Am J Ophthalmology*. 1969;68:474-8.
3. Belkin M, Treister G, Dotan S. Eye injuries and ocular protection in the Lebanon War, 1982. *Israel J Med Sci*. 1984;20:333-8.
4. Steindorf K. Die Kriegschirugie des schorgans. *Berlin Klin Wochensch*. 1914;51:1787-9.
5. Mader TH, Aragones JV, Chandler AC, et al. Ocular and ocular adnexal injuries treated by United States military ophthalmologistsduring Operations Desert Shield and Desert Storm. *Ophthalmology*. 1993;100:1462-1467.
6. Owens BD, Kragh JF jr, Wenke JC, Macaitis J, Wade CE, Holcomb JB. Combat wounds in operation Iraqui Freedom and Operation Enduring Freedom. *J Trauma*. 2006;64:295-299.
7. Lashkari K, Lashkari MH, Kim AJ, Crane WG, Jalkh AE. Combat-related eye trauma: a review of 5, 320 cases. *Int Ophthalmology Clin*. 1995;35:193-203.
8. Cotter F, La Piana FG. Eye casualty reduction for eye armour. *Mil Med*. 1991;156:126-8.
9. Trediche TJ. Management of eye casualties in South East Asia. *Mil Med*. 1968;133:355-62.
10. Gondusky JS, Reiter MC. Protecting military convoys in Iraq: An examination of battle injuries sustained by a mechanised battalion during operation Iraqi Freedom II. *Mil Med*. 2005;170(6):546-549.
11. Lakits A, Prokesh R, Scholda C, Bankier A. Orbital helical computed topography in the diagnosis and management of eye trauma. *Ophthalmology*. 1999;106:2330-2335.
12. Wharton-Young M. Mechanics of blast injuries. *War Medicine*. 1945;8(2):73-81.
13. Chalioulias K, Sim KT, Scott RA. Retinal sequelae of primary ocular blast injuries. *J R Army Med Corps*. 2007;153:124-5.
14. Scott GI, Michaelson le. An analysis and follow-up of 301 cases of battle casualty injuries to eyes. *Br J Ophthalmol*. 1946;30:42-55.
15. Bellows JG. Ocular war injuries. *Am J Ophthalmology*. 1947;30:309-23.
16. Zerihun N. Blast injuries of the eye. *Trop Doc*. 1993;23:76-78.
17. Dalinchuk MN, Lalzoi MN. Eye damage accompanying explosive mine injuries. *Voen Med Zh*. 1989;8:28-30.
18. Bonnet M. *Contribution A L'etude Des Effects Des Explosions De Guerre Sur L'organisme*. Nancy: A Crepin-Leblond; 1918.
19. Kilgore GL. Changes in the ciliary body after contusio bulbi in which only the anterior segment of the eye is affected. Transactions of the Pacific Coast Oto-Ophthalmological Society May 28, 1941. Cal
20. Quere MA, Bouchat J, Cornand G. Ocular blast injuries. *Am J Ophthalmology*. 1969;67:64-69.
21. Sebag 1. Anatomy and pathology of the vitreo-retinal interface. *Eye* 1992;6:541-52, 33. Kaminskaya ZA. Clinical symptoms and therapy of indirect ocular injuries. *Viestnik Oft*. 1943;22:7

22. Elmassri A. Injuries to the posterior segment of the globe. *Bull Ophthal Soc Egypt.* 1970;63: 25-33.

23. Lister WT. War injuries of the eye. *Lancet.* 1918;20:67-71.

24. Margo CE. *Vitreous Haemorrhage,* Diagnostic problems in clinical ophthalmology. Philadelphia: Saunders; 1994:404-15.

25. Hull FE. Management of eye casualties in the Far East Command during the Korean conflict. Transactons of the Joint Committee on Industrial Ophthalmology Oct 14, 1951. Chicago, Ill

26. Kaminskii De. Hole in the macula as a result of ocular contusion by firearms. *Viestnik 01.* 1943;22:25-31.

27. Elmassri A. Injuries to the posterior segment of the globe. *Bull Ophthal Soc Egypt.* 1970;63: 25-33.

28. Lister WT. Huntarian Lecture: Pathological aspects of certain war injuries of the eye. *Lancet.* 1918;20:67-72.

29. Campbell DR. Ophthalmic casualties resulting from air raids. *Br Med J.* 1941;28:966.

30. Margo CE. *Vitreous Haemorrhage,* Diagnostic problems in clinical ophthalmology. Philadelphia: Saunders; 1994:404-15.

31. Mandelcorn MS, Hill JC. Orbital blast injury. *Can J Ophthalmol.* 1973;8:597-9.

32. Cooper GJ., Biological effects of blast. Institute of Explosives Engineers/PSBD Home Office, BCC 1993/MOD.

33. Beiran I, Miller B. Pure ocular blast injury. *Am J Ophthalmol.* 1992;114:504-5.

34. Campbell DR. Ophthalmic casualties resulting from air raids. *Br Med J.* 1941;28:966.

35. Kuhn F, Morris R, Witherspoon CD, Heimann K, Jeffers JB, Treister G. A standardized classification of ocular trauma. *Ophthalmology.* 1996;103:240-243.

36. Wilkins RB, Havins WE. Current treatment of blow-out fractures. *Ophthalmology.* 1982;89(5):464-466.

37. Wilson SA, Last A. Management of corneal abrasions. *Am Fam Physician.* 2004;70:123-128.

38. Kaiser PK, Pineda R 2nd. A study of topical nonsteroidal anti-inflammatory dropsand no pressure patching in the treatment of corneal abrasions. Corneal Abrasion Patching Study Group. *Ophthalmology.* 1997;104:1353-1359.

39. Caspar L. Subepithelial trubungsfiguren der hornhaut, nach verletzungen. *Klin Monatsbl Augenheilkd.* 1916;57:385-90.

40. Monney D. Angle recession and secondary glaucoma. *Br J Ophthalmol.* 1973;57:608-612.

41. Blanton FM. Anterior chamber angle recession and secondary glaucoma. *Acta Ophthalmol.* 1968;46:886-908.

42. Alper MG. Contusion angle deformity and glaucoma: gonioscopic observations and clinical course. *Arch Ophthalmol.* 1963;69:455-467.

43. Sihota RN, Sood NN, Agarwal HC. Traumatic glaucoma. *Acta Ophthalmol Scand.* 1995;73:252-254.

44. Bleiman BS, Schwartz AL. Paradoxical intraocular pressure response to pilocarpine. A proposed mechanism and treatment. *Arch Ophthalmol.* 1979;97:1305-1306.

45. McCannel MA. A retrievable suture idea for anterior uveal problems. *Ophthalmic Surg.* 1976;7:98-103.

46. Demeler U. Surgical management of ocular hypotony. *Eye.* 1988;2:77.

47. Kearns P. Traumatic hyphaema: a retrospective study of 314 cases. *Br J Ophthalmol.* 1991;75:137-141.

48. Lewis H, Aaberg TM, Abrams GW. Causes of failure after initial vitreoretinal surgery for severe proliferative vitreoretinopathy. *Am J Ophthalmol.* 1991;111:8-14.

49. Lewis H, Aaberg TM. Anterior proliferative vitreoretinopathy. *Am J Ophthalmol.* 1988;105:277-284.

50. Mader TH, Carroll RD, Slade CS, George RK, Ritchey JP, Neville SP. Ocular war injuries of the Iraqi insurgency January-September 2004. *Ophthalmology.* 2006;113:97-104.

51. Thach AB, Johnson AJ, Carroll RB, et al. Severe eye injuries in the War in Iraq, 2003-2005. *Ophthalmology*. 2008;115:377-382.
52. Thach AB, Ward TP, Dick SB II, et al. Intraocular foreign body injuries during Operation Iraqui Freedom. *Ophthalmology*. 2005;112:1829-1833.
53. Woodcock MG, Scott RA, Huntbach J, Kirkby GR. Mass and shape as factors in intraocular foreign body injuries. *Ophthalmology*. 2006;113(12):2262-9.
54. Weiss MJ, Hofeldt AJ, Behrens M, Fisher K. *Retina*. 1997;17:105-108.
55. Colyer HH, Weber ED, Weichel ED, et al. Delayed intraocular foreign body removal without endophthalmitis during Operations Iraqi Freedom and Enduring Freedom. *Ophthalmology*. 2007;114:1439-1447.
56. Finkelstein M, Legmann A, Peter R. Projectile metallic foriegn bodies in the orbit: A retrospective study of epidemiologic factors, management and outcomes. *Ophthalmology*. 1997;104:96-103.
57. Adams JH, Brierley JB, Connor RC, Treip CS. The effects of systemic hypotension upon the human brain. Clinical and neuropathological observations in 11 cases. *Brain*. 1966;89: 235-268.
58. Michaelides M, Riordan-Eva P, Hugkulstone C. Two unusual cases of visual loss following severe non-surgical blood loss. *Eye*. 2002;16:185-189.
59. http://thedonovan.com/archives/2006/03/05-week/
60. Özdal MPÇ, Mansour M, Deschênes J. Ultrasound biomicroscopic evaluation of the traumatized eyes. *Eye*. 2003;17:467-472.
61. Carley SD, Mackway-Jones K. The casualty profile from the Manchester bombing 1996: a proposal for the construction and dissemination of casualty profiles from major incidents. *J Accid Emerg Med*. 1997;14:76-80.
62. Mallonee S, Shariat S, Stennies G, Wax weiler R, Hogan D, Jordan F. Physical injuries and fatalities resulting from the Oklahoma City bombing. *JAMA*. 1996;276:382-387.
63. Thach AB, Ward TP, Hollifield RD, Cockerham K, Birdsong R, Kramer KK. Eye injuries in a terrorist bombing: Dharan, Sudi Arabia. *Ophthalmology 2000*. 1996;107:844-847.

Elements of this chapter have been previously published as Scott R. *The Injured Eye Phil. Trans. R. Soc. B* 2011;366:251-260.

# Maxillofacial Ballistic Injuries

# 27

Andrew Martin Monaghan

## 27.1
## Introduction

Military activity in Afghanistan and Iraq, together with terrorist activity in the UK, has resulted in certain UK centers seeing an increase in casualties with ballistic maxillofacial injuries. In general, it is suggested that military head and neck injuries account for 16% of all battlefield injuries,[1] whereas this area accounts for only 12% of the body surface area. Reviews from Iraq and Afghanistan since 2003 have suggested that head and neck injury rates may now exceed 20% of all casualties.[2] Recent analysis of operative data from a Role 3 Hospital in Afghanistan shows that 19% of all operations on trauma patients were on the head and neck.[3] It is suggested that the proportionate increase is due to the effectiveness of body armor and targeting the head and neck by adversaries. However, analysis of cases evacuated to the Role 4 Hospital in Birmingham, reveals that 61% of injuries are due to explosive devices which are non directional, while only 8% were due to gunshot wounds.[4] A similar pattern has been seen in many conflicts including the Second World War.[5]

The facial skeleton supports the muscles of facial expression, protects the globe and neurovascular structures, and maintains the patency of the upper aerodigestive tract. Clearly, damage to the maxillofacial skeleton will have significant impact on a person's ability to interact and even to maintain life.

An understanding of the effects of trauma to the facial skeleton requires knowledge of the surgical anatomy of the region.[6] The mandible comprises the lower third of the facial skeleton and is essentially a contoured long bone with a horizontal body and a vertical ramus. The outer cortex tends to be thick and surrounds cancellous bone through which runs the inferior dental nerve and vessels. The bone articulates with the base of the skull at the temporomandibular joints through the actions of the masticatory muscles. The mid face consists of the nose ethmoids and orbits, zygomatic complexes, and the maxilla. Unlike the lower face, the mid third is predominantly hollow with a series of vertical

A.M. Monaghan
Maxillofacial Surgery, Royal Centre for Defence Medicine,
University Hospital Birmingham Foundation Trust, Edgbaston, Birmingham, UK
e-mail: andrew.monaghan@uhb.nhs.uk

A.J. Brooks et al. (eds.), *Ryan's Ballistic Trauma*,
DOI: 10.1007/978-1-84882-124-8_27, © Springer-Verlag London Limited 2011

buttresses in the piriform, zygomatic, and pterygoid regions. These are strong in a vertical plane but resist horizontal and penetrating forces relatively poorly. The alveolar process of the mandible and maxilla support the dentition.

Blunt trauma to the facial skeleton tends to produce predictable patterns of fracture. In the mandible, linear fractures at right angle to the bone are produced, while in the maxilla the fractures follow the patterns described by Le Fort in 1901; generally, the higher the impact force, the higher the level of fracture. Soft tissue loss and gross contamination is unusual. In contrast, gunshot or fragment injuries produce a penetrating high energy transfer and blast effect to the tissues. In the limb or torso the missile tends to tumble and yaw imparting large amounts of its energy to the tissue, devitalising muscle and sucking debris and bacteria into the wound. In the mid face there is much less mass but comminution of the fine bones and soft tissue loss can be extensive (Fig. 27.1.). The mandible, being denser, provides more resistance and although comminution occurs the fragments are often larger and bone fragments and avulsed teeth may form secondary fragments (Fig. 27.2.). Fractures caused by blast alone have been described as producing inwardly displaced comminution in the maxilla, and shearing horizontal fractures in the mandible.[7] Fractures of the thin floor and medial wall of the orbit may occur without disruption of the rim; such injuries are described as blow-out fractures. Two mechanisms of blow-out fractures have been described; firstly, direct impact on the globe may produce a pulsion effect leading to increased intraorbital pressure and fracture of the thin floor and/or medial wall[8]; secondly, direct impact on the orbital rim may lead to flexion, rather than fracture but the deformation of the thin floor and roof leads to fracture.[9] Recently, bilateral orbital blow-out fractures have been reported in victims of blast injury where there has been no direct impact on the globe or surrounding orbital rim,[10-12] and such cases have been reported in UK

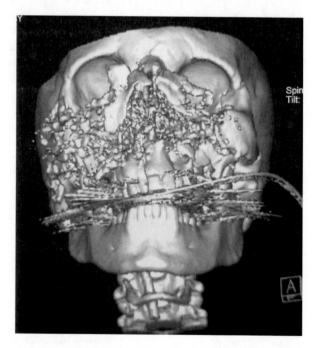

**Fig. 27.1** High velocity injury to the mid-face

**Fig. 27.2** High velocity injury to the mandible

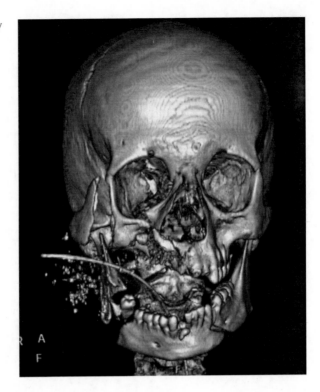

clinical reports from Afghanistan. In our analysis of cases the distribution of facial ballistic fractures is as follows: maxilla 35%; mandible 32%; zygoma/orbit 25%; nose 8%.[4]

Ballistic forces have a much greater effect on soft tissues than blunt trauma. Concurrent cutaneous facial burns are not infrequent. Entry wounds may appear insignificant when compared with the extent of internal soft tissue disruption. The associated soft tissue wounds are heavily contaminated, both at entry and exit, and along the missile tract. In addition, an associated blast effect can produce unseen damage distant from the wound and include vascular structures of not only hard but also soft tissues.[12] These factors should be appreciated if these complex wounds are to be adequately managed.

## 27.2
## Early Care of Patients with Maxillofacial Injuries

### 27.2.1
### Prehospital Care

The aims of early management of casualties with maxillofacial injuries are the preservation of life and to stabilize the patient in preparation for evacuation to a facility providing a higher level of medical care. The principles have been fully developed in ATLS and

BATLS programs. In the last century the greatest advances in survival of such patients were made through improvements in resuscitation and evacuation.

Any patient who has sustained major blunt trauma above the clavicles should be managed as if they have a fractured cervical spine until proven otherwise. Consequently, appropriate precautions must be taken. In unconscious patients with maxillofacial injuries due to blunt trauma the chance incidence of cervical injury has been estimated as 10%.[13] In addition, medical staff should be aware of the risk of concomitant head and or laryngeal injuries. The specific problems of airway control and hemorrhage control in maxillofacial casualties will be discussed further.

Early death in facial ballistic injuries is frequently due to airway obstruction.[14] Airway obstruction may result from a number of factors. Bilateral fractures or comminution of the anterior mandible may lead to poor anterior support for the tongue allowing it to fall back, while maxillary fractures tend to slide back down the skull base, both leading to occlusion of the upper airway, particularly if the patient is supine. The airway may be obstructed by foreign bodies (Fig. 27.3.), fractured teeth and bone fragments, dental prostheses, blood, and secretions. With time oedema will become an increasing problem. In addition, the effect of these factors may be exacerbated by a reduced level of consciousness or airway burns.

Initial management is to clear the airway and give oxygen. A sweep of the finger should remove any solid obstruction in the oral cavity and oropharynx. The airway should be cleared of secretion using suction. If obstruction is due to displaced mandibular or maxillary fragments, these should be pulled forwards, either with a jaw thrust or digital traction

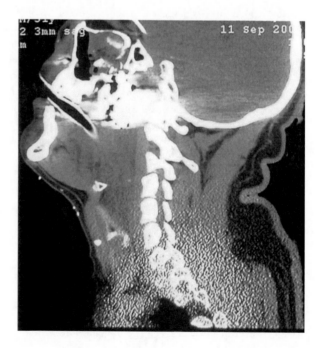

**Fig. 27.3** A large piece of shrapnel which has penetrated the face and lodged in the skull base, leading to upper airway obstruction

on the anterior dental arch. A further maneuver in a posteriorly displaced maxilla is to place a finger behind the hard palate, and again apply traction to pull the fragment forward. The importance of positioning the patient correctly cannot be overestimated in these early stages. There is an old adage that "a patient with facial injuries who is staring to heaven will soon be there." If possible, conscious patients should be sat up leaning forwards, while unconscious or semi conscious patients are best on their sides, or better still prone (Fig. 27.4.). This allows any mobile fragments to fall forwards and any blood or secretions to run from the mouth and not into the airway. In some cases an oral or nasopharyngeal airway may prove a useful adjunct in airway maintenance, if tolerated. In cases where these measures fail, or there is any uncertainty whatsoever about the adequacy of the airway, the patient should be intubated. Cricothyrotomy has an important role in cases where conventional intubation proves impossible. It is recommended that, initially, tracheal intubation tube should be performed rather than a surgical airway under adverse conditions.[15]

Bleeding from the soft tissues of the face and scalp can be profuse. In addition, maxillofacial injuries may produce torrential haemorrhage from inaccessible major vessels, particularly the maxillary and ethmoidal arteries. In the prehospital environment, hemorrhage control is confined to the application of pressure and packing. Scalp wounds can frequently be controlled by repositioning any skin flap and applying a head bandage or placing temporary haemostatic sutures. Digitally reducing a fractured maxilla and applying upward pressure either with a barrel bandage or oral packing may control bleeding. In experienced hands, packing the nose with ribbon gauze or the insertion of proprietary nasal packs (e.g. "Merocel"), together with posterior nasal packs using balloon tamponade with Foley catheters or 'Epistats' can be very effective. Modern battlefield haemostatic agents may be useful in superficial bleeding but, unfortunately, bleeding sources in maxillofacial injuries are often inaccessible. If necessary the whole of the pharynx may be packed to stop deep bleeding; clearly, this is an indication for intubation or tracheostomy.[16] All patients should have intravenous access initiated at an early opportunity and fluid resuscitation commenced.

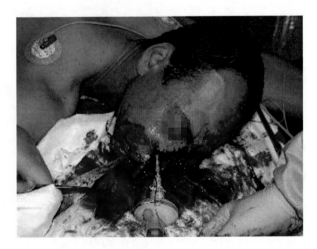

**Fig. 27.4** A patient with a gunshot wound being resuscitated prone. The patient was intubated in this position

## 27.2.2
## Initial Management of the Maxillofacial Wounds at the Field Hospital

Following arrival at a facility providing a higher level of medical care, patients should undergo further reassessment and resuscitation. Patients with maxillofacial injuries who are clinically shocked in the absence of significant hemorrhage, or who are failing to respond to fluid resuscitation should be carefully assessed for hidden injuries in body cavities and limbs. Ballistic injuries can be very disturbing for patients and staff but clinicians should not allow this to distract them from continuing to follow general principles at this stage.

Initially, surgeons should attend to persistent bleeding and provide the patient with a definitive airway. Haemostatic packs may be changed in a more controlled environment and exploration of wounds, with diathermy and ligation of vessels may be undertaken. If uncontrollable life-threatening bleeding occurs, exposure and ligation of the carotid artery and its branches in the neck may be required. If the expertise is available, embolisation is a very effective alternative.

In cases where the airway is compromised by anterior mandibular fracture or comminution, circumfrential interdental wire fixation can produce adequate stabilization until final surgery. A decision will be required on the need for a surgical airway. Data from Vietnam reveals that 17% of facial injuries required tracheostomies,[17] while in a US level 1 trauma center 21% required tracheostomy for civilian gunshot wounds.[18] The indications for tracheostomy in maxillofacial ballistic injuries are as follows[16]:

Obstruction of the airway due to oedema of the tongue (Fig. 27.5.);
Serious and continuing hemorrhage into the tongue base;

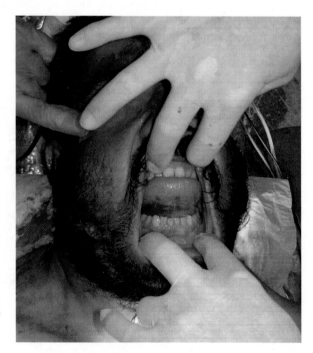

**Fig. 27.5** A high velocity gunshot wound that passed through the mandible and floor of mouth with only small entry and exit wounds. The track can be clearly seen together swelling of the tongue

Risk of secondary infection affecting the upper airway;

Bleeding into the airway requiring packing;

Expectation of multiple general anesthetics as part of treatment;

Aspiration risk;

As required for safe onward evacuation of the patient.

## 27.3
## Management of the Maxillofacial Injury

Ballistic injuries of the facial skeleton provide extreme examples of contaminated compound fractures. The types of wound produced can be described as:

(a) Penetrating: often lower velocity missile; small entry; fragment may be embedded in tissue;

(b) Perforating: often high velocity missile with entrance and exit wounds;

(c) Avulsive: extensive wounds with loss of hard and soft tissue.

Conscious patients should be checked for any neurological deficit of the face and also assessment of vision, globe position, and ocular movements. In addition the tympanic membranes should be examined. Patients should undergo a thorough maxillofacial examination, particularly with regard to steps or mobility of the facial skeleton and disorder of the dental occlusion. Absent teeth should be accounted for to ensure aspiration of fragments has not occurred and checked by chest radiograph. Patients with mid-face injuries should be carefully examined for cerebrospinal rhinorrhoea, indicating an anterior skull base fracture. If available, a head and neck CT should be undertaken. 3 day reconstructions of the facial skeleton simplify the assessment of the bony injuries and aid later surgical planning. Alternatively, a facial and skull radiographic series should be taken.

Previous military conflicts have taught us that ballistic injuries should be managed by thorough irrigation and debridement, leaving wounds open, and, delayed primary closure. In facial wounds, every effort should be made to preserve as much hard and soft tissue as possible. As long ago as the nineteenth century, the Confederate Army Manual of Military Surgery suggested that in maxillofacial trauma no fragments of tooth or bone should be removed unless contamination was great or the fragment completely detached.[19] Consequently, wound management should include thorough irrigation of contaminated tissues; soft tissues with dirty wound edges should be scrubbed to prevent later tattooing. Foreign bodies (if accessible) and detached bone fragments and teeth should also be removed. Periosteal stripping should not be undertaken. Any tissue defects should be packed. Attempts should be made to identify branches of the facial nerve and the salivary ducts; these should be marked with a suture for repair when the wound is clean. Early maxillofacial war surgeons feared secondary infection due to wound infection.[20] Antibiotic therapy has been shown to reduce later wound infection and should be instituted at an early opportunity[12] but should not influence the thoroughness of mechanical cleaning.

Heavily contaminated wounds may require serial debridement and packing.[21] However, experience has shown that in the maxillofacial region, with its excellent blood supply and lack of bulky soft tissue, early definitive soft tissue closure may be undertaken in less contaminated wounds.[22] Soft tissue primary closure should be tension free, and, if uncertainty exists about the health of the tissues, drainage should be instituted.

Where definitive treatment has to be delayed, stabilization of the bone fragments by a combination of interdental wiring, or intermaxillary fixation (IMF) screws[23] or conventional IMF, and external fixation will improve patient's pain control and maintain alignment of the main fragments. Clearly, nasotracheal intubation would normally be required if IMF is placed.

Clearly, the definitive management of ballistic maxillofacial wounds is complex and it is inappropriate for them to be definitively treated by the occasional operator. Defect fractures, in particular, require a mulitidiscilinary approach to care which can only be adequately provided in a specialist center. In particular, speech and language therapy, dietetics, and psychological support are important. However, the importance of the early attention to the wound by the attending surgeons at the previous medical facilities cannot be underestimated, with significant improvement in the condition of the tissues for subsequent reconstruction and the reduction in the incidence of infection and risk of later scarring and contracture. Although a comprehensive discussion of the techniques used in the management of these injuries is outside the scope of this chapter, the basic strategies and principles will be discussed further.

As in the peripheral skeleton, older, traditional methods of maxillofacial fracture fixation used closed methods of reduction and subsequent immobilization. Techniques such as IMF, direct wire osteosynthesis, and external fixation were the standard practice. Over the last few decades open reduction and internal fixation of fractures with plates and screws has become contemporary practice. Techniques have evolved with improved materials and equipment, and a better understanding of the functional anatomy of the facial skeleton and access incisions. In conventional injuries, these open techniques produce anatomical reduction, improved patient function, and less secondary deformity. Much of the work on plate placement in the mandible was done by Champey et al.[24] They described an upper tension zone and a lower compression zone on the mandible which directs strategic plate placement to provide not only fixation, but also allow functional forces to apply compression to the lower border of the mandible. In essence, in uncomplicated fractures, 2 mm plates are required anterior to the mental foramen while one will suffice at the upper tension band more proximally. The success of this approach depends on the fracture bone ends taking some of the functional load. However, in defect or comminuted fractures more robust fixation is required. Access to the mandible is frequently through intra oral incisions at the buccal and labial sulcus. Extra oral incisions are frequently not necessary in uncomplicated fractures. Clearly, in ballistic injuries, lacerations may be utilized as access points.

In the maxilla, the surgical access depends on the level of the fracture. In low level injuries, a horseshoe incision in the upper labial sulcus will suffice. Higher level fractures will require a combination of infraorbital and zygomatic buttress incisions. Access incision around the face should be as cosmetic as possible (large soft tissue loss of the face should not be an excuse for less than optimal surgical technique in other areas) and many clinicians now utilize upper blephoroplasty and transconjunctival approaches. In injuries involving the nasoethmoid complex, frontal sinus, a bicoronal flap gives the optimum access. It also allows access for neurosurgical dural repair in anterior skull base fractures and the harvest of calvarial bone for grafting of the orbits or maxillary buttresses when required. Accurate reduction is guided by the dental occlusion and direct visualization of the fractures at the buttresses. In panfacial fractures it is usually wise to repair the mandible first giving a guide to vertical height of the posterior face and the form of the dental arch. It is important that the reduced maxilla reconstitutes the width, anterior projection, and vertical height of the maxilla if the original facial form is to be created. Miniplates used in the maxilla vary from 1–2 mm depending on the load put upon them and are placed on the buttresses, orbital rims, and zygomatic arches as required.

It has been suggested that all fixation will eventually fail and that fixation is "a race between bone healing and fixation failure." We must, therefore choose fixation that provides adequate stability without over-engineering, particularly if the required extra surgical access risks unnecessary scars on the face. Failures are often due to poor assessment and incorrect treatment rather than failure of hardware.[25] The compromised state of the hard and soft tissues in ballistic injuries compared with conventional blunt trauma must be appreciated if reconstruction is to be successful. In addition, in many ballistic injuries the fractures are often comminuted and of an unusual pattern, making miniplate osteosynthesis more difficult. The excess periosteal stripping required to expose and plate these bony injuries adequately risks devitalisation of bone fragments and their subsequent loss.

Figure 27.6 shows the patient at Fig. 27.1, demonstrating the use of a combination of fixation by miniplate osteosyntheis to the larger fragments on the left side of the maxilla with an external Levant Frame providing craniomaxillary fixation to support the comminuted right side. Note the bicoronal incision to access the displaced nasoethmoidal area. Similarly, Fig. 27.7 shows a high velocity gunshot wound of the mandible showing how external fixation can produce adequate fixation without the need for degloving the comminuted bone (Fig. 27.8). Note the small entry wound in the lip and the use of drainage in the debrided exit wound in the completed case. If required, fixation may be supplemented by IMF.

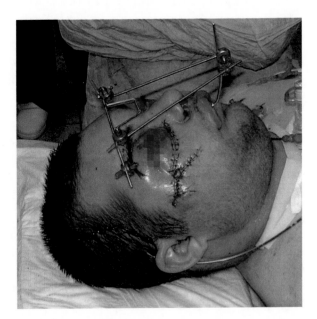

**Fig. 27.6** Fixation of comminited mid-face injury by combination of internal and external fixation to reduce periosteal stripping

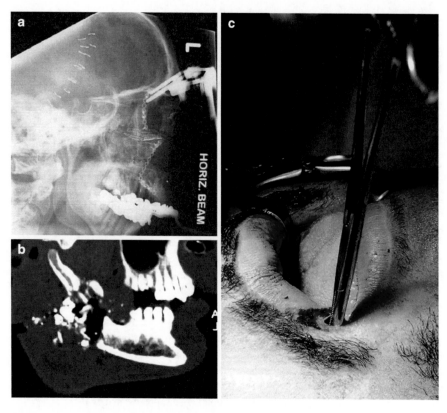

**Fig. 27.7** (**a–c**) Extensive comminution of the mandible in high velocity injury. Note the small entry wound

Avulsive high velocity injuries with loss of large amounts of tissue provide a considerable reconstructive challenge. Many of the techniques have been adapted from the management of defects produced following resection of head and neck malignancies. Authors have discussed the importance of early definitive reconstruction in these ballistic injuries to reduce the risk of contracture distorting the residual soft tissues.[26] However, before embarking on complex forms of reconstruction it is vital to ensure that the remaining tissue bed is free from infection and well vascularised. In particular, where microvascular reconstruction is being used, the presence and patency of residual vessels should be known. It has been demonstrated that ballistic injury in vessels may occur some distance from the obvious wound edges.[27] Where uncertainty exists, angiography or other assessment of the vascular anatomy should be performed.

Every ballistic wound will differ in site and constituent tissue loss. In principle, reconstruction will aim to obliterate any defect with tissues as similar to the original as possible together with producing a functional and aesthetic result. The reconstructive surgeon should have a variety of options available to them so the most appropriate tissue is transferred to close the defect.

**Fig. 27.8** The case at Fig. 27.7 stabilized by an external fixator

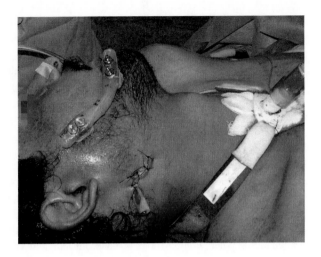

Small areas of soft tissue may be reconstructed by local advancement or rotation flaps. In the past, larger defects were filled by pedicled flaps such as the forehead and axial pectoralis major flaps. These are now less frequently used, being replaced by free tissue transfer. It is worth noting that the pectoralis major is still useful in salvage situations and variations of the forehead flap are a good option for the reconstruction of the dorsum and tip of the nose. The most favored free fascio-cutaenous flaps in our unit include the radial forearm, lateral thigh and, in cases where more bulk is required or multiple paddles, the soft tissue scapula flap.

Defects in the lips produce not only an aesthetic and articulation problems, but are clearly functionally important. Failure to recreate the oral sphincter will affect feeding and, also, incompetence of the lips will lead to drooling. If the commisure is present, every effort should be made retain it as it is impossible to adequately reconstruct. Defects of the upper or lower lips of up to one third may be closed primarily in three layers (mucosa, muscle, and skin) with care to correctly align the vermillion border. Primary closure of larger defects will be under a great deal of tension and prone to dehiscence; also, if the repair does heal there will be a risk of microstomia which can affect later feeding and access for dental rehabilitation. Central upper lip loss can be effectively reconstructed an Abbe flap with rotation of the central part of the lower lip as a pedicled flap; this is extremely good for philtrum reconstruction. Advancement of the remaining upper lip tissue can be improved by crescentic incisions around the lateral part of the nose, allowing further advancement. Large lateral defects may be closed by similar lateral cross lip pedicled flaps. Release of the pedicle is usually at 2–3 weeks subject to the satisfactory appearance of the tissue. Where the commisure is lost the Estlander lateral lip switch flap with a secondary commisuroplasty procedure can be effective. For larger defects, or cases where both lips are affected, various rotation and advancement flaps have been described.[28,29] Where the lip is totally lost a folded free radial forearm flap supported by the palmaris longus tendon,[30] harvested from the same donor site, will allow creation of an oral seal when apposed by the other lip but, clearly, will lack any muscular function and lack the skin match of local tissue.

Bone loss may be replaced by either free or vascularised autogenous grafts. The use of free calvarial bone in the mid face buttresses and orbit has been mentioned previously; free rib is an alternative but is more prone to resorbtion.[31] In the mandible, free iliac crest provides the necessary volume of bone required and is a viable option if the soft tissue bed is good and soft tissue cover available. Vascularised free bone flaps include direct circumflex iliac artery (DCIA) flap, scapula flap, and fibula flap. Each has its advantages, with the DCIA and scapula flaps providing better bone height and are excellent options for both maxillary and mandibular reconstruction, while the fibula provides greater length. All are suitable for implant placement for dental or prosthetic rehabilitation. It is important that grafts are covered by healthy tissue if they are to remain viable. The three flaps discussed can be raised with associated muscle to cover them intraorally, which will later become epithelialised. Where combinations of bone, muscle, and skin are required these can be raised as a single composite flap, particularly in the scapula, giving them great versatility. A reconstruction using free tissue transfer is shown at Fig. 27.9.

Unfortunately, reconstruction of maxillofacial blast injuries may require multiple surgical procedures over months or years. Unfortunately, scar fibrosis and contracture can be increasingly problematic. In later reconstruction, distraction osteogenesis has been successfully used for mandibular reconstruction,[32] including in our own unit. It has the advantage of no donor site being required. In addition, local soft tissue may be increased by the use of balloon expansion.

Techniques for autogenous reconstruction of complex facial units such as the ear[33] and nose[34,35] have been developed but are technically very challenging, multi-stage procedures. In skilled hands they can produce cosmetically good results and have the advantage that they are produced from the patients own tissue and should require little maintenance.

Alloplastic (prosthetic) reconstruction has an important part to play in the management of avulsive ballistic injuries. Although it is possible to recreate the majority of tissues of the

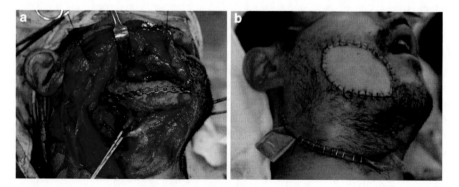

**Fig. 27.9 (a, b)** A large high velocity avulsion injury treated by an iliac crest bone graft and lateral thigh flap. Note the facial artery isolated for anastomosis

face using autogenous tissue, the complexities of the ear, nose, and orbit can often lead the final results to be aesthetically inferior to a specially made prosthesis. In addition, the surgical burden on the patient is often less. However, it may be that free tissue transfer will still be required as a successful prosthesis must be supported by adequate hard and soft tissue if it is to be stable and well retained. Osseointegrated implants have revolutionized alloplastic reconstruction (35%). An implant retained nasal prosthesis is shown at Fig. 27.10. The prosthetic nose is supported by long zygomaticus and conventional osseointegrated implants. The skilful maxillofacial technician is able to produce an almost identical match of the lost tissue from comparison with the opposite ear or orbit, or from old photographs. Patients are often provided with prostheses with differing skin tints to account for tanning of the surrounding skin during summer. Implants require meticulous cleaning by patients and proper maintenance if they are to be viable in the long term. Success rates from our unit for the various prostheses are between 75 and 95% depending on site.

A further important application of prostheses is the obturation persistent fistulae between the oral cavity and nose. Once again these may be implant retained or supported and retained by the local tissues and dentition. Finally, the patient should undergo comprehensive dental rehabilitation.

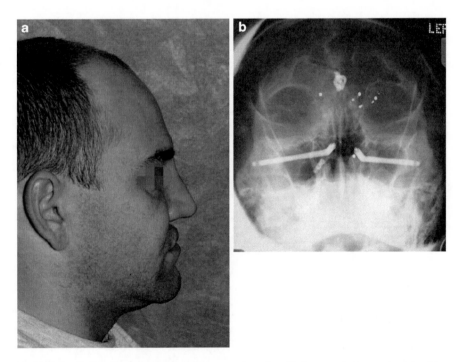

**Fig. 27.10** (**a, b**) Total alloplastic nasal reconstruction of amid face gunshot wound retained by titanium osseointegrated implants

## 27.4
## Summary

The early stages of care of patients with ballistic maxillofacial injuries treatment priorities are aimed at the preservation of life. Subsequently, measures to prevent infection of the wound and production of healthy residual tissues with retention of as much of remaining tissue as possible should be the ultimate goal. Definitive treatment is complex, highly specialized, is often multistage, and requires a multidisciplinary approach to care, which often includes dietetic, speech and language, and psychological support. An overall summary of the maxillofacial management is a follows:

### 27.4.1
### Initial Care

Copious irrigation and debridement with preservation of tissue where possible
Reposition & fixation of main bone fragments
Soft tissue closure and bone coverage
Drainage

### 27.4.2
### Reconstructive Phase

Secondary bony reconstruction
Soft tissue reconstruction including tissue transfer
Correction of any secondary deformity
Prosthetic rehabilitation
Definitive treatment aims to produce a functional result, which is aesthetically and socially acceptable.

**Acknowledgments**   I am grateful to my maxillofacial colleagues at the University Hospital Birmingham Foundation Trust for their help in the management of military casualties with ballistic injuries, particularly to Mr. Ian Sharp and Mr. Tim Martin for the use of their cases in this chapter.

## References

1. Pilcher R. Management of missile wounds of the maxillofacial region during the 20th century. *Injury*. 1996;27:81-88.
2. Xydakis MS, Fravell MD, Casler JD. Analysis of battlefield head and neck injuries in Iraq and Afghanistan. *Otolaryngol Head Neck Surg*. 1995;133:497-504.

3. Breeze J, Monaghan AM, Williams MD, Clark RNW, Gibbons AJ. Five Months of Surgery in the Multinational Field Hospital in Afghanistan with an Emphasis on Maxillofacial Injuries. In print.

4. Opie N, Breeze J, Gibbons AJ, Monaghan A. Military Maxillofacial Injuries Treated at the Royal Centre for Defence Medicine: June 2001 to December 2007. In print.

5. Porritt A. *The Treatment of War Wounds, History of the Second World War (Surgery). 16.* London: HMSO; 1993.

6. Dover MS. Pathophysiology of maxillofacial trauma. In: Alpar KE, Gosling P, eds. *Trauma, a Scientific Basis for Care.* Bath: Arnold; 1998.

7. Shuker ST. Maxillofacial blast injuries. *J Craniomaxillofac Surg.* 1995;23:91-98.

8. Smith B, Reagan WF. Blow-out fracture of the orbit. Mechanism and correction of internal orbital fracture. *Am J Ophthalmol.* 1957;44:733-739.

9. Fujino T, Makino K. Entrapment mechanisms and ocular injury in orbital blowout fractures. *Keio J Med.* 1980;23:115-124.

10. Agir H, Ustundag E, Iscen D. Bilateral isolated orbital blowout fractures among terrorist bombing victims. A very rare entity. *J Plast Reconstr Aesthet Surg.* 2006;59:306-307.

11. Shamir D, Ardekian L, Peled M. Blowout fracture of the orbit as a result of blast injury: case report of a unique entity. *J Oral Maxillofac Surg.* 2008;66:1496-1498.

12. Reed B, Hale RG, Gliddon M, Ericson M. Maximising outcomes for maxillofacial injuries from improvised explosive devices by deployed health care personnel. *ADF Health.* 2008; 9:1-8.

13. Gibbons AJ, Patton DW. Ballistic Injuries of the Face and Mouth in war and Civil Conflict. *Dent Update.* 2003;30:272-278.

14. Demetriades D, Calwan S, Gomez H, Falloballa A, Velmahos G, Yamashita D. *J Trauma.* 1998;45:39-41.

15. Gray RL, Coppel DL. Surgery of violence: III Intensive care patients with bomb blast and gunshot injuries. *Br Med J.* 1975;i:502.

16. Banks P. Gunshot wounds. In: Rowe NL, Williams JL, eds. *Maxillofacial Injuries.* Great Britain: Curchill Livingstone; 1985.

17. Terry BC. Facial injuries in military combat: definitive care. *J Oral Surg.* 1969;27:551.

18. Hollier L, Grantcharova EP, Kattash M. Facial gunshot wounds: a 4-year experience. *J Oral Maxillofac Surg.* 2001;59:277-282.

19. Rowe NL. The history of the treatment of maxillofacial trauma. *Ann R Coll Surg Engl.* 1971;49:329.

20. Kazanjian VH, Burrows H. The treatment of haemorrhage caused by gunshot wounds of the face and jaws. *Br J Surg.* 1918;5:126.

21. Robertson BC, Manson PN. High-energy ballistic and avulsive injuries. A management protocol for the next millennium. *Surg Clin North Am.* 1999;79:1489-1502.

22. Brickler EM. Plastic Surgery: Surgery in World War II. Vol. 2. US Govt Print Off; 1955.

23. Gibbons AJ, Baden JM, Monaghan AM, Dhariwal DK, Hodder SC. A drill-free bone screw for intermaxillary fixation in military casualties. *J R Army Med Corps.* 2003;149:30-32.

24. Champey M, Pape H-D, Gerlach KL, Lodde JP. Mandibular fractures. In: Kruger E, Schilli W, eds. *Oral and Maxillofacial Traumatology.* Berlin: Springer; 1998.

25. Schilli W, Stoll P, Bahr W, Prein J. Mandibular fractures. In: Prein J, ed. *Manual of Internal Fixation in the Cranio-Facial Skeleton.* Berin: Springer; 1998.

26. Eppeley BL, Coleman JJ. Reconstruction of large hard and soft tissue defects of the face. In: Ward Booth P, Eppeley B, Schmeltzeisen R, eds. *Maxillofacial trauma and Esthetic Reconstruction.* Churchill Livingstone: Elsevier; 2003.

27. Tan YH, Zhous S, Liu Y, et al. Small vessel pathology and anastomosis following maxillofacial firearm wounds: an experiment study. *J Oral Maxillofac Surg.* 1991;49:348-352.

28. Karapandzic M. Reconstruction of lip defects by local arterial flaps. *Br J Plast Surg.* 1974;27:93-97.
29. Gillies HD, Millard DR. *The Principles and Art of Plastic Surgery.* Boston: Little Brown; 1957.
30. Jeng SF, Kuo YR, Wei FC, Su CY, Chien CY. Total lower lip reconstruction with a composite radial forearm-palmaris longus tendon flap: a clinical series. *Plast Reconstr Surg.* 2004;113:19-23.
31. Antonyshyn O, Gruss JS, Galbraith DJ, Hurwitz JJ. Complex orbital fractures: a critical analysis of immediate bone graft reconstruction. *Ann Plast Surg.* 1989;22:220-233. discussion 234-5.
32. Shvyrkov MB, Shamsudinov AKh, Sumarokov DD, Shvyrkova II. Non-free osteoplasty of the mandible in maxillofacial gunshot wounds: mandibular reconstruction by compression-osteodistraction. *Br J Oral Maxillofac Surg.* 1999;37:261-267.
33. Nagata S. Total auricular reconstruction with a three-dimensional costal cartilage framework. *Ann Chir Plast Esthét.* 1995;40:371-399.
34. Burget GC, Walton RL. Optimal use of microvascular free flaps, cartilage grafts, and a paramedian forehead flap for aesthetic reconstruction of the nose and adjacent facial units. *Plast Reconstr Surg.* 2007;120:1171-1207.
35. Neukan FW, Girod SC. Reconstruction after tumour ablation; extraoral implants. In: Ward Booth P, Schendel SA, Hausamen J-E, eds. *Maxillofacial Surgery.* New York: Churchill Livingstone; 1999:785-801.

# Neck Injury

28

Matthew J. Borkon and Bryan A. Cotton

## 28.1
## Introduction

"Go for the throat!" "He went straight for the jugular." Such colloquialisms demonstrate even the layperson's appreciation for the vulnerability of the neck. The management of a firearm injury to this area requires an understanding of the trajectory, wound location, and a thorough three-dimensional understanding of the relevant anatomy.[1] Over the last 20 years, trauma surgeons have embraced selective, non-operative management and damage control principles to the severely injured patient. With these new approaches have come dramatic changes in the management algorithms for penetrating neck injuries as well. Prior to this time, mandatory exploration for penetrating neck injuries was deemed standard of care.[2] In the early 1980s, high volume institutions, with considerable experience in firearm injuries, began reporting the selective, non-operative management of patients with Zone II wounds presenting without evidence of vascular or aero-digestive injuries.[3] Several studies over the last decade supported the non-operative approach of these patients after an appropriate diagnostic evaluation had excluded injury.[4,5] More recently, some authors have applied this approach to Zone I as well.[6] With continually improving advances in technology such as helical computerized tomography (CT) and interventional radiology (IR), there exist many options for dealing with specific injuries to the neck.

## 28.2
## Anatomy

The neck contains numerous vital structures in a relatively small area. A surgeon who ventures into this area, whether electively or in a crisis, should have a solid and thorough knowledge of head, neck, and chest anatomy. The central nervous system passes through

B.A. Cotton (✉)
Department of Surgery and Center for Translational Injury Research,
University of Texas Health Science Center, Houston, Texas, USA

A.J. Brooks et al. (eds.), *Ryan's Ballistic Trauma*,
DOI: 10.1007/978-1-84882-124-8_28, © Springer-Verlag London Limited 2011

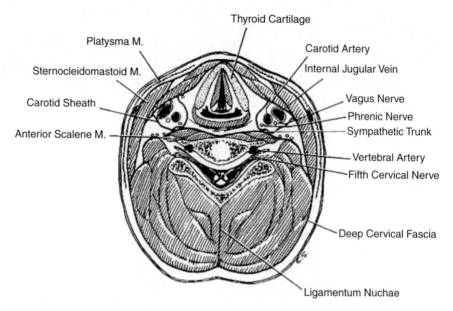

**Fig. 28.1** Operative anatomy of the deep neck space is shown in this illustration (From Ward[7] with permission)

the neck along the protected course of the spinal column, whereas the sympathetic chain, several cranial nerves, and the vagus nerve and its branches remain relatively unprotected. The digestive system, represented by the hypopharynx and the esophagus, are located posteriorly in the neck, lying just anterior to the spinal column (Fig. 28.1). The trachea begins just below the epiglottis at the level of the fifth cervical vertebra. The most vulnerable of all organ systems in the cervical area are the vascular structures. The jugular vessels include the anterior, external, and internal veins. Compared to their arterial counterparts, they lie slightly more superficial in the case of the anterior and external, and more lateral in the case of the internal. The course of the arterial vessels begins at the base of the neck with the aortic arch and its branches. As the common carotid arteries near the thyroid and the hypopharynx, they divide into the internal and external carotid arteries. In addition to the above organ systems, the endocrine system (thyroid and parathyroids) and the skeletal system (cervical vertebrae) are represented.

The classic system of dividing the neck into zones was based on identifying the anatomic region of injury and the appropriate set of diagnostic modalities necessary to evaluate and exclude an injury in that particular area. The most common classification system divides the neck into three zones anterior to the lateral border of the sternocleidomastoid muscle (Fig. 28.2). Zone I begins with the thoracic outlet and clavicles and ends at the cricoid cartilage. Zone II encompasses the area between the cricoid and the angle of the mandible. Zone III contains structures from the angle of the mandible to the base of the skull. More recently, these zones have been utilized as a guide as to the best operative approach to obtain vascular control and exposure for any given cervical wound.

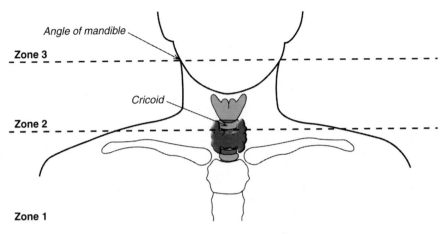

**Fig. 28.2** The neck typically is divided into three zones of injury. Each zone has preferred diagnostic and therapeutic approaches

## 28.3
## Initial Assessment and Management

Despite recent diagnostic and surgical advances, the mortality of firearm injuries to the neck is still greater than 10%. Patients with obvious active bleeding, expanding hematoma, or airway compromise are taken immediately to the operating room for exploration. Patients without these "hard" signs can be managed with appropriate trajectory guided diagnostic studies. Some centers rely solely on the physical exam to guide their decisions for operative or non-operative management, whereas others will employ a cadre of diagnostic tests to definitively exclude injuries to the structures within the neck.[9-12]

### 28.3.1
### Patients Requiring Immediate Exploration

Patients who are hemodynamically unstable from firearm injuries to the neck should be promptly explored in the operating room once a rapid initial assessment is completed and the airway is secured. Nearly 25% of patients with penetrating neck injuries will require urgent intubation.[13] The intubation can be complicated by the associated expanding neck hematoma, laryngotracheal injury, and suspicion of an associated cervical spine injury. Early intubation is the key to control of a situation that can quickly deteriorate into multiple unsuccessful intubation attempts and extremely difficult cricothyroidotomy, often spiraling into anoxia and death. The most experienced person available should be designated for control of the airway.

The patient's Glasgow Coma Scale (GCS) and a brief neurological exam should be quickly obtained and documented. This should be done as early as possible before any sedation or chemical paralysis prevents obtaining an adequate examination. The ability (or inability) of the patient to speak or move his extremities should be assessed and documented as it may later influence the operative management of a vascular injury. As opposed to patients injured by blunt trauma, firearm injuries are more likely to be associated with spinal cord injury. In addition to being a younger population, these patients are more likely to suffer complete spinal cord injury with subsequent paraplegia or tetraplegia than their blunt counterparts.[14]

The existence of cervical spine instability from a firearm injury in a patient who is neurologically intact has been challenged by numerous authors.[15-17] Cervical spine immobilization in this population is equally controversial. The "standard of care" for immobilization of the cervical spine following blunt injury has been extrapolated to the patient with penetrating injury to the neck without any evidence of benefit. The disadvantage of having a collar in place is that life-threatening injuries such as expanding neck hematomas may be overlooked. Barkana and colleagues attributed 22% of deaths in their study to these "overlooked" life-threatening injuries.[17] The authors reviewed all Israeli army soldiers who sustained penetrating neck injuries over a 4 year period. All patients were transported to a trauma center will full cervical spine immobilization. The incidence of cervical spine column injury was approximately 2%, with only 1% of patients having actual spinal cord injury. They found no survivable injury that would have benefited from spine immobilization. This is consistent with the findings of Arishita who evaluated over 4,000 cases of penetrating neck sustained in the Vietnam War.[16] These authors noted that less than 2% of patients with cervical spinal column involvement "might" have benefited from immobilization. They concluded as well that cervical spine immobilization in penetrating neck trauma is "neither prudent nor practical." A recent review by Brywczynski and colleagues noted that the incidence of unstable cervical spine injuries is low and the risks of obscuring an expanding neck hematoma or other hard signs of injury with a cervical collar in the prehospital setting might outweigh the potential benefits of spinal immobilization.[18]

Physical findings such as an expanding neck hematoma, active or pulsatile bleeding, bruit, lateralizing neurological signs, stridor, or obvious laryngo-tracheal injury are considered "hard" signs. These findings are suggestive of major or life-threatening injury and these patients require immediate operative intervention. Active bleeding, if encountered, should be controlled with digital pressure. This should be continued throughout the skin preparation and until proximal and distal control is obtained. Wounds should not be probed, cannulated, or locally explored. These maneuvers can dislodge clot and lead to uncontrolled hemorrhage or embolism. A chest radiograph may demonstrate a life-threatening issue (or cause for the patient's instability) that should be addressed prior to transport to the operating room (i.e., pneumothorax, hemothorax, tracheal deviation, trajectory into the chest).

## 28.3.2
### Patients Requiring Further Diagnostic Evaluation

"Soft" signs include hematemesis, hemoptysis, hoarseness or change in voice, dysphagia, or odynophagia. In the stable patient, these signs mandate further evaluation and exclusion of vascular and aero-digestive injury. Prior to considering non-operative or selective management on a patient with penetrating neck trauma, one must consider the diagnostic modalities that are available and what degree of reliability can be placed on each of them. The initial management of this group of patients should proceed in a similar fashion to that of the unstable patient. Although the sense of urgency may not appear as obvious, these patients have the potential for rapid deterioration and early control of the airway is essential.

## 28.4
## Vascular Evaluation

### 28.4.1
### Physical Examination

In the neck, evaluation of the vascular system begins with a rapid search for pulsatile bleeding, expanding hematomas, and bruits. Once the absence of "hard" signs is noted, vascular assessment of these patients proceeds to an examination for any neurological deficits. The GCS, presence or absence of lateralizing signs, and cranial nerve function should be documented. Neurological deficits that follow a distribution of the carotid vessels (hemiplegia, aphasia, etc.) warrant immediate exploration if the area of injury is surgically accessible. Full exposure of the patient should follow with immobilization of the neck during the course of the log roll. All wounds noted anteriorly should be noted and marked with a radio-opaque marker (e.g., paper clip) prior to rolling the patient (Fig. 28.3). All posterior wounds should also be documented and marked in a similar fashion. The marking of these wounds will aid in trajectory determination on plain radiographs.

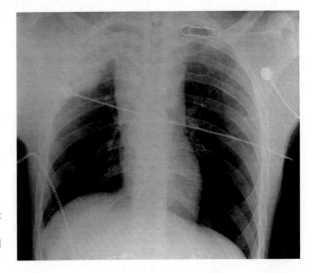

**Fig. 28.3** A chest radiograph in a patient with a gunshot wound to the base of the neck. The paperclip marks the surface wound on the anterior chest. Notice the large pleural cap on the right side as a result of hemorrhage from a proximal right common carotid injury

In the absence of "hard" or "soft" signs of vascular injury, several authors have concluded that penetrating injuries limited to Zone II can be safely triaged by physical exam alone.[5,6,10,11] Atteberry and colleagues evaluated 28 patients without signs of vascular injury and with wounds limited to Zone II.[4] They concluded that physical examination alone was safe and accurate in evaluating this patient population. In a follow-up study from the same institution, Sekharan and colleagues examined 145 patients.[19] Of these, 91 patients had no signs of vascular injury and were observed for 23 h without further diagnostic evaluation. Physical examination had a false-negative rate of 0.7%. The authors concluded that these results were comparable to that of angiography and were much less invasive or costly. However, their follow-up was limited to 2 weeks post-injury. Insull and colleagues conducted a retrospective review of 66 patients with Zone II injuries.[11] In this study, they demonstrated an overall positive neck exploration rate of 25%. 15 of these patients had hard signs of significant injury. Physical examination had a sensitivity of 93% and a positive predictive value of 87%.

In support of the findings of Frykberg and colleagues, both Biffl and Beitsch concluded that asymptomatic patients with Zone II neck injuries could be observed with less than a 1% chance of a missed injury.[9,10] Beitsch and colleagues retrospectively evaluated 178 patients with Zone II injuries, all of which had undergone angiography and operative exploration.[9] Biffl and colleagues extended their policy to Zone III, but continued to recommend that Zone I injuries should receive an arteriogram.[10] Jarvick and colleagues noted physical examination to have 94% sensitivity for detecting all vascular injuries.[12] However, when only considering those injuries that required intervention, sensitivity improved to 100%. In addition, they calculated the cost of using angiography as a screening tool for identifying vascular injury in patients with normal clinical findings. The authors noted the cost to be over three million dollars per central nervous system event prevented.

The Zone I Penetrating Neck Injury Study Group recently published results regarding whether routine angiography is necessary for penetrating injuries to this area of the neck.[20] Eddy and colleagues recently reported the results of a study of five level one trauma centers that examined all Zone I injuries over a 10 year period.[13] They found no arterial injuries in patients with a normal physical examination and normal chest radiograph. With some caution, the authors concluded that this subgroup of patients can be safely managed without angiography.

## 28.4.2
## Angiography

Angiography remains the gold standard for evaluating and excluding arterial injury.[21] Angiography can provide invaluable information in the evaluation and exclusion of injury. In addition, angiography can help in planning the operative approach in the patient with more than one zone involved. In evaluating the patient with penetrating neck injury, an adequate angiogram should visualize the innominate artery, the common, internal, and external carotid arteries, the subclavian arteries, and both vertebral arteries as well. A complete angiogram should also include visualization of the inferior thyroid artery off the cervical trunk.[22]

Zone I and III injuries have traditionally been investigated with angiography because of the greater difficulty of operative exposure relative to Zone II. In fact, as early as 1985, Sclafani and colleagues concluded that angiography is essential in Zone III neck injuries.[21] They cited the ability to facilitate triage decisions and, with the use of various interventional techniques, treat the majority of Zone III injuries without surgical exploration. Until recently, the majority of trauma centers recommend a policy of routine angiography to screen for vascular injury and to minimize non-therapeutic neck explorations.[23] Angiography, however, is an invasive and costly procedure with a yield in most centers of less than 2%.[6]

### 28.4.3
### Computerized Tomographic Angiography (CTA)

With dramatic improvements in image quality and advances in software, helical CT has rapidly gained acceptance in approaching various types of injury mechanisms. Computerized Tomographic Angiography (CTA) is performed using a helical CT scanner (Fig. 28.4). Approximately 100 ml of contrast is injected and the data is acquired after a brief delay of 10–15 s. The data is then reconstructed with 1–3 mm intervals. Munera noted CTA to be a safe alternative to conventional angiography in patients with penetrating neck injuries.[24] The authors conducted a prospective study over 24 months in patients with penetrating neck trauma who were referred for conventional angiography. They found CTA to have a high sensitivity and specificity for detecting major carotid and vertebral arterial injuries from penetrating trauma. CTA had a 100% positive predictive value and a negative predictive value of 98% compared to conventional angiography. In 2002, a study from the same institution found similar results and concluded that CTA could be used as the initial method of evaluation and that conventional angiography could be reserved for those patients with equivocal studies.[25]

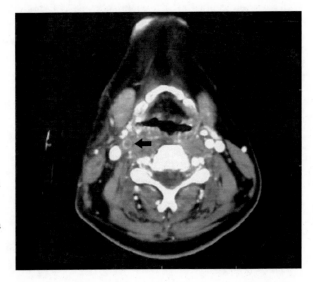

**Fig. 28.4** A CT angiogram image of the neck in a patient with a stab wound. In this case, a right carotid thrombosis (associated with a dissection) can be seen as a filling defect within the lumen of the vessel (*black arrow*)

Other authors have also investigated the role of CTA as a safe and accurate alternative to conventional angiography.[26,27] Ofer and colleagues noted that all CTA obtained were diagnostic and confirmed their findings on surgical exploration.[26] The authors concluded CTA of the carotid arteries may be used as an accurate decisive tool for a needed surgical intervention. This is supported by Stuhlfaut and colleagues who concluded that CTA "allows appropriate triage of patients to conventional angiography or surgery for the appropriate treatment and can guide conservative management when appropriate."[27]

Brywczynski and colleagues advocated that patients with penetrating neck trauma who are hemodynamically stable and exhibit no hard signs of vascular injury may be initially evaluated by MDCT (multi-detector computed tomographic) imaging, even in the presence of platysma violation.[18]

## 28.4.4
### Color-Flow Doppler (CFD)

In the early 1990s, CFD began replacing angiography in the evaluation of atherosclerotic carotid artery disease. Shortly thereafter, Fry and colleagues reported their results on the application of CFD to traumatic carotid injuries.[20] Their prospective study of 100 patients found no false positives or false negatives. They concluded that CFD was as accurate as conventional angiography in diagnosing cervical vascular injuries. These recommendations, however, were based on only eight cervical vascular injuries. Corr and colleagues reported similar findings and made recommendations for utilizing CFD to screen for injury.[28] Their study had only 25 patients and 10 vascular injuries. Montalvo and colleagues were more cautious in their recommendations of CFD replacing angiography in penetrating neck injuries.[29] They evaluated 52 patients prospectively with CFD and compared their findings with angiography or surgery. CFD detected all serious injuries of the carotid arteries and all injuries of the vertebral arteries. Their study was also limited by size with only ten injuries total. Demetriades and colleagues evaluated several diagnostic modalities among a group of 223 patients.[30] After excluding patients with injuries that did not require intervention, CFD had a sensitivity and specificity of 100%. They estimated the financial impact of developing an algorithm based on their findings and noted the cost of evaluating penetrating neck injuries would decrease from 450,000 to 30,000 US dollars. Although CFD is inexpensive and noninvasive, most authors are quick to point out that this test is extremely operator dependent and their studies were interpreted by physicians specializing in sonography.

## 28.4.5
### Magnetic Resonance Angiography (MRA)

The use of MRA has been shown to be accurate in diagnosis of blunt cerebrovascular injury (BCVI).[31-33] MRA allows direct visualization of mural thrombus and determination of the length of the dissection. Dissections are characterized by eccentric hyper-intense signaling on T1-weighted and T2-weighted images. However, Biffl and colleagues have noted the limitations of MRA in detecting lower grade injuries.[31,32] They concluded that MRA should be used as a screening tool for BCVI when conventional angiography is unavailable. In addition, one should remember that the lower grade injuries that are missed by MRA are the types of injuries to the carotid vessels that are noted in most series of penetrating neck injuries. Currently, there is insufficient data to suggest that MRA be used as the definitive evaluation of penetrating neck injuries.

## 28.5
## Esophageal Evaluation

Esophageal injuries are difficult to diagnose pre-operatively. The clinical presentation of patients with vascular or other life-threatening injuries typically obscures the subtle signs of hypopharyngeal or esophageal trauma. Clinical findings suggestive of hypopharyngeal or esophageal penetration include dysphagia, odynophagia, hemoptysis, and subcutaneous emphysema.

### 28.5.1
### Physical Examination

Mandatory exploration for patients with penetrating neck injuries has been advocated, in part, to avoid a missed (and potentially fatal) injury to the hypopharynx and esophagus. Proponents of selective management, however, have argued that the high incidence of negative explorations and the associated morbidity outweigh the small chance of missing a digestive tract injury. Several recent studies have examined the ability of clinical examination to detect injury in these patients.[30,34-37] Investigators at the University of Southern California (USC) have found signs or symptoms suggestive of esophageal injury in over 20% of patients presenting with penetrating neck injuries, but confirmed injuries in less than 3%.[30] However, of the 152 patients without clinical signs or symptoms, none had an injury requiring operation (negative predictive value of 100%). To determine safe criteria for the management of patients with crepitance of the neck, Goudy and colleagues reviewed the charts of 236 patients with the diagnosis of aerodigestive tract injury or subcutaneous emphysema.[36] Nineteen patients were identified with cervical emphysema and or crepitance. Of these, 20% complained of dysphagia and two-thirds had hoarseness or stridor. Diagnostic laryngoscopy identified injuries to the hypopharynx or larynx in 80% of patients.

Other investigators have shown the inaccuracy of clinical findings in predicting penetrating injury to the aerodigestive tract.[35,38] Noyes and colleagues noted that the more common and sensitive physical findings (shock, expanding hematoma, hemorrhage, and subcutaneous crepitance) are not specific for the organ injured and often occur in the absence of serious injury.[38] These authors reported an overall accuracy of 72% when clinical findings were used to predict injuries in penetrating neck wounds. Back and colleagues' evaluation of physical examination was even less promising.[35] Clinical signs or symptoms suspicious for digestive tract injury were present in only three of the eight patients with documented injury. Most of these clinical findings were non-specific and could be attributed to laryngo-tracheal injuries. Despite the promising results from USC investigators, physical examination does not appear reliable in excluding injuries to the esophagus following gunshot wounds.[30,35]

## 28.5.2
## Esophagography Versus Esophagoscopy

As physical exam appears quite unreliable, diagnostic options range from mandatory surgical exploration to various combinations of radiographic and endoscopic inspection to close clinical observation. Much of the ongoing disagreement created by proposed management algorithms is derived from the difficulty in detecting aerodigestive tract injuries relative to vascular injuries caused by penetrating wounds.[38] A retrospective review of 23 cervical esophageal injuries showed that contrast esophagography had only a 62% success rate in identifying cervical esophageal violations, compared to 100% for rigid esophagoscopy.[39] However, rigid esophagoscopy is associated with such serious complications as dental injuries, bleeding, and aspiration. Critics of rigid evaluation also note the need for general anesthesia and poorer image quality as reasons to utilize flexible esophagoscopy.[40]

Flexible endoscopy is being used more often by young surgeons who completed their training with little to no experience with rigid esophagoscopy. Srinivasan and colleagues evaluated 55 patients who underwent emergent flexible endoscopy for the evaluation of penetrating neck injuries in an attempt to determine if flexible endoscopy was safe and what impact it had on the management of the patient with penetrating neck injury.[40]

Flexible endoscopy was performed safely in all patients with a sensitivity of 100% and specificity of 92% for detecting an esophageal injury. The authors concluded that flexible endoscopic examination of the esophagus is safe in the early evaluation of penetrating neck injuries. Their findings are similar to that of Flowers and colleagues who noted 100% sensitivity and 96% specificity for flexible endoscopy.[41] Critics have noted that the "blind passage" of the flexible scope through the hypopharynx increases the risk of missing mucosal defects in the upper cervical esophagus.

Contrast studies require a stable, cooperative patient and are difficult to obtain in agitated or intubated patients. The sensitivity of contrast esophagography in patients with esophageal trauma varies from 48% to 100%.[42,43] The contrast agent and technique employed for esophageal evaluation both have a significant effect on the sensitivity and accuracy of this modality. Water-soluble agents are less viscous and dense and are, therefore, less likely to coat the mucosa adequately. Up to 55% of esophageal perforations will be missed if a water-soluble agent is used alone.[42,43] To slow contrast transit time, and provide a more adequate study, the patient should be placed in the decubitus position. Patients unable to safely swallow should have the contrast agent instilled through a nasogastric tube under pressure. A thorough and properly performed swallow study should detect almost 80–90% of esophageal injuries.[39]

### 28.5.3
### Combined Modalities

When used alone, esophagoscopy and esophagography have sensitivities of 60 – 80%.[39,42,43] Combining the two, however, increases the sensitivity of detecting esophageal injury following penetrating trauma to well over 90%. Demetriades and colleagues noted that physical examination combined with both endoscopy and esophagography detected 100% of penetrating esophageal injuries.[30] Weigelt and colleagues evaluated 118 patients with penetrating neck injuries and no evidence of hard signs.[43] The combination of esophagography with esophagoscopy identified all esophageal injuries. The authors concluded that patients with penetrating neck trauma and minimal clinical findings should be initially evaluated with arteriography and esophagography. Glatterer and colleagues evaluated 21 injuries to the cervical esophagus, all of which underwent surgical exploration.[44] Esophagography was positive in 75% of patients, esophagoscopy was positive in 83%. A combination of the two modalities would have detected all esophageal injuries.

### 28.6
### Laryngo-Tracheal Evaluation

Although injuries to the larynx and trachea are uncommon, they are associated with significant morbidity and mortality. The risk of death and complications associated with these injuries can be minimized by aggressive airway control and an expedient search for occult injuries, respectively. The endotracheal approach to intubation can be safely accomplished in selected patients with laryngo-tracheal injuries.[45] This approach allows for controlled placement of the endotracheal tube, as well as the evaluation of the hypopharynx, larynx, and proximal trachea through direct laryngoscopy. Once the airway is controlled, a careful evaluation of the laryngo-tracheal tree should be undertaken.

### 28.6.1
### Physical Examination

Patients with laryngo-tracheal injury often present with obvious signs of airway injury, such as stridor, dyspnea, or subcutaneous crepitance. As with the digestive tract, physical examination findings are sensitive for detecting airway injury but lack specificity.[35,46] Some authors have suggested that asymptomatic patients could be safely observed regarding potential airway involvement.[46] Others have suggested that patients at risk receive endoscopic evaluation in the form of diagnostic laryngoscopy, tracheobronchoscopy, or both.[35,38]

### 28.6.2
### Diagnostic Laryngoscopy (DL) and Tracheobronchoscopy

Diagnostic Laryngoscopy (DL) is utilized to evaluate the hypopharynx following Zone III injuries, whereas tracheobronchoscopy is better suited for examination of Zones I and II.

Demetriades and colleagues noted that DL detected all major injuries to the laryngo-tracheal region, as well as mild injuries such as pharyngeal edema and submucosal hemorrhage.[46] Other authors have noted that DL detects over 90% of laryngo-tracheal injuries and when combined with tracheobronchoscopy, sensitivity approaches 100%.[35,38] More recently, investigators at the University of Southern California prospectively evaluated 149 patients with penetrating neck injuries using flexible endoscopy. They noted abnormalities in approximately 16% of endoscopies and no missed injuries.[30] They concurred with previous authors that flexible fiberoptic bronchoscopy is the diagnostic modality of choice in detecting laryngo-tracheal injuries.

## 28.7
## Trajectory Determination

As early as 1987, Pass and colleagues noted that findings on plain radiographs (prevertebral soft-tissue swelling, missile fragmentation, missiles adjacent to major vessels) could be useful in predicting anatomic injury.[47] Identifying and marking all wounds (with radioopaque markers such as a paper clip) and assessing possible trajectories with radiographs and or CT, can help define likely anatomic injuries and guide diagnostic evaluations. Nemzek and colleagues noted that clinical findings and plain radiographs lack the specificity necessary to exclude injuries to the neck structures.[48] They concluded that a high index of suspicion, based on the bullet trajectory, is essential for early diagnosis of aerodigestive injuries. Compared to missiles that do not cross the midline, transcervical GSW are twice as likely to injure vital structures in the neck. This has led some authors to suggest that these wounds be considered as a separate category of neck trauma and even advocate mandatory exploration in this special population.[30] Demetriades and colleagues also noted a high incidence of injuries in transcervical GSW, but found that less than one-fourth of patients required exploration. They concluded that a careful clinical examination combined with the appropriate diagnostic tests can safely select the appropriate treatment.

Over the last decade, numerous authors have examined the utility of CT scan in accurately determining the missile trajectory and, therefore, in defining the anatomic injuries in penetrating neck trauma.[49,50] Gracias and colleagues retrospectively evaluated helical CT scan in firearm injuries to the neck. Approximately 60% of patients had "trajectory consistent with injury" excluded by CT scan. 40% underwent angiography because of proximity and less than 10% required endoscopy. They concluded that in stable patients with penetrating neck injuries CT scan can safely and accurately determine "trajectory consistent with injury." A prospective study from Mazolewski and colleagues noted that the sensitivity of CT scan for significant injury was 100% with a specificity of 90%.[50] They concluded that CT scan could help to eliminate the need for mandatory exploration and limit the need for further diagnostic testing (Fig. 28.5).

**Fig. 28.5** A computed tomography image of the neck in a patient with a gunshot wound. In select cases, CT can be used to determine trajectory and screen for possible injuries. White arrows indicate clips used to mark entrance and exit wounds; *black arrow* indicates air in tissue along the bullet path

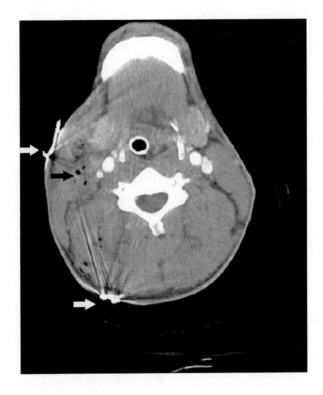

## 28.8
## Operative Approaches

Whereas elective procedures allow the surgeon sufficient time to plan and even discuss with colleagues the best operative approach, patients with penetrating neck injuries offer little time for debate. As previously stated, these injuries require a thorough knowledge of the relevant anatomy, as well as, the optimal approaches for both airway and vascular control. In general, patients should be positioned in the supine position with the arms abducted to 90°. Some surgeons prefer to have the patient's arms tucked and at their sides. This is a reasonable option if the patient's trajectory is determined to be one in which proximal control can be obtained without the need for thoracotomy. Most injuries can be controlled through a sternotomy or anterolateral thoracotomy and arm positioning should not interfere. Unless a cervical spine injury is suspected, the neck should be extended and rotated to the opposite side (15°–20°) (Fig. 28.6). Skin preparation should extend from the ears to the middle of the abdomen with at least one groin prepped out for the possibility of saphenous vein harvest. This coverage area will allow the surgeon access to the neck and chest for proximal and distal vascular control, in addition to an uninvolved limb for harvesting venous conduits.

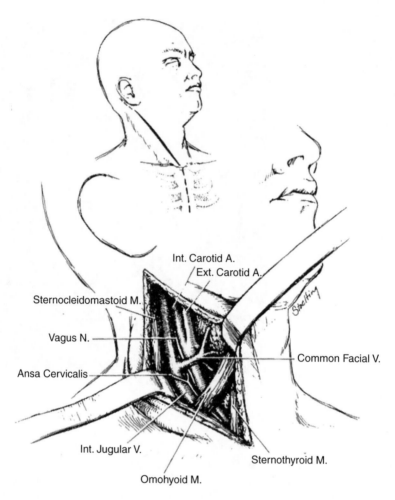

**Fig. 28.6** Operative anatomy of the carotid is shown in this illustration (From Ward[7] with permission)

## 28.8.1
## Zone I

Injuries involving Zone I are usually the most challenging and require the most pre-operative planning. Life threatening injuries usually result from penetrating injuries to Zone I and aggressive management is essential. As with any procedure, exposure is the key to technical success, which typically requires a sternotomy or thoracotomy. A median sternotomy with supraclavicular extension or sternocleidomastoid incision (SCM) is usually the most versatile approach when time does not permit adequate pre-operative evaluation.

In the patient that is unstable or rapidly deteriorating, injuries to the proximal one-third of the left subclavian are best controlled through an anterolateral thoracotomy through the third intercostal space. A supraclavicular counter-incision is then made to achieve distal control. Extension into a "trap-door" sternotomy is rarely necessary to approach or repair any neck injury. To achieve adequate exposure to injuries involving the innominate or common carotid arteries, a median sternotomy provides ample exposure and the ability to achieve proximal (and often distal) control. Utilization of a supraclavicular incision can provide exposure and allow for vascular control of injuries to the right subclavian and distal two-thirds of the left subclavian artery.

Vascular control of the vertebrals arteries is among the most difficult to obtain, especially in the face of active hemorrhage. The majority of the vessel is contained within the foramina, which adds bone to the other structures hindering adequate exposure (venous plexus, brachial plexus, phrenic nerve, and scalene muscles). If one is required to obtain vascular control of a known vertebral artery injury, a supraclavicular incision will provide optimal exposure. This should extend from insertion of the sternoclavicular head to the lateral third of the clavicle. If the area of injury is not known preoperatively, the SCM incision remains the most versatile. The carotid sheath should be identified and retracted laterally. The supraclavicular fat pad should be separated and retracted, exposing the thyrocervical trunk and scalene muscles. Exposure is maximized by ligation of these vessels and division of the anterior scalene. Care should be taken to avoid (and protect the phrenic nerve. The vertebral artery will be noted as the deepest structure lying within the fossa.

## 28.8.2
## Zone II

An anterior sternocleidomastoid (SCM) incision allows for adequate exposure of unilateral neck injuries (Fig. 28.7). For transcervical or bilateral wounds, a transverse (collar) incision can provide adequate exposure for the majority of Zone II injuries. Some surgeons, however, prefer bilateral SCM incisions joined inferiorly or in the mid-portion ("H"- shaped incision). More importantly, both the collar and the SCM incisions can be quickly extended into the chest should a sternotomy be required. Carotid injuries to Zone II can be adequately

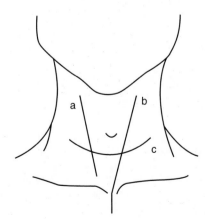

**Fig. 28.7** Operative approaches to the neck include (**a**) the sternocleidomastoid incision, (**b**) the sternocleidomastoid incision with sternotomy extension, and (**c**) the collar incision

visualized through either incision. If the extent of injury extends into either Zone I or Zone III or the point necessary for vascular control lies outside of this area, several maneuvers may be employed. As with Zone I injuries, a sternotomy may be used if more proximal exposure is necessary. For those extending distally (or into Zone III), division of the omohyoids and or digastrics will increase exposure. If necessary, anterior subluxation of the mandible may be utilized for those injuries requiring extreme distal exposure.

### 28.8.3
### Zone III

Due to the inherent difficulty in evaluating and obtaining vascular control in this area, selective management of injuries to Zone III has arisen out of necessity (Fig. 28.8). In addition to subluxation of the mandible, resection of the angle of the mandible or styloid process has also been described. If proximal control can be obtained, distal control of Zone III (and even some Zone II) injuries can be obtained without such morbid maneuvers through the placement and inflation of a Fogarty catheter. This allows for the surgeon to further expose necessary vessels for vascular control or provides control of distal bleeding until interventional radiology or endovascular treatments can be employed. These damage control principles are discussed in further detail below.

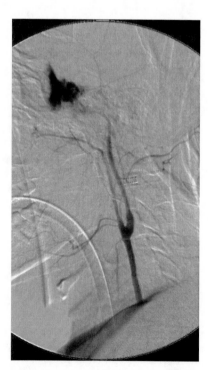

**Fig. 28.8** This cerebral angiogram in a patient with a Zone III neck gunshot wound shows active exsanguination from a very distal carotid injury. The only approach to this injury is by endovascular embolization

## 28.9
## Management Decisions

### 28.9.1
### Vascular Injuries

Carotid artery injuries account for 10–20% of life-threatening injuries that occur in patients with penetrating neck trauma.[51] The primary objective during operative management is to restore antegrade flow to the carotid and preserve neurological function. Carotid injuries should be repaired unless the surgeons is faced with (1) uncontrollable hemorrhage, (2) hemodynamic lability, (3) a comatose patient presenting with no evidence of antegrade flow, or (4) a devastating vessel injury technically impossible to temporize with a vascular shunt. In these circumstances, ligation can and should be employed. Some authors also advocate ligation if there is little to no "back bleeding" from the carotid artery, citing the likelihood of worsening an established ischemic infarct or risk of embolizing a distal clot is increased with attempts at restoring blood flow.[3,51]

Another controversy is whether to use a temporary vascular shunt, as even elective repairs near the carotid bifurcation can be difficult[3,51,52] (Fig. 28.9). While some advocate the routine use of shunts during the repair, others argue that shunts should only be employed if "back" pressures are less than 60 mmHg. If technically possible, a primary repair should be attempted on all common and internal carotid injuries (Fig. 28.10). Those involving the external carotid, however, should be ligated unless they are at or near the bifurcation. Primary repair can be accomplished following debridement of non-viable tissues. This is usually performed in a running fashion using non-absorbable monofilament suture (4-0 to 6-0). If the defect is greater than 2 cm, primary repair should not be attempted due to the excessive amount of tension on the repair. A vein patch can be used for defects involving only one wall of the vessel. Otherwise, saphenous vein from the groin should be used. The jugular vessels should not be utilized for conduit in this setting considering the disruption to venous outflow associated with their harvest.

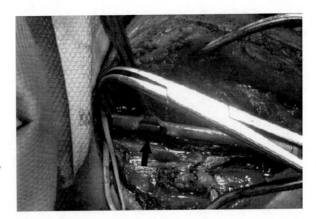

**Fig. 28.9** A gunshot wound to the right common carotid artery with an intraluminal shunt in place (*black arrow*)

**Fig. 28.10** This patient had both a carotid transection and a pharyngeal injury. Note that the sternocleido-mastoid muscle (*thick black arrow*) has been rotated to protect the vascular anastamosis (*thin black arrow*) from the drain exiting superiorly (*white arrow*)

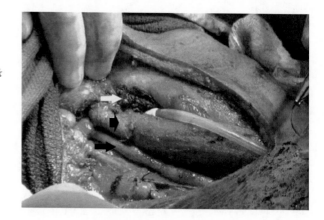

Polytetrafluoroethylene (PTFE) grafts have been employed with increased frequency when primary repair is not possible. Recently, Thompson and colleagues advocated the use of PTFE as the conduit of choice, even in settings where saphenous vein is available.[52] They noted the comparable patency and infection rates with PTFE versus saphenous graft. The majority of studies supporting the use of PTFE, however, have evaluated patency rates following lower extremity re-vascularizations. Vascular principles such as those used in elective procedures ("flushing out" the artery prior to completion of the anastomosis, completion angiography, and systemic heparinization) should be employed.

Repair of the innominate and subclavian arteries can be accomplished using similar principles as those applied to the carotid arteries. When a median sternotomy is used, division of the brachiocephalic vein will allow improved exposure and simplify proximal control of the brachiocephalic, common carotid, and subclavian arteries. Over 30% of patients with these injuries have traditionally had associated brachial plexus injuries.[53,54] Some authors suggest that clavicular resection may have as much to do with this phenomenon as the injuries themselves.[55] Should a supraclavicular approach be chosen and an interposition graft become necessary, the conduit can be tunneled beneath the clavicle without having to resect the clavicle. This can usually be accomplished after "stripping off" the attachments of the pectoralis major and SCM muscles. This avoids the functional difficulties that are often encountered post-operatively following clavicular resection. This also obviates the need for reconstructive surgery in the future.

Vertebral artery injuries may present initially with severe hemorrhage or in a delayed fashion while diagnostic studies are in progress. If the diagnosis is made in a hemodynamically stable patient without active external hemorrhage, the vertebral artery should be embolized in interventional radiology or in an endovascular suite. If, however, the patient presents with active hemorrhage or experienced personnel are not available for angiography and embolization, an attempt at operative control is indicated. Once identified, through a supraclavicular or SCM incision, the vessel should be ligated in the case of a proximal injury. Distal injuries are approached and controlled in a similar fashion. After the artery is ligated proximally, a Fogarty catheter can be passed in an antegrade fashion. The balloon is positioned distal to the point of injury and inflated. Interventional or endovascular assistance should be employed at this time. Following the embolization process, the patient should be monitored closely for evidence of ongoing hemorrhage. Additionally, a follow-up angiogram is usually obtained in the weeks after embolization to demonstrate hemostasis and exclude arteriovenous fistulae (AVF). In institutions without interventional or endovascular support, the Fogarty may be left in place for approximately 72 h. This allows adequate time for thrombosis of the artery, at which point the catheter can be deflated and removed.

Following successful use of endovascular stents in patients with carotid artery disease, Coldwell and colleagues reported on the use of endovascular stents to treat complications following carotid artery injury.[56] Since their report of stent treatment of a carotid pseudoaneurysm after trauma, numerous authors have successfully utilized the endovascular approach to address penetrating cervical vascular injuries.[57,58] Duane and colleagues noted the viable option of endovascular techniques in managing difficult, often inaccessible, vascular injuries of the neck.[57] Stent deployment in their patients allowed non-operative management of Zone III vascular injuries. Strauss and colleagues reported the successful management of subclavian artery injuries through an endovascular approach.[58] The vessels were occluded at the time of evaluation, but underwent thrombectomy and stent deployment without difficulty. Both patients had patency confirmed on 1 year follow-up. Potential additional advantages to the endovascular approach include the ability to embolize those vessels not amenable to stenting, treating traumatic AVF, and addressing occluded vessels in a delayed fashion. The role of endovascular stents in managing cervical vascular injuries continues to evolve.

## 28.9.2
### Esophageal Injuries

The repair of an injury to the cervical esophagus is best approached through an anterior SCM incision. Should there be an associated laryngotracheal injury, however, these combination injuries are best approached through a collar incision. Maximal exposure of the esophagus is achieved through retraction of the trachea and thyroid medially and the carotid sheath laterally. An indwelling nasogastric tube can facilitate not only the localization of the esophagus, but also the identification of the esophageal injury (through the instillation of air or methylene blue). Nonviable edges should be sharply debrided prior to primary repair, which is then carried out in one of two methods. The two-layered repair is performed with an interrupted submucosal (absorbable suture) and a muscular layer (non-absorbable suture). Alternatively, a single layered repair can be performed in an interrupted fashion (non-absorbable suture). Whether a single or two-layered repair is chosen, good mucosal and muscular approximation is necessary to prevent delayed leakage.

Although routine drainage is unnecessary, some principles should be employed to minimize risks of tracheo-esophageal fistula (TEF) formation and in anticipation of anastomotic leaks.[1] Combination injuries, hemodynamic instability, and tracheostomy requirement, place the patient at increased risk of TEF formation. Though the majority of fistulas will heal without surgical intervention, their risk of occurrence can be minimized with a tissue flap or buttress. This can be accomplished by dividing the clavicular head of the SCM muscle and mobilizing the flap between the trachea and esophagus, separating the two structures. The patient should remain NPO until barium swallow (5–7 days post-operatively) has excluded a leak.

A reduction in the number of diagnostic delays has likely accounted for the improvement in survival rates following penetrating esophageal trauma. In the patient without signs of sepsis or clinical deterioration, small injuries detected in a delayed fashion may be managed non-operatively. However, the majority of these patients will require debridement and drainage. Although the management principles are usually centered on creation of a controlled fistula, a buttress repair of the defect should be attempted if possible. Some authors advocate prolonged esophageal "rest" and nasopharyngeal (or T-tube) drainage to decrease the already high risk of fistula formation and anastomotic leaks.[1,46] More devastating wounds may require cervical esophagostomy and parenteral nutrition.

Unlike esophageal injuries, those confined to the hypopharynx can frequently be managed non-operatively. Yugeros and colleagues evaluated 14 patients with penetrating injuries to the hypopharynx that were managed non-operatively.[34] They found no evidence of leaks or fistula formation, and only one patient developed a cervical abscess. They noted non-operative management to be a safe alternative in patients with penetrating injury to the hypopharynx. Shortly thereafter, Stanley and colleagues addressed this issue in a study of 70 patients with hypopharyngeal or cervical esophageal injuries.[59] They noted a significant increase in the number of deep cervical infections and fistulas in patients with injuries below the arytenoids that were managed non-operatively. The authors concluded that patients with injuries above the arytenoids should be managed non-operatively, while those below this level should undergo primary repair. Demetriades and colleagues concurred with these authors, but stated that "major wounds" to the hypopharynx should be managed similarly to those of the cervical esophagus.[46] Finally, despite their widespread use, there is no evidence to support the routine and prolonged use of antibiotics in these patients outside of the immediate post-operative period (first 24 h).

## 28.9.3
### Laryngo-Tracheal Injuries

Patients presenting with low-velocity GSW to the neck will require an urgent airway in 18–44% of cases.[1] Definitive airway control prior to operative exploration may be necessary in the form of endotracheal intubation, cricothyroidotomy, or tracheostomy. In the majority of cases, oral endotracheal intubation will be possible. Either an anterior SCM or collar incision may be utilized to approach these injuries. With combined esophageal injury or transcervical GSW, a collar incision will usually allow improved exposure with fewer struggles than the standard SCM incision. Careful dissection is then carried out, retracting necessary tissues to expose the involved segment. Lateral dissection should be minimized, and if possible avoided, to protect the laterally based blood supply.

Most laryngeal defects from penetrating trauma can be repaired primarily. Small defects noted on endoscopy can usually be managed non-operatively with airway protection, elevation of the head of the bed, and "voice rest." A search for the recurrent laryngeal nerve should be avoided and the dissection minimized. Proper debridement should precede any attempt at primary repair. However, all viable tissues should be spared. Early fracture stabilization (Kirschner wires) of involved components and repair of mucosal lacerations has been associated with improved airway and voice quality. If the cartilaginous framework has been disrupted beyond management with a primary repair, some authors advocate "stenting" the airway with the indwelling endotracheal tube or with the placement of a silicone stent. Tracheostomy should be avoided in the area of injury, but if necessary should be placed distal to the repair to "protect" the anastomosis.

Tracheal injuries are repaired primarily in a single-layer fashion, using an absorbable (3-0) suture. As with laryngeal injuries, viable tissue should be conserved and search for recurrent laryngeal nerves avoided. Large defects (>3 cm) can be repaired primarily after adequate mobilization. This can be accomplished by releasing anterior (thyroid and suprahyoid) attachments and staying clear of the lateral blood supply. Vascularized flaps (SCM muscle) should be employed to buttress the repair, decreasing the risk of fistula formation. The role of tracheostomy in these patients remains controversial. Tracheostomy in this setting has been associated with increased risk of infection, but many advocate its use in "protecting" the proximal repair. Most agree that with very large defects (>6 cm, those requiring vascularized flaps) a tracheostomy should be placed at the time of the initial operation. Avoidance of flexion in the post-operative period (5–7 days) can be achieved with cervical collar immobilization or by suturing the chin to the presternal skin.

## 28.9.4
## Damage Control

The application of damage control principles can be applied to neck injuries as it has been with severe trauma to other body regions. Rotondo and colleagues initially described this concept of "temporary" control of severe injuries in abdominal trauma and its principles have been applied to the management of penetrating neck injury.[60] The rapid control of the patient's airway, followed by packing or employment of catheters for hemorrhage control mirrors that of a damage control laparotomy. The damage control concept centers on the early identification of life-threatening injuries and the decision to avoid complicated, sometimes lengthy, definitive repairs. Recently, Firoozmand and Velmahos reported on the use of these principles to the neck.[61] They described a patient who presented in extremis following a cervical gunshot wound. Direct pressure failed to control hemorrhage from the wound, and Foley catheters were used to cannulate the tracts and tamponade the bleeding. Operative exploration identified several vascular injuries which were amenable to repair, in addition to an inaccessible vertebral artery injury. The patient was packed open and resuscitated in the intensive care unit prior to interventional radiology evaluation for embolization. The damage control approach described here and above should be recognized as an important alternative to attempting definitive repair in the unstable patient.

## References

1. Cotton BA, Pryor JP. Neck Injuries. In: Mahoney PF et al., eds. *Ballistic Trauma: A Practical Guide*. 2nd ed. London: Springer; 2005.
2. Bishara RA, Pasch AR, Douglas DD, Schuler JJ, Lim LT, Flanigan DP. The necessity of mandatory exploration of penetrating zone II neck injuries. *Surgery*. 1986;100(4):655-660.
3. Wood J, Fabian TC, Mangiante EC. Penetrating neck injuries: recommendations for selective management. *J Trauma*. 1989;29(5):602-605.
4. Atteberry LR, Dennis JW, Menawat SS, Frykberg ER. Physical examination alone is safe and accurate for evaluation of vascular injuries in penetrating Zone II neck trauma. *J Am Coll Surg*. 1994;179(6):657-662.
5. Demetriades D, Theodorou D, Cornwell E, et al. Transcervical gunshot injuries: mandatory operation is not necessary. *J Trauma*. 1996;40(5):758-760.
6. Eddy VA. Is routine arteriography mandatory for penetrating injury to zone 1 of the neck? Zone 1 penetrating neck injury study group. *J Trauma*. 2000;48(2):208-213.
7. Ward RE. Injury to the cervical cerebral vessels. In: Blaisdell FW, Turnkey DD, eds. *Trauma Management: Cervicothoracic Trauma*. New York: Thieme; 1986:273.
8. Maxwell RA. Penetrating neck injury. In: Maxwell RA, Peitzman AB, Rhodes M, Schwab CW, Yealy DM, Fabian TC, eds. *The Trauma Manual*. Philadelphia: Lippincott Williams & Wilkins; 2002:192.
9. Beitsch P, Weigelt JA, Flynn E, Easley S. Physical examination and arteriography in patients with penetrating zone II neck wounds. *Arch Surg*. 1994;129(6):577-581.
10. Biffl WL, Moore EE, Rehse DH, Offner PJ, Franciose RJ, Burch JM. Selective management of penetrating neck trauma based on cervical level of injury. *Am J Surg*. 1997;174(6):678-682.
11. Insull P, Adams D, Segar A, Ng A, Civil I. Is exploration mandatory in penetrating zone II neck injuries? *ANZ J Surg*. 2007;77(4):261-264.
12. Jarvick JG, Haynor DR, Longstreth WT Jr. Assessing the usefulness of diagnostic tests. *Am J Neuroradiol*. 1996;17(7):1255-1258.
13. Eggen JT, Jorden RC. Airway management, penetrating neck trauma. *J Emerg Med*. 1993;11(4):381-385.
14. Brywczynski JJ, Barrett TW, Lyon JA, Cotton BA. A structured literature review of penetrating neck injury management in the emergency department. *Emerg Med J*. 2008;25(2):508-513.
15. Apfelbaum JD, Cantrill SV, Waldman N. Unstable cervical spine without spinal cord injury in penetrating neck trauma. *Am J Emerg Med*. 2000;18(1):55-57.
16. Arishita GI, Vayer JS, Bellamy RF. Cervical spine immobilization of penetrating neck wounds in a hostile environment. *J Trauma*. 1989;29(3):332-337.
17. Barkana Y, Stein M, Scope A, et al. Prehospital stabilization of the cervical spine for penetrating injuries of the neck - is it necessary? *Injury*. 2000;31(5):305-309.
18. McKinney J, Brywczynski J, Slovis C. Heart rate: 310. Identifying & treating a rapid wide complex tachycardia. *JEMS*. 2008;33(3):38.
19. Sekharan J, Dennis JW, Veldenz HC, Miranda F, Frykberg ER. Continued experience with physical examination alone for evaluation and management of penetrating zone 2 neck injuries: results of 145 cases. *J Vasc Surg*. 2000;32(3):483-489.
20. Fry WR, Dort JA, Smith RS, Sayers DV, Morabito DJ. Duplex scanning replaces arteriography and operative exploration in the diagnosis of potential cervical vascular injury. *Am J Surg*. 1994;168(6):693-695.
21. Sclafani SJ, Panetta T, Goldstein AS, et al. The management of arterial injuries caused by penetration of zone III of the neck. *J Trauma*. 1985;25(9):871-881.
22. Sclafani SJ, Cavaliere G, Atweh N, Duncan AO, Scalea T. The role of angiography in penetrating neck trauma. *J Trauma*. 1991;31(4):557-562.

23. Demetriades D, Theodorou D, Cornwell E III, et al. Penetrating injuries of the neck in patients in stable condition. Physical examination, angiography, or color flow Doppler imaging. *Arch Surg.* 1995;130(9):971-975.

24. Munera F, Cohn S, Rivas LA. Penetrating injuries of the neck: use of helical computed tomographic angiography. *J Trauma.* 2005;58(2):413-418.

25. Munera F, Soto JA, Palacio DM, et al. Penetrating neck injuries: helical CT angiography for initial evaluation. *Radiology.* 2002;224(2):366-372.

26. Ofer A, Nitecki SS, Braun J, et al. CT angiography of the carotid arteries in trauma to the neck. *Eur J Vasc Endovasc Surg.* 2001;21(5):401-407.

27. Stuhlfaut JW, Barest G, Sakai O, Lucey B, Soto JA. Impact of MDCT angiography on the use of catheter angiography for the assessment of cervical arterial injury after blunt or penetrating trauma. *AJR Am J Roentgenol.* 2005;185(4):1063-1068.

28. Corr P, bdool Carrim AT, Robbs J. Colour-flow ultrasound in the detection of penetrating vascular injuries of the neck. *S Afr Med J.* 1999;89(6):644-646.

29. Montalvo BM, LeBlang SD, Nunez DB Jr, et al. Color Doppler sonography in penetrating injuries of the neck. *AJNR Am J Neuroradiol.* 1996;17(5):943-951.

30. Demetriades D, Theodorou D, Cornwell E, et al. Evaluation of penetrating injuries of the neck: prospective study of 223 patients. *World J Surg.* 1997;21(1):41-47.

31. Biffl WL, Moore EE, Offner PJ, et al. Optimizing screening for blunt cerebrovascular injuries. *Am J Surg.* 1999;178(6):517-522.

32. Biffl WL, Moore EE, Offner PJ, Burch JM. Blunt carotid and vertebral arterial injuries. *World J Surg.* 2001;25(8):1036-1043.

33. Weller SJ, Rossitch E Jr, Malek AM. Detection of vertebral artery injury after cervical spine trauma using magnetic resonance angiography. *J Trauma.* 1999;46(4):660-666.

34. Yugueros P, Sarmiento JM, Garcia AF, Ferrada R. Conservative management of penetrating hypopharyngeal wounds. *J Trauma.* 1996;40(2):267-269.

35. Back MR, Baumgartner FJ, Klein SR. Detection and evaluation of aerodigestive tract injuries caused by cervical and transmediastinal gunshot wounds. *J Trauma.* 1997;42(4):680-686.

36. Goudy SL, Miller FB, Bumpous JM. Neck crepitance: evaluation and management of suspected upper aerodigestive tract injury. *Laryngoscope.* 2002;112(5):791-795.

37. Ngakane H, Muckart DJ, Luvuno FM. Penetrating visceral injuries of the neck: results of a conservative management policy. *Br J Surg.* 1990;77(8):908-910.

38. Noyes LD, McSwain NE Jr, Markowitz IP. Panendoscopy with arteriography versus mandatory exploration of penetrating wounds of the neck. *Ann Surg.* 1986;204(1):21-31.

39. Armstrong WB, Detar TR, Stanley RB. Diagnosis and management of external penetrating cervical esophageal injuries. *Ann Otol Rhinol Laryngol.* 1994;103(11):863-871.

40. Srinivasan R, Haywood T, Horwitz B, Buckman RF, Fisher RS, Krevsky B. Role of flexible endoscopy in the evaluation of possible esophageal trauma after penetrating injuries. *Am J Gastroenterol.* 2000;95(7):1725-1729.

41. Flowers JL, Graham SM, Ugarte MA, et al. Flexible endoscopy for the diagnosis of esophageal trauma. *J Trauma.* 1996;40(2):261-265.

42. Sheely CH, Mattox KL, Beall AC Jr, DeBakey ME. Penetrating wounds of the cervical esophagus. *Am J Surg.* 1975;130(6):707-711.

43. Weigelt JA, Thal ER, Snyder WH III, Fry RE, Meier DE, Kilman WJ. Diagnosis of penetrating cervical esophageal injuries. *Am J Surg.* 1987;154(6):619-622.

44. Glatterer MS Jr, Toon RS, Ellestad C, et al. Management of blunt and penetrating external esophageal trauma. *J Trauma.* 1985;25(8):784-792.

45. Grewal H, Rao PM, Mukerji S, Ivatury RR. Management of penetrating laryngotracheal injuries. *Head Neck.* 1995;17(6):494-502.

46. Demetriades D, Velmahos GG, Asensio JA. Cervical pharyngoesophageal and laryngotracheal injuries. *World J Surg.* 2001;25(8):1044-1048.

47. Pass LJ, LeNarz LA, Schreiber JT, Estrera AS. Management of esophageal gunshot wounds. *Ann Thorac Surg.* 1987;44(3):253-256.
48. Nemzek WR, Hecht ST, Donald PJ, McFall RA, Poirier VC. Prediction of major vascular injury in patients with gunshot wounds to the neck. *AJNR Am J Neuroradiol.* 1996;17(1):161-167.
49. Gracias VH, Reilly PM, Philpott J, et al. Computed tomography in the evaluation of penetrating neck trauma: a preliminary study. *Arch Surg.* 2001;136(11):1231-1235.
50. Mazolewski PJ, Curry JD, Browder T, Fildes J. Computed tomographic scan can be used for surgical decision making in zone II penetrating neck injuries. *J Trauma.* 2001;51(2):315-319.
51. Unger SW, Tucker WS Jr, Mrdeza MA, Wellons HA Jr, Chandler JG. Carotid arterial trauma. *Surgery.* 1980;87(5):477-487.
52. Thompson EC, Porter JM, Fernandez LG. Penetrating neck trauma: an overview of management. *J Oral Maxillofac Surg.* 2002;60(8):918-923.
53. Demetriades D, Chahwan S, Gomez H, et al. Penetrating injuries to the subclavian and axillary vessels. *J Am Coll Surg.* 1999;188(3):290-295.
54. Demetriades D, Charalambides K, Chahwan S, et al. Nonskeletal cervical spine injuries: epidemiology and diagnostic pitfalls. *J Trauma.* 2000;48(4):724-727.
55. Old WL Jr, Oswaks RM. Clavicular excision in management of vascular trauma. *Am Surg.* 1984;50(5):286-289.
56. Coldwell DM, Novak Z, Ryu RK, et al. Treatment of posttraumatic internal carotid arterial pseudoaneurysms with endovascular stents. *J Trauma.* 2000;48(3):470-472.
57. Duane TM, Parker F, Stokes GK, Parent FN, Britt LD. Endovascular carotid stenting after trauma. *J Trauma.* 2002;52(1):149-153.
58. Strauss DC, du Toit DF, Warren BL. Endovascular repair of occluded subclavian arteries following penetrating trauma. *J Endovasc Ther.* 2001;8(5):529-533.
59. Stanley RB Jr, Armstrong WB, Fetterman BL, Shindo ML. Management of external penetrating injuries into the hypopharyngeal-cervical esophageal funnel. *J Trauma.* 1997;42(4):675-679.
60. Rotondo MF, Schwab CW, McGonigal MD, et al. 'Damage control': an approach for improved survival in exsanguinating penetrating abdominal injury. *J Trauma.* 1993;35(3):375-382.
61. Firoozmand E, Velmahos GC. Extending damage-control principles to the neck. *J Trauma.* 2000;48(3):541-543.

# Damage Control

**29**

Benjamin Braslow, Adam J. Brooks, and C. William Schwab

## 29.1
## Introduction

Massive hemorrhage is a major cause of trauma-related mortality and is the second most common cause of death after central nervous system injuries in the prehospital setting.[1] Moreover, uncontrolled bleeding is the most common cause of early in-hospital mortality (first 48 h) due to major trauma.[2] During the last two decades, advances in prehospital care and trauma bay efficiency (especially in busy urban trauma centers) have led to more severely injured trauma patients surviving to the point of operative intervention. Regarding penetrating-trauma patients, the increasing use of powerful semiautomatic firearms by the civilian population has manifested in patients arriving with multiple penetrations and more severe tissue destruction. These patients often are wounded in multiple body cavities, suffering massive hemorrhage and both physiological and metabolic exhaustion.

A combination of profound acidosis, hypothermia, and coagulopathy, also known as the "lethal triad," is commonly noted in these patients. The "traditional surgical approach" to such patients, in which surgeons would repair all identified injuries at the initial operation, often led to patient demise despite control of anatomic bleeding.

During the peak of American gun violence in the late 1980s and early 1990s, urban trauma centers accumulated a wealth of experience in treating these severely injured patients and the concept of "Damage Control" surgery was born.

Damage control is a traditional Navy term[3] that refers to keeping a badly damaged ship afloat after major penetrating injury to the hull so as to maintain mission integrity. Typical procedures for temporary righting and stabilizing the vessel classically involved stuffing mattresses into gaping holes in the ship's hull, extinguishing local fires, and "dogging down" watertight doors to limit flooding and spread of damage.[4] These measures, which keep the ship afloat, allow for the assessment of other damage and afford time to establish a feasible plan for definitive repair. The analogy to the care of the seriously injured is obvious.

A.J. Brooks (✉)
Emergency Surgery and Major Trauma, Nottingham University NHS Trust,
Nottingham, UK and
Academic Department of Military Surgery and Trauma, Royal Centre for
Defence Medicine, Birmingham, UK
e-mail: adam.brooks@nuh.nhs.uk

A.J. Brooks et al. (eds.), *Ryan's Ballistic Trauma*,
DOI: 10.1007/978-1-84882-124-8_29, © Springer-Verlag London Limited 2011

For the trauma surgeon, damage control describes the technique of abbreviated laparotomy, with rapid and precise containment of hemorrhage and contamination and temporary intra-abdominal packing for initial injury control. Following this, the patient is transferred to the surgical intensive care unit (ICU) for physiologic resuscitation. Subsequently, the patient returns to the operating room for definitive repair of all injuries and, if possible at that time, abdominal wall closure. This approach must not be deemed as surgical failure or an abandonment of proper surgical technique. Instead, it has proven to be an aggressive, deliberate strategy to combat the pattern of physiologic failure that accompanies major blunt and penetrating trauma.

## 29.2
## History

The history of present-day damage control surgery is grounded in the early successes realized with hepatic packing for uncontrolled hemorrhage.[5]

Pringle, in 1908, first described the concept of hepatic packing in patients with portal-venous hemorrhage.[6] In 1913, Halstead went on to modify this technique by suggesting that rubber sheets be placed between the packs and the liver to protect the parenchyma.[7]

As surgical techniques, instruments, and materials improved, packing for control of hepatic hemorrhage fell from favor, and by the end of the Second World War (WW II), primary repair re-emerged as the preferred approach. This continued through the era of the Vietnam war.

The technique started to re-emerge when, in 1976, Lucas and Ledgerwood described a prospective 5-year evaluation of 637 patients treated for severe liver injury at the Detroit General Hospital. Three patients underwent perihepatic packing, and all three survived.[8]

In 1979, Calne and colleagues reported four patients in whom massive hemorrhage from severe hepatic trauma was managed initially by conservative surgery and packing. The patients then were transferred by ambulance for definitive surgery. All of these patients survived.[9] Two years later, at the Ben Taub General Hospital, Feliciano and colleagues reported a 90% survival in ten patients in whom intra-abdominal packing for control of exsanguinating hepatic hemorrhage was used. These authors noted that this technique appeared to be lifesaving in highly selected patients in whom coagulopathy, hypothermia, and acidosis made further surgical efforts likely to increase hemorrhage.[10]

In 1983, Stone and colleagues described a stepwise approach to the exsanguinating, hypothermic, and coagulopathic trauma patient that included abbreviated laparotomy and extensive intra-abdominal packing (beyond the scope of just hepatic injuries). They made suggestions for temporizing maneuvers for other injured organs, such as the intestines and urinary tract. Once hemodynamic stability was achieved and the coagulopathy corrected, the patient was returned to the operating room (OR) for definitive surgical repairs and abdominal closure. Eleven of 17 patients, deemed to have a lethal coagulopathy, survived as a result of this strategy.[11] In this landmark study, the three phases of present-day damage control were defined.

Over the next decade, the concept and its application continued to evolve. In 1993, Rotondo and Schwab coined the term "Damage Control" and detailed a standardized three-phase approach that yielded a 58% survival rate.[12] When applied to select cohorts of patients, that is, a maximum injury subset with major vascular injury and two or more visceral injuries, survival increased further to 77%.

As outlined in their paper:

- Part one (DC I) consists of immediate exploratory laparotomy with rapid control of bleeding and contamination, abdominal packing, and abbreviated wound closure.
- Part two (DC II) is the ICU resuscitative phase where physiologic and biochemical stabilization is achieved and a thorough tertiary examination is performed to identify all injuries.
- In part three (DC III), re-exploration in the OR is undertaken and definitive repair of all injuries is performed.

In 2001, Johnson and Schwab introduced a fourth component to the damage control sequence, "Damage Control Ground Zero" (DC 0)[13] (Fig. 29.1). This represents the earliest phase of the damage control process that occurs in the prehospital setting and continues

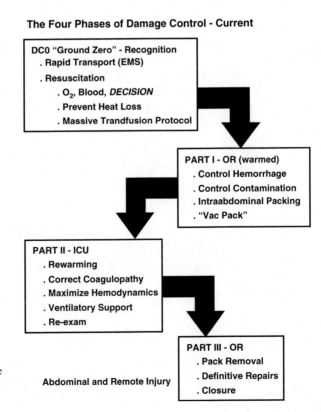

**The Four Phases of Damage Control - Current**

DC0 "Ground Zero" - Recognition
. Rapid Transport (EMS)
. Resuscitation
  . O$_2$, Blood, *DECISION*
  . Prevent Heat Loss
  . Massive Trandfusion Protocol

PART I - OR (warmed)
. Control Hemorrhage
. Control Contamination
. Intraabdominal Packing
. "Vac Pack"

PART II - ICU
. Rewarming
. Correct Coagulopathy
. Maximize Hemodynamics
. Ventilatory Support
. Re-exam

PART III - OR
. Pack Removal
. Definitive Repairs
. Closure

Abdominal and Remote Injury

**Fig. 29.1** The four components of the Damage Control Sequence[13] (Hoey and Schwab[14])

into the trauma bay. Here the emphasis is on injury-pattern recognition for potential damage control beneficiaries. This manifests in truncated scene times for emergency medical service (EMS) and abbreviated emergency department resuscitation by the trauma team. Rapid-sequence intubation, early rewarming maneuvers, immediate blood product resuscitation, and expedient transport to the OR are the key elements of "DC 0" in the trauma bay.

As reported survival rates in this maximally injured subset of patients has continued to rise, so has the popularity of the damage control approach. A recent collective review by Shapiro and colleagues of over 1,000 damage control patients revealed an overall 50% survival.[15] The high morbidity rates (overall morbidity 40%) are not surprising and include wound infection (5–100%), intra-abdominal abscess (0–80%), dehiscence (9–25%), bile leak (8–33%), enterocutaneous fistula (2–25%), abdominal compartment syndrome (2–25%), and multisystem organ failure (20–33%). Other common morbidities in damage controlled patients include hepatic necrosis, intestinal obstruction or prolonged ileus, anastomatic leak, and pancreatic fistula.

The damage control philosophy stresses survival as the ultimate goal. Means to achieve this goal in this unique patient population are aggressive and prolonged ICU stays and multiple operations are often unavoidable.[16]

## 29.3
## Indications for Damage Control

Although major liver injury and progressive coagulopathy remain the most frequent indications for damage control, the list has continued to expand. Because of the associated morbidity that often accompanies the process, patient selection and proper timing is crucial.

Early identification of patients who require damage control promotes optimal results. Inappropriate use of this strategy on more stable patients subjects them to associated morbidities.

Rotondo and colleagues defined a "maximal injury subset" of patients suffering penetrating injuries that clearly benefit from the damage control procedure.[10] These are patients with a major vascular injury, two or more hollow viscus injuries, and profound shock. In their initial damage control series, patients with this complex of injuries who underwent definitive laparotomy had an 11% survival rate compared with 77% for those in whom damage control was employed. Later, Rotondo and Zonies[17] expanded upon and organized the "key" factors in patient selection for damage control (Table 29.1).

Moore and colleagues[18] have also published their major indications for abbreviated laparotomy/damage control. In their estimation, the decision to proceed with damage control usually is based on a combination of these factors and may be influenced additionally by the resources available (e.g., inadequate blood products, limited surgical expertise, multiple casualties).

Table 29.2 is a comprehensive list of damage control triggers used at the University of Pennsylvania for initiating the damage control pathway. In general, the decision to proceed with damage control ultimately must be made when the surgeon recognizes a trend towards physiologic exhaustion.

**Table 29.1** Key factors in patient selection for damage control[17]

| |
|---|
| *Conditions* |
| High energy blunt torso trauma |
| Multiple torso penetrations |
| Hemodynamic instability |
| Presenting coagulopathy and/or hypothermia |
| *Complexes* |
| Major abdominal vascular injury with multiple visceral injuries |
| Multifocal or multicavitary exsanguination with concomitant visceral injuries |
| Multiregional injury with competing priorities |
| *Critical factors* |
| Severe metabolic acidosis (pH < 7.30) |
| Hypothermia (temperature < 35°C) |
| Resuscitation and operative time >90 min |
| Coagulopathy as evidenced by development of nonmechanical bleeding |
| Massive transfusion (>10 units packed red blood cells) |

*Source*: With permission Hoey and Schwab[14]

**Table 29.2** Triggers used at the University of Pennsylvania for initiating the damage control pathway

| |
|---|
| Severe shock with: |
| • Hypothermia (<95°F or 35°C), acidosis, coagulopathy |
| • Suboptimal response to resuscitation |
| • Inability to perform definitive repair: physiologic, equipment[a], judgement[a] |
| • Inaccessible major anatomic injury (IVC, intrahepatic, retroperitoneal, pelvis) and demand for nonoperative control[a] (vascular control best accomplished by angiographic embolization) |
| • Need for time consuming procedure(s)[a] (Whipple, etc.) |
| • Indeterminate serious injury[a] (pancreatic head/duct) |
| • Need to reevaluate abdominal contents (intestinal ischemia) |

[a] Shock may be absent

Since this is often an intraoperative decision based on the severity of injuries identified at exploration, constant communication between the anesthesiologist and the surgeon regarding the patient's response to ongoing resuscitation is essential.

## 29.4
## The Damage Control Sequence

### 29.4.1
### Damage Control: Ground Zero

Damage Control Ground Zero is the earliest phase of the damage control process and occurs in the prehospital setting and continues into the trauma bay. The emphasis is on injury pattern recognition for patients likely to benefit from damage control.

- For the EMS providers, this manifests in truncated scene times and early notification of the trauma response team.
- For the trauma team, abbreviated emergency-department resuscitation is the goal. Gaining large-bore intravenous (IV) access, rapid-sequence intubation, chest tube placement if indicated, early rewarming maneuvers, immediate blood product resuscitation, and expedient transport to the OR are the key elements of DC 0 in the trauma bay. For the rapid workup of penetrating trauma in the unstable patient, minimal diagnostic X-rays are required. A chest X-ray following intubation is imperative to confirm tube placement and identify hemo- and/or pneumothorax that might compromise the patient during transport to the OR. If blunt trauma also is suspected, spinal precautions must be observed, including the placement and/or continuation of a cervical collar. A pelvic X-ray is required to rule out pelvic ring instability and the need for a temporary stabilization device to reduce the pelvic volume and tamponade bleeding. The blood bank needs to be made aware that there is the potential for massive transfusion requirement. Additionally, a cell-saver device should be mobilized to the OR for the collection and reinfusion of shed blood intraoperatively. It is in this phase of the damage control sequence that broad-spectrum intravenous antibiotics and tetanus prophylaxis should be administered.

### 29.4.2
#### Damage Control Part I: The Initial Laparotomy

The primary objectives of the initial laparotomy are control of hemorrhage, limiting contamination and the secondary inflammatory response, and temporary abdominal wall closure to protect viscera and limit heat loss. All of this is done by the most expedient means possible.

### 29.5
### Preparation

The operating room should be warmed to approximately 27°C before the patient's arrival, and the anesthesiologists should prepare their circuit to deliver warmed oxygen and anesthetic agents. As the patient is transferred onto the operating room table, the nursing team prepares the instrument trays, which should consist of a standard laparotomy set and vascular and chest instruments, including a sternal saw. A large supply of laparotomy pads must be immediately available for the initial packing. It is useful to have a cart stocked with damage control equipment (Table 29.3) available in the room, thus reducing the time OR personnel are away.

The patient is placed in a supine position on the table with upper extremities abducted at right angles on arm boards. Positioning of the electrocardiogram (ECG) leads and monitoring equipment must not limit the options for surgical exposure. In anticipation of the need for a median sternotomy, resuscitative left thoracotomy, or bilateral tube

**Table 29.3** Damage control essential equipment

Basic:
- Abdominal, vascular, and chest instruments (including sternal saw)

Damage control essentials:
- Packs
- Shunts (sterile plastic conduits)
- Balloon catheters (large Foley of various sizes with 30 cc balloons)
- Sterile silastic bags
- Adhesive plastic
- Hemostatic agents
- Benzoine
- Suction drains

thoracostomy, no leads or tubing should be present on the anterior or lateral chest wall. The patient is prepped from chin to mid thighs, extending down to the table laterally should thoracotomy be necessary. A urinary catheter and nasogastric tube are inserted during the prep if not already performed in the trauma bay.

Surgery should not be delayed while waiting for the insertion of invasive monitoring devices, that is, arterial lines or central venous lines. These can be placed during the procedure, either by the anesthesiologists or members of the surgical team if in the prepped region.

## 29.6
## Incisions

The most expeditious incision for abdominal exploration is the vertical midline extending from the xiphoid process to the pubic symphysis. In the setting of a suspected severe pelvic fracture, the inferior limit of this incision initially might be curtailed to just below the umbilicus, allowing for continued tamponade of a potential large pelvic hematoma.

If the patient has had a previous midline incision, a bilateral subcostal incision can be employed. This allows for rapid access to the peritoneal cavity away from the expected midline adhesions involving bowel and omentum. These adhesions then can be divided rapidly under direct vision.

## 29.7
## Hemorrhage Control

Once the peritoneum is entered, the next steps need to be performed in a rapid but orderly fashion. Large clots are removed manually. A large hand-held abdominal wall retractor is used sequentially around the periphery of the abdomen to provide space for the packing of all four quadrants. Surgeons on opposite sides of the table trade retraction and packing as appropriate. The falciform ligament is divided to prevent iatrogenic injury to the liver during pack placement in the right upper quadrant. The cell-saver suction should be in place to maximize autologous blood capture and return. While packing the abdomen, the surgeon is assessing the degree and location of the most significant injuries.

Knowledge of the trajectory of the projectiles may aid in assessing potential sites of major bleeding or organ injury. Next, a large self-retaining abdominal retractor is placed to free up the surgeons and provide maximal exposure.

Once the peritoneum is opened, any tamponade effect that had been provided by the abdominal wall is lost immediately. This may induce abrupt and severe hypotension. If the patient remains profoundly hypotensive after packing, control of aortic inflow should be obtained. Manual occlusion of the aorta at the diaphragmatic hiatus can be performed quickly to control abdominal exsanguination and give the anesthesia team some time to catch up with volume replacement. This maneuver also has been shown to augment cerebral and myocardial perfusion.[19] It is performed by passing the hand anterior to the stomach and posterior to the left hepatic lobe. In this position, the abdominal aorta can be palpated immediately to the right and posterior to the esophagus. Control is obtained by compressing it between the thumb and the index finger or by compression against the vertebral column with the hand or an aortic occlusion device.

If prolonged occlusion is necessary, or if surgical hands need to be freed up, a vascular clamp can be placed on the aorta after minimal dissection is performed. First, the diaphragmatic attachments of the left hepatic lobe are divided and the lobe is retracted to the right. Next, a longitudinal incision is made in the hepatogastric ligament approximately one centimeter medial to the esophagus. The muscle fibers of the right crus of the diaphragm then can be split longitudinally by blunt finger dissection to fully expose the aorta and allow for the placement of a large, curved vascular clamp (Fig. 29.2).

Between occlusion of the aorta and intra-abdominal packing, the majority of significant bleeding should be controlled temporarily. Next, packs are removed in a sequential fashion, beginning in the areas least likely to harbor the source of major hemorrhage. This will provide space to pack the bowel away from the areas of hemorrhage and create maximal exposure.

Initial control of major vascular hemorrhage is performed rapidly using a variety of techniques. If an injury is amenable to rapid arteriorraphy or venorrhaphy, this is the treatment of choice. Simple lateral repairs are performed immediately utilizing appropriate vascular clamps for proximal and distal control.

Definitive reconstruction of complex arterial injuries, however, should be delayed unless the surgeon is confident that placing a prosthetic interposition graft [i.e., woven Dacron or polytetrafluoroethylene (PTFE)] can be done rapidly and there is not significant contamination present from concomitant bowel injury.

The placement of temporary intravascular shunts (i.e., thoracostomy tubes, silastic catheters, or commercially available heparin-bonded devices) in the more critical vessels [abdominal aorta, superior mesenteric artery (SMA), iliac and common femoral arteries, etc.] has been well described.[20,21] This technique is an excellent rapid alternative to arterial ligation, which often can put end organ and limb viability in jeopardy.

Experience with prolonged use of intravascular shunts in humans is limited. Johansen and colleagues reported three patients with lower-extremity intravascular shunts in place

**Fig. 29.2** Application of a vascular clamp on the aorta at the diaphragm (Hoey and Schwab[14])

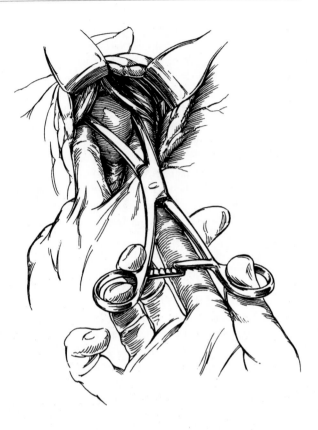

that underwent air transfer to a Level I trauma center for definitive care. Shunt times ranging from 12 to 17 h were well tolerated and extremity ischemia minimized. No anticoagulation was used and no evidence of shunt thrombosis or distal emboli was observed.[22]

Experimentally, Aldridge and colleagues found that heparin-bonded polyvinylchloride intravascular shunts remained patent in the arterial circulation for a 24-h period without evidence of distal embolization and no increase in coagulation factor or platelet consumption or red blood cell destruction. In that same model, venous shunts often were noted to be partially lined with mural thrombus. One of ten venous shunts thrombosed within 24 h.[19] The value of major abdominal and pelvic vein shunting in critically injured patients is controversial, as published patency rates are low. However, it has been proposed that temporary shunting may help control short-term edema during acute high-volume resuscitation.

If no significant intra-abdominal bleeding has been identified, a retroperitoneal source should be considered and explored. This begins with the evisceration of the small bowel to inspect the aorta, iliac arteries and veins, and inferior vena cava. Next, retroperitoneal viscera (i.e., colon, kidneys, and duodenum) are mobilized.

Prolonged repair for bleeding from solid organ injuries must be avoided. Splenic and renal hemorrhage is managed best with resection. Bleeding from liver parenchyma is dealt with by manually displacing the liver inferiorly, followed by packing over the dome with multiple laparotomy pads. The space between the diaphragm and the liver is obliterated.

Here the initial ligation of the falciform ligament helps prevent iatrogenic injury as the liver is mobilized. Next, the inferior surface of the liver is also tightly packed.

Ongoing bleeding from deep parenchymal injury then is controlled by the Pringle maneuver (temporary hepatic vascular inflow occlusion by compression of the Porta Hepatis within the lateral edge of the gastrohepatic ligament) followed by finger fracture to expose deep intraparenchymal bleeding vessels for suture ligation or clip application.[23]

More complex injuries (such as transhepatic gunshot wounds with long narrow columns of shredded hepatic parenchyma and active bleeding) require more innovative techniques. Insertion and inflation of a Foley catheter balloon or the use of an inflated Penrose drain over a red rubber catheter is a useful technique.[24,25]

Other strategies can be employed to deal with larger, actively bleeding liver parenchymal disruptions. Placement of hemostatic agents, such as microfibrillar collagen, cellulose sheets, or even fibrin glue within the liver wound itself, may provide additional hemostatic support.[26]

We have had anecdotal success with the "liver tampon." This consists of a sausage-sized piece of absorbable gelatin sponge (Gelfoam™) cut into two centimeter by eight centimeter strips, soaked in thrombin solution, stacked to appropriate width, and wrapped in a sheet of oxidized cellulose (Surgicell™). It is stuffed into the parenchymal defect, followed by additional packing to effectively tamponade the bleeding and provides a hemostatic milieu.

In all cases of complex hepatic injury, we immediately follow the completion of DC I with angiography. Even in those cases where hemostasis seemingly is achieved, we have been surprised at the high incidence of intrahepatic arterial bleeding or arterio-venous fistula revealed by angiogram, which require therapeutic embolization. The care of the patient while in interventional radiology (IR) will be discussed in the DC II section.

## 29.8
## Controlling Contamination

The second priority in a damage control laparotomy, following hemorrhage control, is to control the spillage of intestinal contents or urine from hollow viscus injuries.

Simple bowel perforations that are limited in size and number are repaired using a single-layer continuous suture and then tagged for later reinspection. More extensively injured bowel segments can be either isolated (using cotton umbilical tapes passed through the mesentery) or stapled across (using a linear stapler) on both sides of the wound. To save time, formal resection and reconstruction are avoided, as is stoma creation and feeding tube placement.

With high-velocity penetrating wounds, the extent of bowel wall edema and blast injury effects often are underappreciated at the initial operation; this can cause delayed bowel ischemia and threaten anastamoses and stomas. Therefore, bowel continuity is deferred until DC III following reevaluation of bowel viability.

Biliary tract and pancreatic injuries can be controlled temporarily by intra- or extraluminal tube drainage. This is important because of the damaging effects of the pancreatic enzymes and bile on surrounding tissues. Definitive repair or resection is delayed until physiologic restoration is achieved. Drains are brought out laterally through the flank at the mid-axillary line and intra-abdominal packs are carefully placed so as not to cause kinking of these tubes. Adjunctive studies, including endoscopic retrograde cholangiopancreatography (ERCP) or intraoperative distal pancreatography can be obtained prior to definitive repair if pancreatic and/or bile duct anatomy remains in question.[27]

Once all vascular and bowel injuries have been controlled, intra-abdominal packing is performed. This technique is especially important when coagulopathy is recognized and extensive retroperitoneal or pelvic dissection has been performed.[28,29] Folded laparotomy pads are placed over any solid organ injury and all dissected areas. Packing should be tight enough to provide adequate tamponade without impeding venous return or arterial blood supply.

## 29.9
## Abdominal Closure

Abdominal closure is the final step prior to transport to the ICU. In all damage control cases, fascial closure is not recommended at the initial laparotomy. Secondary to reperfusion injury and ongoing capillary leakage during resuscitation, intestinal and abdominal wall edema will continue and potentially cause intra-abdominal hypertension, abdominal compartment syndrome, and fascial necrosis if there is not adequate provision for volume expansion. Skin-only closures allow for considerable expansion of the abdominal contents and wall while maintaining an insulating protective environment.

One of the most rapid methods of closing the abdomen is to place towel clips in the skin. Alternatively, a simple running nonabsorbable suture placed in the skin is adequate and has the added advantage of allowing ancillary studies (i.e., arteriogram) without radiopaque clamps obstructing the view.

At times, even skin closure is not possible because of massive bowel edema (i.e., bowel protrudes above the abdominal wall when viewed horizontally across the abdomen). In this situation, our practice has evolved from temporary silo-type devices (i.e., the Bogotá bag) to the placement of a vacuum pack (vac-pac) dressing (Figs. 29.3–29.6). This dressing allows rapid temporary abdominal coverage and considerable increase in

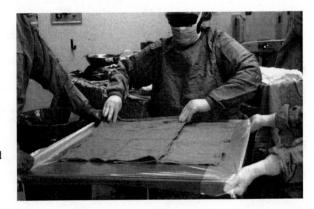

**Fig. 29.3** A sterile towel is covered on one side with adhesive plastic dressing and placed over the intestines and tucked under the fascial edges (Hoey and Schwab[14])

**Fig. 29.4** Closed suction drains are placed above the towel in the subcutaneous gutters and brought out superiorly through long subcutaneous tunnels (Hoey and Schwab[14])

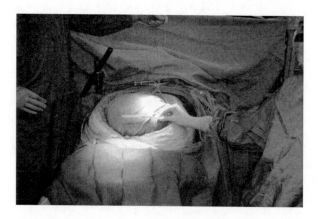

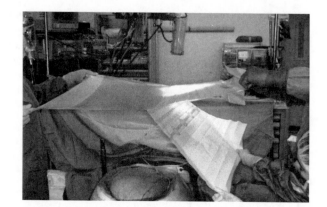

**Fig. 29.5** A second large adhesive drape is placed over the entire abdomen (Hoey and Schwab[14])

**Fig. 29.6** The drains are placed on continuous low suction, creating a vacuum effect; the wound is sealed (Hoey and Schwab[14])

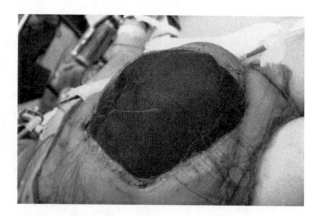

abdominal volume. Controlled egress of fluid from the abdomen is permitted and a sterile barrier is maintained while providing a durable dressing for possible prone-position ventilation.

First, the omentum, if present, should be used to drape the small bowel. Then a large Ioban™ (3M, St. Paul, MN) sheet is held adherent-side up as a sterile blue surgical towel is placed on top. The edges then are folded in and the completed pack is placed over the intestines and tucked beneath the fascia with the Ioban™ side in contact with the bowel to create a nonadherent surface. Two flat Jackson Pratt drains are laid alongside the pack and their ends brought out through separate skin stab wounds cephalad to the upper apex of the incision. A second large Ioban™ sheet then is placed adherent-side down over the abdomen and the intra-abdominal pack. To ensure that the Ioban™ sticks securely to the skin, all abdominal hair, especially in the groin and the suprapubic areas, is shaved and the skin is painted with a thin layer of benzoin. No effort is made to approximate skin edges or force the abdominal wall edges together. The drains are placed on low-pressure, continuous wall suction, creating a vacuum. The drains allow controlled egress of fluid and blood, and the layered plastic dressing maintains a sterile, waterproof barrier.

## 29.10
## Further Procedures

Damage Control Part I cannot be considered complete until all surgical bleeding is arrested, and occasionally a patient will require an interventional radiology procedure to achieve or prolong hemodynamic stability.

Uncontrolled surgical bleeding may not respond to packing alone, and often interventional radiology techniques are necessary to halt bleeding that could not be addressed adequately in the OR. This is particularly true for complex hepatic, retroperitoneal, pelvic, or deep muscle injuries that, because of location, are not amenable to surgical control or would require lengthy surgical exploration, often in the setting of coagulopathy.

Aberrant hepatic arterial anatomy is fairly common and branches arising from the SMA or celiac trunk are difficult to identify intraoperatively, but readily are seen on angiography. This also is true of bleeding lumbar arteries, as well as deep pelvic arterial bleeds.[30]

It is essential that DC II strategies be initiated and maintained during the time the patient spends in the interventional suite. Appropriate monitors, suction devices, respiratory support, patient and fluid warming devices, as well as capable nursing personnel must be available as the IR suite is transformed into an extension of the surgical ICU.

### 29.10.1
### Damage Control Part II: ICU Resuscitation

The goal of DC II is to reverse the sequelae of shock-related metabolic failure and support physiologic and biochemical restoration. Here, simultaneous treatment of all physiologic abnormalities is essential. Preparations for this phase should begin prior to the completion of the initial laparotomy: warming the room, setting up appropriate hemodynamic monitoring devices, ventilator placement, preparing patient and IV fluid warming devices, communication with the blood bank, and assuring adequate nursing availability. The first several hours in the ICU are extremely labor intensive and often require the collaborative efforts of multiple nurses and ancillary staff.

One of the keys to physiologic restoration is the establishment of adequate oxygen delivery to body tissues. Invasive monitoring devices are used to direct this maximization of hemodynamics. In our practice, femoral artery catheters are preferred, as Dorman and colleagues showed that they provided more accurate measures of systolic and mean arterial pressures than radial artery catheter measurements if a patient required high vasopressor support during volume resuscitation.[31]

The use of the pulmonary artery catheter remains controversial. Although it has never been proven to enhance patient outcome in the critically ill, in the damage control subset of injured patients, the volumetric oximetry pulmonary artery catheter is a useful tool to assist in guiding resuscitation based on parameters of preload[32] and oxygen delivery.[33]

To date, the exact hemodynamic endpoints that patients must attain following severe injury in order to reliably survive remain controversial. Moreover, resuscitating patients to arbitrary endpoints of normal or supranormal hemodynamic and oxygen transport variables has not been shown to predict survival. Abramson and colleagues, however, did show that serum lactate clearance correlates well with patient survival and that the ability to clear lactate to normal levels within 24 h was paramount to ensuing patient survival.[34]

Immediate and aggressive core rewarming not only improves perfusion, but also helps reverse coagulopathy. All of the warming maneuvers initiated in the trauma bay and operating room are duplicated in the ICU. These include increasing ambient room temperature, use of a turban or heating device on the patient's head, the application of a convective warm-air blanket or fluid-circulating heat blanket over the trunk and extremities, use of a heating cascade on the ventilator, administration of all resuscitative fluids and blood products through a high-flow warming system, and pleural, gastric, or bladder lavage with warmed fluids.

Occasionally, extracorporeal circulation devices such as veno–venous bypass and arterial–venous bypass via femoral vessel cannulation are necessary for rapid correction of severe hypothermia (core temperature 28–32°C). Rewarming rates of 2°C to 3°C per hour can be achieved with these devices. The limitations of veno–venous bypass include the need for systemic anticoagulation while arterial–venous bypass can be maintained with a heparin-bonded system.[35] However, this requires a normal systolic blood pressure to drive the flow. Gentilello and colleagues showed that failure to correct a patient's hypothermia after a damage control operation is a marker of inadequate resuscitation or irreversible shock.[36]

An aggressive approach to correction of coagulopathy is paramount in DC II. Standard therapy to correct coagulopathy includes reversal of hypothermia and administration of fresh frozen plasma (FFP), which is rich in factors V and VIII. Repletion of clotting factors with FFP continues until laboratory values of the PTT and international normalized ratio (INR) are normalized. Platelet levels also should be followed and corrected accordingly. Likewise, fibrinogen levels should be assessed and, if necessary, cryoprecipitate infused. All blood products should be warmed prior to infusion.

Throughout DC II, the patient should remain sedated and receive complete ventilatory support. Arterial blood gases are used to guide ventilator adjustments.

## 29.11
## Tertiary Survey

During this phase, a complete physical examination or "tertiary survey" of the patient should occur. Appropriate radiographs should be obtained to evaluate for additional skeletal injuries based on physical findings.

Immobilization and/or traction devices are applied when indicated. In the case of associated blunt mechanism, completion of the spine survey is imperative. Peripheral wounds are addressed and vascular integrity of all injured limbs is assessed frequently.

Adjunctive studies such as computed tomography (CT) scanning should be obtained at this time unless the patient is too unstable for travel.

Recruitment of consultants for all definitive repairs should occur early in this phase, and both the extent and priority of repairs must be established.

## 29.12
## Unplanned Reoperation

Two subgroups of patients emerge who require "unplanned" reoperation during DC II prior to achieving physiologic restoration.

The first is the group of patients who continue to require packed red blood cell transfusions despite a corrected coagulopathy and normalized core temperature. These patients usually are found to have ongoing surgical bleeding from a vascular site that was not treated adequately during the initial damage control operation. Once recognized, immediate operative re-exploration to localize and stop the bleeding must occur. These patients have a very high mortality rate.[12,16]

The second group requiring unplanned return to the operating room have developed abdominal compartment syndrome (ACS). This syndrome, first suggested in 1863 by Marey, is a term used to describe a constellation of physiologic sequelae of increased intra-abdominal pressure (IAP) or intra-abdominal hypertension (IAH). It is characterized clinically by a tensely distended abdomen, elevated intra-abdominal pressure and peak airway pressure, impaired ventilation associated with hypoxia and hypercarbia, decreased urine output, increased systemic vascular resistance (SVR), and decreased cardiac output.[37]

Abdominal compartment syndrome has a reported incidence of 6% in patients with severe abdominal and/or pelvic trauma undergoing emergency damage control laparotomy.[38]

These patients are at high risk for the development of IAH from several causes: the use of bulky abdominal packs, continued bleeding into the abdominal cavity from uncorrected coagulopathy; bowel distension and edema from extensive resuscitation volumes (>10 L), or mesenteric vascular injuries and abdominal wall edema.

Management of the open abdomen with the vacuum pack closure technique does not obviate the development of ACS.[39] This may be due to the efficiency with which the vac-pac dressing is able to contain the abdominal volume and allow subsequent intra-abdominal pressure increases to continue.

Vigilant monitoring of intra-abdominal pressure is mandatory in this patient population to recognize IAH and treat it expediently before ACS develops. This is done by intermittently transducing a urinary bladder pressure through the urinary catheter as described by Kron and colleagues.[40]

The technique consists of instilling 50 mL of saline into the urinary bladder via the Foley catheter. The tubing of the collecting bag is clamped and a needle is inserted into the specimen-collecting port of the tubing proximal to the clamp. This needle is attached to tubing that leads to a monitoring device (i.e., a central venous pressure monitor). Bladder pressures above 25 mmHg signify intra-abdominal hypertension. Patients who develop intra-abdominal hypertension must be treated immediately to prevent ACS and its associated extreme mortality.[41]

Treatment consists of opening the patient's abdomen to relieve the pressure. If ongoing blood loss is suspected as the cause of the increased intra-abdominal pressure, this best is performed in the operating room, where lighting and equipment availability is maximized as long as the patient can tolerate the necessary transport. The alternative is to open the abdomen at the bedside in the ICU under sterile conditions. Occasionally, adequate decompression can be achieved without extensive operative intervention by incising the external Ioban™ drape of the vacuum pack to allow for further expansion of the neoabdominal wall prior to placement of a new sterile Ioban™ cover.

## 29.13
## Damage Control: Beyond the Abdomen

More and more case reports are being generated describing the adaptation of damage control principals to severely injured patients with single or multiple injuries to regions of the body other than the abdominal cavity.

Damage control orthopedics describes caring for the patient with severe extremity injury in "extremis." The goal is hemorrhage control and maintenance of flow to distal tissues of the affected limb(s). External fixation of long bone and pelvic ring fractures is performed as an emergency procedure. Formal vascular repair occurs only if simple, otherwise temporary shunts are utilized. Rapid debridement and dressing placement then is performed and the patient is resuscitated in the ICU. This approach has been shown to minimize the duration of initial surgery, hypothermia, and additional blood loss. Formal internal fixation is delayed until the patient's physiology is restored.[42-44]

Damage control surgery principles have been applied selectively in the chest. In the physiologically exhausted patient, the definitive operation is abandoned in favor of an abbreviated thoracotomy.

In an unstable patient with a penetrating lung injury, stapled, nonanatomic wedge resection or pulmonary tractotomy with direct suture ligation of bleeding vessels can be performed. The latter technique works well when the site of hemorrhage is secondary to a deep through and through stab wound or gunshot wound. Here, the pulmonary parenchyma bridging the wound tract is divided using a linear stapling/cutting device. This permits direct inspection of the tract, with selective ligation of bleeding points and control of air leaks.[45]

Although packing of the pleural cavity is an option to temporarily control bleeding, it has obvious physiological consequences related to compression of the heart, great vessels, and viable lung tissue.

A recent case report out of Ben Taub General Hospital describes the "pulmonary hilum twist" as a thoracic damage control technique to control hemorrhage for severe lung trauma when a suitable hilar clamp is unavailable or if hilar control is particularly difficult with instrumentation. This procedure involves division of the inferior pulmonary ligament, then anterior rotation of the lower lobe over the upper lobe, achieving vascular occlusion. This occlusion can be maintained during resuscitation, and definitive resection can follow once physiologic parameters have improved.[46]

A report from Los Angeles described extending damage control principals to the neck.[47] In this report, bleeding in an unstable patient who had sustained a gunshot wound to zone II of the neck initially was controlled by insertion of two Foley catheters into the wound tract and inflation of the balloons. Uncontrollable hemorrhage from the vertebral vessels was encountered intraoperatively during exploration. Standard operative techniques to control bleeding only led to more hemorrhage as the patient became acidotic, hypothermic, and coagulopathic. The decision to damage control was made and the wound was packed tightly and the patient taken to the ICU for resuscitation, followed by the interventional radiology suite for embolization.

## References

1. MacKenzie EJ, Fowler CJ. Epidemiology. In: Mattox KL, Feliciano DV, Moore EE, eds. *Trauma*. 4th ed. New York: McGraw-Hill; 2000:21-39.
2. Sauaia A, Moore FA, Moore EE, et al. Epidemiology of trauma deaths: a reassessment. *J Trauma*. 1995;38:185-193.
3. Gaynor F. *The New Military and Naval Dictionary*. New York: Philosophical Library Publishers; 1951.
4. Department of Defense. Surface Ship Survivability. Washington, DC: Department of Defense; 1996. Naval War Publication 3-20.31.
5. Richardson JD, Franklin GA, Lukan JK, et al. Evolution in the management of hepatic trauma: A 25-year perspective. *Ann Surg*. 2000;232:324-330.
6. Pringle J. Notes on the arrest of hepatic hemorrhage due to trauma. *Ann Surg*. 1908;48: 541-549.
7. Halsted W. Ligature and suture material: the employment of fine silk in preference to catgut and the advantages of transfixing tissues and vessels in controlling hemorrhage—also an account of the introduction of gloves, gutta-percha tissue and silver foil. *JAMA*. 1913;LX: 1119-1126.
8. Lucas C, Ledgerwood A. Prospective evaluation of hemostatic techniques for liver injuries. *J Trauma*. 1976;16:442-451.
9. Caln R, McMaster P, Pentlow B. The treatment of major liver trauma by primary packing with transfer of the patient for definitive treatment. *Br J Trauma*. 1978;66:338-339.
10. Feliciano D, Mattox K, Jordan G. Intra-abdominal packing for control of hepatic hemorrhage: a reappraisal. *J Trauma*. 1981;21:285-290.
11. Stone H, Strom P, Mullins R. Management of the major coagulopathy with onset during laparotomy. *Ann Surg*. 1983;197:532-535.

12. Rotondo M, Schwab CW, McGonigal, et al. Damage control: an approach for improved survival in exsanguinating penetrating abdominal injury. *J Trauma*. 1993;35:373-383.

13. Johnson JW, Gracias VH, Schwab CW, et al. Evolution in damage control for exsanguinating penetrating abdominal injury. *J Trauma*. 2001;51(2):261-271.

14. Hoey BA, Schwab CW. Damage control surgery. *Scand J Surg*. 2002;91:92-103.

15. Shapiro MB, Jenkins DH, Schwab CW, et al. Damage control: collective review. *J Trauma*. 2000;49:969-978.

16. Morris J, Eddy V, Blinman T, et al. The staged celiotomy for trauma: Issues in unpacking and reconstruction. *Ann Surg*. 1993;217:576-584.

17. Rotondo MF, Zonies DH. The damage control sequence and underlying logic. *Surg Clin North Am*. 1997;77:761-777.

18. Moore EE, Burch JM, Franciose RJ, et al. Staged physiologic restoration and damage control surgery. *World J Surg*. 1998;22(12):1184-1190.

19. Garcia-Rinaldi R et al. Unimpaired renal, myocardial, and neurologic function after cross clamping of the thoracic aorta. *Surg Gyn Obstetr*. 1976;143:249-252.

20. Reilly PM, Rotondo MF, Carpenter JP, et al. Temporary vascular continuity during damage control: intraluminal shunting for proximal superior mesenteric artery injury. *J Trauma*. 1995;39:757-760.

21. Aldridge SD, Badellino MM, Malaspina PJ, et al. Extended intravascular shunting in an experimental model of vascular injury. *J Cardiovasc Surg*. 1997;38(2):183-186.

22. Johansen KH, Hedges G. Successful limb reperfusion by temporary arterial shunt during a 950-mile air transfer. *J Trauma*. 1989;29:1289-1291.

23. Pachter HL, Spencer FC, Hofstetter SR, et al. Significant trends in the treatment of hepatic trauma. Experience with 411 injuries. *Ann Surg*. 1992;215:492-502.

24. Poggetti RS, Moore EE, Moore FA, et al. Balloon tamponade for bilobar transfixing hepatic gunshot wounds. *J Trauma*. 1992;33:694-697.

25. Demetriades D. Balloon tamponade for bleeding control in penetrating liver injuries. *J Trauma*. 1998;44:538-539.

26. Shen GK, Rappaport W. Control of nonhepatic intra-abdominal hemorrhage with temporary packing. *SGO*. 1992;174:411-413.

27. Carrillo C, Folger RJ, Shaftan GW. Delayed gastrointestinal reconstruction following massive abdominal trauma. *J Trauma*. 1993;34:233-235.

28. Feliciano DV, Mattox KL, Burch JM, et al. Packing for control of hepatic hemorrhage. *J Trauma*. 1986;26:738-743.

29. Saifi J, Fortune JB, Graca L, et al. Benefits of intra-abdominal pack placement for the management of nonmechanical hemorrhage. *Arch Surg*. 1990;125:119-122.

30. Kushimoto S, Arai M, Aiboshi J, et al. The role of interventional radiology in patients requiring damage control laparotomy. *J Trauma*. 2003;54:171-176.

31. Dorman T, Breslow MJ, Lipsett PA, et al. Radial artery pressure monitoring underestimates central arterial pressure during vasopressor therapy in critically ill surgical patients. *Crit Care Med*. 1998;26:1646-1649.

32. Cheatham ML, Safcsak K, Block EF, et al. Preload assessment in patients with an open abdomen. *J Trauma*. 1999;46:16-22.

33. Bishop MH, Shoemaker WC, Appel PL, et al. Prospective, randomized trial of survivor values of cardiac index, oxygen delivery, and oxygen consumption as resuscitation endpoints in severe trauma. *J Trauma*. 1995;38:780-787.

34. Abramson D, Scalea TM, Hitchcock R, et al. Lactate clearance and survival following injury. *J Trauma*. 1993;35:584-589.

35. Gentilello LM, Cobean RA, Offner PJ, et al. Continuous arteriovenous rewarming: rapid reversal of hypothermia in critically ill patients. *J Trauma*. 1992;32:316-325.

36. Gentilello LM. Practical approaches to hypothermia. In: Maull KI, Cleveland HC, Feliciano DV, Rice LL, Trunkey DD, Wolfoth CC, eds. *Advances in Trauma and Critical Care*. Vol 9. St. Louis: Mosby; 1994:9.

37. Ivatury RR, Sugerman HJ. Abdominal compartment syndrome: a century later, isn't it time to pay attention? *Crit Care Med*. 2000;28:2137-2138.

38. Ertel W, Oberholzer A, Platz A, et al. Incidence and clinical pattern of the abdominal compartment syndrome after "damage control" laparotomy in 311 patients with severe abdominal and/or pelvic trauma. *Crit Care Med*. 2000;28:1747-1753.

39. Gracias VH, Braslow B, Johnson J, et al. Abdominal compartment syndrome in the open abdomen. *Arch Surg*. 2002;137:1298-1300.

40. Kron IL, Harman PK, Nolan SP. The measurement of intra-abdominal pressure as a criterion for exploration. *Ann Surg*. 1984;199:28-30.

41. Rowlands BJ, Flynn TC, Fischer RP. Temporary abdominal wound closure with a silastic "chimney". *Contemp Surg*. 1984;24:17-20.

42. Przkora R, Ulrich B, Zelle B, et al. Damage control orthopedics: a case report. *J Trauma*. 2002;53:765-769.

43. Nowotarski PJ, Turen CH, Brumback RJ, et al. Conversion of external fixation to intramedullary nailing for fractures of the shaft of the femur in multiply injured patients. *J Bone Joint Surg Am*. 2000;82:781-788.

44. Scalea TM, Boswell SA, Scott JD, et al. External fixation as a bridge to intramedullary nailing for patients with multiple injuries and femur fractures: damage control orthopedics. *J Trauma*. 2000;48:613-621.

45. Wall MJ, Villavicencio RT, Miller CC, et al. Pulmonary tractotomy as an abbreviated thoracotomy technique. *J Trauma*. 1998;45:1015-1023.

46. Wilson A, Wall MJ, Maxson R, et al. The pulmonary hilum twist as a thoracic damage control procedure. *Am J Surg*. 2003;186:49-52.

47. Firoozmand E, Velmahos G. Extending damage-control principals to the neck. *J Trauma*. 2000;48:541-543.

# Management of Vascular Trauma

# 30

Kate Brown and Nigel Tai

## 30.1
## Introduction

Uncontrolled hemorrhage is the cause of up to 40% of deaths in civilian trauma and over half of combat deaths.[1,2] Truncal hemorrhage has been identified as the leading cause of potentially survivable deaths in combat casualties, irrespective of injury severity.[3] The combat environment provides a difficult working environment with possibilities for delayed patient transport, limitations on resources, and surgeons who lack vascular expertise. The significant advances made in vascular surgery over the course of the last century are closely related to the experience obtained during military conflict. Ligation - being the method of choice in both World Wars - resulted in an amputation rate of mangled extremities with vascular injuries of 50%.[4] However, surgeons mobilized during the Korean War had the benefit of new understanding in surgical physiology and improved instrumentation that heralded restorative techniques, a reduction in the amputation rate to 13%, and the modern era of vascular surgery.[5]

Vascular injuries are particularly intolerant of suboptimal technique; repair can be lengthy (2–9 h),[6] especially if the operating team lacks day-to-day familiarity with vascular exposures, vessel handling, and repair skills. Furthermore, attempting limb salvage carries an appreciable mortality risk in both civilian and combat trauma.[7]

## 30.2
## Epidemiology

Vascular injuries in conflict are not overly common. In combat trauma, they account for 4.8–7% injury rate,[8,9] although this is higher than the 2–3% rate observed during the Vietnam War. This may be a reflection of the improvement of body armor leading to an

K. Brown (✉)
Trauma and Orthopaedics, Royal College of Defence Medicine, Birmingham, UK
e-mail: katevbrown@aol.com

A.J. Brooks et al. (eds.), *Ryan's Ballistic Trauma*,
DOI: 10.1007/978-1-84882-124-8_30, © Springer-Verlag London Limited 2011

increase in casualties reaching the higher echelons of care with complex extremity injuries.[10] In fact, a 5% extremity vascular injury rate in UK military personnel has been recently reported. Central vascular injuries are less common (<2% abdominal vascular injuries) and are highly lethal.[4,5,11]

In comparison, there is a much higher incidence of abdominal vascular injuries in civilian trauma - up to 30% - possibly because of the more modest wounding capacity of handguns and sharp implements, and reduced pre-hospital timelines.

## 30.3
## Pathophysiology

Conflict wounds differ vastly from civilian trauma due to the prevalence of high energy missile and blast injury. Civilian ballistic trauma is mostly low energy, with less soft tissue destruction. Missiles and fragments can strike the vessel directly, or the vessel can be injured by energized secondary bone fragments from an adjacent fracture site. Vessels may be traumatized indirectly by high energy missiles due to propagation of the shock wave front across the vessel axis, with intimal disruption. Total energy transfer to the soft tissues determines wounding power, which depends upon the kinetic energy of the missile (weight, velocity), the profile of the missile as it travels through tissue, and the retarding force exerted by the tissue on that missile (tissue density). Low energy transfer wounds are associated with confinement of the injurious effect to the wound track; high energy transfer wounds may be associated with damage beyond the immediate axis of the missile's track due to the associated shock wave and cavitational effects observed with higher velocity missiles. Whatever the weapon, the surgeon must base treatment on the nature of the wound before him or her.

Blast injuries have been generally categorized as primary, secondary, tertiary, or quaternary.[12,13] Primary blast injuries are caused by the sudden change in environmental pressure called the blast wave. Secondary blast is resultant from objects sufficiently energized by the explosion to become projectiles. Tertiary blast trauma occurs when the casualty is thrown against the ground or an object. Quaternary or miscellaneous causes include inhalational and thermal injury. The instantaneous pressure change injures tissue through spalling, implosion, acceleration-deceleration, and pressure differential phenomena, any of which may disrupt the vessel wall.

Penetrating trauma causes free bleeding either from complete or partial transection. Complete transection allows for vessel retraction and spasm, which may mitigate against on-going hemorrhage, whereas partial transection does not. Vessel contusion without penetration may, despite axial continuity, lead to intimal flap, dissection, thrombosis, and end-organ ischaemia.

Repair of arterial structures and restoration of flow should be completed within a 6-h period or irreversible tissue change will occur. This time window has been cited since the landmark paper by Miller and Welch, which showed unacceptable levels of infection, anastomotic failure, and muscular contracture, resulting in reduced function and limb loss, in extremities that underwent ischaemic episodes of more than 6 h.[14] This was confirmed by Malan's histological studies on critical warm ischaemia time for striated muscle.[15] Six hours represents the maximal distal time-point for flow restoration: muscle necrosis may occur in as little as 3 h[16]; nervous tissue – which exhibits a higher basal metabolic rate – is more vulnerable still to ischaemia. Minimisation of warm ischaemia time is essential in securing favorable outcomes.

## 30.4
## Clinical Features

The key to diagnosing peripheral vascular trauma is a careful, thorough physical examination. On going hemorrhage and ischaemia is classically indicated by the presence of the "hard signs" of vascular injury - these mandate urgent intervention and repair (Table 30.1). The utility of these signs – in determining need for surgery – is widely accepted in ballistic trauma patients, but validation is restricted to non-ballistic series looking at popliteal trauma in relation to knee dislocation (100% negative predictive value and a 94.3% positive predictive value).[17] In ballistic patients the possible presence of confounding factors (global shock as the cause of diminished pulses, or direct damage to the peripheral nerves as the cause of neurological deficit) must be taken in to consideration. The so-called "soft signs" of vascular injury (Table 30.2), if found, necessitate further investigation to rule out vascular trauma. When vascular injury is suspected, compartment syndrome must be sought for and addressed – if necessary by prophylactic fasciotomy. Wounds should be objectively classified according to the International Committee of the Red Cross wound classification.[18]

Hard and soft signs are less applicable to major vascular trauma within the trunk, when rapid onset of severe shock is the usual presentation. Wounds to the neck can be usefully be classified as Zone I (from suprasternal notch to cricoid cartilage), Zone II (cricoid to angle of jaw) or Zone III (angle of jaw to base of skull) – although this categorisation makes the assumption that the site of skin breach correlates to the site of vessel damage.

**Table 30.1** The hard signs of vascular injury

| |
|---|
| 1. Active hemorrhage |
| 2. Expanding/expansile haematoma ± bruit |
| 3. Distal ischaemia (Pallor, Pulselessness, Paraesthesia, Pain, "Perishingly" cold, Paralysis) |

**Table 30.2** The soft signs of vascular injury

| |
|---|
| 1. Peripheral nerve deficit |
| 2. History of hemorrhage at the scene |
| 3. An injury in proximity to a major artery |

## 30.5
## Investigations

Plain radiographs are useful as fracture patterns give useful clues as the likelihood of injury to adjacent vessels. Common examples would be the association between supracondylar humeral fractures and brachial artery injuries or tibial plateau fractures and popliteal injuries. Visualization of retained fragments or rounds allows estimation of wound track and at-risk vessels.

The simplest adjunct to diagnosis of peripheral vascular trauma is the Ankle: Brachial Pressure Index (ABPI). This is measured by obtaining the highest arterial occlusion pressure using a manual blood pressure cuff at the ankle and hand-held Doppler probe placed over the dorsalis pedis and the posterior tibial arteries. This pressure value is divided by the highest brachial systolic blood pressure.

ABPI = Ankle systolic blood pressure/highest brachial systolic blood pressure

An abnormal ABPI is signified by any value <0.9. A pressure deficit of >10% or 20 mmHg compared to the contralateral uninjured limb is a "soft sign" of arterial injury and mandates confirmation with further investigations. In the absence of obvious signs of arterial injury, the arterial pressure index has been shown in civilian trauma to have a high sensitivity and specificity for arterial disruption[19-21] thus avoiding the need for more time consuming and invasive investigations.

The latter include formal contrast angiography, computed tomographic (CT) angiography and duplex. Typically, these modalities will be employed when the level of injury is unknown because of multiple fragmentation or spalling levels. Formal angiography with a view to intervention (embolisation, stent placement) is aided by involvement of an interventional radiologist working in a dedicated angiography suite. Diagnostic angiography does not necessarily require these assets, and may be undertaken in the operating theater using either C-Arm image intensification or a toweled plain X-Ray cassette beneath the patients' extremity. The required elements are a 14 gauge IV, a three-way stopcock, two 20–30 mL syringes and intravenous contrast media. The upstream uninjured vessel is exposed, controlled, and a proximal clamp applied prior to cannulation and injection of contrast and image acquisition. One syringe is used for aspiration and flushing with heparinised solution and the other is used to inject full strength contrast. Failure to visualize the vessel axis must be correlated with the injury track and the patient's condition, recognizing that vessel visualization may be difficult in the shocked, cold patient. However, observed cut-offs in contrast filling should never be dismissed as "spasm" – especially if the casualty has been appropriately resuscitated.

Multi-detector CT angiography (CTA) now rivals contrast angiography in terms of injury detection (contrast "blush," pseudo-aneurysm, luminal filling defects), is non-invasive, can delineate non-vascular injury, and is particularly useful in truncal and neck trauma.[22] CTA allows judicious selection of patients for appropriate endovascular techniques such as embolisation in hard-to access vessels (such as the intra-cervical vertebral artery and in pelvic hemorrhage). One shortfall is the degradation of image from metallic artifact – making formal angiography a necessity in such cases. Color flow duplex is accurate in the delineation of pseudo-aneurysms and arteriovenous fistula in non-acute

**Table 30.3** Principles of management of injury to root of neck

| |
|---|
| 1. Nurse head down (prevent air embolus) |
| 2. Effective pressure/Foley catheter |
| 3. Securing of airway |
| 4. Contralateral venous access |

cases, but limited out-of-hours availability restricts overall utility in most trauma-receiving centers.

As explained above, neck wound classification (Zone 1–III) is a useful adjunct in guiding investigation and management: Zone II wounds are more amenable to surgical exploration via a standard axial neck incision (made anterior to sternocleidomastoid), whilst Zone I and III wounds require a more cautious approach because of potential difficulty in getting proximal and distal control respectively. Assuming patient stability, further investigation with angiography or CTA may be rewarded with information that guides the surgeon to a more proximal incision (thoracotomy, median sternotomy), or to employ an endovascular approach (vertebral artery embolisation) (Table 30.3).

## 30.6
## Management

The management of ballistic trauma follows the <C>ABC systemic approach to minimize blood loss, maximize tissue oxygenation, and optimize outcome. It aims to achieve and conclude an operative procedure before the physiologic point of no return is reached - an irreversible progression of the deadly triad of hypothermia, metabolic acidosis, and coagulopathy.

Victims of improvised explosive devices may present with catastrophic injury patterns including traumatic amputation, mangled extremity, and torso trauma. Control of bleeding can be achieved with firm digital pressure following removal of the bandages and elevation of the limb (particularly effective with venous injuries). Care should be taken if a tourniquet is already in-situ and bleeding has been controlled. The decision to release the tourniquet in the ED depends upon the time the tourniquet has been in place, the clinical state of the extremity and the decision as to the immediacy of transfer of the casualty to the operating theater. Haemostatic adjuncts (such as QuikClot or HemCon) should generally be left in-situ until the patient is in the theater and take-down can be performed under controlled circumstances. Fluid therapy should follow the principles of haemostatic resuscitation and permissive hypotension to minimize the development of coagulopathy.[6,23,24] Haemostatic resuscitation has not been associated with subsequent graft thrombosis.

Where pressure alone is not efficacious, balloon tamponade can be employed to control a bleeding wound track using a Foley catheter. The classic indication for this technique is juxta-thoracic outlet trauma where the subclavian artery has been injured and there is an associated haemothorax. Following careful insertion, the balloon is inflated, and the outflow lumen clamped. A second catheter is then introduced superficially and inflated to control the external bleeding. Placement requires careful technique in order to reduce the chance of iatrogenic injury.

Explosive munitions and even civilian firearms cause contaminated wounds and therefore antimicrobial (and tetanus prophylaxis in vulnerable populations) is essential.

Rapid surgical planning and communication between the ED, attendant orthopedic and general surgeons and theater will expedite patient transfer for definitive intervention. The theater team should be pre-briefed as to what instruments are required, patient and table positioning, and the basic operative plan. Where the vascular injury occurs in the context of polytrauma, a multi-team, parallel approach has obvious advantages in reducing total surgical time.

## 30.7
## Operative Management

The principle objective in theater is to gain control of the bleeding. The patient should be adequately prepared and draped with full exposure of the wound site and anticipation as to the necessity for proximal and distal extension of incisions. With extremity injuries, the entire limb and adjacent torso area should be prepped (including an uninvolved lower limb to allow for harvesting of autologous graft). Upper extremity or neck injuries require preparation of the chest to allow for rapid median sternotomy or thoracotomy. Abdominal injuries mandate preparation of the entire torso; lower extremity injury necessitates abdominal preparation.

Incisions should be centered on the observed wound and extended axially, following the line of the neurovascular bundle and using natural anatomical planes. The initial sequence of maneuver should allow proximal then distal vascular control, followed by adequate tissue debridement (removal of debris, foreign objects, detached bone, and contaminated tissue) prior to carefully definition of the vascular injury. Thrombi are removed by the careful passage of a Fogarty balloon catheter in a retrograde and antegrade direction, whilst avoiding over inflation of the balloon to prevent intimal damage. Inflow and backflow should be assured prior to heparinised saline flush, both proximally and distally (Table 30.4).

**Table 30.4** Principles of surgical wound management

| |
|---|
| 1. Excision of all foreign material and devitalised tissue |
| 2. Copious wound irrigation |
| 3. Stabilization of associated fractures (splintage, external fixation) |
| 4. Leave wounds opens |
| 5. Targetted antimicrobial therapy of short duration |

## 30.8
## Intra-Operative Decision Making

Once vascular control and injury definition has been achieved, a critical decision must be taken as to whether a strategy of damage control or definitive repair is to be undertaken. This decision is dependant upon a number of factors including: the patient's overall injury burden, the number of casualties waiting to be treated, and the skill set of the surgeon. However, patient physiology (temperature, acid-base status, haemodynamic profile, and coagulation parameters) is the governing influence on whether a damage control procedure is required.

## 30.9
## Damage Control

### 30.9.1
### Ligation

Ligation does not necessarily lead to limb loss. Whilst popliteal artery ligation is associated with subsequent amputation in three-quarters of cases, ligating arteries in well collateralized vascular beds such as the upper arm (brachial artery) or upper thigh (superficial femoral artery) carries less risk of limb loss. It is acceptable to ligate one of the two forearm arteries, or two of the three distal arteries in the acute setting, as this does not generally influence limb loss rates.[4]

### 30.9.2
### Shunting

Whilst this technique has found contemporary favor in Iraq and Afghanistan, the use of temporary vascular shunts for battlefield injury is not a new phenomenon : shunts were utilized to restore perfusion prior to fracture fixation in combined vascular/orthopedic injury during the Algerian War, Northern Ireland and Vietnam.[25] Used in this way, shunt insertion allows orthopedic management (accurate fracture reduction and fixation) to precede definitive vascular repair – a previously contentious issue of prioritization.[26,27] When used in unstable patients, shunts reduce the time to flow restoration by negating the need to harvest vein and suture the anastomoses. Shunts may be used in both the venous and arterial circulations where there is co-existent damage - diminishing venous hypertension, bleeding, and perhaps enhancing patency of the arterial shunt. Additionally, shunts may favorably temporize and compensate for lack of vascular expertise in the forward or austere setting, permitting flow restoration and casualty evacuation to a more stable and sophisticated surgical center.

Practically, it seems that shunt use is best confined to above-elbow or above-calf vessel repair, since patency in distal injuries is poor (12%) although this has not been observed to

**Table 30.5** Principles of techniques for use of shunts

| |
|---|
| 1. Distal fasciotomy |
| 2. Re-establishment venous outflow before arterial shunting |
| 3. Avoidance of looping |
| 4. Appropriate shunt diameter |
| 5. Avoidance external angulations of extremities |
| 6. Distal monitoring with ultra sound |
| 7. Briefing of "actions on" to clinical and nursing staff |

adversely affect early limb loss rates. Patency in proximal vascular injuries approaches 90%[28] in combat casualties and duration of use for up to 52 h has been reported in a civilian context.[29] Shunt selection is largely dependant on availability and surgeon preference. The most commonly used commercial shunts are the Javid, Argyll, Sundt, and Pruitt-Inhara,[30] originally designed to provide carotid bypass for the cerebral circulation during endart-erectomy. Shunts can also be fashioned from sterile medical tubing such as intravenous tubing, nasogastric tubes, endotracheal suction catheters, ventriculoperitoneal shunts, and thoracostomy tubes. In general, it is preferable to have the shunt placed in-line with the vessel, secured with a simple snugging ligature at each end, with minimal looping/redun-dancy of shunt. The shunt should be long enough to counter the risk of dislodgement, but short enough such that distal vessel curvature does not cut across the end-face of the shunt lumen and obstruct outflow (Table 30.5).

Dislodgment is rare and usually secondary to inadequate fixation.[31] Critical care medi-cal staff, nurses, and others involved in the ICU management or evacuation of shunted patients should be briefed about the warning signs of shunt dislodgement or thrombosis. Dislodgement is usually marked by sudden wound swelling and bleeding between the wound sutures. The immediate action is to take the patient back to theater for wound exploration, control of hemorrhage, and re-siting of the shunt. Occlusion is manifested as an alteration in limb color, temperature, and capillary return. An unviable limb mandates return to theater, and should the patient's condition allow it, definitive reconstruction. Although a historical series of single system/vessel trauma has reported benefit with post-reconstruction systemic heparinisation,[32] the latter may exacerbate traumatic coagulopathy in those with multi-system injury (the cohort in which a shunt is likely to be needed) and is therefore to be avoided.[29]

### 30.9.3
### Fasciotomy

All patients undergoing shunting or ligation for peripheral vascular trauma should undergo an appropriate fasciotomy to the limb compartments supplied by the injured vessel.

Four-compartment fasciotomy via full length medial and lateral incisions is the stan-dard default procedure in lower-limb vascular trauma, and should be considered prior to exploration of the vascular injury when ischaemic times are prolonged. Aggressive prophylactic fasciotomy is justifiable when the patient has combined venous and arterial trauma, co-existent shock, a prolonged ischaemic time, or when the patient is sedated, obtunded, or due to be dispatched in to an evacuation chain.

## 30.9.4
## Amputation

Limb amputation is a serious and irreversible procedure and should not be undertaken lightly. The decision should, in ideal circumstances, be made by two senior surgeons. It is indicated if the patient is judged to be too unwell to tolerate revascularisation, or has experienced prolonged ischaemia making functional recovery very unlikely, or because the limb is unsalvageable due to the extent of damage to cutaneous, musculo-skeletal, nervous, and vascular structures. Whilst useful in comparing populations, limb trauma scoring systems are not sufficiently sensitive or specific to select individual patients for amputation[33-36] and have not been validated in either civilian[37] or combat casualties.[38]

   Guillotine sections through the obviously viable tissue above the injury risk unnecessary loss of length; flap formation at the initial surgery risks subsequent flap failure and necessity for re-formation later – again with loss of length. Instead, the amputation should be considered a form of debridement, with the goal being preservation of limb length through the use of creative planes of tissue section, preservation of potentially salvageable tissues, and washout of the stump prior to light packing of tissue planes and careful dressing with gauze and crepe. Serial re-inspection allows further post resuscitation tissue inspection, debridement, washout, and eventual closure.

## 30.9.5
## Torso Vascular Damage Control

The major vascular structures in the abdomen are located within the retroperitoneal tissues; damage to these structures presents as a retroperitoneal haematoma (central, lateral, pelvic). Initial abdominal packing and suction followed by evisceration, sequential pack removal, and classification of the site of the haematoma is the prelude to the key maneuvers needed to expose the bleeding vessels. In *in-extremis* patients, the supra-coeliac aorta should be compressed whilst haemostatic resuscitation is delivered. Definitive aortic occlusion can be obtained by clamping the supracoeliac segment. The liver is retracted toward the right shoulder and the stomach toward the left hip, tensing the lesser omentum, through which a window is made to reach the posterior peritoneum overlying the diaphragmatic crura. The peritoneum is divided and the crura split along the line of its fibers to reach the pearly-white aorta, lying to the left of the midline. A plane is developed around the aorta's lateral borders in order to allow application of a straight aortic clamp. Failure to recover a blood pressure is usually associated with futility.

   Central haematomata - secondary to significant damage to the aorta or its visceral branches, or injury to the inferior vena cava or portal circulation - must be explored.

The key maneuvers are extended medial visceral rotation –left, right, or combined – in order to gain proximal control. Lateral haematomata – seen in penetrating kidney trauma – must also be explored in the context of ballistic injury – with control of the hilum achieved via medial visceral rotation or central trans-mesenteric dissection. Pelvic haematomata caused by penetrating mechanisms should also be explored, using a "walk the clamps" approach to progressively isolate the bleeding pelvic vessel prior to repair, shunting, or ligation. Ligation of abdominal vasculature for damage control is a feasible tactic - with the exception of suprarenal IVC injury or trauma to the proximal portion of the superior mesenteric artery - due to the high incidence of renal failure and intestinal infarction respectively. As for any other damage control laparotomy, the abdomen should be left unclosed to offset development of abdominal compartment syndrome.

Injury to the aortic arch vessels – heralded by a Zone 1 neck injury - is classically approached via initial median sternotomy in order to get proximal control, although a high, 3rd intercostal space clamshell thoracotomy is a quicker incision to expedite in peri-arrest patients. Supraclavicular incision, division of the anterior scalene -sparing the phrenic nerve - and access to the 2nd and 3rd parts of the subclavian artery can be combined with median sternotomy for additional control. The axillary artery may be approached via an infraclavicular counter-incision and exposed once the overlying fibers of pectoralis major have been split and the tendon of pectoralis minor divided. The subclavian and axillary arteries can be ligated judiciously with little risk of limb loss. In the neck, the external carotid and internal jugular can be unilaterally ligated with few sequelae.[22] However, the internal carotid artery (ICA) and common carotid artery should be repaired if possible to offset the chance of stroke due to an incomplete circle of Willis. The use of shunts in this situation is controversial; but the only way to ensure that pro-grade hemispherical flow is maintained during repair is to deploy a by-pass shunt to aid cerebral circulation. When ICA repair is not possible the vessel should be ligated, clipped, or if there is insufficient stump to work with, "embolised" using a size 3 Fogarty catheter placed and inflated within the vessel lumen a centimeter beyond the injury. The balloon can be left in-situ, having clipped the inflation channel of the catheter and sutured the catheter shaft into position to prevent distal dislodgement.

## 30.10
## Definitive Management and Repair

Assuming that a damage control approach is not required, the next step following vascular control, injury definition, inspection, debridement, and Fogarty sweep is to make an appraisal of the type of repair required. Minor and transverse lacerations may be primarily sutured – with sutures placed along the axial length of the vessel to prevent luminal narrowing. Such injuries are comparatively rare in ballistic trauma; and patch angioplasty or interposition grafting is usually required. The former is applicable when, following meticulous and thorough debridement, greater than 50% of the lacerated vessel's circumference remains. More extensive loss or vessel transection typically requires grafting. The conduit of choice in extremity injury is autologous reversed long saphenous vein (assuming that the venous drainage of the ipsilateral lower limb is not threatened). Synthetic grafts are acceptable in civilian, low energy wounds, although use in combat wounds carries a high risk of infection and complication due to wound contamination.[28] The wound bed surrounding and covering the graft must be viable – muscle flaps can be swung over or behind the graft if there is an insufficient soft tissue envelope, or the graft can be laid in an extra-anatomic position away from the wound cavity in order to prevent "spanning" – a prelude to thrombosis. Where possible, venous injuries should be repaired, particularly in combat trauma where destruction of venous collateral circulation is more prevalent due to the higher energy mechanisms.

It is essential to warn the anesthetist that flow is about to be restored prior to final release of clamps, in order that the local and systemic sequelae of wash-out from an ischaemic tissue bed are mitigated by appropriate fluid and ventilatory maneuvers. The surgeon should actively consider prophylactic fasciotomy in limbs where a vascular repair has been necessary, even when the compartments are initially flaccid, as peak elevation in compartmental pressure is often delayed.

## 30.11
## Endovascular Management

Although increasingly used in the early management of blunt traumatic disruption of the thoracic aorta,[39] endovascular techniques have yet to win similar favor in the acute management of acute ballistic vascular injury. Temporary balloon occlusion or trans-catheter embolisation of difficult-to-access vessels in deep muscle beds, junctional areas, or bony canals is the most advantageous interventions. Covered stent deployment across a transected vessel is dependent on the necessity to successfully traverse the gap with a guide wire – a challenging procedure; once deployed stents may become infected,[40] thrombose or embolise. Long-term data are non-existent as follow-up is not possible in many ballistic-injury patients. Chronic traumatic pseudo-aneurysms and arteriovenous fistula lend themselves better to elective endovascular treatment. The array of specialist personnel and equipment required for most endovascular procedures weighs against utilization in the forward or austere setting, although advances in equipment design and training may make this a more practical proposal in the future.

## 30.12
## Summary

Vascular trauma remains an uncommon but important injury pattern in patients wounded by ballistic mechanisms. Proximal and distal control, meticulous debridement, and painstaking repair: the individual surgical techniques and maneuvers required for successful restoration of vascular anatomical integrity have remained largely unchanged for four decades. Modern advances include multidetector CTA, which is reducing the need for formal angiography in many patients; the acceptance of the damage control approach in the operative treatment of the critically injured; and the possible reduction in need for damage control techniques as haemostatic resuscitation extends the operative window of opportunity. Endovascular techniques have yet to usurp conventional surgery in the management of the majority of casualties, but technological advances may make this modality more applicable in the future.

## References

1. Sauaia A, Moore FA, Moore EE, et al. Epidemiology of trauma deaths: a reassessment. *J Trauma*. 1995;38(2):185-193.
2. Bellamy RF. The causes of death in conventional land warfare: implications for combat casualty care research. *Mil Med*. 1984;149(2):55-62.
3. Kelly JF, Ritenour AE, McLaughlin DF, et al. Injury severity and causes of death from operation iraqi freedom and operation enduring freedom: 2003–2004 versus 2006. *J Trauma*. 2008;64(2 Suppl):S21-S26. Discussion S26-S27.
4. Debakey ME, Simeone FA. Battle injuries of the arteries in world war II: an analysis of 2,471 cases. *Ann Surg*. 1946;123(4):534-579.
5. Hughes CW. Arterial repair during the korean war. *Ann Surg*. 1958;147(4):555-561.
6. Fox CJ, Gillespie DL, Cox ED, et al. The effectiveness of a damage control resuscitation strategy for vascular injury in a combat support hospital: results of a case control study. *J Trauma*. 2008;64(2 Suppl):S99-S106. Discussion S106-S107.
7. Bondurant FJ, Cotler HB, Buckle R, Miller-Crotchett P, Browner BD. The medical and economic impact of severely injured lower extremities. *J Trauma*. 1988;28(8):1270-1273.
8. Clouse WD, Rasmussen TE, Peck MA, et al. In-Theater management of vascular injury: 2 years of the balad vascular registry. *J Am Coll Surg*. 2007;204(4):625-632.
9. Fox CJ, Gillespie DL, O'Donnell SD, et al. Contemporary management of wartime vascular trauma. *J Vasc Surg*. 2005;41(4):638-644.
10. Starnes BW, Beekley AC, Sebesta JA, Andersen CA, Rush RM. Extremity vascular injuries on the battlefield: tips for surgeons deploying to war. *J Trauma*. 2006;60(2):432-442.
11. Rich NM. Vascular trauma in Vietnam. *J Cardiovasc Surg (Torino)*. 1970;11(5):368-377.
12. Leibovici D, Gofrit ON, Stein M, et al. Blast injuries: bus versus open-air bombings–a comparative study of injuries in survivors of open-air versus confined-space explosions. *J Trauma*. 1996;41(6):1030-1035.
13. Stapczynski JS. Blast injuries. *Ann Emerg Med*. 1982;11(12):687-694.
14. Miller HH, Welch CS. Quantitative studies on the time factor in arterial injuries. *Ann Surg*. 1949;130(3):428-438.
15. Malan E, Tattoni G. Physio- and anatomo-pathology of acute ischemia of the extremities. *J Cardiovasc Surg (Torino)*. 1963;4:212-225.
16. Vaillancourt C, Shrier I, Vandal A, et al. Acute compartment syndrome: how long before muscle necrosis occurs? *CJEM*. 2004;6(3):147-154.
17. Miranda FE, Dennis JW, Veldenz HC, Dovgan PS, Frykberg ER. Confirmation of the safety and accuracy of physical examination in the evaluation of knee dislocation for injury of the popliteal artery: a prospective study. *J Trauma*. 2002;52(2):247-251. discussion 251-252.
18. Coupland RM. The red cross classification of war wounds: the E.X.C.F.V.M. Scoring system. *World J Surg*. 1992;16(5):910-917.
19. Lynch K, Johansen K. Can doppler pressure measurement replace "exclusion" arteriography in the diagnosis of occult extremity arterial trauma? *Ann Surg*. 1991;214(6):737-741.

20. Johansen K, Lynch K, Paun M, Copass M. Non-Invasive vascular tests reliably exclude occult arterial trauma in injured extremities. *J Trauma*. 1991;31(4):515-519. Discussion 519-522.

21. Mills WJ, Barei DP, McNair P. The value of the ankle-brachial index for diagnosing arterial injury after knee dislocation: a prospective study. *J Trauma*. 2004;56(6):1261-1265.

22. Fox CJ, Gillespie DL, Weber MA, et al. Delayed evaluation of combat-related penetrating neck trauma. *J Vasc Surg*. 2006;44(1):86-93.

23. Brohi K, Singh J, Heron M, Coats T. Acute traumatic coagulopathy. *J Trauma*. 2003;54(6): 1127-1130.

24. Holcomb JB. Damage control resuscitation. *J Trauma*. 2007;62(6 Suppl):S36-S37.

25. Eger M, Golcman L, Goldstein A, Hirsch M. The use of a temporary shunt in the management of arterial vascular injuries. *Surg Gynecol Obstet*. 1971;132(1):67-70.

26. Freischlag JA, Sise M, Quinones-Baldrich WJ, Hye RJ, Sedwitz MM. Vascular complications associated with orthopedic procedures. *Surg Gynecol Obstet*. 1989;169(2):147-152.

27. O'Donnell TF, Brewster DC, Darling RC, Veen H, Waltman AA. Arterial injuries associated with fractures and/or dislocations of the knee. *J Trauma*. 1977;17(10):775-784.

28. Rasmussen TE, Clouse WD, Jenkins DH, Peck MA, Eliason JL, Smith DL. The use of temporary vascular shunts as a damage control adjunct in the management of wartime vascular injury. *J Trauma*. 2006;61(1):8-12. Discussion 12-15.

29. Granchi T, Schmittling Z, Vasquez J, Schreiber M, Wall M. Prolonged use of intraluminal arterial shunts without systemic anticoagulation. *Am J Surg*. 2000;180(6):493-496. Discussion 496-497.

30. Ding W, Wu X, Li J. Temporary intravascular shunts used as a damage control surgery adjunct in complex vascular injury: collective review. *Injury*. 2008;39(9):970-977.

31. Aucar JA, Hirshberg A. Damage control for vascular injuries. *Surg Clin North Am*. 1997;77(4):853-862.

32. Daugherty ME, Sachatello CR, Ernst CB. Improved treatment of popliteal arterial injuries using anticoagulation and extra-anatomic reconstruction. *Arch Surg*. 1978;113(11):1317-1321.

33. Johansen K, Daines M, Howey T, Helfet D, Hansen ST. Objective criteria accurately predict amputation following lower extremity trauma. *J Trauma*. 1990;30(5):568-572. Discussion 572-573.

34. Howe HR, Poole GV, Hansen KJ, et al. Salvage of lower extremities following combined orthopedic and vascular trauma. A predictive salvage index. *Am Surg*. 1987;53(4):205-208.

35. McNamara MG, Heckman JD, Corley FG. Severe open fractures of the lower extremity: a retrospective evaluation of the mangled extremity severity score (MESS). *J Orthop Trauma*. 1994;8(2):81-87.

36. Russell WL, Sailors DM, Whittle TB, Fisher DF, Burns RP. Limb salvage versus traumatic amputation. A decision based on a seven-part predictive index. *Ann Surg*. 1991;213(5):473-480. Discussion 480-481.

37. Bosse MJ, MacKenzie EJ, Kellam JF, et al. A prospective evaluation of the clinical utility of the lower-extremity injury-severity scores. *J Bone Joint Surg Am*. 2001;83-A(1):3-14.

38. Pringle JHV. Notes on the arrest of hepatic hemorrhage due to trauma. *Ann Surg*. 1908;48(4):541-549.

39. Alsac JM, Boura B, Desgranges P, Fabiani JN, Becquemin JP, Leseche G, for the PARIS-VASC. Immediate endovascular repair for acute traumatic injuries of the thoracic aorta: a multicenter analysis of 28 cases. *J Vasc Surg*. 2008, Sep 18.

40. Fox CJ, Starnes BW. Vascular surgery on the modern battlefield. *Surg Clin North Am*. 2007;87(5):1193-1211. xi. Nov;70(6):372–376.

# Damage Control Part III: Definitive Reconstruction

**31**

Steven R. Allen, Adam J. Brooks, Patrick M. Reilly, and Bryan A. Cotton

## 31.1
## Introduction

The concept of damage control resuscitation encompasses multiple phases of care: the prehospital and trauma bay resuscitation (DC 0), the initial surgical exploration via laparotomy, thoracotomy, or sternotomy with exsanguination and contamination control (DC I) and further resuscitation within the surgical intensive care unit (DC II). All of this leads up to definitive organ repair and abdominal closure, termed damage control phase III (DC III). Timing of this particular stage is critical as it will likely have the most impact on achieving traditional measures of "successful outcomes" (e.g.- hospital length of stay, surgical site infections, anastomotic leaks, etc.). Prior to transitioning to DC III, the team should ensure that adequate resuscitation and physiological optimization has been achieved; i.e.; normothermic, normal coagulation studies as well as a normal pH and lactate. With focused, aggressive critical care management and resuscitation one may obtain this physiologic state within 24–36 h.[1,2]

Circumstances which may influence the timing of definitive repair include: re-operation to salvage an ischemic limb due to shunt occlusion or suboptimal vascular repair following restoration of a normal coagulation profile; early re-operation is advisable for bowel that has been interrupted at several sites, resulting in a closed-loop obstruction that threatens bowel viability; and early re-exploration required to address suboptimal control of spillage at the initial laparotomy from packed or drained duodenal, kidney, or bladder disruption.

S.R. Allen (✉)
Surgery Department, Traumatology and Surgical Critical Care,
Hospital of the University of Pennsylvania, Philadelphia, PA, USA
e-mail: steve.allen@uphs.upenn.edu

A.J. Brooks et al. (eds.), *Ryan's Ballistic Trauma*,
DOI: 10.1007/978-1-84882-124-8_31, © Springer-Verlag London Limited 2011

## 31.2
## Operative Game Plan

As trauma teams have evolved to meet the challenges of resident work-hour restrictions and increased patient volumes from trauma center regionalization, the delivery of care and surgeon coverage has changed dramatically as well. As such, in those situations in which the initial operative team is different from the team performing the re-exploration, a thorough discussion and detailed "hand-off" should occur prior to DC III. In the operating room, the patient is prepped and draped appropriately for the definitive repairs ahead. The temporary abdominal dressing is prepped into the field prior to removal and subsequent exposure of the abdominal contents.

All packs are irrigated copiously and removed carefully; teasing them slowly away from all surfaces to avoid clot disruption. As with DC I, the surgeon must be prepared to accept failure if bleeding is encountered on pack removal. When repeated attempts to control the bleeding using local hemostatic measures fail, immediate repacking is the safest course of action to prevent massive blood loss and recurrent physiologic deterioration. Alternatively, during the initial and subsequent explorations, the packs may be wrapped in a material such as Ioban to prevent adherence and therefore obviate the need for "teasing" them off clot, bowel serosa, or liver parenchyma.

Following successful pack removal, a complete re-examination of the abdominal contents should occur, with particular attention paid to any previous repairs made during DC I. Significant injuries are often overlooked, or only partially defined, during the rapidly performed initial laparotomy in an exsanguinating, unstable patient. Additional sites of bleeding are controlled, vascular repairs are performed, and intestinal continuity is restored using standard anastomotic techniques. Any bowel anastomosis should be protected with omentum and/or tucked under mesentery to provide protection.

If fascial closure is not possible, percutaneous feeding tubes and stomas should be avoided, as they are associated with a high leak rate and make subsequent mobilization and separation of abdominal wall components difficult when closure eventually is performed. Instead, primary anastomoses should be created for gastrointestinal continuity, and both naso-gastric tubes and naso-duodenal tubes should be placed and directed into position intra-operatively for proximal decompression and feeding, respectively. If creation of a stoma is necessary, it should be placed laterally (lateral to the rectus muscles) through the oblique muscles. Ideally, a stoma should lie between the anterior and mid-axillary line of the abdominal wall.

## 31.3
## Liver Injuries

While peri-hepatic packing is frequently necessary to control exsanguination from the liver, reoperation for definitive management is eventually required. Frequently haemostasis will be complete when the packs are removed and drainage of the liver injury for potential bile leaks is all that is required. Multiple techniques may be employed to repair the injured liver when required. Hepatorrhaphy with a running or interrupted mattress suture using absorbable sutures may be adequate to repair the bleeding liver. Hepatotomy via finger fracture technique may also be an ideal option for those with a normal coagulation profile in order to control bleeding vessels deep in the liver parenchyma. Anatomic hepatic resection is an option in the face of major hepatic disruption but should only be undertaken by those experienced in both trauma surgery and elective liver resection.

## 31.4
## Duodenal and Pancreatic Injuries

During the initial operation, injuries to the stomach, duodenum, and pancreas are handled expeditiously. Injuries to the stomach and duodenum are sewn or stapled closed to control contamination while those to the pancreas are widely drained without any anatomic resection of the pancreas. At the time of re-operation, definitive repair of gastrotomies and enterotomies may be performed in the standard fashion. In the case of multiple injuries or a significant injury to a particular portion of the bowel, resection with anastomosis may be favored over primary repair. In the case of duodenal injuries, pyloric exclusion may be considered with subsequent gastrojejunostomy. Pancreatoduodenectomy may be performed for devastating injuries to the pancreas and duodenum. The resection portion of this procedure may be performed at the time of the initial operation however the reconstruction should be delayed until the patient has improved physiologically.

## 31.5
## Abdominal Closure

Once all of the repairs are completed, formal abdominal closure without tension is the challenging final step in the planned reoperation sequence. An initial assessment to evaluate the potential to formally approximate the fascial edges should be performed with towel clamps. If gentle adduction allows the fascial edges to approximate, a standard fascial closure should be possible. However, persistent edema within the retroperitoneum, bowel wall, and abdominal wall often renders primary closure impossible at this time.

As a general rule, when the abdomen is viewed from across the operating table and the bowels are above the level of the skin, a low-tension primary closure is unlikely. Should the peak airway pressure rises more than 10 cm $H_2O$ during temporary fascial approximation, then the fascia should be left open and the temporary abdominal closure device replaced.

The patient is returned to the ICU where aggressive diuresis is implemented in an attempt to decrease bowel and body wall edema as hemodynamically tolerated. During this period, the patient undergoes daily abdominal washouts, re-inspection, and careful replacement of the abdominal closure device to prevent fistula formation. This may occur at the bedside if personnel and resources are available. The majority of damage controlled open abdomens can be closed primarily within 1 week, especially if there is no sign of intra-abdominal infection.

## 31.6
## Delayed Fascial Closure

Multiple techniques have been developed in the case of delayed fascial closure. Devices including the Whitman Patch™ have been developed to serially re-approximate the fascial edges. Additionally, techniques including the use of vicryl mesh and split-thickness skin grafts have been utilized to temporarily cover the viscera until the abdomen is able to be closed primarily months down the line.

The Whitman Patch™ (Star Surgical Inc., Burlington, WI) is often employed to assist in stepwise fascial closure during the period of diuresis. This device consists of two thin sheets of semi-rigid material comprised of a non-adherent undersurface with a Velcro-like material on the outer surface. Tiny perforations are present over the sheets to allow for the egress of third-space fluids. These sheets are sutured to the fascia on both sides of the abdominal wound, and when overlapped with slight tension, allow for partial fascial approximation without threat of loss of domain. The fascia is gently approximated with minimal tension. The gap between its edges is slowly reduced with each daily abdominal washout. The non-adherent smooth undersurface reduces fistula formation, as the bowel wall is not irritated by contact. The patch is removed prior to definitive fascial closure.[3] A limiting factor in the decision to use this device is its relatively high cost ($1,000–$1,200 per device).

Alternatively, a stepwise silo-type closure can be performed with a durable non-adherent material (i.e., an opened 3-l intravenous bag sewn to the fascial edges) in a manner similar to that described in the pediatric surgical literature for neonates with an omphalocoele or gastroschisis.[4] Gradual reduction in the size of the silo, and hence the wound, is achieved as the bag is incised, trimmed, and sutured closed during subsequent abdominal washouts.

If fascial closure is not achieved after 7 days, the surgeon faces a number of alternatives to cover the abdominal defect, but will leave the patient with a large ventral hernia. The first of these involves closing the skin with no attempt at fascial approximation. The patient would then undergo repair of the abdominal wall defect several months later. This often is not possible, as the gap is too wide. Despite skin flap mobilization, the edges cannot be approximated. Alternatively, a vicryl (polyglycolic acid) mesh is placed over the entire abdominal wall defect and sutured to the fascial edges. The omentum, if available, should be draped over the bowel to reduce the risk of enteric fistula formation.

Meticulous daily dressing changes with saline-soaked gauze are performed over this mesh. This allows the wound to granulate through the material. Once a smooth bed of granulation tissue is established, usually in 2–3 weeks, a split-thickness skin graft is applied to the granular bed. The skin graft will mature, separate, and develop a thin layer of connective tissue or fat between the underlying viscera over the next 6–12 months. One may utilize the "pinch test" to determine whether the skin graft has "matured" enough to allow the abdominal viscera to separate from the abdominal wall. At this point, the patient is ready for excision of the skin graft and definitive reconstruction.

Many reconstructive techniques have been described in the literature and include the use of preoperative tissue expanders,[5] as well as abdominal wall component separation with bilateral rectus sheath release. This allows one to achieve primary component closure with extra-fascial mesh support. The involvement of a plastic surgeon at this step is advisable.

## 31.7
## Damage Control: Beyond the Abdomen

More and more reports are being generated describing the adaptation of damage control principals to severely injured patients with single or multiple injuries to regions of the body other than the abdominal cavity.

## 31.8
## Thoracic Injury

Damage control surgery principles have been applied selectively in the chest. In the physiologically exhausted patient, the definitive operation is abandoned in favor of an abbreviated thoracotomy or sternotomy. Packs placed in the thoracic cavity may be an option to temporarily control bleeding, but may have significant physiologic consequences related to compression of the heart, great vessels, and viable lung tissue. Therefore damage control for thoracic injuries often involves definitive surgery using rapid, non traditional surgical techniques. When the chest is packed for significant chest wall bleeding, timing of pack removal, definitive repair and closure of the chest is critical. This should be undertaken once the patient has been physiologically optimized.

In an unstable patient with a penetrating lung injury, stapled, non-anatomic wedge resection or pulmonary tractotomy[6] with direct suture ligation of bleeding vessels may be performed. The latter technique works well when the site of hemorrhage is secondary to a deep through and through stab wound or gunshot wound. Here, the pulmonary parenchyma bridging the wound tract is divided using a linear stapling/cutting device. This permits direct inspection of the tract, with selective ligation of bleeding points and control of air leaks.

In DCIII of the thoracic cavity, care must be taken to soak the previously placed packs to avoid further injury to the delicate pulmonary parenchyma. Once the packs are out a thorough investigation of the damage is required. Often the techniques such as non-anatomic wedge resection or pulmonary tractotomy, as described above, are sufficient to repair the injured lung. However at the time of the DCIII one must be prepared to further debride the injured lung and possibly perform an anatomic resection such as a lobectomy or pneumonectomy.[7]

Chest wall closure, either of a thoracotomy or sternotomy, is often achieved early in relation to the initial injury. In the case of a thoracotomy, the ribs are approximated with heavy suture and the muscles and soft tissues closed in layers. Due to swelling of the heart from fluid overload or injury sustained to the heart, one may experience hemodynamic instability while closing an open sternum. In this case the chest should be closed temporarily. Diuresis and further physiologic improvement will allow for delayed closure of the sternum during a subsequent visit to the operating room.

## 31.9
## Vascular Injury

Vascular injuries may be amenable to damage control techniques as well with the use of temporary intravascular shunts (TIVS's). Typically used in large, proximal vessels TIVS's allow perfusion of distal tissues which may not have adequate collateral circulation. TIVS's have shown good patency rates when left in place up to 24 h, however, there are case reports of temporary shunts left in place for up to 72 h prior to definitive vascular repair with the longest reported time of 10 days in an axillary artery.[8] Retrospective reviews have demonstrated an improved rate of survival in the face of extensive vascular injury as well as improved limb survival. In one retrospective review the shunt thrombosis rate was 5% with an overall survival of 88% and combination of limb/patient survival rate of 73%.[9]

In the case of a vascular repair which requires a TIVS, the shunt and distal perfusion must be monitored closely. Should the patient show signs of distal ischemia they should be taken to the operating room for repair sooner than originally planned. Repair of any orthopedic repairs must be coordinated with the final repair/construction of a vascular anastomosis so as to not disrupt the final repair with bony manipulation. Standard vascular techniques such as saphenous vein grafts as well as Dacron or PTFE grafts should be utilized as indicated based on the injury location and extent of tissue destruction. Patients with vascular injury that require shunting followed by definitive vascular repair in either the upper or lower limb should have full length, all compartment fasciotomies.

## 31.10
## Controversies of Damage Control III

Damage control surgical and resuscitation strategies have improved survival from major traumatic injuries (both penetrating and blunt mechanisms). While it has gained wide popularity for the care of the physiologically devastated patient, controversy still exists as to other patient populations in which it may be beneficial. Other controversies include the timing of DCIII reconstruction, creation of a primary anastomosis versus the creation of a stoma or colostomy and the best method of abdominal coverage and subsequent closure if primary closure is not possible.

Damage control strategies have proven life saving in maximally injured patients. Early indications for damage control included a major vascular injury, two or more visceral injuries and profound shock. Survival was 77% in the damage control group compared to 11% in those undergoing laparotomy with primary repair and closure.[1] The concern for overuse of damage control techniques is one to consider. Damage control principles in those who do not need it from a physiologic standpoint are at risk of many of the known complications which include wound infections, intra-abdominal sepsis, and abscess formation, enteroatmospheric fistulae, abdominal wall necrosis, and multi-system organ failure.

Timing of DCIII reconstruction and incisional closure is dependent on the individual patient. The goal is to resuscitate the patient to within normal physiologic parameters. For some patients this may only require 12 h while many more will require 24–36 h of ongoing resuscitation. One should keep in mind that if a patient does not normalize hemodynamically or lactic acid or base deficit fail to improve, the patient should be taken back to the operating room earlier for re-exploration. Ongoing hemorrhage or missed visceral injuries will compromise these efforts.

The decision to perform a primary anastomosis or create a stoma or colostomy has been a point of controversy. Historically, for colonic injuries, colostomies were the treatment of choice. Multiple recent studies have demonstrated improved outcomes and lower morbidity with primary colonic anastomosis compared to those who received colostomies.[10] In the setting of damage control, the bowel injuries are stapled or sewn closed to minimize and control contamination. The bowel should not be anastomosed while hypothermia, coagulopathy, or hypotension remains.

The decision to sew or staple anastomoses in the face of traumatic injury has been at the center of much controversy. Previous studies in elective surgery have shown no difference in the incidence of complications between sewn and stapled anastomoses. However, one single center retrospective review and another multi-center retrospective cohort study have demonstrated an increased incidence of clinically significant anastomotic leaks in those which are stapled compared to hand sewn anastomoses.[11,12] For this reason, once the patient is in condition for DC III reconstruction, one should consider a hand sewn anastomosis.

## 31.11
## Conclusions

The concepts of damage control surgery and resuscitation have led to significant improvement in survival for the severely injured trauma patient. An abbreviated operation to attain control of hemorrhage and enteral contamination as well as aggressive resuscitation allows one to improve the patients physiology. Damage control principles may be utilized in abdominal, thoracic, or even vascular trauma. Once the patient has improved hemodynamically, damage control III should be instituted for definitive repair. Decisions such as the time to definitive repair, primary anastomosis vs. stoma and type of abdominal closure are difficult ones that must be tailored to each patient and their respective injury pattern.

# References

1. Rotondo MF, Schwab CW, McGonigal MD, et al. "Damage Control": an approach for improved survival in exsanguinating penetrating abdominal injury. *J Trauma*. 1993;35:375-382.
2. Johnson JW et al. Evolution in damage control for exsanguinating penetrating abdominal injury. *J Trauma*. 2001;51(2):261-269. discussion 269-271.
3. Hadeed JG et al. Delayed primary closure in damage control laparotomy: the value of the Wittmann patch. *Am Surg*. 2007;73(1):10-12.
4. Rowlands BJ, Flynn TC, Fischer RP. Temporary abdominal wound closure with a silastic "chimney". *Contemp Surg*. 1984;24:17-20.
5. Livingston DH, Sharma PK, Glantz AI. Tissue expanders for abdominal wall reconstruction following severe trauma: technical note and case reports. *J Trauma*. 2002;32:82-86.
6. Wall MJ Jr et al. Pulmonary tractotomy as an abbreviated thoracotomy technique. *J Trauma*. 1998;45(6):1015-1023.
7. Wall MJ Jr, Soltero E. Damage control for thoracic injuries. *Surg Clin North Am*. 1997;77(4):863-878.
8. Feliciano D, Accola KD, Burch JM, Spjut-Patrinely V. Extraanatomic bypass for peripheral arterial injuries. *Am J Surg*. 1989;158:506-510.
9. Subramanian A, Vercruysse G, Dente C, Wyrzykowski A, King E, Feliciano DV. A decade's experience with temporary intravascular shunts at a civilian level I trauma center. *J Trauma*. 2008;65(2):316-326.
10. Bowley DM et al. Evolving concepts in the management of colonic injury. *Injury*. 2001;32(6):435-439.
11. Brundage SI et al. Stapled versus sutured gastrointestinal anastomoses in the trauma patient. *J Trauma*. 1999;47(3):500-507. Discussion 507-508.
12. Brundage SI et al. Stapled versus sutured gastrointestinal anastomoses in the trauma patient: a multicenter trial. *J Trauma*. 2001;51(6):1054-1061.

# Penetrating Genitourinary Trauma

# 32

Jay J. Doucet and David B. Hoyt

## 32.1
## Introduction

The genitourinary system lies in the retroperitoneal space and shares the perineum with the rectum and major neurovascular structures. As a result, penetrating trauma to the genitourinary system usually is associated with injury to multiple organ systems and requires a multidisciplinary effort with an organized and thorough evaluation of all injuries.

Eight percent of civilian gunshot wounds include the kidney. Fifty-six percent of stab wounds and 96% of gunshot wounds to the kidney have associated injuries, most commonly the liver, small bowel, stomach, and colon.[1] In the United States, 20% of renal penetrating injury results in renal loss.

## 32.2
## Mechanisms of Penetrating Genitourinary Trauma

Stab wounds of the genitourinary system are low-energy wounds where the injury is confined to the wound tract. Such wounds may be minor lacerations, such as a superficial parenchymal laceration as classified by the renal injury scheme shown in Table 32.1. Major lacerations into the medullary portion of the kidney may involve the collecting system and lead to urinary extravasation. About 20% of stab wounds cause vascular injuries to a main or segmental renal vein.

Gunshot wounds are more likely to cause major lacerations. The deposition of energy by a projectile is determined by the viscoelastic properties of the tissues. The kidney is a relatively dense, non elastic structure with a capsule suspended in the Gerota's fascia of

J.J. Doucet (✉)
Division of Trauma, Burns and Critical Care,
University of California Medical Center, San Diego, CA, USA

A.J. Brooks et al. (eds.), *Ryan's Ballistic Trauma*,
DOI: 10.1007/978-1-84882-124-8_32, © Springer-Verlag London Limited 2011

**Table 32.1** Kidney organ injury scoring system

| Grade | Type of injury | Injury description | AIS-90 |
|-------|---------------|--------------------|--------|
| I | Contusion | Microscopic or gross hematuria, urological studies normal | 2 |
| | Hematoma | Subcapsular, nonexpanding without parenchymal laceration | 2 |
| II | Laceration | <1 cm parenchymal depth of renal cortex without urinary extravasation | 2 |
| | Hematoma | Nonexpanding perirenal hematoma confined to renal retroperitoneum | 2 |
| III | Laceration | >1 cm depth of renal cortex, without collecting system rupture or urinary extravasation | 3 |
| IV | Laceration | Parenchymal laceration extending through the renal cortex, medulla, and collecting system | 4 |
| | Vascular | Main renal artery or vein injury with contained hemorrhage | 5 |
| V | Laceration | Completely shattered kidney | 5 |
| | Vascular | Avulsion of renal hilum that devascularizes kidney | 5 |

*Source*: Moore et al.[14]. With permission, Lippincott Williams and Wilkins 2003

Advance one grade for bilateral injuries up to and including Grade III

elastic fat and connective tissue. Similarly, the testicle is a dense, encapsulated structure suspended in elastic aerolar tissue and skin. Missiles decelerate more rapidly and deposit energy more rapidly in denser tissue. High-velocity missiles may pass through the relatively elastic connective tissues with little effect, but can cause extensive destruction to these solid organs by the effects of cavitation and fragmentation.

War or terrorist events tend to be dominated by wounds caused by fragment and by blast injury instead of gunshot wounds.[2–4] Sixty-eight percent of genitourinary injuries in combat are to the external genitalia.[5,6] Blast injuries can cause genitourinary injuries by the externally applied acceleration from the blast wave. These blast injuries frequently are accompanied by fragment injuries.

Antipersonnel mines are a particular threat for genitourinary injury.[7] During the recent war in Bosnia, one field hospital's review of 136 casualties with genitourinary injuries revealed 40% had injuries to the external genitalia, about two-thirds of which were thought to be due to mines.[8] When stepped on, small buried mines typically explode and direct fragments upward to cause severe extremity trauma in addition to missile injuries to the external genitalia and perineum. Bounding mines, those designed to jump into the air before detonating, typically detonate at a height that will cause severe penetrating injury to the abdomen and genitalia.

## 32.3
## Penetrating Renal Injuries

### 32.3.1
### Diagnosis

Penetrating renal trauma is diagnosed by clinical, laboratory, and medical imaging. In the hemodynamically unstable patient who must undergo laparotomy to assess abdominal penetration, the evaluation of the genitourinary system may be completed intraoperatively.

### 32.3.2
### Clinical Findings

After ensuring that the patient's airway and ventilatory status is satisfactory, the patient's hemodynamic status is assessed. In one series, 29% of stab wounds and 52% of gunshot wounds to the kidney presented with a systolic blood pressure less than 90 mmHg.[1] While resuscitating the patient, a history of the wounding is obtained. Clinical examination of the abdomen should include careful examination of the skin of the back and flanks for multiple penetrations, which may be small and nonbleeding, as well as the skin folds of the perineum and buttocks. Clinical assessment determines those patients who require immediate surgery and those who need further investigation.

### 32.3.3
### Laboratory Findings

Hematuria is defined as microscopic if there is more than five red blood cells per high powered field in apparently clear urine, or gross hematuria if blood stained urine is readily visible in the Foley catheter drainage bag. Hematuria of any degree in penetrating injury should raise suspicion of genitourinary injury and mandates investigation. The degree of hematuria does not correlate with the severity of injury. Approximately 18% of stab wounds and 6.8% of gunshot wounds did not have hematuria in the University of California, San Francisco (UCSF) series.[1] Thirty-three percent of patients with penetrating injuries severe enough to require nephrectomy did not have gross hematuria.

### 32.3.4
### Radiological Findings

The intravenous pyelogram (IVP) or excretory urogram is the most thoroughly investigated imaging mode in penetrating renal injury, but it is being replaced at many centers by contrast-enhanced computed tomography (CT) scanning.

The hemodynamic stability of the patient should be considered carefully in choosing imaging modalities. An unstable patient should not be placed in the CT scanner, but may have a one-shot IVP in the resuscitation area or in the operating room prior to laparotomy. The recommended dose is of two milligrams per kilogram of a 50% iodinated contrast material, such as diatrizoate (Hypaque, Amersham Health, Princeton, NJ). This is given at wide open drip, followed by an X-ray in 10 min. This can determine bilateral renal function and detect some ureteral injuries.

The utility of the routine use of one-shot IVP before laparotomy in the stable penetrating injury patient has been questioned by Nagy and colleagues, who noted in a study of 240 patients that the prevalence of a unilateral nonfunctioning kidney was less than 1%.[9] In addition, the IVPs were of suboptimal quality in 22% of cases. The IVP was normal in 59% of patients with a proven renal injury, regardless of grade of injury. Nagy and colleagues concluded that the IVP should not be used to exclude renal injuries, but only should be used when the wound trajectory was near the kidney or with gross hematuria.

Patel and colleagues reviewed 40 patients with penetrating abdominal trauma who received one-shot IVP for injuries with proximity to the kidney before laparotomy.[10] Only two of ten patients with proven urologic injuries had positive one-shot IVPs. Seven had renal injuries and 3 had bladder injuries. Two of nine patients with gross hematuria had a positive IVP, but urologic injuries were found at laparotomy in six out of nine patients. There were eight false-positive and six false-negative one-shot IVPs in this study, yielding a positive predictive value of 20%. The decision of whether or not to perform laparotomy was not influenced in any case. Given the unilateral nonfunctioning kidney rate of less than 1%, Patel and colleagues concluded that one-shot IVP did not influence management of any patient, but did delay definitive management.

It should be noted that concern over the function of a contralateral kidney can be addressed in the operating room after control of bleeding has been obtained by the use of intraoperative IVP or injection of vital dyes such as indigo carmine or methylene blue.

Computed tomography scanning provides superior visualization of renal anatomy and perfusion.[11] Computed tomography scanning also can identify injury to adjacent viscera and the renal vasculature and has eliminated the need for renal angiography. Computed tomography scanning facilitates the nonoperative management of penetrating renal injury.[12] Computed tomography scanning is indicated only in patients who have been hemodynamically stable and without an indication for immediate laparotomy. Delayed images taken 2–5 min after the initial injection can provide evidence of renal function with contrast seen in the renal pelvis and ureter. Extravasation of contrast aids detection of extravasation of blood and urine.

## 32.3.5
### Nonoperative Management

Nonoperative management of renal injury has been driven by the finding of a higher nephrectomy rate with exploration of blunt kidney injuries versus nonoperative management. Concern exists that opening Gerota's fascia and releasing a perinephric hematoma leads to a higher nephrectomy rate.[13] It has not been possible to determine precisely an American Association for the Surgery of Trauma (AAST) Grade of renal injury that mandates surgical exploration (Table 32.1).[14] Minor injuries such as Grade I and II traditionally have been managed conservatively. Grade IV (renal vascular, pedicle injury) and Grade V (avulsion) injuries usually have been managed operatively. Blunt Grade III injuries (major lacerations) have been managed successfully in a nonoperative manner for three decades.[15]

Gunshot wounds to the abdomen traditionally have been managed by abdominal exploration at laparotomy. Zone I hematomas are explored in blunt or penetrating trauma due to the possibility of abdominal vascular, duodenal, or pancreatic injury. Zone II perinephric nonexpanding retroperitoneal hematomas caused by penetrating injuries found at laparotomy routinely have been explored, whereas in blunt trauma they were not explored (Fig. 32.1). However, stable, lateral perinephric Zone II hematomas that have been staged by CT scanning do not require exploration.[16]

Shaftan introduced the concept of "selective conservatism" in the 1960s, which was validated by Nance in later studies.[17,18]

The nonoperative management of penetrating wounds to the kidney is becoming practiced more widely with the use of CT scanning.[19–21] Wounds can be marked with a metallic marker at the wound on the skin or by insertion of a contrast-soaked sponge in the wound. Computed tomography scanning can delineate the tract and can exclude injury to the retroperitoneum in tangential wounds.

In the context of the Level 1 trauma center with an in-house trauma team, selective nonoperative management of civilian abdominal gunshot wounds has been described by

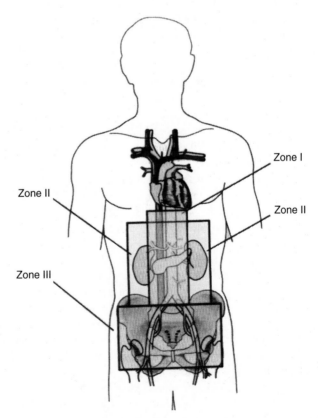

**Fig. 32.1** Anatomic zones of retroperitoneal hematomas. Zone I = periaortic; Zones II = perinephric; Zone III = pelvic (From Hoyt[75] with permission)

several authors. Velmahos and colleagues reported on selective nonoperative management in 1,856 patients with abdominal gunshot wounds.[22] Patients who were hemodynamically stable, had no evidence of peritonitis, and who had a reliable clinical examination were observed. Computed tomography scanning was carried out increasingly in all patients undergoing nonoperative management for the first 5 years of the study and in all patients undergoing nonoperative management by the last 3°years of the study. Seven hundred and ninety-two (42%) patients were selected for nonoperative management. Thirty-four percent of the patients had anterior wounds and 68% had posterior wounds. Eighty (4%) patients failed nonoperative management, no patient died as a result of the delayed laparotomy. Patients with posterior gunshot wounds were more likely to have nonoperative management, but had the same rate of delayed laparotomy and negative delayed laparotomy as anterior abdominal gunshot wounds.

Velhamos and colleagues earlier described the nonoperative management of gunshot wounds to the back.[23] Two hundred and three patients with gunshot wounds were subject to selective nonoperative management. Of the 130 (69%) selected for nonoperative management, four (3%) underwent laparotomy for increasing abdominal tenderness; none of those laparotomies were deemed therapeutic.

Velmahos reported on selective nonoperative management of 52 consecutive renal gunshot wound patients.[19] Patients underwent laparotomy if there was evidence of continued bleeding or a renal hilar injury. Only four patients were managed nonoperatively, three Grade II injuries and one Grade III injury. Of the 48 patients undergoing laparotomy, 32 had Gerota's fascia opened. Two of the two Grade I and two of the five Grade II injuries were deemed to have undergone unnecessary renal exploration. Reconstruction of the kidney was carried out in six of seven Grade III explorations, one Grade III injury underwent nephrectomy, and one Grade III injury did not undergo renal exploration at laparotomy. All grade IV (14 of 52) and V (6 of 52) wounds were explored. Ten of 14 Grade IV injuries were reconstructed. Four Grade IV and all six Grade V injuries underwent nephrectomy. Patients who underwent nephrectomy were more likely to have presented with a systolic blood pressure below 90, a hematocrit less than 30%, an Injury Severity Score greater than 20, or with Grade IV or V injuries.

Santucci and colleagues correlated AAST grade and mechanism of injury (blunt trauma, stab wound, gunshot) in 2,467 patients at the UCSF.[24] Grade III stab wounds had an exploration rate of 78% compared to a 93% exploration rate and nephrectomy rate for Grade III gunshot wounds. Grade IV stab wounds had an exploration rate of 94% compared to a 100% exploration rate for Grade IV gunshot wounds. All Grade V penetrating injuries were explored.

These reports of nonoperative management of renal injuries come from major trauma centers. Nonoperative management of penetrating renal trauma appears only to be an option in a defined setting of a hemodynamically stable patient with a CT scan demonstrating a Grade I–III injury with a reliable clinical abdominal exam which can be followed closely in the trauma center. There are limited numbers of patients with Grade IV or Grade V penetrating injuries reported as undergoing nonoperative management. Nonoperative management of such patients only would be appropriate in the setting of a clinical trial.

Before World War I, penetrating torso wounds were managed expectantly. During that conflict, the 53% mortality of abdominal wounds spurred development of abdominal surgery.[25] There are no modern reports on nonoperative management of abdominal gunshot wounds in the austere or conflict environment, where CT scanning, a dedicated trauma team, and skilled nursing units usually are lacking. Occasionally, forward-located military surgeons may have the option of rapid evacuation of a stable penetrating abdominal casualty to a larger rear area hospital, but this not an alternative for humanitarian and developing world surgeons. More often, laparotomy and intraoperative evaluation of the genitourinary tract and associated abdominal injuries will be the prudent action.

## 32.3.6
## Operative Management

Absolute indications for exploration of the kidney are hemodynamic instability due to renal injury, expanding perinephric hematoma, and incomplete radiological assessment of a renal injury. Relative indications include urinary extravasation, nonviable renal parenchyma with a large laceration, and renal vascular injury.

The technique of abdominal exploration requires a midline trans-abdominal incision. This allows prompt access to the intra-abdominal viscera to allow complete examination and rapid access to the central vasculature of the abdomen, including the renal vessels.

Controversy exists in the need to routinely control the renal pedicle before renal exploration. Carroll and McAnnich obtained vascular control of the renal pedicle before opening Gerota's fascia to reduce the rate of nephrectomy due to uncontrolled hemorrhage.[26,27] They reported that renal pedicle clamping was required in 12% of explorations which resulted in a three-fold increased rate of renal salvage.

If vascular control is desired, the renal pedicle may be accessed anteriorly by reflecting the transverse colon and small intestine superiorly and exposing the retroperitoneum. A vertical incision is made in the peritoneum over the aorta and extended superiorly to the ligament of Treitz. A large retroperitoneal hematoma may obscure these landmarks; however, the inferior mesenteric vein usually is visible, in which case the incision is made medial to that vein. The anterior surface of the aorta is identified and dissection proceeds superiorly to identify the left renal vein, which crosses anterior to the aorta. The vessels ipsilateral to the injured kidney then can be dissected out posteriorly. Vessel loops then can be applied to the renal artery and vein. Gerota's fascia then can be opened lateral to the kidney. Should the release of the tamponade provided by the perinephric hematoma cause uncontrolled bleeding, vascular clamps can be applied to the vessels loops and the injuries identified.

Some surgeons prefer a lateral approach instead of preliminary vascular control in all explorations, believing it saves time without increasing nephrectomy rates.[28,29]

In the unstable patient, a rapid or "scoop" nephrectomy may be required to control exsanguinating hemorrhage. This is accomplished rapidly by incising the peritoneal surface lateral to the injured kidney and then entering Gerota's fascia. The plane behind the kidney is developed with the surgeon's hand and the kidney is reflected anteriorly and medially to allow the renal pedicle to be controlled with digital pressure and vascular clamps.

Renal vascular injuries can be challenging. The kidney cannot tolerate more than an hour of warm total ischemic time, although there may be partial flow from small adrenal and ureteric collaterals. Associated injuries occur in most cases; mortality in a recent series ranged from 2.4%[39] to 54%.[30]

The renal pedicle lies in Zone I along with the renal pelvis and proximal ureter, abdominal aorta, vena cava, duodenum, pancreas, and celiac and superior mesenteric arteries and their branches and tributaries. A small incision in the retroperitoneum directly over the renal vessels may not allow adequate examination of these structures in the setting of a large hematoma or active hemorrhage. Wide access to this area can be obtained by incising the lateral peritoneum widely and performing left or right visceral rotations (Figs. 32.2 and 32.3).

Renorrhaphy requires adequate mobilization and exposure of the kidney. Injuries to the parenchyma should have their edges debrided. Bleeding vessels in the renal parenchyma can be ligated with suture ligatures. Injuries in the collecting system should be repaired with continuous fine absorbable suture. Isolated renal lacerations can be repaired by placing an absorbable hemostatic bolster within the laceration. The renal capsule is then loosely

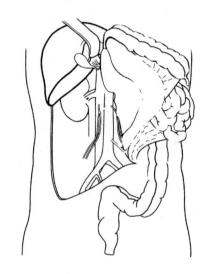

**Fig. 32.2** *Left* visceral rotation to expose the *right* kidney, renal vessels, and aorta (From Hoyt[75] with permission)

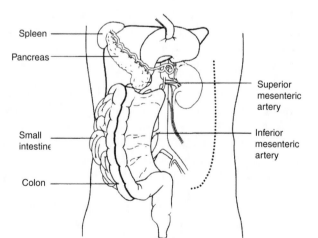

**Fig. 32.3** *Right* visceral rotation to expose the *left* kidney, renal vessels, and vena cava (From Hoyt[76] with permission)

approximated over a second bolster. Omental or peritoneal flaps can be mobilized to cover extensive defects or to separate the injury from an associated visceral injury. Partial nephrectomy can be used in cases where the pole of the kidney is injured. Drains are used when injuries are extensive or involve the collecting system. Gerota's fascia is left open.

Lacerations of the renal vessels may be repaired with fine vascular suture. The left renal vein may be ligated proximal to the vena cava, with the gonadal and adrenal veins acting as collateral venous drainage. Segmental veins also can be ligated safely due to collaterals, but ligation of segmental arteries will result in ischemia to a segment of parenchyma. Associated abdominal injuries, an unreconstructable renal pedicle or kidneys, shock, difficulty in obtaining adequate exposure, and the risk of renovascular hypertension with a stenotic arterial repair are factors that lead to a significant failure rate in repairing renal arterial injuries. Ivatury reported that nephrectomy is the usual outcome in half of renal vascular injuries.[31]

A review of renal vascular injuries by the Western Trauma Association (WTA) described 30 penetrating Grade IV injuries and 14 penetrating Grade V injuries with renal vascular injuries.[32] Penetrating injuries tended to have better outcomes than blunt trauma. Vein repairs had better outcomes than arterial repairs. Hypertension ensued in 4.5% of renovascular repairs, typical of reported rates in recent literature.[33,34] The WTA study suggested that the best outcomes were obtained in penetrating Grade IV injuries with immediate exploration and repair and in Grade V injuries with immediate nephrectomy.

Patients with a solitary kidney or with bilateral injuries require aggressive management to preserve renal function. In the case of bilateral injuries, the less injured kidney usually is explored, first to reduce the risk of attempting salvage, then performing nephrectomy on a badly injured kidney, and then discovering the contralateral kidney requires considerable time to salvage. Autotransplantation may be required in rare cases.[35,36]

## 32.3.7
### Associated Injuries

Associated injuries to adjacent viscera such as the pancreas or colon may complicate 80% of penetrating renal injury. Patients with combined injuries have a higher rate of complications, including abscess, fistula, urinoma, sepsis, and death. However, the decision whether to perform nephrectomy or renal salvage in these patients should be determined by the nature of the renal injury and the patient's overall condition, rather than by the presence of fecal contamination.

Wessels reported on 62 cases of combined penetrating colon and renal injury with 23% stab wounds and 52% gunshot wounds.[37] Exploration was carried out in 58% of cases and nephrectomy resulted from 16% of those explorations. Twenty-five percent of patients suffered postoperative complications, including abscesses (15%) and one late nephrectomy in a patient with a delayed diagnosis of a colon injury due to blast injury with subsequent abscess after an explored gunshot wound to the kidney. Fecal spillage had no effect on patient outcome or likelihood of urologic complication, nephrectomy, or survival. Despite the higher complication rate in these cases, the rate of renal salvage was felt to justify managing the renal injury based on the degree of renal trauma only.

## 32.3.8
## Outcome and Complications

Complications include delayed bleeding, urinoma and urinary extravasation, perirenal abscess, hypertension, renal failure, and death.

Delayed bleeding occurs in about 18% of nonoperatively managed renal stab wounds.[38] The delayed bleeding rate in nonoperative gunshot wounds is undetermined. The delayed bleeding rate in surgically operated penetrating renal injury is 3.7%.[39]

Computed tomography scanning is sensitive for urinary extravasation. Massive extravasation extending medially (from the renal pelvis) or from a lacerated pole of the kidney suggests a major injury unlikely to stop spontaneously and is managed best with operative repair. Urinomas are large collections of urine in the retroperitoneal space surrounded by a pseudocapsule, best seen on CT scan. They form 14 days to 30 years after injury. Image-guided percutaneous drainage is an effective and safe therapy.[40]

Perirenal abscesses occur when bacteria invade the hematoma, urine, and injured kidney in the perinephric space. The postoperative incidence is low, about 1.5%.[41]

These present about 5–7 days after injury with spiking fever, ileus, and flank tenderness. Computed tomography scan is diagnostic and percutaneous image-guided drainage is safe and effective.

The most common delayed complication is hypertension, seen in about 5% of renal injuries. Hypertension usually has its onset within 6 months of injury, with some presentation in days and some as late as 20 years.[42] Hypertension may be due to parenchymal ischemia secondary to compression or vascular injury and stenosis. Patients with vascular injuries (Grade IV) appear to be at highest risk. The WTA study noted 15 of 21 renal vascular repairs had poor outcome on follow-up renal scans and recommended obtaining follow-up renal nucleotide scans to screen for poor function that may lead to hypertension and renal failure.[32]

## 32.4
## Penetrating Ureteral Injuries

Ureteral injuries from non-iatrogenic trauma are rare, comprising about 1% of all genitourinary injuries and about 2–4% of all gunshot wounds to the abdomen.[43–45] A recent report from the conflict in Croatia indicated a relatively high incidence of ureteric injury (9.6%) in genitourinary injury, mostly from penetrating fragments.[46] The ureter is small and lies in a relatively protected location. However, it need not be struck directly by a missile to be injured; the cavitation and fragmentation effect by close missile passage may cause significant injury, including disruption or obstruction.

## 32.4.1
## Clinical Findings

There are no classical signs or symptoms in ureteric injury. Frequently, the injury is unrecognized at presentation, and the late signs of flank pain, fever, and fistula formation from urinary leakage prompt investigation. Delay in diagnosis occurs in up to 57% of cases and leads to urinoma, infection, urinary sepsis, and prolonged hospital stays.[43,44,47,48] Ureteric injury must be suspected in all patients with penetrating abdominal injury, and a gunshot wound in proximity to the ureter warrants exploration.

### 32.4.2
### Laboratory Findings

Hematuria is absent in 30–47% of cases.[45,47,49]

### 32.4.3
### Radiological Findings

The "complete" IVP (instead of the one-shot IVP) may demonstrate extravasation, delayed function, or ureteral dilation proximal to the injury. There is a significant rate of nondiagnostic studies, which has been reported as about 33–37%.[44,47] Computed tomography scanning can be helpful, although the exact sensitivity has not been reported and there is still a significant nondiagnostic study rate. Retrograde pyelogram can be done if time and the patient's condition permits; however, there are cases of nondiagnostic studies reported.[50] The majority of ureteral injuries are diagnosed intraoperatively.[49]

### 32.4.4
### Associated Injuries

Associated injuries are seen in about 97% of ureteric trauma.[51,52] The most common sites are the small intestine, colon, iliac vessels, liver, and stomach. Missed ureteric injuries are seen more commonly in the upper third of the ureter.[53] Missed injuries often are associated with a large retroperitoneal hematoma that may inhibit full exploration of the ureter at laparotomy.

### 32.4.5
### Classification

The ureter is divided into three components according to location:

- Upper, from the pelvic junction to the level of the iliac crest
- Middle, overlying the pelvic bones
- Lower, the segment lying below the pelvic brim to the bladder

The AAST Organ Injury Scale categorizes ureteric injuries as contusions, partial transections, complete transections, and devascularization (Table 32.2).

The most common penetrating injury is a partial transection of the ureter in the middle third.[43,44,54]

**Table 32.2** Ureteric organ injury scoring system

| Grade | Type of injury | Injury description | AIS-90 |
|-------|----------------|--------------------|--------|
| I | Hematoma | Contusion or hematoma without devascularization | 2 |
| II | Laceration | <50% transection | 2 |
| III | Laceration | >50% transection | 3 |
| IV | Laceration | Complete transection with 2 cm devascularization | 3 |
| V | Laceration | Complete transection with >2 cm devascularization | 3 |

*Source*: Moore et al.[79]. With permission, Lippincott Williams and Wilkins 2003
Advance one grade for multiple injuries

## 32.4.6
## Immediate Management

Most patients with ureteral injury require laparotomy for the associated injuries. Preoperative imaging cannot be relied upon to confirm or exclude the diagnosis.[53] Missile injuries can be associated with cavitation with a blunt ureteric injury. The contusion from gunshot injuries may appear minor, but can progress to subsequent ischemic necrosis.[55] Ureteric contusions from shrapnel injury also have a high incidence of subsequent ureteral stenosis if neglected.[46,56] During laparotomy, the ureter must be identified and visualized for evidence of injury, including contusion, discoloration, or lack of bleeding, suggesting devascularization. In cases where exploration of the ureter is unsatisfactory, indigo carmine or methylene blue has been used intraoperatively, although there are cases where injuries were missed despite their use. The appropriate management of an injury depends on the site and severity of injury, delay in diagnosis, the patient's condition, and the surgeon's experience.

Ureteric injuries in an unstable patient in which the time cannot be taken for a careful mucosa-to-mucosa repair over a double-J stent may be managed by cutaneous ureterostomy or exteriorization of a stent passed into the proximal transected ureter and postoperative percutaneous nephrostomy. Poor outcomes and dehiscence of the ureteral repair is more likely in patients presenting with shock, intraoperative bleeding, or associated colon injury. In these patients, temporization is preferable to a lengthy reconstructive procedure. Concomitant renal, ureteric, and associated intra-abdominal injuries may warrant nephrectomy. In a severe life-threatening situation where an expedient damage control approach is indicated, the ureter can be ligated until a subsequent laparotomy is performed in more favorable conditions. Operative nephrostomy is not used in management of ureteric trauma.

## 32.4.7
## Ureteral Reconstruction

Urologic consultation should be sought. There are a variety of techniques for reconstruction, all require careful debridement, a watertight, spatulated, and tension-free repair, and adequate ureteral and periureteral retroperitoneal drainage (Fig. 32.4).[57]

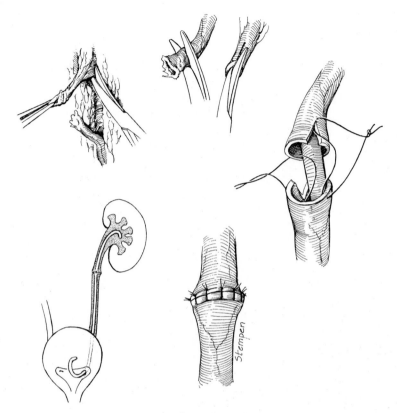

**Fig. 32.4** Ureteroureterostomy showing proximal and distal ureteral segment mobilization, debridement, spatulation, and anastomosis over a double J stent (From Presti[78] with permission)

Injuries in the lower third usually are managed by reimplantation into the bladder, either directly or by mobilizing the bladder with a psoas hitch or Boari flap. The ureter is tunneled through the submucosal tunnel with a length three times the ureters diameter and a mucosa-to-mucosa repair is carried out at the neoureterocystostomy. Absorbable sutures (4–0) are used and the anastomosis is stented.

Injuries in the middle and upper thirds usually are managed with a primary ureteroureterostomy over a double-J stent. Five to seven centimeters of additional ureteric length can be obtained by mobilization of the kidney. Associated intra-abdominal injury or a tenuous repair may require interposition of omentum to isolate the repair.

Long segmental defects may require transureteroureterostomy, autotransplantation, or interposition with an ileal graft.

All repairs are drained by stents and external drains. Anastomoses can be bolstered by the application of omental flaps. Stents typically are left in for 6 weeks. Tenuous repairs, and especially those made in the presence of renal, colon, or pancreatic injury, should be protected by percutaneous nephrostomy.[58] A Foley catheter is left in the bladder for 5–7 days to avoid backpressure on the anastomosis.

## 32.4.8
## Outcome

Complications after ureteral repair for gunshot wounds occur in 20–25% of patients.[53,59,60] Patients with missed ureteric injuries or with ureteric anastomotic dehiscence present with evidence of urinary extravasation with flank pain, fevers, and ileus. Computed tomography scanning is preferred to IVP for diagnosis. Management is with percutaneous nephrostomy, retrograde ureteric stenting, and/or operative repair. Nephrostomy was a definitive treatment in 44% of cases in a report of 63 neglected ureteric injuries in the conflict zone.[61]

Healing is documented by IVP at 6 and 12 weeks. Delay in diagnosis leads to additional morbidity and cost, and a high index of suspicion is warranted in any patient with penetrating abdominal injury. Dehiscence of the repair is more likely in patients presenting with shock, intraoperative bleeding, or with associated colon injury.

## 32.5
## Penetrating Bladder Injuries

Penetrating injury to the bladder accounts for 4–25% of bladder injuries and is usually the result of gunshot wounds.[62,63] Extraperitoneal penetration is more common than intraperitoneal penetration.

## 32.5.1
## Clinical Diagnosis

The injury is suggested by the location of the wound. Stab or gunshot wounds to the lower abdomen, pelvis, or perineum may injure the bladder. Patients may have lower abdominal pain or tenderness and guarding on palpation.

## 32.5.2
## Laboratory Diagnosis

Gross hematuria is seen in 95% of cases of penetrating bladder injury.

## 32.5.3
## Imaging

Cystography is the most accurate method; it is done by completely distending the bladder via a Foley catheter with 350 ml of contrast material and taking an X-ray. The bladder then is emptied and a postdrainage film obtained. The second film is important in that 13% of retroperitoneal extravasations are detected only with this film.[64]

Computed tomography cystography has been reported to have similar predictive value to plain film cystography in blunt trauma, but there are no series evaluating its use in penetrating trauma.

### 32.5.4
### Associated Injuries

Mortality usually is due to associated injuries. The small intestine, colon, rectum, and ureter are commonly involved. Women should have a speculum exam to exclude vaginal injury.

### 32.5.5
### Classification

Bladder injuries can be classified by the AAST Bladder Organ Injury Scale (Table 32.3). In a series of 23 patients by Cass, contusions (Grade I) consisted of about 17% of penetrating injuries. Extraperitonal ruptures were most common at 43%; these are Grade II when less than 2 cm and Grade III when 2 cm or more.[65] Intraperitoneal lacerations comprised 21%; they are Grade III when less than 2 cm and Grade IV when 2 cm or more. Grade V lacerations extend into the bladder neck or ureteral orifice (trigone).

### 32.5.6
### Management

Small bladder penetrations can be difficult to find during laparotomy. Hemodynamically stable patients with penetrations in proximity to the bladder should have cystography

**Table 32.3** Bladder organ injury scoring system

| Grade | Type of injury | Injury description | AIS-90 |
|-------|----------------|--------------------|--------|
| I     | Hematoma       | Contusion, intramural hematoma | 2 |
|       | Laceration     | Partial thickness  | 3 |
| II    | Laceration     | Extraperitoneal bladder wall laceration <2 cm | 4 |
| III   | Laceration     | Extraperitoneal (>2 cm) or intraperitoneal (<2 cm) bladder wall lacerations | 4 |
| IV    | Laceration     | Intraperitoneal bladder wall laceration >2 cm | 4 |
| V     | Laceration     | Laceration extending into bladder neck or ureteral orifice (trigone) | 4 |

*Source*: Moore et al.[79]

Advance one grade for multiple injuries

preoperatively. Care must be taken to look under abdominal retractors during abdominal exploration to examine the bladder adequately.

Contusions can be managed by catheter drainage alone. Intraperitoneal and extraperitoneal penetrating injury should be managed by surgical exploration and primary repair. Nonoperative management of extraperitoneal bladder rupture is well described, but there is limited experience in nonoperative penetrating injury.

Once intra-abdominal injury has been excluded at laparotomy, the space of Retzius is opened and the anterior bladder dissected away from the pubis. The bladder is opened via an anterior cystostomy to allow examination of the entire interior surface. The ureteric orifices must be examined for injury. Trial insertion of a ureteric stent or use of methylene blue or indigo carmine can ensure ureters are intact.

Extraperitoneal ruptures are closed with absorbable sutures in one or two layers. Intraperitoneal ruptures are closed in two layers, with the peritoneal and muscular bladder wall in one layer and the bladder mucosa in another layer. Injuries extending into the trigone require careful reconstruction of the sphincter or risk incontinence or contracture.

A large suprapubic tube traditionally is used in conjunction with a urethral catheter, especially with a large or tenuous repair, but may not be necessary in many cases.[66] The urethral catheter is removed with the clearing of gross hematuria. The suprapubic catheter is removed at 8–10 days after a cystogram is done to ensure bladder integrity.

### 32.5.7
### Outcome and Complications

Morbidity is related more closely to the associated injuries than to the bladder injury. Infection and continued bleeding are early complications. Long-term complications are uncommon and include incontinence.

### 32.5.7.1
### Penetrating Genital Injuries

Genital injuries comprised about 68% of genitourinary injuries from combat versus 7% of civilian injuries.[6,58] High-velocity injuries are common in combat; civilian injuries more commonly are low-velocity gunshot wounds than stab wounds. In a civilian series of genital gunshot wounds, the penis was injured most frequently, followed by the testicles and the scrotum only.[67] Thirty percent of civilian patients have multiple gunshot wounds.

### 32.5.8
### Clinical Findings

The external location of the genitalia lends ready inspection. However, associated injuries are seen in over 75% of penetrating genital trauma, including urethra, thigh, buttocks, and hand.[68,69] Injuries to the rectum, iliac vessels, bony pelvis, and hip joint also are possible.

Fifty percent of penile gunshot wounds involve the urethra. Most of theses injuries are in the distal, "pendulous" urethra versus the bulbous or proximal urethra. The perineum should be examined for signs of ecchymosis or urinary extravasation.

## 32.5.9
### Radiological Findings

Patients with penetration of the genitalia with blood at the meatus, gross, or microscopic hematuria or inability to void should be suspected of having a urethral injury and require a retrograde urethrogram (RUG). This is done by placing a small Foley catheter just past the meatus and using a Brodny clamp to ensure a seal. 30–50 cm$^3$ of contrast is infused and radiographs taken. If a Foley catheter has already been successfully placed, a small feeding tube can be placed adjacent to the Foley catheter to obtain a useable RUG.

Suspected bladder injuries should be addressed with a static and postdrainage cystogram.

Scrotal injuries should be investigated with ultrasonography to evaluate testicular integrity.[70] Rupture of the testicle reveals an abnormal echo pattern associated with tubular extrusion or contusion with hemorrhage. Color flow Doppler imaging available on most ultrasound machines provides evidence of testicular perfusion.

## 32.5.10
### Management

All penetrating injuries to the genitalia should be explored. Wounds that are seen to be superficial can be debrided and irrigated. Wounds, including high-velocity penetrations, can be closed after exploration.[58]

Penetrating penile injuries require surgical exploration. A circumferential subcoronal incision is made and the skin retracted down the shaft. The rich vascular supply to the area lessens the risk of infection and dehiscence, and therefore does not require extensive debridement, which can impair erectile function. Injuries to the corpora, Bucks fascia, and tunica albuginea are repaired precisely with interrupted absorbable sutures after minimal debridement. Associated urethral injuries are repaired with interrupted fine absorbable sutures and the urethra stented with a silicone Foley catheter. Long segmental defects can be managed by insertion of a suprapubic bladder catheter and delayed urethral reconstruction by a variety of specialized techniques.

Penetrating injury to the testes require surgical exploration via a midline scrotal incision. Hematomas are evacuated and the testes, epididymis, and spermatic cord are inspected. Debridement of devitalized tissue or extruded tubules is carried out and hemostasis obtained. The tunica albuginea is reapproximated with absorbable suture. Hematomas in the spermatic cord are associated with arterial injury and require exploration and inspection to obtain hemostasis. A small Penrose drain is left to drain the scrotum, which is closed with absorbable interrupted sutures. Extensive destruction of the testicle or cord requires orchiectomy.

Large skin defects in the perineum may require skin grafting; this can be carried out at the first exploration if the wound is clean and without contamination or devitalized tissue. Otherwise the wound is dressed until delayed grafting is possible onto a granulating wound bed. Loss of the scrotum with viable testicles may require the testes to be placed in skin pockets made through the skin into the subcutaneous tissue of the medial thigh. Thin split-thickness skin grafts are appropriate except on the penis. If the patient is potent, and skin contracture of the graft will complicate erection, then thick split-thickness or full-thickness grafts are appropriate.[71]

Large defects of the perineum may require myocutaneous flaps rotated from the posterior or lateral thigh or from the rectus abdominus.[72]

## 32.5.11
### Outcome and Complications

The external genitalia can be assessed easily and rapidly for injury. Penetrations in this area require exploration after appropriate imaging. Associated injuries are common in genital gunshot wounds and must be considered with a high index of suspicion. The excellent vascular supply of the genitalia ensures rapid healing and the likelihood of acceptable healing and function.[73,74]

## References

1. McAninch JW, Carroll PR, Armenakas NA, Lee P. Renal gunshot wounds: methods of salvage and reconstruction. *J Trauma*. 1993;35(2):279-283.
2. Spalding TJ, Stewart MP, Tulloch DN, Stephens KM. Penetrating missile injuries in the Gulf war 1991. *Br J Surg*. 1991;78(9):1102-1104.
3. Lovric Z, Kuvezdic H, Prlic D, Wertheimer B, Candrlic K. Ballistic trauma in 1991/92 war in Osijek, Croatia: shell fragments versus bullets. *J R Army Med Corps*. 1997;143(1):26-30.
4. Ilic N, Petricevic A, Radonic V, Biocic M, Petricevic M. Penetrating thoraco-abdominal war injuries. *Int Surg*. 1997;82(3):316-318.
5. Cass AS, ed. *Genitourinary Trauma*. Boston, MA: Blackwell Scientific; 1988.
6. Cass AS. Male genital trauma from external trauma. In: Cass AS, ed. *Genitourinary Trauma*. Boston, MA: Blackwell Scientific; 1988:141.
7. Coupland RM, Korver A. Injuries from antipersonnel mines: the experience of the International Committee of the Red Cross. *BMJ*. 1991;303(6816):1509-1512.
8. Hudolin T, Hudolin I. Surgical management of urogenital injuries at a war hospital in Bosnia-Hrzegovina, 1992 to 1995. *J Urol*. 2003;169(4):1357-1359.
9. Nagy KK, Brenneman FD, Krosner SM, et al. Routine preoperative "one-shot" intravenous pyelography is not indicated in all patients with penetrating abdominal trauma. *J Am Coll Surg*. 1997;185(6):530-533.
10. Patel VG, Walker ML. The role of "one-shot" intravenous pyelogram in evaluation of penetrating abdominal trauma. *Am Surg*. 1997;63(4):350-353.
11. Bretan PN Jr, McAninch JW, Federle MP, Jeffrey RB Jr. Computerized tomographic staging of renal trauma: 85 consecutive cases. *J Urol*. 1986;136(3):561-565.

12. Meredith JW, Trunkey DD. CT scanning in acute abdominal injuries. *Surg Clin North Am.* 1988;68(2):255-268.

13. Holcroft JW, Trunkey DD, Minagi H, Korobkin MT, Lim RC. Renal trauma and retroperitoneal hematomas—indications for exploration. *J Trauma.* 1975;15(12):1045-1052.

14. Moore EE, Shackford SR, Pachter HL, et al. Organ injury scaling: spleen, liver, and kidney. *J Trauma.* 1989;29(12):1664-1666.

15. Cass AS, Ireland GW. Trauma to the genitourinary tract: evaluation and management. *Postgrad Med.* 1973;53(7):63-68.

16. Feliciano DV. Management of traumatic retroperitoneal hematoma. *Ann Surg.* 1990;211(2):109-123.

17. Shaftan GW. Indications for operation in abdominal trauma. *Am J Surg.* 1960;99:657-664.

18. Nance FC, Wennar MH, Johnson LW, Ingram JC Jr, Cohn I Jr. Surgical judgment in the management of penetrating wounds of the abdomen: experience with 2212 patients. *Ann Surg.* 1974;179(5):639-646.

19. Velmahos GC, Demetriades D, Cornwell EE III, et al. Selective management of renal gunshot wounds. *Br J Surg.* 1998;85(8):1121-1124.

20. Renz BM, Feliciano DV. Gunshot wounds to the right thoracoabdomen: a prospective study of nonoperative management. *J Trauma.* 1994;37(5):737-744.

21. Wessells H, McAninch JW, Meyer A, Bruce J. Criteria for nonoperative treatment of significant penetrating renal lacerations. *J Urol.* 1997;157(1):24-27.

22. Velmahos GC, Demetriades D, Toutouzas KG, et al. Selective nonoperative management in 1,856 patients with abdominal gunshot wounds: should routine laparotomy still be the standard of care? *Ann Surg.* 2001;234(3):395-402.

23. Velmahos GC, Degiannis E. The management of urinary tract injuries after gunshot wounds of the anterior and posterior abdomen. *Injury.* 1997;28(8):535-538.

24. Santucci RA, McAninch JW, Safir M, Mario LA, Service S, Segal MR. Validation of the American Association for the Surgery of Trauma organ injury severity scale for the kidney. *J Trauma.* 2001;50(2):195-200.

25. Rignault DP. Abdominal trauma in war. *World J Surg.* 1992;16(5):940-946.

26. McAninch JW, Carroll PR. Renal trauma: kidney preservation through improved vascular control—a refined approach. *J Trauma.* 1982;22(4):285-290.

27. Carroll PR, Klosterman P, McAninch JW. Early vascular control for renal trauma: a critical review. *J Urol.* 1989;141(4):826-829.

28. Atala A, Miller FB, Richardson JD, Bauer B, Harty J, Amin M. Preliminary vascular control for renal trauma. *Surg Gynecol Obstet.* 1991;172(5):386-390.

29. Gonzalez RP, Falimirski M, Holevar MR, Evankovich C. Surgical management of renal trauma: is vascular control necessary? *J Trauma.* 1999;47(6):1039-1042.

30. Asensio JA, Chahwan S, Hanpeter D, et al. Operative management and outcome of 302 abdominal vascular injuries. *Am J Surg.* 2000;180(6):528-533.

31. Ivatury RR, Zubowski R, Stahl WM. Penetrating renovascular trauma. *J Trauma.* 1989;29(12):1620-1623.

32. Knudson MM, Harrison PB, Hoyt DB, et al. Outcome after major renovascular injuries: a Western trauma association multicenter report. *J Trauma.* 2000;49(6):1116-1122.

33. Montgomery RC, Richardson JD, Harty JI. Posttraumatic renovascular hypertension after occult renal injury. *J Trauma.* 1998;45(1):106-110.

34. Watts RA, Hoffbrand BI. Hypertension following renal trauma. *J Hum Hypertens.* 1987;1(2):65-71.

35. Wazzan W, Azoury B, Hemady K, Khauli RB. Missile injury of upper ureter treated by delayed renal autotransplantation and ureteropyelostomy. *Urology.* 1993;42(6):725-728.

36. Angelis M, Augenstein JS, Ciancio G, et al. Ex vivo repair and renal autotransplantation after penetrating trauma: is there an upper limit of ischemic/traumatic injury beyond which a kidney is unsalvageable? *J Trauma.* 2003;54(3):606-609.

37. Wessells H, McAninch JW. Effect of colon injury on the management of simultaneous renal trauma. *J Urol.* 1996;155(6):1852-1856.

38. Bernath AS, Schutte H, Fernandez RR, Addonizio JC. Stab wounds of the kidney: conservative management in flank penetration. *J Urol.* 1983;129(3):468-470.

39. Carroll PR, McAninch JW. Operative indications in penetrating renal trauma. *J Trauma.* 1985;25(7):587-593.

40. Peterson NE. Complications of renal trauma. *Urol Clin North Am.* 1989;16(2):221-236.

41. McAninch JW, Carroll PR, Klosterman PW, Dixon CM, Greenblatt MN. Renal reconstruction after injury. *J Urol.* 1991;145(5):932-937.

42. Monstrey SJ, Beerthuizen GI, vander Werken C, Debruyne FM, Goris RJ. Renal trauma and hypertension. *J Trauma.* 1989;29(1):65-70.

43. Rober PE, Smith JB, Pierce JM Jr. Gunshot injuries of the ureter. *J Trauma.* 1990;30(1):83-86.

44. Bright TC III, Peters PC. Ureteral injuries due to external violence: 10 years' experience with 59 cases. *J Trauma.* 1977;17(8):616-620.

45. Brandes SB, Chelsky MJ, Buckman RF, Hanno PM. Ureteral injuries from penetrating trauma. *J Trauma.* 1994;36(6):766-769.

46. Tucak A, Petek Z, Kuvezdic H. War injuries of the ureter. *Mil Med.* 1997;162(5):344-345.

47. Campbell EW Jr, Filderman PS, Jacobs SC. Ureteral injury due to blunt and penetrating trauma. *Urology.* 1992;40(3):216-220.

48. Peterson NE, Pitts JC III. Penetrating injuries of the ureter. *J Urol.* 1981;126(5):587-590.

49. Presti JC Jr, Carroll PR, McAninch JW. Ureteral and renal pelvic injuries from external trauma: diagnosis and management. *J Trauma.* 1989;29(3):370-374.

50. Mendez R, McGinty DM. The management of delayed recognized ureteral injuries. *J Urol.* 1978;119(2):192-193.

51. Carlton CE Jr, Scott R Jr, Guthrie AG. The initial management of ureteral injuries: a report of 78 cases. *Trans Am Assoc Genitourin Surg.* 1970;62:114-122.

52. Holden S, Hicks CC, O'Brien DP, Stone HH, Walker JA, Walton KN. Gunshot wounds of the ureter: a 15-year review of 63 consecutive cases. *J Urol.* 1976;116(5):562-564.

53. Medina D, Lavery R, Ross SE, Livingston DH. Ureteral trauma: preoperative studies neither predict injury nor prevent missed injuries. *J Am Coll Surg.* 1998;186(6):641-644.

54. Liroff SA, Pontes JE, Pierce JM Jr. Gunshot wounds of the ureter: 5 years of experience. *J Urol.* 1977;118(4):551-553.

55. Cass AS. Ureteral contusion with gunshot wounds. *J Trauma.* 1984;24(1):59-60.

56. Selikowitz SM. Penetrating high-velocity genitourinary injuries. Part I. Statistics mechanisms, and renal wounds. *Urology.* 1977;9(4):371-376.

57. Presti JC Jr, Carroll PR. Ureteral and renal pelvic trauma: diagnosis and management. In: McAninch JW, ed. *Traumatic and Reconstructive Urology.* Philadelphia: WB Saunders; 1996:171-179.

58. Selikowitz SM. Penetrating high-velocity genitourinary injuries. Part II: ureteral, lower tract, and genital wounds. *Urology.* 1977;9(5):493-499.

59. Perez-Brayfield MR, Keane TE, Krishnan A, Lafontaine P, Feliciano DV, Clarke HS. Gunshot wounds to the ureter: a 40-year experience at Grady Memorial Hospital. *J Urol.* 2001;166(1):119-121.

60. Azimuddin K, Milanesa D, Ivatury R, Porter J, Ehrenpreis M, Allman DB. Penetrating ureteric injuries. *Injury.* 1998;29(5):363-367.

61. al Ali M, Haddad LF. The late treatment of 63 overlooked or complicated ureteral missile injuries: the promise of nephrostomy and role of autotransplantation. *J Urol.* 1996;156(6):1918-1921.

62. Carroll PR, McAninch JW. Major bladder trauma: mechanisms of injury and a unified method of diagnosis and repair. *J Urol.* 1984;132(2):254-257.

63. Brosman SA, Fay R. Diagnosis and management of bladder trauma. *J Trauma.* 1973;13(8):687-694.

64. Carroll PR, McAninch JW. Major bladder trauma: the accuracy of cystography. *J Urol.* 1983;130(5):887-888.
65. Cass AS, Luxenberg M. Management of extraperitoneal ruptures of bladder caused by external trauma. *Urology.* 1989;33(3):179-183.
66. Parry NG, Rozycki GS, Feliciano DV, et al. Traumatic rupture of the urinary bladder: is the suprapubic tube necessary? *J Trauma.* 2003;54(3):431-436.
67. Gomez RG, Castanheira AC, McAninch JW. Gunshot wounds to the male external genitalia. *J Urol.* 1993;150(4):1147-1149.
68. Campos JA, Gomez-Orta F. Continent diversion vesicoplasty for the treatment of the irreparable, multi-operated urethral stricture patient. *Arch Esp Urol.* 1993;46(3):255-260.
69. Miles BJ, Poffenberger RJ, Farah RN, Moore S. Management of penile gunshot wounds. *Urology.* 1990;36(4):318-321.
70. Fournier GR Jr, Laing FC, McAninch JW. Scrotal ultrasonography and the management of testicular trauma. *Urol Clin North Am.* 1989;16(2):377-385.
71. McAninch JW. Management of genital skin loss. *Urol Clin North Am.* 1989;16(2):387-397.
72. Schlossberg SM, Jordan GH, McCraw JB. Myocutaneous flap reconstruction of major perineal and pelvic defects. In: McAninch JW, ed. *Traumatic and Reconstructive Urology.* Philadephia: WB Saunders; 1996:715-725.
73. McAninch JW. *Traumatic and Reconstructive Urology.* Philadephia: WB Saunders; 1996.
74. Bandi G, Santucci RA. Controversies in the management of male external genitourinary trauma. *J Trauma.* 2004;56(6):1362-1370.
75. Hoyt DB, Coimbra R, Potenza BM, Rappold JF. Anatomic exposures for vascular injuries. *Surg Clin North Am.* 2001;81(6):1317-1318.
76. Hoyt DB, Coimbra R, Potenza BM, Rappold JF. Anatomic exposures for vascular injuries. *Surg Clin North Am.* 2001;81(6):1322.
77. Armenakas NA, McAninch JW. Genitourinary tract. In: Ivatury RR, Cayten CG, eds. *The Textbook of Penetrating Trauma.* Media, PA: Williams and Wilkins; 1996:684-685.
78. Presti JC, Carroll PR. Intraoperative management of the injured ureter. In: Schrock TR, ed. *Perspectives in Colon and Rectal Surgery.* St Louis: Thieme; 1998:98-106.
79. Moore EE, Cogbill TH, Jurkovich GJ, et al. Organ injury scaling. III: chest wall, abdominal vascular, ureter, bladder, and urethra. *J Trauma.* 1992;33(3):337-339.

# Burns

Alan Kay

## 33.1
## Introduction

Burn injury is seen with ballistic trauma both in isolation and as part of multiple injuries. It is important that those dealing with victims of ballistic trauma understand the nature of burn injury and can manage it effectively.

Although modern definitive burn care is based on large multidisciplinary expert teams working in centers of excellence, much of the success in treating burn injury is dependant on the adequacy of initial management performed before arrival at a definitive care facility. Burn injured casualties are trauma victims and early care does not deviate from ATLS principles. Lack of familiarity with burns and the unpleasant nature of the injury, however, often distract the carer from following these basic management techniques.

This chapter aims to provide a framework for assessment and initial management, guidelines for who requires transfer to a specialist facility and an overview of the principles of definitive care.

In all environments, treating a severe burn draws heavily on resources and a small number of casualties can stretch the capability of any facility. Unlike many other types of trauma injury, burn victims can become progressively more unstable for several days even with appropriate management. This on-going burden needs to be appreciated in circumstances where resources are constrained. Triage decisions can be difficult.

## 33.2
## Epidemiology

The pattern of burn injury related to ballistic weaponry is very variable. Traditional munitions use an explosive charge to create the energy to injure, which, by its nature, produces

A. Kay
Academic Department of Military Surgery and Trauma,
Royal Centre for Defence Medicine, Birmingham, UK
e-mail: alankay@doctors.org.uk

A.J. Brooks et al. (eds.), *Ryan's Ballistic Trauma*,
DOI: 10.1007/978-1-84882-124-8_33, © Springer-Verlag London Limited 2011

heat. The energy is often transferred to the victim via a projectile. If a casualty is close enough to the detonation to sustain serious burns, they are normally killed. Where dismounted infantry alone are used, the incidence of burns is low. This changes with the use of vehicles, aircraft, and ships. Weapon systems designed to defeat armor again will not normally primarily cause significant burns in survivors. The predominant cause of burn injury is the secondary ignitions of fuel and munitions in the vehicle. The incidence of burns is, therefore, higher in armored, air and sea warfare.

There has been little published data about the incidence of burns in terrorist bomb attacks. Atrocities in Omagh, Northern Ireland 1998, and Bali 2002 seemed to have a larger proportion of significant burns. Victims from the latter overwhelmed the burn services of Australasia.

There are of course weapons that are, by their nature, designed to inflict burns such as Napalm, phosphorus, and flame-throwers.

The perception from a historical look at the latter half of the twentieth Century is that the majority of burns encountered in conflicts will be accidental. Fifty eight percent of all burn injuries sustained by US Forces in the Vietnam War were not related to fighting. The background incidence of non-combat related burns in the civilian population may rise as normal social habits are changed, for example; the use of kerosene to cook when electricity supplies are disrupted. Combatants are particularly at risk of accidental burns in transition to war due to lack of familiarity and incorrect use of equipment and ignoring safety procedures. The type of injuries will be similar to those seen in normal civilian practice where there is a low incidence of concomitant non-burn injury.

In war fighting, burn injury rates vary significantly with the type of conflict. In the 1982 Falklands conflict, 34% of those injured on ships sustained burns compared to 14% of total UK casualties. Burns were seen in 10% of injured troops in the 1973 Yom Kippur war but in up to 70% of Israeli tank casualties. Up to 50% of battlefield burn casualties may have concomitant non-burn injury.

Looking more broadly across all wars and conflicts, a fairly consistent finding is that between 5% and 10% of all casualties have a burn injury. Another recurring finding is that 80% of burn injuries are less than 20% total body surface area. This tradition pattern seems to be continuing during the most recent conflicts in Iraq and Afghanistan. As these campaigns have matured, however, it has been noted that the incidence of combat related burns now exceeds non-combat burns.

Thermonuclear detonations will cause large numbers of burns. Radiation doses sufficient to cause cutaneous burns will generally be fatal. Combined thermal burns and radiation exposure reduces chances of survival but the poor outcome from burns in Hiroshima and Nagasaki would have had as much to do with the massive degradation of the health services.

Newer enhanced blast weapons, such as thermobaric explosives, produce significantly higher amounts of heat but their impact on survivable burn incidence has yet to be seen.

## 33.3
## Pathophysiology

Thermal injury causes burns to the skin and upper airway. This is associated with inflammation that can be systemic. Inhalation of the products of combustion can injure the lungs and cause systemic toxicity.

### 33.3.1
### Systemic Injury

Direct thermal injury causes cell death progressively with temperatures over 45°C and almost instantaneously above 60°C. Heat is also conducted into surrounding tissues causing injury. Tissues non-fatally injured by heat exhibit very marked inflammation with increased capillary permeability and loss of fluid from the intravascular space. The clinical impact of the inflammation evolves for several hours and is related to the total volume of tissue injured. This is best expressed as the percentage of total body surface area burned (% TBSAB).

The most superficial of burns cause only erythema with no effect on capillary leakage and as such should not be considered when calculating the % TBSAB.

Injuries above about 15% TBSAB in adults and 10% in children cause sufficient loss of intravascular fluid for physiological signs of hypovolaemia to be seen. Additional fluids need to be administered to prevent shock developing.

Injuries above about 25–30% TBSAB cause massive activation of inflammatory mediators and a potentially fatal Systemic Inflammatory Response Syndrome (SIRS) develops. This is a progressive process and the clinical signs of SIRS can be delayed for several hours after the burn. Toxins released from the burn wound further stimulate the SIRS.

### 33.3.2
### Inhalation Injury

This consists of a variable combination of:

### 33.3.2.1
### The True Airway Burn

This is caused by inhalation of hot gases be the flame, smoke, or steam. The resulting injury is thermal in nature and normally only affects the supraglottic airway. The initial manifestation is upper airway oedema which develops over a period of hours and is maximal between 12 h and 36 h. The oedema can be severe enough to obstruct the airway.

### 33.3.2.2
### Lung Injury

The upper airways are efficient at dissipating heat and, along with reflex laryngeal closure, protect the lower airways from direct heat injury. If, however, the products of combustion are inhaled into the lower airways, they dissolve into the fluid lining the bronchial tree and alveoli. This leads to a chemical injury to the lungs which causes: hyperaemia, mucosal ulceration and sloughing, increased mucous production, and a protein rich transudate, all combining to the production of obstructing casts and increased lung water. The clinical manifestations of the resultant pulmonary failure is often delayed by hours or even days. The pulmonary complications of SIRS adds a further insult to the inhalation injury.

### 33.3.2.3
### Systemic Toxicity

Absorption of the products of combustion into the circulation through the alveoli leads to systemic toxicity. The most important agents are carbon monoxide and cyanides. This is the most common cause of death due to fires in enclosed spaces. Carbon monoxide competes with oxygen for binding to hemoglobin, having 240 times the affinity. It therefore displaces oxygen, effectively causing hypoxaemia. It also binds to the intracellular cytochrome system causing abnormal cellular function. A low level of carboxyhemoglobin (<10%) causes no symptoms and can be found in heavy smokers. Above 20% feelings of fatigue and nausea can start and higher mental functions are impaired. Levels above 40% lead to progressive loss of neurological function, and death occurs with levels over 60%. Note that in the presence of carboxyhemoglobin, pulse oximeter readings are unreliable indicators of oxygen saturation (% $SaO_2$).

There is no measure to quantify the severity of an inhalation injury but its presence significantly worsens the prognosis following a burn.

Blast Lung is an injury secondary to the passage of a shock wave through the lungs and, although in some ways clinically similar, is not part of inhalation injury.

### 33.3.3
### Cutaneous Injury

The severity of a cutaneous burn is difficult to qualify. The % TBSAB will be reflected by the degree of systemic inflammation and will dictate resuscitative needs. The depth of burn has less of an effect on the systemic response but dictates wound management needs. The extent and distribution of any residual burn scarring can have devastating social and psychological effects. The personal impact of burn scarring on an individual is very variable and has been shown to be not related to the size or location of scars. The interactions of the burn survivor in society are complex.

Classification of the burn wound is purely descriptive and indicates the % TBSAB and depth involved. Methods of calculating % TBSAB are described later.

With respect to depth, burns either involve the full thickness of the skin and are called full thickness burns or involve only part of the thickness of the skin and are called partial thickness burns. Partial thickness burns are sub-classified depending on which parts of the skin are involved.

### 33.3.3.1
### Epidermal Burns

These cause local inflammation of the epidermis leading to erythema alone, like sunburn. No blistering is seen. They can be extremely painful. Spontaneous resolution in about 48 h is expected. They are not included when calculating % TBSAB.

### 33.3.3.2
### Partial Thickness Burns

These are sub-divided into:

Superficial dermal: The skin blisters and oozes clear fluid. When the blisters are removed, the underlying surface has marked erythema which blanches on pressure and has an intact capillary refill. The deeper skin adnexal structures survive providing a source of epithelial cells for healing. If managed correctly these burns should heal in less than 2 weeks.

Deep dermal: When the blisters are removed, the underlying surface has a darker red color which does not blanch. This "fixed staining" is caused by damage to deeper blood vessels. There is no visible capillary refill. Due to loss of deeper epithelial elements, these burns rarely heal in 2 weeks and often require skin grafting.

### 33.3.3.3
### Full Thickness Burns

The thermal damage causes total destruction of dermis leaving a firm leathery necrotic layer known as eschar. This can be waxy white or have lobster red fixed staining. Soot or charred tissue may mask the true appearance and needs to be cleaned off. Surgery is required except for very small areas.

The level of pain from a wound and the pinprick test of sensation are poor discriminators of depth and should not be relied on.

Burn wounds are not homogenous and a mixed pattern may be seen.

The inflammation surrounding the burn wound alters the local circulation and can lead to further necrosis. This burn wound progression can account for the deepening seen in some wounds originally thought to be superficial. Early cooling of a burn wound can reduce the magnitude of the local inflammatory injury and lower the chance of progression.

Deep dermal and full thickness burns can constrict deeper structures, particularly if circumferential. Around the torso this can restrict respiration. In the limbs a similar picture to compartment syndrome will be seen. In these situations, surgical release of the constriction (escharotomy) is indicated.

### 33.4
### Managing the Burn Victim

Burn victims are trauma victims and the initial assessment is the same as for any other seriously injured patient. There may be injuries other than the burn and these must be treated or excluded. Some common sense should prevail and not every patient needs to be treated as a major trauma case. As a general principle though, any burn involving greater than 10% of the total body surface area should be regarded as significant.

Whatever the cause of the burn, the severity of the injury is proportional to the volume of tissue damage. In terms of survival, the % TBSAB is the most important factor. Functional outcome is more often dependant on depth and site of the burn.

At all levels of care the broad principles of management are: anticipate and pre-empt any potential of airway problem, estimate likely fluid requirements and administer them to prevent burn shock, monitor the adequacy of fluid replacement, perform initial burn wound care, prevent hypothermia, and transfer appropriate cases for definitive care.

Burns are painful and the victims often terrified. With large burns, there are tangible levels of anxiety in carers, even those familiar with such cases. Relatives and friends of the victim are usually distraught. The whole atmosphere surrounding the initial care of a burn injured patient is frequently highly charged. It is vital that the patient receives early adequate analgesia, anxiolitics and sedation. Intravenous opiates are the obvious choice. This should be supported by the professional staff acting in a manner that will instill confidence.

## 33.5
## First Aid

With safety of the rescuer in mind, the immediate priority is to stop the burning process. This is best achieved by dousing the effected area in cold water and removing smoldering clothes and those soaked in scalding fluids. All constricting items such as jewelery, watches, and tight clothing should be removed. The apocryphal teaching of leaving adherent clothing on the burn in an attempt to reduce infection is erroneous – it should be removed.

Carry out any necessary standard Basic Life Support first aid.

There is evidence that immediate cooling of the burn wound modifies local inflammation and reduces progressive cell necrosis. This is best achieved by the topical application of cool water, preferably flowing. Proprietary wet gels may have a role in this respect. Cooling the wound also has a beneficial analgesic effect. Very cold water and ice cause local vasoconstriction and are to be avoided.

Ideally the cooling should be started immediately and continue for about 20 min. It is uncertain if there is any benefit beyond this time. Protracted cooling and cooling large areas may lead to systemic hypothermia, particularly in small children and a degree of common sense should prevail. The maxim "cool the burn but warm the patient" is true but difficult to achieve in large burns.

A clean non-stick dressing can then be placed on the burn. Clingfilm is ideal and there are also several proprietary "first burn dressings" available. The dressing does not need to be sterile and clean moistened linen is a satisfactory alternative. Air movement over a fresh burn causes pain and this initial dressing removes that stimulus. Do not wrap the burn as this can lead to constrictions, merely lay the dressing on.

Give adequate analgesia as soon as possible.

Further management at the scene or in transit depends on the local capabilities and proximity of the medical facility. For burns over about 20% in adults and 10% in children, administer oxygen if possible and obtain intravenous access if feasible.

If a significant delay in arrival at a medical facility is anticipated, commence an intravenous infusion of crystalloid to run at 100 mL/h. Give 250 mL boluses as required if signs of hypovolaemic shock become apparent.

## 33.6
## Initial Medical Care

On arrival at a medical facility, the burn victim should be assessed by standard trauma management principles.

Perform a primary survey using the ABCDE approach. If the history indicates there is the possibility of other injuries, these must be excluded or, if identified, treated appropriately. The events around the incident, the painful nature of the injury and staff unfamiliar with burns can lead to significant other injuries being overlooked. Catastrophic hemorrhage needs urgent attention. In line spinal immobilization must be maintained until the spine is cleared.

### 33.6.1
### A: Airway

Airway swelling occurs progressively for many hours following inhalation injury and may not be evident when the casualty is first seen. It is important to anticipate those at risk of developing airway obstruction.

The presence of any of the following indicates the possibility of an inhalation injury:

- A history of exposure to fire and smoke in an enclosed space.
- Exposure to blast.
- Collapse, confusion, or restlessness at any time.
- Hoarseness or any change in voice.
- Harsh cough.
- Stridor.
- Flame or steam burns to the face.
- Singed nasal hairs.
- Soot in saliva or sputum.
- An inflamed oropharynx.

Oxygen should be administered in the highest concentration feasible, preferably humidified.

It can be very difficult to decide on how severe an upper airway burn is. Experienced senior help should be sort as soon as possible.

If any degree of upper airway obstruction is present, endotracheal intubation is mandatory. Remember, the swelling is likely to be increasing. The majority of cases will be conscious and intubation will be impossible without first anesthetising the patient.

In areas where anesthetic expertise may not be available, judgement is required in cases where there is a high suspicion of inhalation injury but without evidence of upper airway obstruction. If it is considered safe to observe a casualty with a possible inhalation injury unintubated, they should be nursed sitting up. In high risk cases, it may be necessary to perform a surgical airway on an awake patient. If there is any doubt, endotracheal intubation (by whichever route) should be performed.

## 33.6.2
## B: Breathing

The pulmonary manifestations of burn injuries rarely occur early. If the airway is clear, the only likely effect of a burn that will cause compromise of respiration in the first few hours is a restriction of chest excursion by a deep circumferential torso burn. This is an indication for emergency escharotomy (see below).

## 33.6.3
## C: Circulation

Hypovolaemic shock secondary to a burn takes some time to produce measurable physical signs. If the burn victim is shocked soon after injury, other causes should be excluded. A history of a blast, vehicle collision or a fall whilst escaping the fire should raise suspicion of other injuries.

If the patient has hypovolaemic shock, this should be treated according to current shock protocols independent of the severity of burn.

Establish intravenous access with two large bore cannulae. It is possible to cannulate through burnt skin but this should be avoided if possible. If necessary use cut-downs, intraosseous or, as a last resort, central routes. Commence an intravenous infusion of crystalloid.

## 33.6.4
## D: Disability

A reduced level of consciousness, confusion, or restlessness normally indicates hypoxia and in the burn victim this can be secondary to an inhalation injury. Do not, however, overlook the possibility of other injuries. Drug and/or alcohol ingestion should be considered.

## 33.6.5
## E: Exposure/Environment

The entire body surface area should be inspected for burns and other injuries, but care should be taken to avoid hypothermia. Unwrap one limb at a time to avoid excessive cooling. It may be possible to assess the burn without removing previously applied cling film. Ensure no constricting items of clothing remain. If possible, keep the ambient temperature high.

## 33.6.6
### Other Initial Interventions

Ensure the casualty has received adequate analgesia.

If the facilities are available, measure the full blood count, urea and electrolytes, and blood gases. If there is a suspicion of inhalation injury, obtain a chest X-ray and measure carboxyhemoglobin levels. Even in severe inhalation injury, the chest x-ray and blood gases may be normal initially.

In burns over 20% TBSA in an adult and 10% in a child, insertion of a nasogastric tube and urinary catheter will be required.

Reassess the patient's ABCD and perform a full secondary survey.

## 33.7
### Initial Specific Burn Management

## 33.7.1
### Inhalation Injury

Regularly reassess those with suspected inhalation injury. Beyond keeping a patent airway and delivering the maximally achievable oxygen concentration, there is little that can be done without critical care intervention. Any patient with a suspected inhalation injury should be closely observed in an area equipped for intubation. If there is a definite inhalation injury then the patient should be managed by an experienced anesthetist before and during transfer.

Remember to interpret pulse oximetry readings with caution.

There is no evidence that administration of steroids is beneficial (although pre-injury users should continue their steroids).

There should be an extremely low threshold for elective intubation if the patient is going to be transferred to another hospital.

## 33.7.2
### Establish the Size of the Burn

Accurate assessment of the size of burn can be difficult. When seen early, it may not be possible to tell whether or not areas of erythema will progress to blistering. Soot may mask an underlying burn. Initially an estimate should be made upon which to base the fluid requirements.

**Fig. 33.1** The rule of nines – for estimating the % TBSAB

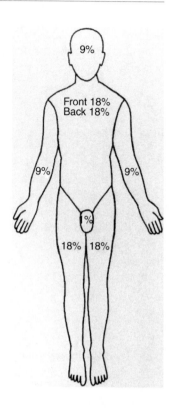

Aids to estimating the % TBSAB are serial halving (see box) and "Rule of Nines" (Fig. 33.1). In very large burns it is often easier to work out how much is not burnt. The palmar surface of the patient's hand including the fingers equates to 1% TBSA and can be used to estimate small areas of burn.

---

*Serial halving*

This is designed to be a quick method of triaging the burn victim into one of four groups to describe the size of the burn.

Look at the front of the patient. This represents half of their TBSA. Estimate if more or less than half of the front is burned. If it is less than half, is it more or less than half of a half? Repeat the same for the rear of the patient.

You can then describe the burn as being:

More than half of the body (>50% TBSAB)

Between a quarter and a half (25–50% TBSAB)

Between an eighth and a quarter (12.5–25% TBSAB)

Less than an eighth (<12.5% TBSAB)

---

At this stage it is not necessary to evaluate burn depth apart from identifying circumferential deep burns. Consideration should be given for the need of emergency escharotomies (see below).

As soon as is possible, an accurate assessment of the burn should be made. For this a Lund and Browder chart should be used (Fig. 33.2). If there is to be no undue delay in transfer, this can safely be left until arrival at a definitive care facility.

**Fig. 33.2** Lund and Browder chart – for accurate assessment of the % TBSAB (Lund and Browder 1944)

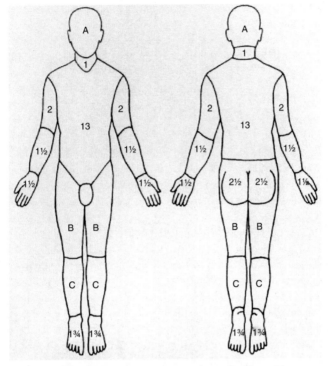

Relative Percentage of Areas Affected by Growth

| Age in Years | 0 | 1 | 5 | 10 | 15 | Adult |
|---|---|---|---|---|---|---|
| A – ½ of head | 9½ | 8½ | 6½ | 5½ | 4½ | 3½ |
| B – ½ of one thigh | 2¾ | 3¼ | 4 | 4¼ | 4½ | 4¾ |
| C – ½ of one leg | 2½ | 2½ | 2¾ | 3 | 3¼ | 3½ |

## 33.7.3
## Calculate the Fluid Requirements

Prophylactic intravenous fluids above normal requirements should be administered to prevent burn shock in injuries greater than 15% TBSAB (10% in children). The fluid calculations are based on an assumption that the need for additional fluids starts at the time of injury, not the time of assessment. Several formulae have been developed over the years, all based on retrospective analysis of fluids administered. It should be remembered that all formulae provide only an estimate of needs and the ultimate guide to adequacy is the patient's physiological response. The most widely used formula at present estimates the likely volume of crystalloid needed in the first 24 h.

Volume of crystalloid needed in first 24 h (mL) = 2 × weight (kg) × % TBSAB

In children this should be; 3 × weight (kg) × % TBSAB

Half this volume is given in the first 8 h from injury then the second half in the following 16 h.

Hartmann's/Ringer's Lactate solution is recommended. Normal saline can be used if necessary but in large volumes produces a hyperchloraemic acidosis.

The rate of administration must take in to account that the requirement of fluids starts at the time of injury.

Other fluid requirements are not accounted for in this regime. Administer additional fluids where indicated for losses due to other injuries and normal daily maintenance.

### 33.7.4
### Monitor

The calculated volume for fluid administration is an initial guide only. The individual's physiological response should be monitored to assess its adequacy. Large full thickness burns and those with an inhalation injury often require very large volumes of fluid over what is expected. An accurate fluid balance record should be maintained and updated at least hourly.

The simplest guide to adequacy of fluid administration is urine output. Aim to keep the urine output between 0.5 and 1 mL/kg body weight/h in adults and double this for children. Do not be afraid to adjust the fluid input to keep the urine output within these limits. It is equally as important to reduce fluid administration when indicated. Full blood count and urea and electrolytes should be measured at least twice in the first 24 h.

In children, a reduced capillary refill time and tachypnea are also good indicators of inadequate perfusion.

Use pulse oximetry to monitor % $SaO_2$ and pulse rate. Carbon Monoxide poisoning can give anomalously high % $SaO_2$ readings.

### 33.7.5
### The Burn Wound

Apart from small superficial burns, wound management needs to be supervised by experienced surgeons. Beyond stopping the burning process and cooling the burn as described above, there is rarely any indication for the initial team to interfere with the burn wound.

If the patient is going to be transferred to another facility, Clingfilm is a more than adequate dressing. Do not apply ointments or creams as this can make later accurate wound assessment more difficult. If there is to be a delay in planned arrival at definitive care beyond about 12 h then the burn wound should be thoroughly cleaned as described below.

Burns are usually sterile initially and infection is uncommon for the first few days. In uncomplicated civilian type burns, there is no requirement for antibiotic prophylaxis. In the battlefield situation, wound contamination is assumed and antibiotics should be administered. Make sure the casualty is tetanus immune.

A circumferential full thickness burn can act like a tourniquet and compromise circulation. Division of the constriction is known as escharotomy. This is not a straight forward undertaking and should be performed in an operating theater by skilled persons. There is rarely a need to perform an escharotomy within the first few hours. The exception is full thickness burns of the entire trunk that are compromising respiration by restricting chest

**Fig. 33.3** Lines of election of escharotomies

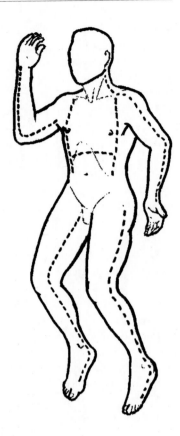

excursion. This constitutes a surgical emergency and in this situation it is appropriate to perform torso escharotomies in any setting (Fig. 33.3).

## 33.8
## Transfer to Definitive Care

Burns are complex injuries and the occasional burn practitioner will not be in a position to achieve optimal recovery.

### 33.8.1
### Referral Criteria

The following injuries should be referred to a facility able to provide definitive burn care:

- Presence of an inhalational injury
- Burns greater than 10% TBSA in an adult

- Burns greater than 5% TBSA in a child
- Full thickness burns greater than 1% TBSA
- Burns of special areas; face, hands, feet, genitalia, major joints
- Electrical burns
- Chemical burns
- Circumferential burns (except where superficial)
- Burns in the very young and very old
- Burns associated with any condition that may impact on outcome such as pre-existing disease, other injuries, social circumstances, non-accidental injury

Early contact with a burn center should be made. Further advice on initial management and transfer will be given. There may be specific local guidelines that need to be followed.

## 33.8.2
## Preparation for Transfer

All patients at this stage will have had a primary survey with appropriate resuscitative interventions, an assessment of the burn and initial burn management as outlined above commenced. Before transfer it is important to ensure the following:

- A thorough secondary survey has been performed and any other injuries identified be appropriately managed.
- Oxygen is being administered.
- If there is any suspicion of an inhalational injury, the patient has been assessed by an experienced anesthetist and intubated if necessary.
- Adequate intravenous access is secured and appropriate fluid resuscitation has started.
- The burn wound is covered appropriately and the patient is being kept warm.
- There is adequate analgesia.
- There is a urinary catheter in place.
- There is a free draining nasogastric tube in place.
- All findings and interventions, including fluid balance, are clearly and accurately documented.

With the interventions described above, a burn casualty should remain stable and fit for transfer for about 12 h. In many areas of the world, arrival at a definitive care facility within this time is unlikely. If it is likely that transfer will exceed this time then the situation needs to be discussed further with the receiving burn center. In this circumstance it may be deemed necessary for:

- Escharotomies to be performed
- The burn wound to be cleaned and a specific dressing applied
- The commencement of maintenance intravenous fluids and/or nasogastric feeding

All patients should be transferred with appropriately trained escort staff.

Experience has shown that burn injured casualties tolerate long distance aeromedical transfer satisfactorily if carried out early. As the SIRS evolves, such transfers become more complicated. This becomes very significant progressively beyond 48 h.

## 33.9
## Principles of Definitive Care

Definitive burn care should be delivered by a multidisciplinary team in a facility capable of providing all aspects of care simultaneously. The process of full rehabilitation of the burn survivor back in to society can be long and complicated.

The initial goal, though, is to achieve burn wound healing whilst managing any systemic response. Deep dermal and full thickness burns need surgery and the management of SIRS requires critical care facilities. Inhalation injury will normally be managed in intensive care. Ideally all these capabilities should be found within a burn center.

A full description of the definitive management of burn care is beyond the scope of this chapter. Below is a summary of important aspects that those providing care outside of specialized facilities may need to consider.

## 33.9.1
## On-going Care

Using the system of care described above with good monitoring and fine adjustment of the advocated fluid regime where appropriate, the majority of cases up to about 40% TBSAB will pass through the phase of systemic inflammation fairly smoothly. Burn injury does produces changes in normal physiology that do not resolve even with adequate management. These include a tachycardia, pyrexia of up to 38.5°C and a leucocytosis and can persist for several days even in uncomplicated burns.

Deep burns cause loss of red blood cells and transfusion may be required. Breakdown products of the lost red cells are excreted in the urine and increase the risk of acute tubular necrosis. If dark red pigmentation of the urine is seen, increase fluid input to achieve a urine output of 1.5–2 mL/kg/h.

Nasogastric feeding should be started as early as possible, ideally immediately on admission. This helps maintain gut function, lowers the risk of peptic ulceration and may have a benefit in reducing bacterial translocation. If it is not possible to start nasogastric feeding, give either a $H_2$ antagonist or proton pump inhibitor to prevent peptic ulceration.

The patient should be nursed partially sitting up with arms elevated on pillows to help reduce oedema. Physiotherapy should start early with the aim of maintaining the range of motion of all joints. This may need to be compromised to avoid damage to recent skin grafting.

Once a casualty's burns are dressed, analgesia requirements decrease. High levels of anxiety remain though and good psychological support is important. Anxiolytics can help along with a balanced analgesia regime. NSAIDs should be avoided in the first 24 h.

Additional fluid requirements extend beyond the first 24 h. With nasogastric feeding, a standard regime will provide for the majority of cases. 500 mL boluses of colloid (10 mL/kg for children) should be used if hypovolaemia becomes apparent. Again, the patient's physiological response is the main indicator of fluid requirement. In general, a low urine output is an indicator of hypovolaemia and diuretics should not be used unless it is certain that there is sufficient intravascular volume.

In large burns and those with inhalation injury, the SIRS can be severe and management becomes complicated. The general strategies of intensive care become necessary. The balance between giving sufficient fluids to maintain renal perfusion without causing excessive pulmonary fluid is difficult to achieve.

## 33.9.2
## Inhalation Injury

The management of inhalation injury requires experience in respiratory intensive care.

Actual upper airway oedema is an indication for endotracheal intubation. High risk cases not yet showing signs should be nursed sitting up in a high dependency area equipped for intubation. Supplementary oxygen should be administered as necessary to keep the $PaO_2$ above 10 kPa.

Even in severe injuries, initial blood gas and chest X-ray results may be normal. The normal clinical picture is that of deterioration up to several days following injury.

Fiber-optic bronchoscopy is the investigation of choice.

The general strategy for treatment is; reducing the obstructive element of airway casts, reducing secondary lung injury by use of "gentle" mechanical ventilation, and avoidance of fluid overload. The use of pulmonary toilet, nebulised therapies, and various ventilation strategies will depend on the experience of clinicians and equipment available. Chest physiotherapy should be commenced early in all cases.

Systemic intoxication is treated with general supportive measures and administration of 100% inspired oxygen until signs resolve or carboxyhemoglobin levels fall below 15%.

Current practice suggests there is no role for prophylactic antibiotics, steroids, or hyperbaric oxygen in inhalation injury, apart from the latter in isolated, non-burn carbon monoxide poisoning.

## 33.9.3
## Accurate Assessment of the Burn

To do this properly causes pain and adequate analgesia will normally need to be supplemented with sedation. In large burns a general anesthetic is appropriate and the best environment is in a warm (30°C) operating theater.

Thoroughly clean all involved areas with copious volumes of warm aqueous based antiseptic solution. All blister roofs, loose skin, debris, and soot should be removed. This has to be a vigorous process using large gauze swabs. Gentle wiping of the burn is ineffectual. There are now devices available to assist in this procedure, such as Versajet™.

Once cleaned, the full extent of the burn will be clear. Draw the burn areas on a Lund & Browder chart (see Fig. 33.2) and calculate the % TBSAB. Do not include simple erythema. Re-calculate expected fluid requirements if this accurate assessment is widely different from a previous estimate but at this stage, it is the patient's physiological response that is the primary guide to fluid administration rates.

Identify deep areas that may cause circumferential constriction. This is the time to perform escharotomies (see below). The need for accurate assessment of burn depth depends on the surgical strategies to be used.

## 33.9.4
## Escharotomies

The necrotic layer of firm and unyielding deeply burnt skin is known as eschar. As oedema forms in the deeper tissues, the eschar resists swelling and tissue pressure rises. When circumferential this can compromise perfusion and in the torso restrict ventilation. Surgical division of the eschar, escharotomy, is then indicated.

The restriction of chest excursion constitutes a surgical emergency. It is unusual, however, for there to be a need for escharotomies of the limbs within the first couple of hours. It is best to perform the procedure under controlled conditions in an operating theater. To adequately relieve the constriction it is necessary to extend the incisions just into unburnt tissue and the procedure, therefore, does cause pain and bleeding. A general anesthetic is indicated.

The lines of election for escharotomies are shown in Fig. 33.3. As much normal ventilation is performed diaphragmatically, it is important to ensure the horizontal torso release is over the upper abdomen. There is a risk of damaging the ulnar nerve at the elbow and common peroneal nerve around the fibular head. Deep burns to the hands do require dorsal hand releases but escharotomies to the fingers is of uncertain benefit and it is easy to cause iatrogenic injuries.

Cutting diathermy should be used to carefully incise down until the constriction is released along the full length of the deep burn. Slashing down into unburnt fat is not required. As with letting down a tourniquet, a period of local hyper-perfusion follows and significant bleeding can occur. It is important to ensure good haemostasis.

When there has been prolonged delay in performing escharotomies, compartment syndrome may be encountered necessitating fasciotomies.

## 33.9.5
## Achieving Burn Wound Healing

Following a basic surgical premise that dead tissue needs to be debrided, necrotic burnt skin should be removed. In deep dermal and full thickness burns this requires surgical excision and takes the form of tangential shaving. It is now recognized that leaving necrotic burn provides a stimulus for SIRS and early excision (certainly within the first couple of days) is advocated. Indeed in the case of life threatening SIRS it should be the view that debridement is essential rather than that the patient is too sick for surgery. In extensive very deep burns, it is sometimes more practical to excise the burnt areas straight down to (but not including) the fascia, even if this involves taking unburnt fat.

The resultant post-excision wound is closed by various strategies depending on its extent. Autologous split skin grafting is the mainstay. Once the excised burn area exceeds about 40%, it is very difficult to obtain enough autograft to achieve straight forward closure. Other techniques then need to be used, including allograft, synthetic temporary wound covers, cultured and artificial skin components.

In superficial dermal burns, where it is anticipated uncomplicated wound healing will be achieved within 2 weeks, the vigorous cleaning described above should suffice as debridement. Various dressings can be applied to maintain an optimum healing environment.

Between the obvious superficial and deep burns lies the common situation of the "indeterminate depth" burn. In this situation, newer biologically active dressings are used (following vigorous cleaning) to try and achieve as much healing as possible without surgery.

Where it is not possible to excise deep burns, the use of topical agents can help reduce the risk of wound infection and possibly diminish the effect on SIRS. Examples are; cerium in silver sulphadiazine cream (Flammacerium®), normal silver sulphadiazine cream (Flammazine®) and mafenide acetate. Burn wounds produce a large volume of exudate. The dressings need to be changed when soaked through or, if possible, at least daily.

### 33.9.6
### Infections in Burns

Burn wounds are initially sterile but become progressively contaminated increasing the risk of invasive infection. In large burns there is marked immunosupression. Several of the traditional signs of infection are also seen as part of the normal systemic response to burn injury (tachycardia, pyrexia, and leucocytosis). Positive surface wound cultures do not necessarily indicate invasive infection. It can therefore be difficult to diagnose infection in burn injury.

With a lack of any clear evidence of benefit and the risk of resistance emergence, it is not normal practice to use prophylactic antibiotics in uncomplicated civilian type burn injuries. Where wounding is secondary to ballistic trauma, contamination is potentially significant and prophylaxis is indicated. Early burn wound excision and the antimicrobial activity of the topical agents is the main strategy for reducing infection.

Streptococcal and Staphylococcal infections predominate in the first 5 days with gram negative organisms becoming evident beyond this time.

If infection is apparent, antibiotics should be given according to microbiological culture results. In cases of extremis, blind therapy should be based on knowledge of local prevalent pathogens and any resistance patterns.

### 33.10
### Special Burns

### 33.10.1
### Phosphorus Burns

These are almost exclusively a military phenomenon. The metal spontaneously ignites in air and is prevented from doing so by immersion in water. The majority of phosphorus burns are caused by secondary ignition of clothing and are treated as normal.

To prevent further ignition of phosphorus imbedded in wounds, visible lumps should be removed and the area irrigated with water. Soaking dressings are then applied and kept wet until arrival at a surgical facility.

To help identify further particles during wound debridement an ultraviolet lamp will highlight phosphorescence. Debrided particles must be immersed in water to prevent ignition in the operating theater.

## 33.10.2
### Vesicant Burns

Various chemical warfare agents cause cutaneous burns. The main aim of these agents is to produce large numbers of surviving casualties who require significant medical input. Typically irritation and erythema appear several hours after exposure followed by blistering. Wound healing is significantly slower than with a comparable thermal injury. There may be associated pulmonary, systemic, and ocular injury.

Full decontamination procedures must be carried out before admission to any medical facility.

Thorough cleaning with removal of all blisters is performed. There is usually no active agent in blister fluid. The exception is Lewisite but this is easily neutralized by using a weak hypochlorite solution.

Dressings and fluid resuscitation are then the same as for thermal burns. The loss of fluid can be delayed in vesicant burns and the need for replacement starts when blisters appear as opposed to the moment of exposure.

Pulmonary involvement is treated as for an inhalation injury. Sulfur mustard causes bone marrow suppression increasing the risk of infection. British anti-Lewisite (BAL) is a specific antidote for systemic Lewisite toxicity.

Despite the long healing time, vesicant burns will often do well without skin grafting. Debridement of the wound using either dermabrasion or laser has been shown to experimentally accelerate healing.

## 33.11
### Burns in Mass Casualty Scenarios

With optimal care, survival with good quality of life can be achieved even in massive burn injury. It is no longer appropriate to arbitrarily choose a certain % TBSAB above which it is assumed care is futile. The high demand of burn care, however, necessitates careful use of triage when resources are stretched.

The factors that significantly reduce survival rates are:

- Inhalation injury (except isolated oropharyngeal swelling)
- Deep burns over 80% TBSA
- Age over 60
- Significant concomitant illness or injury

Burns that need skin grafting of over about 40% TBSA require a very high level of surgical input and will draw heavily on time and manpower.

In mass casualty scenarios, the prime importance of a Burn Assessment Team consisting of an experienced surgeon, anesthetist, and nurse is in making the appropriate triage decisions, not just delivering care.

Oral fluid therapy can be used for burns at least up to 20% TBSA and may be even higher if the nasogastric route is used. Moyer's solution or proprietary oral rehydration formulae can be used. A normal diet with extra water to drink is probably as efficacious.

## Further Reading

Herndon DN. *Total Burn Care*. 3rd ed. London: Saunders Elsevier; 2007.

## Specific Papers

Alvarado R, Chung KK, Cancio LC, Wolf SE. Burn resuscitation. *Burns*. 2009;35:4-14.

Arturson G. The pathophysiology of severe thermal injury. *J Burn Care Rehabil*. 1985;6:129-146.

Bellamy RF. The medical effects of conventional weapons. *World J Surg*. 1992;16:888.

Baxter CR. Fluid volume and electrolyte changes in the early post-burn period. *Clin Plast Surg*. 1974;1:693-703.

Chapman P. Operation corporate – the Sir Galahad bombing. Woolwich burns unit experience. *J R Army Med Corps*. 1984;130(2):84-88.

Jackson DM. The diagnosis of the depth of burning. *Br J Surg*. 1953;40:588-596.

Jandera V, Hudson DA, de Wet PM, Innes PM, Rode H. Cooling the burn wound: evaluation of different modalities. *Burns*. 2000;26:265-270.

Leonard LG, Scheulen JJ, Munster AM. Chemical burns: effect of prompt first aid. *J Trauma*. 1982;22:420-423.

Levine BA, Petroff PA, Slade CL. Prospective trials of dexamethasone and aerosolized gentamicin in the treatment of inhalational injury in the burned patient. *J Trauma*. 1978;18:188-193.

Lund CC, Browder NC. The estimate of area of burns. *Surg Gynecol Obstet*. 1944;79:352-358.

Moritz AR, Henriquez FC. Studies of thermal injury II. The relative importance of time and surface temperature in the causation of cutaneous burns. *Am J Pathol*. 1947;23:695-720.

Pruitt BA Jr. Fluid resuscitation of extensively burned patients. *J Trauma*. 1981;21(Suppl):690-692.

Richard T. Medical lessons from the Falklands. *Br Med J*. 1983;286:790.

Renz EM. Thermal injuries in operations Iraqi and enduring freedom (OIF and OEF). *J Trauma*. 2007;62(6 Suppl):S22.

Scheinkestel CD, Bailey M, Myles PS, et al. Hyperbaric or normobaric oxygen for acute carbon monoxide poisoning: a randomised controlled clinical trial. *Med J Aust*. 1999;170:203-210.

Smith JJ, Scerri GV, Malyon AD, Burge TS. Comparison of serial halving and rule of nines as a pre-hospital assessment tool. *J Emerg Med*. 2002;19(suppl):A66.

# Management of Extremity Injuries

# 34

David E. Hinsley and Jon Clasper

## 34.1
## Introduction

Limb wounds are the most common injuries seen during military conflict, accounting for up to 80% of all wounds, with the lower limb most commonly involved. In general, the majority of penetrating injuries are due to fragments although in some conflicts, such as in recent years in Northern Ireland, bullet wounds predominate. The wounds can range in severity from superficial low-energy wounds from fragments, some of which can be managed conservatively, to high-energy bullet wounds when as many as half of the injuries are associated with a fracture, and complex surgical reconstruction may be required. In addition the recent conflicts in Iraq and Afghanistan have been characterized by the use of improvised explosive devices (IEDs), which have resulted in devastating limb trauma.

The predominance of extremity injury is related to the survivability of these injuries, relative to head and thoraco-abdominal injuries. Femoral fractures and junctional trauma (groin/axillary) may be associated with significant vascular injury and consequently may be life threatening. In addition, multiple limb injury may result in cumulative blood loss. As a result, all limb injuries can be associated with considerable morbidity and therefore adequate early assessment and appropriate treatment is necessary. This applies not only to military injuries, but also to civilian ballistic trauma that is being increasingly seen worldwide.

It is important to realize that the true assessment of most wounds can only be made at the time of surgery, and cannot be made on external appearances, particularly if there are no exit wounds. Figure 34.1 shows a high-energy wound to the upper arm from several bullets; the skin wounds are small, but despite the external appearance an extensive soft-tissue and bony wound is present (Fig. 34.2) and the outcome was relatively poor. Figure 34.3 illustrates an apparently more severe wound and yet there is a simple fracture (Fig. 34.4), relatively minimal soft-tissue damage and early internal fixation and flap coverage was possible (Fig. 34.5), with a good functional outcome.

D.E. Hinsley (✉)
Trauma and Orthopaedics, Frimley Park Hospital, Wakefords Park, Church Crookham, Fleet, Surrey GU52 8EZ, UK
e-mail: dehinsley@aol.com

A.J. Brooks et al. (eds.), *Ryan's Ballistic Trauma*,
DOI: 10.1007/978-1-84882-124-8_34, © Springer-Verlag London Limited 2011

**Fig. 34.1** Multiple gunshot wounds to the upper arm; despite the small wounds extensive soft tissue and bony damage is present

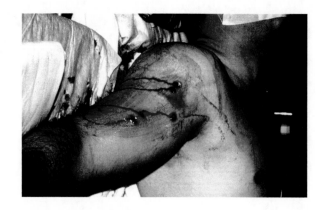

**Fig. 34.2** Radiograph of the humerus of Fig. 34.1; extensive fracture stabilized by external fixation

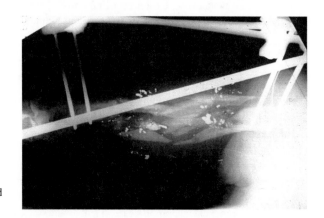

**Fig. 34.3** Shotgun wound to the upper arm; despite the appearances relatively little soft tissue or bony damage is present

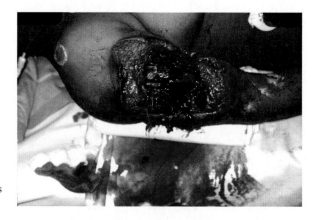

**Fig. 34.4** Radiograph of the humerus of Fig. 34.3 demonstrating a simple complete fracture

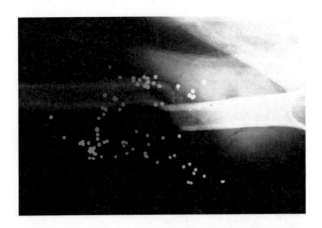

**Fig. 34.5** Patient shown in Fig. 34.3 (upper arm at *top* abducted away from the side) showing early closure using a local (latisimus dorsi) flap

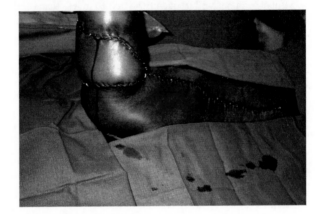

## 34.2
### Differences Between Military and Civilian Injuries

As well as the extensive soft-tissue damage and the multi-fragmentary nature of high-energy ballistic fractures, the morbidity is also due to the highly contaminated nature of some (particularly military) wounds. Although ballistic injuries are being increasingly seen in the civilian environment these injuries usually differ considerably from military injuries. These differences include:

*Military wounds are more heavily contaminated.* Reports from the Second World War, Korea, and Vietnam have documented that military wounds are more heavily contaminated than civilian wounds, with three to four different species of bacteria isolated from most military wounds, and up to six different species in some reports. This compares to only 1 species from most civilian wounds, even when the wounds have been caused by gunshots. The species of aerobic bacteria appear to be very similar, however, anaerobic bacteria contaminate most military wounds but are rarely isolated from acute civilian wounds. The only civilian equivalent of military wounds, are those injuries occurring in agricultural or sewage settings. The subsequent infection rate is also much higher with military wounds, with UK, US, and Israeli papers reporting rates of 30–50%, especially when bony injury is present.

*Delays in evacuation*, which averaged 10 h between wounding and starting appropriate care during the Gulf War. It has been stated that wounds can be considered contaminated for up to 6 h, but after this the bacteria are actively dividing and have spread via the lymphatic system. However recent civilian reports have questioned the need to operate within 6 h, and reported no increase in infection rates when surgery was delayed for up to 24 h. Provisional results from the UK suggest the same may be true for military wounds, and it is possible that time to initial surgery is not a significant factor.

Military wounds are more likely to be associated with penetrating trauma to the torso, which may be associated with the *spillage of abdominal contents*. This is due to the multiple penetrating wounds seen during conflict. Civilian wounds, in contrast, are associated with far fewer wounds. Abdominal injuries may result in further contamination with Gram negative pathogenic bacteria.

Military wounds will frequently be treated in less than ideal circumstances, with *limited resources* and *possible mass casualties*. This may impose further delays on the initiation of treatment.

This means that although the principles in the management of military and civilian ballistic injuries are the same, in general, military wounds probably require more radical local surgery in an attempt to reduce the infection rate.

## 34.3
## Management

### 34.3.1
### Overview

The principles of treatment for ballistic injuries remain the same as any trauma, with the initial aim being to identify and treat any life-threatening injuries. Unless there is an obvious source of major hemorrhage, limb wounds will not be dealt with until the secondary survey, after the patient has been stabilized.

The principles of wound care are also similar to the civilian environment, surgical debridement and adequate lavage, stabilization of the limb, and the use of appropriate antibiotics. Of these adequate surgery is by far the most important factor. Antibiotics, although an important factor, are secondary to early surgery and should not be considered as an alternative form of treatment.

### 34.3.2
### Resuscitation

According to Advanced Trauma Life Support (ATLS) protocols, the priorities in the management of any casualty are the ABCs:

- The airway must be secured, with cervical spine control if required.
- Adequate breathing confirmed, with the application of dressings and chest drains as appropriate.

- External bleeding should be stopped, usually by compressive dressings, and intravenous fluids started as necessary.

Although this principle is accepted, for military casualties, it has been recognized that they are far more likely to die of hemorrhage than airway problems and so the priorities are changed to C<>ABC, with the control of catastrophic hemorrhage performed before airway management. In addition, it is unlikely that control of the cervical spine is necessary if the casualty has only sustained penetrating trauma.

Most bleeding from the limbs can be controlled by local pressure and appropriate dressings. Occasionally a tourniquet may be required, particularly when under fire. Although the use of tourniquets has lead to much debate, they are now carried by both US and UK service personnel, however, these tourniquets are relatively narrow bands and unlike pneumatic tourniquets the pressure they exert on the limb cannot be measured. This may cause local tissue damage under the tourniquet or conversely inadequate pressure to prevent arterial inflow to the distal limb. In this situation, a venous tourniquet effect occurs where venous outflow is obstructed whilst arterial inflow is permitted. This may result in increased bleeding. It demonstrates the importance of ensuring that distal pulses are checked following tourniquet application and only applying tourniquets when they are necessary.

Fasciotomy is advised following prolonged ischaemia which includes the application of tourniquets. In order to minimize this requirement, tourniquets should be released after they have been in place for approximately 2 h. They should remain off for 15 min prior to being reapplied. Combat tourniquets should be replaced by a broader tourniquet as soon as is practicable, preferably a pneumatic tourniquet.

The majority of patients with limb injuries, however, will not have major life-threatening injuries, will usually be conscious, and some may even be able to walk. All wounds should be covered with a sterile dressing, appropriate antibiotics should be commenced, and tetanus prophylaxis considered. Although heavily contaminated wounds can be superficially washed, the majority of wounds should be left until the patient has been anesthetised.

If clinically, there is suspicion of a fracture the limb should be reduced and immobilized as appropriate. The diagnosis of a fracture will often be straightforward as the limb will be flail at the site of the wound, however, incomplete fractures can occur (see below).

### 34.3.3
### Surgical Treatment

The aim of local surgery is reduce the risk of infection, one of the most important factors in the morbidity after ballistic injuries. All military bullet wounds must be formally explored to reduce the infection risk, although civilian trauma centers have reported the successful non-operative management of bullet wounds. These were, however, low-energy wounds, evacuated rapidly to a hospital and not associated with the factors discussed above.

When small fragment wounds, particularly multiple wounds, are present not all need debridement. If wounds are small, there is no evidence of fracture or joint penetration and they appear to be superficial and low-energy, then a conservative approach can be adopted provided regular review is possible.

### 34.3.4
### Surgical Technique

The principle of debridement is to remove all foreign and non-viable tissue.

Debridement starts with the skin, and often excision of the skin margins is all that is required; degloving injuries may require more extensive debridement of skin. Although minimal excision is required the wound should be extended to allow its full extent to be visualized. For high-energy wounds considerable extension may be required. This should be in the long axis of the limb, with the exception of the flexor surface of a joint, when oblique incisions should be used.

Subcutaneous fat should be excised, but additional areas of degloving must not be created by over generous debridement.

The deep fascia should be incised along the complete length of the wound, including any extensions. Fasciotomies with complete longitudinal division of the deep fascia along the full length of the compartment should be carried out in most high-energy wounds, particularly if there has been associated ischaemia.

Adequate debridement of muscle is essential, and often a large amount of necrotic muscle may have to be excised. The aim is to remove all non-viable tissue, with the aim of leaving only pink, healthy-looking, contractile muscle. Lack of capillary bleeding or contractility, color, and consistency (the 4 Cs) are guides, but experience is the best way of judging viability of muscle. Debridement of muscle may result in considerable bleeding from the wound, and both the surgeon and anesthetist should be prepared for this.

Nerves and patent blood vessels should be left, as can tendons in continuity with muscles. Often, however, the tendons may be become desiccated and may have to be excised at a later date (Fig. 34.6). Divided nerves ends can be marked with a non-absorbable monofilament suture.

Difficulties can often occur in the debridement of bone, particularly the fate of the many small fragments. Bone fragments without any soft tissue attachments are avascular and should be removed. Often, however, periosteal and other soft tissue attachments are present and the viability of the fragment can be difficult to determine. Experience is probably the most important factor in deciding the viability of a bone fragment or muscle. Experimental work has suggested that there is the limited spread of contamination beyond the fracture site and, therefore, exposure of intact bone beyond the fracture site is not necessary. However, the fracture site itself must be well visualized and washed out (Fig. 34.7).

All wounds should be washed with copious amounts of fluid. It has been recommended that 9 L are used for open fractures. In a military environment, it may impossible to use this quantity of sterile fluids, but potable water can be used with a final washout of 1 L of sterile saline. With high-energy transfer wounds contamination can be spread along tissue planes, and these should be thoroughly irrigated. Antiseptic solutions can be used, but these may be toxic to local tissues, in addition soap solutions have also been shown to reduce the bacterial count, probably by reducing bacterial adherence. Much of the evidence for

**Fig. 34.6** Desiccated non-viable tendon at second debridement, it had been viable during the initial operation

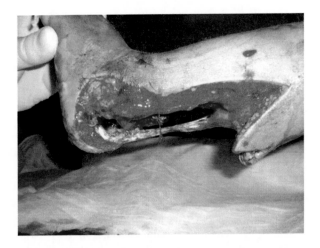

**Fig. 34.7** Open fracture after debridement with all dead and foreign material excised and the fracture site fully exposed

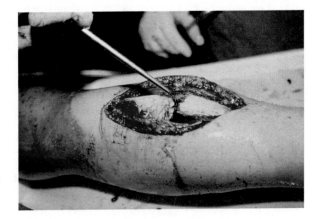

different lavage solutions is based on experimental work, and this may not translate, clinically, to a lower wound infection rate.

## 34.3.5
## Amputation

Primary amputation may be required as part of the initial debridement. Although the decision may be easy with a limb that is hanging off and obviously non-viable, the viability of less severe injuries can be difficult to determine. The following criteria can be used in deciding when to amputate:

- The presence of a large bony defect.
- Extensive skin wounds that will require flap coverage.

- Soft tissue including vein injuries that will impair function.
- Vascular injury that requires repair.
- Neurological injury, particularly involving the hand or sole of the foot.
- Local national with unreconstructable (in host nation hospital) limb injury

In practice, however, the decision with military casualties is commonly determined by the presence of a vascular injury that requires repair to save the limb, whether the casualty is medically stable enough for the prolonged procedure required, and whether local conditions will allow the reconstruction.

Even if bone loss is present, the limb can be allowed to heal short, soft tissue loss can be managed in prolonged plaster, and even a poorly functioning limb may be better than no limb, particularly if local limb fitting services are poor. It should be remembered that a limb can always be amputated at a latter date, but cannot be re-planted at a later date!

Although scoring systems have been developed for civilian limb injuries, there is still no reliable predictor of the need for amputation. There has been a recent consensus paper produced by the Army Medical Services in order to guide the operating surgeon. Even in the military environment, a second opinion should be obtained, if possible, prior to amputation. If the viability of the limb cannot be determined initially, it may be reassessed after 48 h. However, with military casualties a return to the operating theater cannot be guaranteed, as problems with evacuation or mass casualty situations may occur. The decision to perform bilateral or upper limb amputations injuries will often be delayed, but infection may threaten the life of the casualty and this must be considered.

## 34.3.6
### Closure of the Wound

Delayed primary closure of ballistic wounds is the rule. Wounds are left open to allow for swelling, and to prevent raised tissue pressures, which will impair microcirculation and lead to further tissue death, predisposing to infection. Although certain injuries, such as wounds to the face or genitals may need to be closed primarily, this should be the exception. High-energy transfer wounds, with comminution of the bone should never be closed primarily, and will often require plastic surgical techniques several days after the initial debridement (see Fig. 34.5). Delayed primary closure can be carried out between 2 and 14 days after initial surgery, depending on the nature of the wound, evacuation of the casualty and available resources and casualty numbers. Heavily contaminated wounds and limbs that may require amputation can be reassessed at 48 h, but for most wounds 4–5 days is the optimum period until the wound is closed.

Low energy injuries are associated with small wounds and require minimal debridement. Often they can be left to close by secondary intention, but should not be closed primarily.

Intra-articular fractures are associated with a poor outcome. Exposed joint surfaces should probably be covered at the initial operation to protect the articular surface and reduce the risk of infection. Ideally this should be achieved by closure of the joint capsule, but in cases of tissue loss, part of the skin wound can be closed. Although the wound has been sutured the patient should still be returned to the operating theater after several days for a further inspection and washout. Exposed bone or tendon does not have to be covered at the initial operation, but consideration should be given to early closure of these wounds to prevent desiccation. Bone or tendon that is left exposed for long periods will usually require further debridement despite appearing viable at initial surgery (see Fig. 34.6).

Wounds can be dressed with plain gauze, which can be fluffed up, but the wound should not be packed. The purpose of the dressing is to allow absorption of fluid, and not to hold the wound open. Tight packing will increase wound pressure leading to further tissue death.

Following debridement, antiseptic soaked dressings should not be used. If debridement has been adequate antiseptics are unnecessary, and are potentially toxic particularly to bone cells. Bandages and tape can be used to secure the dressing but must not be allowed to encircle and constrict the limb.

### 34.3.6.1
### Vacuum (VAC) Assisted Negative-Pressure Topical Dressings

VAC dressings are widely used for the management of soft tissue defect with or without infection. The perceived advantages are increasing vascularity, decreasing defect size, sterility and decreasing dead-space. Early results in the military environment have been encouraging, but it too early to define its role. Similarly novel wound dressings, such as silver are also being assessed, and may have a role.

### 34.3.7
### Use of Tourniquets

For wounds of the forearm, hands, and feet a pneumatic tourniquet should be used if possible (Fig. 34.8). Home made or non-pneumatic devices (such as the CAT or other pre-hospital tourniquets) should not be used due to the inability to control the pressure and possible local tissue damage. A pressure of approximately 250–300 mmHg should be used and the tourniquet should not be inflated for longer than 90 min.

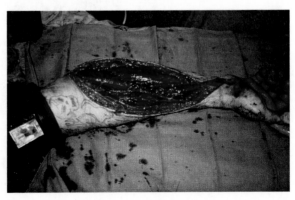

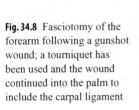

**Fig. 34.8** Fasciotomy of the forearm following a gunshot wound; a tourniquet has been used and the wound continued into the palm to include the carpal ligament

## 34.3.8
## Extent of Bony Injury

Bone is less elastic than skin and muscle. This rigidity produces a greater resistance and results in greater energy transfer, and commonly bone fracture is a sequel to ballistic injury. In addition to the soft tissue injury, instability of the limb may occur, requiring stabilization of the fracture site.

Fractures can be divided into complete or incomplete, depending on whether some continuity of the bone is maintained.

Complete fractures further can be divided into:

- Simple – when only two main fragments are present (Fig. 34.9).
- Comminuted – when multiple fragments are present (Fig. 34.10).

Incomplete fractures can also be subdivided into:

- Drill hole type – when a channel is created through the bone (Fig. 34.11).
- Divot or chip type – when part of the cortex is removed, but no channel exists (Fig. 34.12).

High-energy weapons such as military or hunting rifles usually result in complete fractures, which are often comminuted (multifragmentary). Low-energy weapons, such as handguns, often result in incomplete fractures and even when complete, are not usually

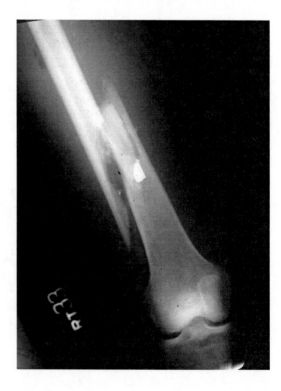

**Fig. 34.9** Complete simple fracture

**Fig. 34.10** Complete multifragmentary fracture

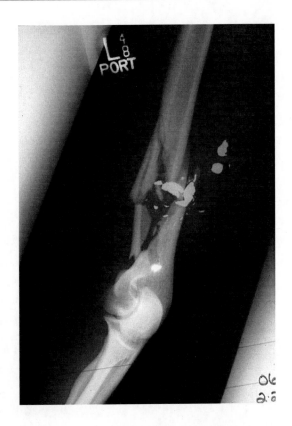

**Fig. 34.11** Incomplete drillhole fracture of the elbow; the channel and bullet communicated with the joint and had to be removed

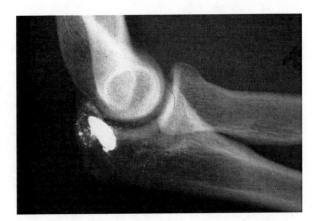

multifragmentary. High-energy wounds are also more likely to have greater contamination and it these unstable, highly contaminated injuries that have to managed appropriately.

Newer mechanisms such as the IEDs can result in significant injuries, often involving several bones (Fig. 34.13).

**Fig. 34.12** Incomplete divot fracture; the bullet "bounced off" the upper cervical vertebrae and passed further down the neck – no major structure was damaged and the patient survived

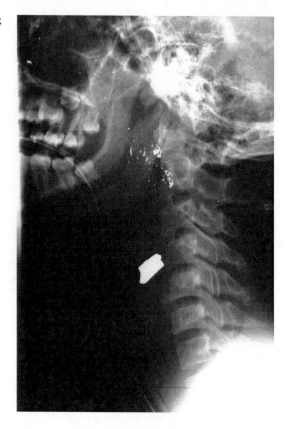

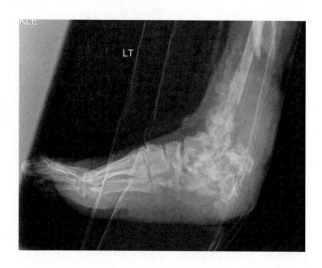

**Fig. 34.13** Radiograph of complex fracture following explosion

## 34.3.9
## Stabilization of the Fracture

The majority of fractures, and all extensive soft tissue wounds should be splinted. Stabilization of fractures provides pain relief, and helps to prevent further bone and soft tissue injury. Stabilization, with the fracture reduced, allows functional use of the limb and this of particular concern during war, as it may allow casualties to help to care for themselves. Despite debates on the pros and cons of the various methods of splinting, adequate local surgery is more important than the method of stabilization.

## 34.3.9.1
## Plaster

Plaster was originally developed for use on the battlefield, and remains the best method of splinting limb injuries. Little additional equipment is required, and personnel can be readily trained in its use. Although plaster is often considered inadequate for extensive wounds, the technique of encasing the wound in plaster and allowing the wound to heal on its own was used extensively during the Spanish Civil War, with a good outcome reported. In addition plaster can be combined with other external splints and has been used to facilitate evacuation of casualties with fractures of the femur (see below).

Plaster backslabs should be used, and these can be supplemented with lateral slabs when used in the lower limb, particularly with the knee and ankle joints. In the acute situation, or after initial debridement, plaster must not be allowed to encircle the limb. If cylinders are used they must be split down to skin along their complete length. Tight dressings are one of the commonest causes of severe post-operative pain and this must be avoided, particularly as patients may undergo prolonged evacuation with limited medical care available.

The disadvantages of plaster are its inability to control movement at the fracture site, and shortening and malunion are common with multifragmentary fractures. This would be a particular problem with high-energy wounds, but plaster is certainly suitable for low-energy wounds. Difficulty of access to the wounds can also be a problem with the use of plaster.

## 34.3.9.2
## Other External Splints

The Thomas splint has been used in the management of patients with ballistic fractures of the femur since the First World War. With the increased use of intramedullary nailing of civilian femoral fractures, its use has diminished. It remains a useful method of stabilizing fractures in the military environment, either alone or in combination with plaster, and can be used in the definitive management of military fractures. The disadvantages of the Thomas splint are related to the prolonged immobilization necessary, and the difficulty with access to wounds.

Other splints are available, including malleable wire and inflatable devices, but their main role is the short-term stabilization of fractures treated in civilian hospitals.

### 34.3.9.3
### Traction

Prior to the advances in both internal and external fixation, traction was used widely to control fractures that were difficult to manage in plaster, particularly unstable or open fractures. It still has a place in the management of fractures when limited resources are available, and has been used extensively by the Red Cross. However, it is less than ideal when rapid, prolonged, or repeated evacuation is necessary. To obtain good results experience in the use of traction, and regular adjustments may be required, and this may be difficult to achieve in the military environment. It does, however, have potential in both the initial, and the definitive treatment of ballistic fractures.

### 34.3.9.4
### Internal Fixation

#### *Plates*

The advantages of internal fixation with plates and/or screws are the accurate reduction, and rigid fixation that can be achieved. However, internal fixation of ballistic fractures can be technically demanding and has been associated with a high infection rate. Delayed internal fixation has been shown to have a lower complication rate than acute plating, however, despite this, the complication rate of both infection and delayed healing is still high. With the other advances that have been made, internal fixation probably has little place in the acute management of most ballistic fractures, especially the lower limb. Plate fixation of upper limb fractures has been used for civilian injuries, and is suitable particularly when the fracture is near a joint (Fig. 34.14).

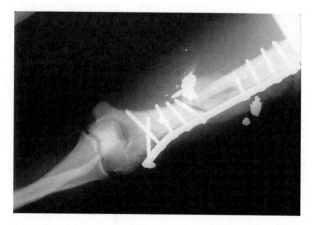

**Fig. 34.14** Ballistic fracture of the humerus (as shown in Fig. 34.9) stabilized by internal fixation with a plate; the fragments of the bullet did not need to be removed

### 34.3.9.5
### Intramedullary Fixation

Intramedullary (IM) fixation with a nail is currently considered to be the method of choice for the stabilization of open tibial and femoral fractures in the civilian environment. The advantages of IM nailing are the high rates of healing for both wound and fracture. No additional splints are necessary, and this allows full access to the wound for inspection, dressings, or plastic surgical procedures.

Its main disadvantage is that the operation is technically very demanding. It requires even more equipment than plating, including image intensification, making it relatively unsuitable for use in most military facilities. However, as a conflict matures, and stable base hospitals are established, such as the current situation in Iraq and Afghanistan IM nailing becomes a very useful technique, however, time may tell if the secondary infection rate is prohibitively high.

In a report from the Vietnam War, the results of open fractures that required a vascular repair were discussed, and the method of stabilization of the fracture analyzed. It was reported that when IM nailing was used, 50% of the nails required removal for complications directly related to the implant. The most common complication was infection, and the authors concluded that, in the military environment, external splints with the use of transfixion pins was a safer option for the stabilization of fractures associated with vascular injuries. The possible reasons for the high infection rate are discussed above. In the civilian environment, particularly in the United States, IM nailing is used extensively in the treatment of ballistic long bone fractures (Fig. 34.15) but these are low-energy, minimally contaminated fractures are usually treated within 6 h of wounding.

### 34.3.9.6
### External Fixation

External fixation (Fig. 34.16), together with plaster, is one of the main methods of stabilizing military ballistic fractures. Indications for external fixation rather than plaster include:

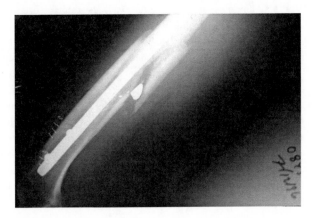

**Fig. 34.15** Ballistic fracture of the femur (as shown in Fig. 34.8) stabilized by internal fixation with an IM nail; the fragments of the bullet did not need to be removed

**Fig. 34.16** Ballistic fracture of the elbow stabilized by a bridging external fixation

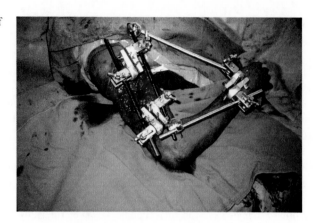

- Extensive bone loss
- Large soft tissue wounds
- Vascular injuries that require repair
- Fractures in association with burns
- Multiple injuries
- Facilitate casualty evacuation

External fixators are often considered easy to apply, but for ballistic injuries, they may be technically difficult to apply well due to the multifragmentary nature of many of the fractures, and will be associated with a high complication rate.

### Technique of External Fixation

If possible, pins should be inserted into the subcutaneous surface of a bone. Although the pins can be inserted through "stab" incisions, these should be at least 1 cm in length. One of the complications of external fixation is damage to adjacent structures, and larger incisions should be used, if necessary, to ensure safe insertion of pins. Open insertion should be used for distal humeral and distal radial pins.

It may be advisable to apply an external fixator before a fasciotomy is carried out to avoid compromising skin incision or closure options.

Bicortical pin placement, where the pin passes through the medullary canal, prior to penetrating the far cortex, must be ensured. With many fixators, predrilling is essential, however, with the British military pattern fixators, the pins have been designed to be self-drilling and self-tapping.

Ideally all pins should be connected to the same bar. This can be achieved by inserting the most proximal and distal pins first. These are connected to a single bar and the fracture reduced as accurately as possible. Further pins can than be inserted by connecting pin-to-bar connectors to the bar and using these as guides for further pin insertion. In most circumstances a second bar should also be used to increase the stability of the frame. Following fracture reduction, the skin wounds should again be checked, and any tenting of the skin released.

Inserting pins in the proximal and distal fragment and then reducing the fracture may result in tenting of the skin and compromise the result, and so the fracture should be reduced before the pins are inserted.

## 34.4
## Specific Injuries

### 34.4.1
### Upper Limb

#### 34.4.1.1
#### Upper Arm

This has two compartments, the flexor, containing the biceps and related muscles, and extensor containing the triceps. Both can be decompressed by longitudinal incisions, which may be possible through the wound.

If exposure of the vessels is also required, the incision can be placed medially. A lateral incision can be used to avoid exposing the artery, but if external fixation is also required, closure of a lateral wound may be compromised.

Extensive soft-tissue wounds and all fractures of the humerus must be splinted, usually with the elbow at 90°. Plaster is ideal, but simple splints, particularly when worn under the clothes are also very effective. Following debridement plaster should be used for the majority of fractures, avoiding external fixation unless there are specific indications.

If external fixation is considered necessary:

- Pins should not be inserted into the proximal humerus; there is a poor hold and significant risk of neurovascular damage.
- There is no proven benefit of bridging the shoulder joint with pins in the clavicle or scapula, compared with leaving the proximal humerus un-splinted, and there are significant risks with scapula or clavicle pins and the large lever arm that results.
- In the shaft they should be inserted through the lateral aspect of the bone, with particular care to avoid the anteromedial neurovascular bundle.
- Distal pins should also be inserted laterally, but under direct vision, through an open incision, to avoid the radial nerve.

For distal fractures, or severe soft tissue injuries around the elbow joint, a bridging fixator, with pins inserted into the distal humerus and ulna shaft should be considered (see Fig. 34.16). With low-energy wounds, particularly in the civilian environment, internal fixation with plates (see Fig. 34.14) or even an IM nail may be considered.

If the initial treatment is with external fixation, later conversion to internal fixation may be considered, although continuing with plaster or external fixation may be appropriate. Early bone grafting should be considered for fractures with bone loss.

The current UK experience would support the use of splints and plaster in the initial stabilization of these injuries followed by internal fixation with plate and screws following evacuation to the base hospital.

### 34.4.1.2
### Forearm

Surgical debridement of the forearm should be carried out with care due to the close proximity of neurovascular structures, but excision of all non-viable tissue must be carried out.

Although the forearm also has a flexor and extensor compartment, release of individual muscle may be required at the time of fasciotomy. If fasciotomy is required, consideration should also be given to releasing the carpal tunnel.

Both soft tissue and bony injuries can be splinted with plaster, which should include the wrist and, for proximal injuries, the elbow.

Definitive stabilization with plates may be considered for civilian injuries, or as a secondary procedure at a base hospital for military injuries. External fixation will rarely be required in the civilian environment due to the availability and safety of internal fixation techniques. Even in the military environment it will seldom be utilized as vascular injuries in the forearm are unlikely to be repaired at a forward surgical facility, and for severe soft tissue and bony injuries, primary amputation may be required.

If required, pins should be inserted through the subcutaneous border of the ulna and only the distal radius should be considered for pin placement, and then only using an open technique.

However, having said that there is such a wide spectrum of injuries that each case should be considered on an individual basis (Fig. 34.17). Internal fixation is probably the best method of definitive stabilization following evacuation to a base hospital.

### 34.4.1.3
### Hand

Ballistic injuries to the hands can be complex and the cause of significant morbidity. Adequate conditions are essential, appropriate anesthesia, good light, tourniquet, and experience. All injuries must be fully assessed, and many require exploration under an anesthetic. Although this is not life-saving surgery, it should be carried early to optimize functional recovery. Skin excision should be kept to the minimum and extensive debridement is usually not necessary. In particular skin flaps should be preserved even if they appear degloved; they may be required for wound closure.

Compartment syndrome of the hand is rare except for crush injuries. The techniques of release are not within the scope of this chapter and with the possible exception of carpal tunnel release should only be carried out by surgeons with experience in hand trauma.

All injuries should be splinted by plaster; with the wrist slightly extended, the MCP joints at 90° and the interphalangeal joints extended. The hand *must* be elevated in a sling to reduce swelling, and the tips of the fingers should be visible.

Early expert input must be obtained.

**Fig. 34.17** Complex segmental forearm fracture

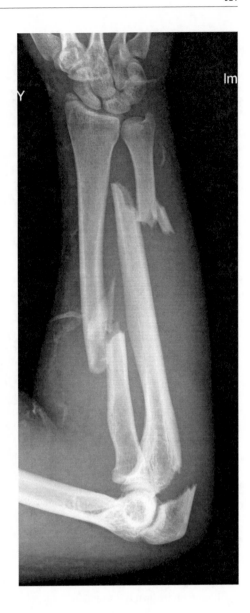

## 34.4.2
## Lower Limb

### 34.4.2.1
### Thigh

Casualties with extensive thigh wounds will have lost a considerable amount of blood, particularly if associated with a fracture. Although these patients may appear to be stable initially, they may deteriorate, particularly if there were delays in evacuation. All patients must be adequately assessed and resuscitated as appropriate (Fig. 34.18).

**Fig. 34.18** Gunshot wound to
the femur; despite a small
entrance wound the patient
was profoundly shocked and
there was an extensive
soft-tissue, bone, and vascular
injury

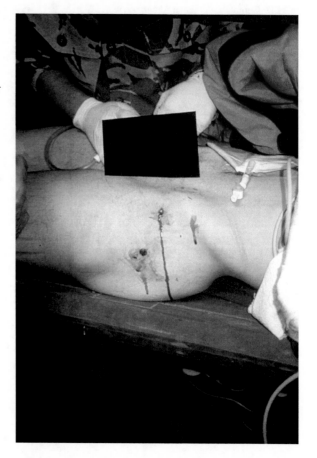

The thigh contains three compartments, flexor, extensor, and a medial adductor compartment. In civilian practice release of anterior and posterior compartments, through a single lateral incision, may be sufficient, but penetrating injuries to the thigh may require release of the medial compartment, particularly when associated with a vascular injury. This will require a separate incision.

Extensive soft tissue wounds and fractures of the femur should be managed by splinting. Plaster on its own is unsuitable, but can be used in combination with a Thomas splint, also known as a Tobruk splint.

External fixation should be avoided unless there are specific indications. Although it is a satisfactory method of stabilizing femoral fractures (providing sufficient bone is present both proximally and distally), there is a high complication rate due to the amount of soft-tissue that must be traversed by the fixator pin. Movement at the soft-tissue/pin interface is associated with increase in fluid and consequently infection which, in time, contaminates the medullary cavity.

Three good pins must be inserted into each segment, and at least two and preferably 3–4 bars should be used to connect the pins. The pins can be inserted through the anterior, lateral, or postero-lateral surface of the bone, but pins above the lesser trochanter or below the flare of the distal femur should be avoided.

The initial stabilization of proximal fractures is controversial. Bridging external fixation is commonly carried out, but there is a significant risk with pins in the pelvis due to the relatively poor hold and the long lever arm. In addition transport and nursing may be compromised; it may be better to use skeletal traction initially, which shouldn't compromise later reconstruction.

Injuries around the knee can also be immobilized in a Thomas splint, but plaster is also effective. For extensive injuries bridging external fixation, with pins in the distal femur and proximal tibia, can be very effective.

For civilian low-energy injuries IM nailing has been widely used with low complication rates. It is likely that an IM nail is the method of choice for definitive stabilization of military fractures, following evacuation to a base hospital, but longer term follow-up of recent casualties from Iraq and Afghanistan is required to confirm this.

### 34.4.2.2
### Lower Leg

This is the most common site of injury during war and is frequently seen in civilian practice. The prognosis for open fractures of the tibia is worse than that of other long bones and, therefore, adequate local treatment of these injuries must be carried out as soon as practicable.

There are four compartments anterior and lateral, and superficial and deep posterior compartments. Failure to release the deep posterior compartment is the most common error in lower limb fasciotomy, and occurs when releasing the soleus muscle from the posterior aspect of the tibia is mistaken for releasing the compartment. The posterior tibial artery is located between the two posterior compartments, and this can be used as a landmark during surgery. A two incision technique should be used in the lower limb, decompressing the posterior compartments through an incision just posterior to the medial border of the tibia. An incision too posterior will damage the perforators and may compromise soft tissue closure.

The anterior and lateral compartments can be decompressed through an incision between the lateral border of the tibia and the fibula.

Plaster provides sufficient stabilization for many fractures, although external fixation is commonly required, particularly for gunshot or explosive injuries.

Pins should be inserted into the subcutaneous surface of the bone. Care should be taken to ensure bicortical placement due to the triangular shape of the tibia.

The method of secondary stabilization following initial external fixation is still unclear. Previous conversion to an IM nail was considered the method of choice, but this has been associated with high infection rates, probably related to the injury itself rather than the technique. It may be more appropriate to continue with external fixation, probably with conversion to a hybrid or multi-planar device.

### 34.4.2.3
### Foot Injuries

Although these are not life-threatening, but should never be dismissed as minor injuries. Significant injuries can occur (Fig. 34.19) and inadequate management will cause later morbidity and functional limitations.

The principles of management remain the same, but stabilization of severe foot injuries can be difficult. Plaster is inadequate for severe injuries, except in the short term and external fixation or wire fixation should be considered (see Fig. 34.19).

External fixator pins can be inserted into the tibial shaft, a transfixion pin can be inserted through the calcaneus, and pins inserted into the great toe metatarsal and the fifth toe metatarsal. This triangulation frame as well as stabilizing fractures, maintains the foot at 90° to

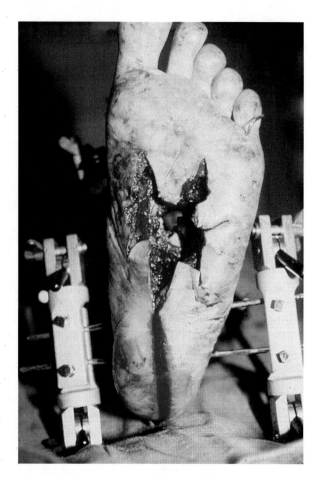

**Fig. 34.19** High-energy gunshot wound to the foot with significant soft-tissue and bony damage; extensive local surgery with external fixation was necessary to avoid amputation

the leg, preventing an equinus deformity, which can be a cause of significant later morbidity.

As with hand injuries the foot must be elevated to reduce swelling.

The later management of severe foot injuries is not within the scope of this chapter. Flap coverage may be required as may bone grafting, local fusions, and partial amputations. In addition the severe injuries from IEDs are a cause of significant morbidity and late amputation.

## 34.5
## Miscellaneous Issues

### 34.5.1
### Radiographs

Plain radiographs should be obtained for all ballistic limb injuries in the civilian environment, and although not essential in the management of military limbs, are very useful. With direct, high-energy fractures endosteal spread is universal, and the spread of infection is more extensive than with indirect fractures. As the fracture pattern is different, the extent of contamination can be estimated on radiographs prior to debridement. In addition, the extent of the fracture can be assessed, and this may determine the technique of stabilization. External fixator pins should not be inserted within 2–3 cm of a fracture. Not only is there a risk of propagating cracks from the fracture site but also this region will be contaminated, predisposing to a pin tract infection.

The extent of the bony injury is also a reflection of the energy transfer and can give an indication of prognosis. The initial radiograph may be helpful in determining the need for amputation (see Fig. 34.13).

If used, however, radiography must not be allowed to delay the management of patients, particularly in a mass casualty situation.

### 34.5.2
### Retained Fragments

Many bullet wounds will be associated with an entrance and exit wound, and the issue of retained fragments will not arise. Most of the remaining fragments will be removed at the time of initial debridement, but some will be left behind, and are often diagnosed on later radiographs.

Retained metal fragments can usually be left, with only a small risk of subsequent infection. If the wound does develop an infection, secondary surgery will often be required, and the fragments can be removed at this stage. Consideration must be given, however, to the removal of retained bullets.

Civilian data suggests that intra-articular and intra-bursal bullets should be removed due to the risk of lead arthropathy. This can, however, be delayed, and arthroscopic techniques can be used.

Bullets retained in soft tissues including muscle can be observed, and the current evidence would also suggest that bullets retained in bone can also be treated conservatively (see Figs. 34.14 and 34.15).

### 34.5.3
### Non-operative Management of Ballistic Fractures

Whilst it is true that in certain circumstances low-energy missile wounds involving bone can be treated non-operatively, much of the data derives from American trauma centers. As discussed above there are significant differences between civilian wounds, and those seen during military conflicts and the infection rate with military wounds is higher than with civilian wounds. However, a recent study of extremity trauma due to hunting rifle wounds demonstrated a similarly high rate of infection.

### 34.5.4
### Secondary Management of the Fracture

*Initial treatment in plaster* – For fractures treated by plaster, if a satisfactory position is confirmed on subsequent radiographs, plaster can be used as the definitive treatment. If any delay in healing occurs, early bone grafting with or without appropriate internal fixation should probably be carried out.

*Initial treatment by external fixation* – For the more complex injuries an external fixator may have been applied. However the short-term outcome is often poor and long term outcome of external fixation in the treatment of military fractures is not known, and complications do occur with the civilian use of external fixators. Many of the problems associated with external fixation are due to the prolonged use of a uniplanar frame, and it is possible that initial external fixation should be used followed by conversion to a different method of stabilization at a later date, when better facilities are available.

*Fractures with joint involvement* – If the fracture involves a joint surface, and the fragments are displaced, plaster, external fixation, and IM nailing are not suitable methods of definitive treatment. If reconstruction is possible and suitable facilities are available, early fixation with screws and/or plates should be carried out. If reconstruction of the joint is not possible, the position should be accepted and early mobilization carried out. Fusion of the joint is an alternative for some joints, particularly the ankle and wrist but should be avoided at the hip and knee, and particularly the elbow if possible.

### 34.5.5
### Red Cross Wound Classification

The International Committee of the Red Cross (ICRC) has developed a scoring system to allow the classification of military wounds. This classification was designed, not only to permit wound assessment, but also to allow surgical audit, and to attempt to determine the relationship of war wounds to experimental ballistic injuries. The grading is based on the size of both entry and exit wounds, as well as the presence of a fracture, cavity, metallic fragments, or damage to a vital structure. This allows a grading and subtyping of wounds and can be used to help in the treatment as well as an outcome measure it has been validated in several studies. Further information can be found in specific ICRC publications. Unfortunately, the usefulness of fracture classifications, in guiding the operating surgeon, has been questioned and consequently decision making is based on the surgeons judgement.

## Further Reading

Clasper J. The interaction of projectiles with tissues and the management of ballistic fractures. *J R Army Med Corps*. 2001;147(1):52-61.

Clasper J. Amputations of the lower limb: a multidisciplinary consensus. *J R Army Med Corps*. 2007;153(3):172-174.

Coupland RM. Technical aspects of war wound excision. *Br J Surg*. 1989;76(7):663-667.

Coupland RM. The Red cross classification of war wounds: the E.X.C.F.V.M. scoring system. *World J Surg*. 1992;16(5):910-917.

Rich NM, Metz CW Jr, Hutton JE Jr, Baugh JH, Hughes CW. Internal versus external fixation of fractures with concomitant vascular injuries in Vietnam. *J Trauma*. 1971;11(6):463-473.

Trueta J MD. The classic: the treatment of war fractures by the closed method. *Clin Orthop Relat Res*. 1981;156:8-15.

# Ballistic Trauma in Children

**35**

Graeme Pitcher

## 35.1
## Epidemiological Background

The natural inquisitiveness and vulnerability of early life predispose children to penetrating injury; varying in severity from a minor laceration or foreign body penetration to life-threatening impalement, stab wound, or missile injury. Ballistic injuries, defined as injuries caused by thrown or projected missiles, comprise an important proportion of pediatric penetrating injury. Penetrating injuries are responsible for approximately 15% of pediatric trauma deaths in developed countries.[1] Injury patterns differ widely between different communities, socioeconomic groups, cities, countries, and cultures. Such injuries are also more common during times of revolution or sociopolitical change.

Missile injuries may be intentional (homicidal or suicidal intent) or unintentional. In younger children, most are unintentional or homicidal. Suicidal attempts are confined mainly to adolescence. In developed countries, most children are injured unintentionally, occurring as a result of the child playing with the firearm or during firearm sports. These injuries appear to be declining in incidence, but they are still a prominent cause of death in the pediatric population.[2] In 1988, gunshot wounds were the eighth leading cause of unintentional injury deaths among persons in all age groups in the United States, and the third leading cause of such deaths among children and teenagers aged 10–19 years.[3] This underscores the importance of educating gun owners in the safe use and storage of their weapons, as this has been shown to be a contributory factor in the decline of this type of injury.[4]

The incidence of serious penetrating injuries, and of gunshot wounds in particular, seems to be on the increase worldwide.[5-7] The incidence of pediatric gunshot injuries varies according to the number and availability of firearms in the community, with the United States having the greatest incidence amongst developed countries.[8,9] Homicide and suicide in pediatric age groups appears to be increasing in incidence in most countries worldwide.

G. Pitcher
General Surgery Department, Division of Pediatric Surgery,
University of Iowa Hospitals and Clinics, 200 Hawkins Drive, Iowa, IA, USA
e-mail: graeme-pitcher@uiowa.edu

A.J. Brooks et al. (eds.), *Ryan's Ballistic Trauma*,
DOI: 10.1007/978-1-84882-124-8_35, © Springer-Verlag London Limited 2011

From 1950 through 1993, the overall annual death rate for US children aged less than 15 years declined substantially, primarily reflecting decreases in deaths associated with unintentional injuries, pneumonia, influenza, cancer, and congenital anomalies. However, during the same period, childhood homicide rates tripled and suicide rates quadrupled. In 1994, among children aged 1–4 years, homicide was the fourth leading cause of death; among children aged 5–14 years, homicide was the third leading cause of death, and suicide was the sixth.[6] In America, the factors that have been identified with increased risk of intentional injury include: urban resident, age group 10–16 years, male gender, lower socioeconomic group, poor family support systems, and African-American race.[10,11] In male adolescents, gang activities with alcohol and drug abuse account for the bulk of injuries in many cities.[2,12] The emergence in the last few decades of the phenomenon known as "family murders" – where an adult member of the family, usually the father executes the entire family and then commits suicide – has perhaps also contributed to this disturbing trend. In general, the perpetrator of firearm injuries in young children tends to be an adult, whereas in adolescents, peers are usually responsible. Overall, the child's status as a protected and cherished member of the community appears to be increasingly threatened.

In developing countries, particularly in times of social instability and change, children too young to be able to participate in crime and violence are frequently shot as innocent bystanders or in retaliation for the perpetrator's grudge against a parent. These patients often suffer severe injuries, and almost inevitably, there is a delay in reaching the hospital, with resultant high mortality rate and significant long-term major morbidity.[13]

In Cape Town, South Africa, homicide is the single leading cause of non-natural death in the under-19 age group.[12] An exponentially increasing incidence of childhood gunshot wounds over the last 20 years has been reported from another South African province – KwaZulu-Natal. The mean age of pediatric gunshot victims in that province is 6.4 years. Experience here also shows that for every child admitted to hospital with a gunshot wound, four were delivered to police mortuaries in the province during the same period. This statistic underscores the wounding and killing potential of modern weapons when used against children.

It is abundantly clear that urgent preventative measures are required in all communities to protect children from this senseless litany of violence.

## 35.2
## Weapons and Patterns of Penetrating Injury

Ballistic weapons are designed to inflict bodily damage to adult victims. The severity of injury sustained by the pediatric victim is therefore not unexpectedly much higher. This is particularly true for the soft and vulnerable tissues of the neonate and infant. In addition, the bony skeleton is incompletely mineralized, providing less resistance to the passage of missiles. A positive effect of this is that injury due to secondary bony missiles is rarely seen. Anecdotal experience on the effect of high-velocity military weapons such as rifles, grenades, and fragments, on children is that these weapons have extraordinary wounding and killing potential in the young child. During times of war, these injuries are particularly devastating and have a high mortality, particularly in young children. The tragedy of large populations of amputees, many of whom are children, in countries such as Angola and Mozambique is well known. They are the victims of antipersonnel mines laid in times of civil conflict. Some areas still have a multitude of unexploded mines lying in wait for innocent civilian victims. These weapons usually are designed to maim an adult soldier, but not necessarily to kill. Their effect on a young child is devastating and often fatal – for every amputee consigned to a life of disability in these under-resourced countries, there are many unpublicized fatalities.

In peacetime, children are often injured by air-powered missiles such as air rifle pellets. The wounding potential of these has become apparent. They frequently are responsible for injuries to the globe of the eye and have been documented to cause body cavity penetration, head injury, major vascular injury, and death. A significant number of patients experience long-term morbidity.[14-16] The ability of these weapons to inflict serious injury should not be overlooked. In the urban environment, especially in high-risk areas, children are usually injured by handguns. Shotgun wounds are not infrequently seen in both urban and rural areas. They are associated with high mortality rates.[17] High-velocity rifle injuries are uncommon, usually occurring in rural areas and usually as a result of hunting accidents. Children are frequently injured by arrows, crossbow bolts, darts, marine spearguns, and a miscellany of other penetrating missiles due to their intrinsic inquisitiveness and desire to experiment. Home-made bombs are well known to cause bizarre missile injuries, as well as thermal and chemical burns.

## 35.2.1
### Prehospital Care and Resuscitation

Much debate still continues regarding the optimum approach to the prehospital care of trauma victims. Proponents of the "scoop and run" approach maintain that prolonged efforts at on-scene treatment only delays the arrival of the patient at the definitive care establishment and are deleterious, particularly in the patient with penetrating thoracic injury.[18] Most formal studies evaluating the efficiency of pediatric prehospital care have contained an overwhelming majority of blunt trauma victims.[19] Major penetrating injury in early life is frequently associated with hypovolemia and severe instability. It is precisely this group of patients who require rapid definitive surgical hemostasis for a successful outcome. On-scene fluid resuscitation has never been shown to be of value in this group of patients, and may indeed be detrimental. Venous access by any technique other than intraosseous puncture is difficult and likely to delay hospital transfer. In most areas, experience shows that effective prehospital care of children is only provided by personnel with advanced training who have the opportunity to regularly practice and update their skills. In many developed countries, prehospital personnel attend to severely injured children infrequently so that the individual practitioner has difficulty developing the necessary experience.[20]

In the case of the child with life-threatening penetrating injury, the prehospital staff should be able to provide airway interventions, effectively control external hemorrhage, establish venous access (with the use of intraosseous infusion if necessary), initiate *appropriate* fluid resuscitation, and rapidly transfer the patient safely to an appropriate "child capable" institution. The on-scene time should not exceed 10 min. If the above cannot be achieved for whatever reason, a "scoop and run" approach will probably ensure a better outcome, particularly if the transport time to a surgical facility is short.

The concept of delayed or hypotensive resuscitation for adult patients with penetrating truncal trauma is currently being investigated. In patients with ongoing blood loss requiring surgical hemostasis (e.g., major vascular injuries), the endpoints of resuscitation are not clear. It has been suggested recently that minimal volume resuscitation prior to surgical hemostasis in adults with penetrating abdominal trauma or ruptured abdominal aortic aneurysms may be beneficial.[21-24] It appears as if prolonged fluid resuscitation to attempt to produce hamodynamic normality – particularly if this resuscitation delays definitive surgical repair – is deleterious to the patient and is associated with a greater incidence of coagulopathy, hypothermia, and a poorer outcome. This approach may be unsuitable to blunt trauma patients with head injury, as it may decrease critical cerebral perfusion during the period of delay; conventional endpoint resuscitation is currently recommended in this group.[25] Prospective trials researching minimal volume resuscitation in the pediatric trauma population need to be done before any firm conclusion can be reached. In the patient with ongoing massive bleeding (without head injury) where it is clear that surgery will be required for hemostasis, resuscitation should probably be of *minimal duration*, with a goal of ensuring adequate venous access and the administration of sufficient fluid or blood to ensure adequate end organ perfusion. This patient should be transferred to the operating room without delay, where definitive hemostasis and further resuscitation can occur concurrently.

## 35.3
## Ballistic Head Injury

This is fortunately a rare injury in childhood. The prehospital mortality of cranial gunshot wounds in children is high. Pellet penetrations occur more commonly, and even these have been associated with fatal outcomes. Resuscitation of the severe cases should proceed along normal lines and often will include endotracheal intubation and ventilation. In the young baby with a compliant skull, life-threatening hypovolemia can ensue from intracranial bleeding. Vigorous arterial bleeding from injuries at the base of the skull often portends a poor prognosis.

After stabilization, all cases should be investigated by an emergency cranial computed tomography (CT) scan (Fig. 35.1). This will provide important prognostic information and guide surgical intervention. Cranial arteriography is used less frequently today and is usually reserved for specific circumstances when deemed necessary by the attending neurosurgeon. Examples include deep-seated hematomas, traumatic arteriovenous fistulae or false aneurysms, and prior to the removal of retained blades or large missiles.

Children are uniquely susceptible to raised intracranial pressure caused by progressive cerebral edema with blunt injury. The role of intracranial pressure monitoring is well

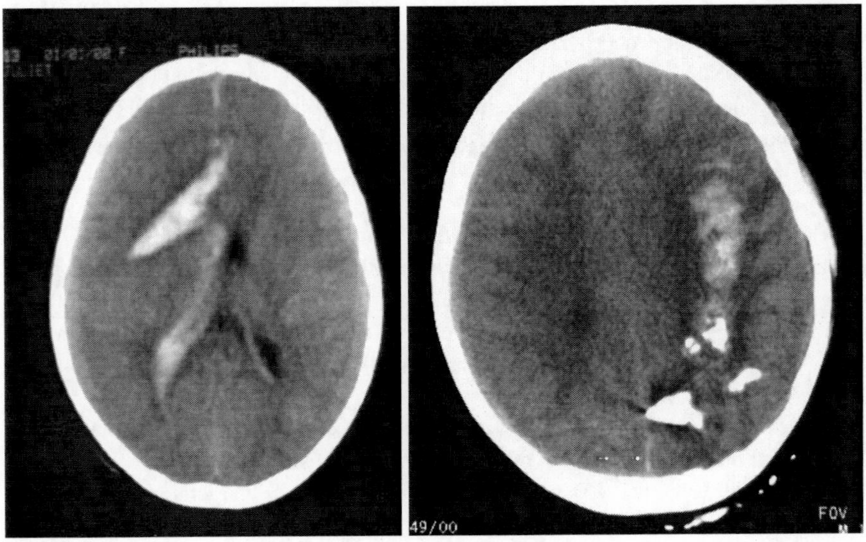

**Fig. 35.1** *Left*: A CT scan showing a linear intracerebral hemorrhage with intraventricular hemorrhage after an assault with a broad bladed knife (panga). *Right*: the bullet tract created by a 9 mm bullet traversing the left cerebral hemisphere of a 3-year-old boy who was the victim of a family murder

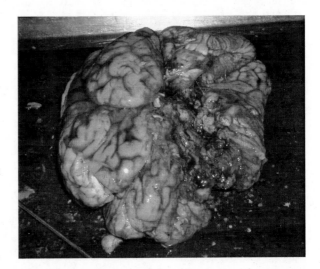

**Fig. 35.2** Autopsy findings in five-year-old sibling of patient B in Fig. 19.1 showing massive damage to the frontal and temporal lobes after passage of a 9 mm missile

established in this situation, although its impact on survival remains unproven. Transhemispheric wounds commonly cause massive brain destruction, especially in young children, often causing death (Fig. 35.2). In survivors, cerebral edema can occur and appears to be more frequently seen with higher-velocity missile injuries. It is currently recommended that intracranial pressure transducers be used whenever cerebral edema requires active treatment.[26] The development of posttraumatic hydrocephalus, although rare, should always be sought in the recovery period. Prophylactic antibiotics are used universally and should be of a broad spectrum. Anticonvulsant medication should be used to treat convulsions, but there is little evidence for their use prophylactically beyond the second week post injury. Specifically, they have not been shown to reduce the risk of post-injury epilepsy in the long term.

The surgical management of penetrating brain injury is controversial. In many instances the first decision to be taken is whether the patient's prospects for meaningful neurological recovery warrant aggressive surgery. Some patients with a poor neurological prognosis after thorough assessment are best treated by minimal local wound care. Generally accepted factors associated with a poor prognosis are presented in Table 35.1.

For civilian injuries, there is a tendency towards less-aggressive debridement without an apparent increase in infective complications. The decision to operate is best left to the attending neurosurgeon. Most will operate for significant intracranial hematomata, severely depressed skull fractures, and large open wounds with brain and dura exposed. The principles of wound debridement and cleaning, dural closure, and primary or flap closure are usually adhered to. For children with small penetrating wounds without severe tissue destruction, simple closure appears adequate. Prophylactic broad-spectrum antibiotics should be used. In most instances, no attempt is made to remove bullets during the acute phase, as this can result in worse cerebral edema and can be harmful. Bullets causing symptoms or seizures can be removed later as the clinical situation demands it.

**Table 35.1** Poor prognostic factors in patients with cranial gunshot wounds

| Type of variable | Variable |
| --- | --- |
| Demographics | Younger age |
| Epidemiology | Suicide attempt<br>Military injury<br>High-caliber and -velocity weapon<br>Perforating (through and through) injury |
| Systemic secondary insults | Hypotension<br>Hypoxia<br>Coagulation abnormalities |
| Neurological assessment | Level of consciousness (GCS 3–5)<br>Fixed dilated or unequal pupils<br>Raised intracranial pressure |
| Imaging features | Missile track through both hemispheres<br>Passage through ventricle<br>Evidence of raised intracranial pressure<br>Hemorrhage or lesion with mass effect |

Modified from Florin RE J Trauma. 2001;51:S44–S86

## 35.4
## Neck Injury

Selective conservatism of cervical stab injury is becoming increasingly more common in adult patients. The safety of this approach has been documented for Zone II stab injuries in children.[27] Its safety for gunshot and other missile injuries has not been satisfactorily ascertained and the clinician should use their discretion tempered with common sense. The proximity of vital structures in the small child's neck rarely permits its safe application in this group. If a conservative approach is adopted, angiography, endoscopy, and contrast esophagography should be used liberally (Fig. 35.3). Angiography is recommended for Zone I and Zone III injuries, including in stable patients where surgery is planned. The need for angiography to assess the vasculature in patients with Zone II injuries being treated conservatively who do not have clinical signs of vascular injury is controversial. The approach should be individualized in each case, bearing in mind the risk of iatrogenic vascular injury that is present in young children and CT angiography may be a safer alternative. Air rifle pellet injuries, even those involving the retropharyngeal space, have successfully been treated conservatively.[28]

Penetrating vascular injuries in the cervical area generally require surgical exploration and repair. Venous injuries are treated by direct repair or ligation, and injuries to the carotid

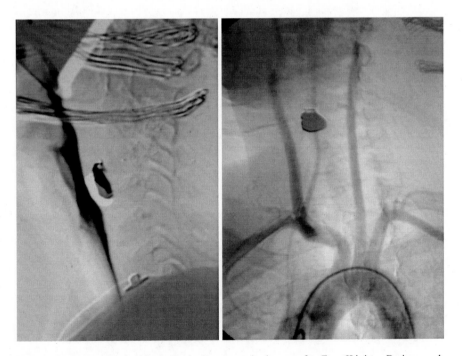

**Fig. 35.3** Ten-year-old boy with a bullet in the prevertebral space after Zone II injury. Barium swallow and angiogram performed as part of nonoperative management

artery complex are treated by repair whenever feasible. Patency rates for arterial repairs and grafts of the internal carotid artery in children under 5 years of age are not good. In stable patients, repair using the operating microscope is an option if the injury lends itself to this. Most young healthy children have adequate vertebrobasilar collateral flow, allowing ligation as a safe, more practical alternative.

Spinal cord injury is not uncommon after gunshot wounds in the neck and torso. In the absence of other indications for cervical exploration, these patients are investigated by magnetic resonance scanning. Usually, direct cord injury is confirmed to be the cause of neurological deficit, but rarely an intraspinal hematoma is shown to be present, which should be decompressed. Unstable cervical bony injuries are rare and usually can be treated in a traction device at this age.

The use of methylprednisone therapy in these injuries is not supported by any evidence and is not recommended.

The recommended incisions for exploration of the child's neck are as follows:

1. Anterior sternomastoid incision as the standard incision, especially where the need for exploration of the vascular structures of Zone I and III is anticipated. This incision affords optimal exposure of the internal carotid artery at the base of the skull and can easily be extended to a median sternotomy for control of mediastinal vascular structures.
2. Transverse collar incision is useful for transverse injuries in Zone II, especially where through-and-through injury exists to the upper trachea, larynx, and pharynx. Most concurrent vascular injuries are easily dealt with through such an incision, but it should be used with caution and is not advised in patients suspected of having vascular injuries of the skull base or root of the neck.

## 35.5
## Thoracic Injury

Penetrating thoracic injuries carry a mortality of approximately 15% in early life and the thoracic injury is directly responsible for the death.[29] The small size of the child and the proximity of organs in the abdomen and chest make thoracoabdominal injuries more common in the younger age groups. High-velocity missile wounds to the chest can be devastating in early life, but these patients rarely reach the hospital alive. With the increasing incidence of pediatric gunshot wounds, the spectrum of injuries seen in childhood mirrors that seen in the adult population.

## 35.5.1
## Technique of Insertion of a Chest Drain

The standard position recommended for intercostal drain placement is the fifth intercostal space in the anterior axillary line. It can be expected that the young child will be

**Table 35.2** Recommended chest drain sizes by age

| Age | Size (Fr) |
|---|---|
| 0–3 months | 10–12 |
| 3–18 months | 12–16 |
| 18–24 months | 18 |
| 2–4 years | 20–22 |
| 4–6 years | 22–24 |
| 6–8 years | 24–28 |
| 8–12 years | 28–30 |
| 12–16 years | 30–34 |

uncooperative with regard to the drain during the recovery period. For this reason, the drain should be well secured by both suture and skin strapping to ensure that the patient does not remove it prematurely. The skin incision should be placed one intercostal space below the intended space of chest entry to ensure a tunneled subcutaneous tract. This facilitates removal of the drain later to allow for direct pressure on the subcutaneous tract, thereby preventing air entering the pleural space and causing iatrogenic pneumothorax in a crying child. The drain should be placed primarily by blunt dissection; trocars are not used to avoid iatrogenic injury. The recommended size of intercostal drains at various ages is shown in Table 35.2.

## 35.5.2
### Special Investigations Required

Every patient should have a chest X-ray in the erect position, if possible. The use of radiopaque markers (Fig. 35.4) on any entrance or exit wounds facilitates interpretation of the films. In the unstable patient with clear signs of thoracic injury, chest decompression should be performed for a suspected tension pneumothorax and a chest drain can be placed without radiological confirmation of the presence of an injury. For stable patients, treatment should be delayed until a chest X-ray can be obtained.

If the chest X-ray or the patient's clinical signs are suggestive of specific organ injury, further investigations may be needed. Sometimes thoracic ultrasonography is helpful to detect small collections of blood in the pleural space. Echocardiography is requested whenever there is a possibility of cardiac injury in a stable patient. Liquid-soluble contrast swallows and esophagoscopy are used to diagnose suspected esophageal injury and bronchosopy is used to diagnose major airway injury.

**Fig. 35.4** Four-year-old male with gunshot wound right lower chest showing use of radiopaque markers

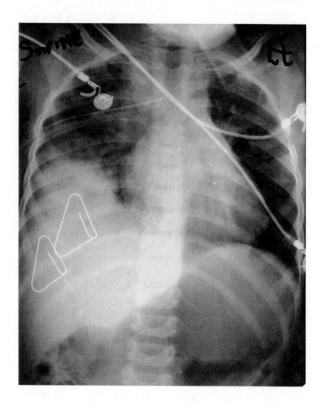

### 35.5.3
### Thoracoscopy

Thoracoscopy is increasingly being used to assess the diaphragm or intrathoracic structures after penetrating injury in children. It should be reserved for those patients without clinical indications for emergency thoracotomy (see below), and only in stable patients. Studies in adult patients have indicated that the use of thoracoscopy may exclude injuries and reduce the need for formal thoracotomy in equivocal cases.[30] It is probably the most efficient modality to assess the diaphragm for injury, which can be easily repaired using a stapling device[31] or intracorporeal suturing. In this situation, there is always the risk of a missed abdominal injury. Either the abdomen can be assessed concurrently by laparoscopy or the thoracoscopy can be used as a screening test, mandating an exploratory laparotomy when a diaphragmatic injury is found. Laparoscopy has its advocates, and in skilled hands is an option for stable patients without a large hemoperitoneum. In most, a laparotomy seems the safest and simplest option.

In our environment, a sterilized fiberoptic gastroscope has been used to assess the integrity of the diaphragm in cases of blunt and penetrating trauma. The intercostal drain is removed and the scope is passed through the drain tract into the chest. This allows any residual hemothorax to be evacuated by suction and the lung can be collapsed by air insufflation and the diaphragm inspected. The procedure is well tolerated and can be performed without general anesthesia in the emergency room.[32]

## 35.5.4
## Indications for Thoracotomy

### 35.5.4.1
### Resuscitative Thoracotomy

The place of emergency department thoracotomy is one of the ongoing controversies in the management of the injured patient. It is probably better termed resuscitative thoracotomy (RT), indicating its role as an adjunct to resuscitation when the patient does not respond to conventional resuscitation. A number of studies have addressed the role of RT in pediatric trauma.[33-36] Previously, children were assumed to have greater physiological reserve and hence RT was applied liberally in an attempt to salvage desperate situations. Cumulative experience to date indicates that RT should be reserved for the following categories of pediatric patients after penetrating trauma:

1. Penetrating thoracic injury with deterioration or poor response despite vigorous resuscitation
2. Patients with penetrating thoracic injury who present with no signs of life to the emergency room but with a recently witnessed cardiac arrest

Under these circumstances, salvage rates of between 4% and 26% can be expected depending on the mechanism of injury and local circumstances.[33-35] Children with penetrating abdominal trauma who do not respond to resuscitation should be transferred immediately to the operating room where the operation and prompt surgical hemostasis can be carried out concurrently with further fluid resuscitation. Results of RT for patients with penetrating abdominal injuries who present without vital signs are so dismal that it cannot be advocated.

## 35.6
## Definitive Thoracotomy

Most (approximately 80%) penetrating thoracic injuries in children can be satisfactorily managed by placement of an intercostal drain alone.[37] Patients with gunshot injuries may require surgery more frequently, especially in the younger age groups.[38,39] Accepted indications for emergency thoracotomy include:

1. Brisk thoracic hemorrhage and ongoing hemodynamic instability or deterioration
2. Evidence of cardiac tamponade or posttraumatic pericardial effusion
3. Evidence of major airway injury
4. Evidence of esophageal injury

Ongoing bleeding requiring blood transfusion of greater than 50% of blood volume or at a rate of greater than 1–2 mL/kg/h may be an indication for thoracotomy depending on the circumstances.

### 35.6.1
### Incisions for Access

Children tolerate all types of incisions for thoracic access better than their adult counterparts. Their inherent good health and cardiopulmonary reserves mean that postoperative ventilation is usually not necessary and intensive care stays are much shorter. Complications related to the wound, pleural fluid collections, and atelectasis occur infrequently, and children can usually be mobilized out of bed as early as the first postoperative day without any difficulty. Pain is easily controlled by a combination of intercostal nerve blocks and opiate analgesia.

The incision used for access to the chest varies depending upon the side of injury and the anticipated surgery required.

## 35.7
## Resuscitative Thoracotomy

Performed by a left anterolateral thoracotomy through the fifth intercostal space. If there is a penetrating injury to the right hemithorax with obvious bleeding from that cavity, then a right anterolateral thoracotomy is preferred. The anterolateral approach gives adequate emergency room access to the heart, aorta, and pulmonary hilum, and can always be extended posteriorly for better definitive access in the operating room.

## 35.8
## Definitive Thoracotomy

Is usually performed through a sixth or seventh intercostal space approach in the posterolateral position.

## 35.9
## Median Sternotomy

In the young child with flexible ribs, the degree of exposure that can de achieved gives excellent access to the heart, major vessels, trachea, both lungs, and pleural cavities. The sternum can quickly and easily be divided by using a pair of Mayo-type scissors in the younger child or osteotomy shears in the older child. Sternotomy is therefore an excellent incision for general access to the child's chest in the trauma situation and should always be used if there is a suspicion of cardiac or major vessel injury, or if the side of the injury is not clinically obvious.

## 35.10
## "Clam Shell" Incision

Extending an anterolateral thoracotomy transversely across the sternum and through the opposite intercostal space (sometimes referred to as a sternothoracotomy) gives excellent exposure to the chest contents, with the possible exception of the mediastinal great vessels. This option can be used in instances where a resuscitative anterolateral thoracotomy suggests an injury such as a cardiac or contralateral pulmonary hilar injury that cannot comfortably be dealt with through the initial incision. This situation is not encountered commonly, but the incision is becoming increasingly popular for elective surgical procedures such as bilateral pulmonary metastasectomy and lung and heart transplantation,[40,41] and it has been used in children and infants for cardiac surgery with good results.[42] Care must be taken when closing the incision to achieve careful approximation of the sternum by using K-wires or stainless steel wires, otherwise unsightly overlapping of the sternum may result.

## 35.11
## Abdominal Injury

No specific distinction is made between high-velocity gunshot wounds and low-velocity injuries sustained typically from handgun injuries except to recognize the devastating wounding potential of the former weapons in small children. High-velocity injuries from weapons such as military assault rifles and hunting rifles are fortunately rare in children, but carry a high mortality, with most patients dying at the scene of injury. Clinical experience is therefore mainly derived from the management of civilian handgun injuries.

In adults, the policy of selective conservative management for penetrating abdominal stab wounds and other low-velocity penetrating injuries is well established.[43] Data documenting the safety of selective conservative treatment strategies for penetrating injuries in children are sparse. This is probably a result of the relative rarity of these injuries and the inability of single centers to compile a sufficient number of cases in order to construct prospective controlled trials. With bullet wounds, fragment injuries, and other high-velocity missiles that penetrate the peritoneal cavity, the chance of visceral injury requiring operative intervention is much greater and exploratory laparotomy is mandatory.

### 35.11.1
### Diagnostic Peritoneal Lavage

Diagnostic peritoneal lavage (DPL) has little role in the assessment of the child with suspected penetrating abdominal injury. It requires a general anesthetic in the conscious child and compromises the clinical assessment of the abdomen by virtue of the associated pain thereafter. Two potential indications for DPL in penetrating injury in children are the assessment of the diaphragm and the assessment of peritoneal penetration. Thoracoscopy and laparoscopy, respectively, are superior in this situation and provide more specific information.

### 35.11.2 Incisions

The infant and young child (up to 3 years of age) has a round abdomen. The transverse supra-umbilical laparotomy incision serves very well as the standard incision for access to the abdomen for non-trauma surgery in this age group. It suffers from two main disadvantages in the trauma situation when the nature of the required surgery is notoriously unpredictable:

1. It does not allow for extensions of the incision in a cranial or caudal direction to gain access to the pelvic area and epigastrium, if required. Exposure of the bladder and rectum can be awkward in a child outside the neonatal period.
2. It cannot be extended directly into a median sternotomy to allow for direct cardiac massage, deal with any unexpected cardiac injury, or allow access to the great vessels. If a transverse laparotomy is extended upwards into a sternotomy, this results in a cosmetically unsatisfactory wound and the problem of having to close the abdominal wall at the junction of the two incisions.

For these reasons, one should consider the use of a midline incision as the standard access to deal with penetrating and ballistic injuries in children (Fig. 35.5).

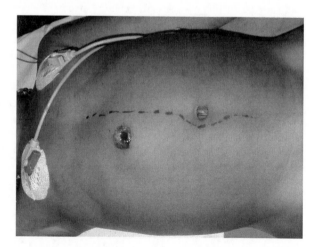

**Fig. 35.5** Two-year-old girl with epigastric gunshot wound illustrating the use of the midline incision

### 35.11.3
### Special Situations for Consideration

### 35.11.3.1
### The Patient Presenting in Shock

Children presenting with penetrating abdominal injury and shock should be prepared for immediate exploratory laparotomy. Blood should be urgently crossmatched, initial venous access obtained, and the patient transferred as rapidly as possible to the operating room. Where surgical hemostasis and further resuscitation should occur together. There should be no undue delays for X-rays or ultrasound investigations. These patients should always be sent to the nearest capable institution and never spend prolonged time in transportation and transfer between hospitals, if at all possible.

### 35.11.3.2
### Workup of Penetrating Injuries with Hematuria

*Stable patients* with hematuria and penetrating abdominal injuries are investigated by contrast studies of the lower tract or emergency room excretory urography, or both if deemed clinically relevant. The information obtained is useful to plan operative strategy and to localize the site of injury; it also confirms the function and position of the contralateral kidney in case nephrectomy is required.

## 35.12
## Peripheral Vascular

Gunshot wounds causing major peripheral vascular injury are an unusual clinical problem in children. The challenges of vascular repair procedures in the under-five age group are significant, with poor patency rates being the historical norm. The ongoing evolution of microvascular techniques has resulted in recent improvements in results in small children.

### 35.12.1
### The Role of Angiography

The diagnosis of a vascular injury usually is clinically evident, presenting with vigorous bleeding, an expanding hematoma or false aneurysm, or signs of vascular insufficiency. In general, clinical examination is sufficient to make the diagnosis and to decide on the need for operative intervention.[44] The use of Ankle:Brachial Artery Pressure Index (the systolic arterial pressure measured by Doppler in the injured limb divided by the systolic pressure in the uninjured limb) has been shown to reliably exclude extremity major vascular injury in adults.[45] A threshold of 0.9 is used to indicate a probable arterial injury. This technique is simple, quick, and inexpensive, and it should be a routine part of the vascular assessment of any limb in which an arterial injury is not clinically evident but needs to be ruled out.

In specialized centers, arteriography can be safely performed with low complication rates, even in young children. It is associated with higher complication rates when performed by the inexperienced or occasional operator and should only be performed when the presentation is atypical or the physical signs are equivocal. The role of angiography to detect arterial injury when a penetrating injury is anatomically in proximity to the vascular structures, but in the absence of signs of vascular injury, has largely been discredited in adult trauma practice,[46,47] and studies have confirmed this for the pediatric population as well.[48] The reason for this is that injuries are rarely found and are usually not of sufficient severity to require repair. There is some controversy as to whether it is important to detect such minor arterial injuries in children[49] (where their presence may result in growth retardation), but these are usually treated conservatively in any event. There are no long-term follow-up studies to give guidelines for the management of these occult arteriographically detected lesions in children. The current practice in most units is to keep the patient under surveillance and to intervene if patients experience claudication or growth retardation in the affected limb.

## 35.12.2
### Conservative Management

It is generally accepted that all major vascular injuries in childhood are treated by prompt exploration and repair with revascularization. This is true for all cases of penetrating trauma where there are signs of ischemia or where the surgeon needs to control bleeding or repair traumatic arteriovenous fistulae.

The generally excellent cardiovascular status of the young child provides for the establishment of an efficient collateral circulation after acute injury. Even when complete vascular occlusion has occurred, there may be no signs of acute ischemia. This is particularly true in the axillary and brachial arteries. Many children present with clear signs of an arterial injury, but with no evidence of ischemia or limb threat. If these patients are operated on in an attempt to restore flow, the surgeon may do harm by interfering with the collateral circulation and converting a stable situation where neither the limb nor patient is threatened to one of limb threat. This is particularly likely in the young child, where the vascular anastamosis is most technically challenging. It is recommended that under these circumstances, if there is no other urgent need for operation, that the patient be observed.[50] The Ankle:Brachial Arterial Pressure Index (API) is helpful under these circumstances. An index of greater than 0.6 indicates sufficient arterial perfusion by collaterals. These patients must be carefully followed. If the patient develops claudication or growth retardation of the affected limb, elective vascular repair can be performed at a later date. In the small number of patients that we have treated in this way, chronic ischemia has not occurred.

### 35.12.3
### Arterial Spasm

Arterial spasm is said to occur with greater frequency in pediatric arterial injury than in the adult. The frequency with which it is reported varies from series to series. It is usually reported to be present in patients with blunt trauma where arteriography demonstrates an abnormality, but where, at exploration, there is narrowing of the vessel but no macroscopically visible injury.[44] Vasospasm is thought to occur when there is a shear injury or contusion to a blood vessel. This results in anatomical or functional separation of the endothelium and the media. The constant vasodilatory effect maintained by endothelial production of nitric oxide is therefore lost and the vessel goes into prolonged spasm.[51] The small caliber of pediatric vessels makes them particularly vulnerable to spasm.[52] The role of spasm in penetrating arterial trauma is less clear. Generally, exploration for penetrating injury reveals a clearly injured vessel. Spasm certainly occurs in the artery being anastamosed, but this usually resolves after successful anastamosis or can be diminished by the topical application of papaverine.

It is important that all patients with clinical or arteriographic signs of a vascular injury after penetrating injury are assumed to have a vascular injury and treated appropriately. If signs of ischemia are present, the area of injury must be promptly explored. It is dangerous and usually erroneous to assume that the condition is due to spasm and therefore self-limiting. This may delay exploration and repair of the vessel and decrease the chances of successful revascularization (Fig. 35.6).

### 35.12.4
### Techniques of Repair and Revascularization

Many injuries can be managed by mobilization of the vessel ends, excision, and primary end-to-end anastamosis. If this is not possible without tension, then bypass grafting should

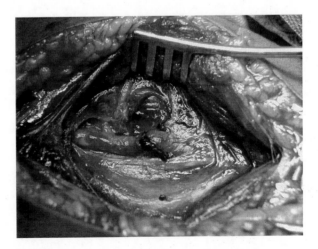

**Fig. 35.6** Injury to the superficial femoral artery in an 8-year-old boy. Appearance at the time of exploration for "spasm"

be performed. Reversed vein grafts are preferred because they have better patency rates in small vessels and have the potential to grow with the patient. Anastamoses in children should be performed by using an interrupted suture technique to allow for an increase in the vessel diameter with growth. Most peripheral vessels are best sutured with 6-0 or 7-0 polypropylene and the use of magnification is mandatory. Systemic heparinization generally is not used.

Venous injuries when encountered are treated by simple repair if this is feasible without significant narrowing of the vein. In most peripheral venous injuries, there is an excellent system of venous collaterals, which makes complex repairs of venous injuries unnecessary. The superior vena cava and the suprarenal inferior vena cava are the only veins that should always be repaired. The injured vein should be ligated if repair with a reasonable chance of success cannot be achieved without compromising the patient (by excessive blood loss and prolonged operating time). Any postoperative venous engorgement that ensues will be manageable by supportive treatment. One notable exception is the popliteal artery and vein injury where, like in adults, every attempt should be made to restore both arterial and venous flow because of the well-known risks of venous hypertension in this situation.

## 35.13
## Fetal Injury

Occasionally, the surgeon is called upon to treat a preterm baby injured during penetrating maternal trauma. This situation is typically seen in the third trimester, is usually a stabbing injury, and the mother often knows the perpetrator. Although pregnant mothers do suffer abdominal gunshot wounds, the survival prospects for these fetuses are slim.

## References

1. Vane D, Shedd FG, Grosfeld JL, et al. An analysis of pediatric Trauma deaths in Indiana. *J Pediatr Surg.* 1990;9:955-960.
2. From the Centers for Disease Control. Unintentional firearm-related fatalities among children, teenagers – United States, 1982–1988. *JAMA.* 1992;268:451-452.
3. Unintentional firearm-related fatalities among children and teenagers – United States, z1982–1988. *MMWR Morb Mortal Wkly Rep.* 1992 Jun;41(25):442-5, 451.
4. Cummings P, Grossman DC, Rivara FP, Koepsell TD. State gun safe storage laws and child mortality due to firearms. *JAMA.* 1997;278:1084-1086.
5. Powell EC, Tanz RR. Child and adolescent injury and death from urban firearm assaults: Association with age, race, and poverty. *Inj Prev.* 1999;5:41-47.
6. Nance ML, Stafford PW, Schwab CW. Firearm injury among urban youth during the last decade: An escalation in violence. *J Pediatr Surg.* 1997;32:949-952.
7. Copeland AR. Childhood firearms fatalities: The Metropolitan Dade County experience. *South Med J.* 1991;84:175-178.
8. Rates of homicide. Suicide, and firearm-related death among children – 26 industrialized countries. *MMWR Morb Mortal Wkly Rep.* 1997;46:101-115.

9. Krug EG, Dahlberg LL, Powell KE. Childhood homicide, suicide, and firearm deaths: an international comparison. *World Health Stat Q*. 1996;49:230-235.

10. Patterson PJ, Holguin AH. Firearm-related deaths among children in Texas: 1984–1988. *Tex Med*. 1990;86:92-97.

11. Dowd MD, Knapp JF, Fitzmaurice LS. Pediatric firearm injuries, Kansas City, 1992: A population-based study. *Pediatrics*. 1994;94:867-873.

12. Wigton A. Firearm-related injuries and deaths among children and adolescents in Cape Town – 1992–1996. *S Afr Med J*. 1999;89:407-410.

13. Hadley GP, Mars MS. Gunshot injuries in infants and children in KwaZulu-Natal – an emerging epidemic? *Afr Med J*. 1998;88:444-447.

14. Scribano PV, Nance M, Reilly P, Sing RF, Selbst SM. Pediatric nonpowder firearm injuries: outcomes in an urban pediatric setting. *Pediatrics*. 1997;100:E5.

15. Bratton SL, Dowd MD, Brogan TV, Hegenbarth MA. Serious and fatal air gun injuries: more than meets the eye. *Pediatrics*. 1997;100:609-612.

16. Bhattacharyya N, Bethel CA, Caniano DA, Pillai SB, Deppe S, Cooney DR. The childhood air gun: serious injuries and surgical interventions. *Pediatr Emerg Care*. 1998;14:188-190.

17. Nance ML, Sing RF, Branas CC, Schwab CW. Shotgun wounds in children. Not just accidents. *Arch Surg*. 1997;132:58-62.

18. Ivatury RR, Nallathambi MN, Roberge RJ. Penetrating thoracic injuries: In field stabilisation vs prompt transport. *J Trauma*. 1987;27:1066-1072.

19. Paul TR, Marias M, Pons PT, Pons KA, Moore EE. Adult vs paediatric prehospital trauma care. Is there a difference? *J Trauma*. 1999;47:455-459.

20. Gaffney P, Johnson G. Paediatric prehospital trauma care. *Trauma*. 1999;1:279-284.

21. Bickell WH, Wall MJ Jr, Pepe PE, et al. Immediate versus delayed fluid resuscitation for hypotensive patients with penetrating torso injuries. *N Engl J Med*. 1994;331:1105-1109.

22. Bickell WH, Barrett SM, Romine Jenkins M, Hull SS Jr, Kinasewitz GT. Resuscitation of canine hemorrhagic hypotension with large-volume isotonic crystalloid: impact on lung water, venous admixture, and systemic arterial oxygen saturation. *Am J Emerg Med*. 1994;12:36-42.

23. Bickell WH, Bruttig SP, Millnamow GA, O'Benar J, Wade CE. Use of hypertonic saline/dextran versus lactated Ringer's solution as a resuscitation fluid after uncontrolled aortic hemorrhage in anesthetized swine. *Ann Emerg Med*. 1992;21:1077-1085.

24. Bickell WH. Are victims of injury sometimes victimized by attempts at fluid resuscitation? *Ann Emerg Med*. 1993;22:225-226.

25. Wright JL, Patterson MD. Resuscitating the pediatric patient. *Emerg Med Clin North Am*. 1996;14:219-231.

26. Sarnaik AP, Kopec J, Moylan P, Alvarez D, Canady A. Role of aggressive intracranial pressure control in management of pediatric craniocerebral gunshot wounds with unfavorable features. *J Trauma*. 1989;29(10):1434-1437.

27. Hall JR, Reyes HM, Meller JL. Penetrating zone-II neck injuries in children. *J Trauma*. 1991;31(12):1614-1617.

28. Mitchell RB, Pereira KD, Younis RT, Lazar RH. The management of asymptomatic firearm injuries in children. *J R Coll Surg Edinb*. 1997;42(6):418-419.

29. Cooper A, Barlow B, Di Scala C, String D. Mortality and truncal injury: the pediatric perspective. *J Pediatr Surg*. 1994;29:33-38.

30. Mineo TC, Ambrogi V, Cristino B, Pompeo E, Pistolese C. Changing indications for thoracotomy in blunt chest trauma after the advent of videothoracoscopy. *J Trauma*. 1999;47:1088-1091.

31. Chen MK, Schropp KP, Lobe TE. The use of minimal access surgery in pediatric trauma: a preliminary report. *J Laparoendosc Surg*. 1995;5:295-301.

32. Pitcher GJ. Fiber-endoscopic thoracoscopy for diaphragmatic injury in children. *Semin Pediatr Surg*. 2001;10:17-19.

33. Powell RW, Gill EA, Jurkovich GJ, Ramenovsky ML. Resuscitative thoracotomy in children and adolescents. *Am J Surg.* 1988;54:188-191.

34. Rothenberg SS, Moore EE, Moore FA, Baxter BT, Moore JB, Cleveland HC. Emergency department thoracotomy in children – a critical analysis. *J Trauma.* 1989;29:1322-1325.

35. Beaver BL, Moore VL, Peclet M, Haller JA, Smialek J, Hill JL. Efficacy of emergency room thoracotomy in paediatric trauma. *J Pediatr Surg.* 1987;22:19-23.

36. Sheikh AA, Culbertson CB. Emergency department thoracotomy in children: rationale for selective application. *J Trauma.* 1993;34:323-328.

37. Inci I, Ozcelic C, Nizam O, Eren N, Ozgen G. Penetrating chest injuries in children: a review of 94 cases. *J Pediatr Surg.* 1996;31:673-676.

38. Nance ML, Sing RF, Reilly PM, Templeton JM, Schwab CW. Thoracic gunshot wounds in children under 17 years of age. *J Pediatr Surg.* 1996;31:931-935.

39. Peterson R, Tepas JJ 3rd, Edwards FH, Kissoon N, Pieper P, Ceithaml EL. Pediatric and adult thoracic trauma: Age-related impact on presentation and outcome. *Ann Thorac Surg.* 1994;58:14-18.

40. Bains MS, Gisnberg RJ, Jones WG 2nd, et al. The clamshell incision: An improved approach to bilateral pulmonary and mediastinal tumor. *Ann Thorac Surg.* 1994;58(1):30-33.

41. Shimizu J, Oda M, Morita K, et al. Evaluation of the clamshell incision for bilateral pulmonary metastases. *Int Surg.* 1997;82(3):262-265.

42. Luciani GB, Starnes VA. The clamshell approach for the surgical treatment of complex cardiopulmonary pathology in infants and children. *Eur J Cardiothorac Surg.* 1997;11(2):298-306.

43. Shorr RM, Gottlieb MM, Webb K, Ishiguro L, Berne TV. Selective management of abdominal stab wounds: importance of the physical examination. *Arch Surg.* 1988;123:1141-1145.

44. Mills RP, Robbs JV. Paediatric arterial injury: management options at the time of injury. *J R Coll Surg Edinb.* 1991;36:13-17.

45. Johansen K, Lynch K, Paun M, Copass M. Non-invasive vascular tests reliably exclude occult arterial trauma in injured extremities. *J Trauma.* 1991;31:515-522.

46. Gahtan V. The role of emergent arteriography in penetrating limb trauma. *Am Surg.* 1994;60:123-127.

47. Weaver FA, Yellin AE, Bauer M, et al. Is arterial proximity a valid indication for arteriography in penetrating extremity trauma? A prospective analysis. *Arch Surg.* 1990;125:1256-1260.

48. Reichard KW, Hall JR, Meller JL, Spigos D, Reyes HM. Arteriography in the evaluation of penetrating pediatric extremity injuries. *J Pediatr Surg.* 1994;29:19-22.

49. Itani KM, Rothenberg SS, Brandt ML, et al. Emergency center arteriography in the evaluation of suspected peripheral vascular injuries in children. *J Pediatr Surg.* 1993;28:677-680.

50. Frykberg ER, Crump JM, Dennis JW, Vines FS, Alexander RH. Nonoperative observation of clinically occult arterial injuries: a prospective evaluation. *Surgery.* 1991;109:85-96.

51. Kuo PC, Schroeder RA. The emerging multifaceted roles of nitric oxide. *Ann Surg.* 1995;221:220-235.

52. Reichard KW, Reyes HM. Vascular trauma and reconstructive approaches. *Semin Pediatr Surg.* 1994;3:124-132.

# Ballistic Trauma in Pregnancy

# 36

Michael J. Socher and Peter E. Nielsen

During peacetime, trauma is consistently listed as the most common cause of nonobstetric complications of pregnancy leading to some degree of morbidity and regrettably mortality in approximately 7% of all pregnancies.[1,2] The maternal mortality from penetrating injuries is less in pregnancy-4% as compared with 13% in the nonpregnant state.[2] Fetal mortality, however, is high approaching 42–71%, depending on penetrating mechanism of stab versus missile, respectively.[3,4] This is due in part to shielding of maternal viscera. This number undoubtedly increases in war-torn regions of the world such as the Middle East. Ballistic trauma is challenging to study in western societies thanks to relative peace. The nearest to ballistic trauma that Western physicians face is with firearms. In 2005, The United States reported 30,694 persons died from firearm injuries, accounting for 17.7% of all injury deaths. Pregnant women are an increasing part of that statistic. Firearm suicide and homicide, the two major component causes, accounted for 55.4% and 40.2% of these deaths, respectively.[1]

The management of the gravid trauma patient is equitant to management of nonpregnant patients. However, the surgeon must keep in mind the significant and at times profound changes in anatomy and physiology that accompany pregnancy, particularly in the latter half of pregnancy, as well as the fact that one's management decisions affect not only the mother but the life of the unborn child. Additionally, management timelines, gestational ages for prediction of maturity, statistical analyses of neonatal well-being after traumatic injuries taken from data in western society as well as management criteria used in tertiary medical centers all fall short where resources are scarce (such as on the battlefield, natural disasters, terrorism). In this chaotic arena, the surgeon is faced with a plethora of decisions wrapped in a multitude of uncertainties whose consequences can be far-reaching and are often unpredictable (Fig. 36.1).

Management decisions are made through the standard trauma assessment with slight modifications. Clearly, no matter how valiant the efforts at saving the fetus are, they are lost if the mother dies. Care of the gravid patient suffering from ballistic trauma is facilitated by knowledge of the anatomical and physiological changes associated with

M.J. Socher(✉)

Obstetrics and Gynecology, Uniformed Services University of the Health Sciences,
Walter Reed Army Medical Center, Washington DC, USA
e-mail: michael.socher@us.army.mil

A.J. Brooks et al. (eds.), *Ryan's Ballistic Trauma*,
DOI: 10.1007/978-1-84882-124-8_36, © Springer-Verlag London Limited 2011

**Fig. 36.1** Picture of
pregnant trauma patient.
Photo courtesy of
Michael J. Socher, MD

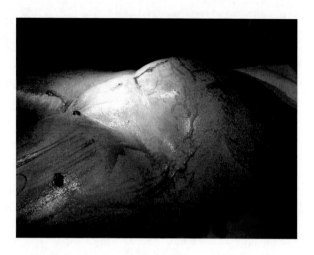

pregnancy, the mechanism of the injury, and ultimately a candid assessment of limits of
care that can safely and effectively be rendered to the mother and (potential) neonate.

## 36.1
## Anatomy and Physiology

By the end of the 1st trimester of pregnancy, many physiologic changes have already taken
place in the gravida. To the surgeon caring for the pregnant trauma patient, arguably the
most significant is related to the circulation[5] (Table 36.1).

She has decreased total peripheral resistance due to progesterone-related smooth muscle
relaxation. Blood pressure and central venous pressure both start to decline reaching nadirs
in the beginning of the 3rd trimester (approximately 28 weeks). Due mostly to increased
heart rate, cardiac output increases to nearly 50% above baseline in the 2nd trimester. Blood
volume also increases during the 2nd trimester to add nearly a 50% increase to her normal
volume. However, the hematocrit decreases to a mild anemia of 32% due to disproportion-
ate rise in blood plasma over red cell mass, the latter only increasing by roughly 30%. The
plasma is enriched with coagulation factors, stimulated through enough estrogen production for three women over their entire lifetime. This "hypercoagulable state" is protective,
and in fact she is an organism prepared for the increased metabolic demands of the fetus as
well as the bleeding experienced in labor and the puerperium. However, she is also at-risk
for postoperative complications related to venous thromboembolic events.

In the usual healthy woman, the circulatory changes of the gravida lead to a situation
where moderate hemorrhage (approximately 25% of blood volume or 1,500 mL)[6] is well-
tolerated, and is usually clinically unnoticed except in laboratory evaluation. Indeed, the
normal patient undergoing spontaneous vaginal delivery experiences average blood loss of
500 mL. Cesarean section doubles this loss. Hemorrhage after delivery is controlled by the
immediately effective coagulation cascade, as well as contraction of the uterus. The uterus

**Table 36.1** Physiological changes during pregnancy (Adapted from Clark et al.[5])

| | 11–12 Weeks postpartum | 36–38 Weeks gestation | Change from nonpregnant state |
|---|---|---|---|
| Cardiac output(L/min) | 4.3±0.9 | 6.2±1.0 | +43% |
| Heart rate (bpm) | 71±10.0 | 83±10.0 | +17% |
| Systemic vascular resistance (dyne·cm·s$^{-5}$) | 1,530±520 | 1,210±266 | −21% |
| Pulmonary vascular resistance (dyne·cm·s$^{-5}$) | 119±47.0 | 78±22 | −34% |
| Colloid oncotic pressure (mmHg) | 20.8±1.0 | 18±1.5 | −14% |
| Mean arterial pressure (mmHg) | 86.4±7.5 | 90.3±5.8 | NS |
| Pulmonary capillary wedge pressure (mmHg) | 3.7±2.6 | 3.6±2.5 | NS |
| Central venous pressure (mmHg) | 3.7±2.6 | 3.6±2.5 | NS |
| Left ventricular stroke work index (g·m·m$^{-2}$) | 41±8 | 48±6 | NS |

Data are presented as mean±standard deviation$^{-2}$

rapidly decreases in size to the level of the umbilicus after delivery of the placenta. During this phase, uterine artery vasoconstriction and myometrial contraction, mediated by oxytocin, leads to an autotranfusion, augmenting cardiac preload. For example, uterine contractions have been demonstrated to increase left ventricular stroke volume by 16% and cardiac output by 11% during labor.[7] In trauma, uterine artery vasoconstriction, similar to splanchnic constriction in the nongravid state, is preservative of the mother at the expense of the fetus. There is no autoregulation of the uterine bloodflow.[8] The surgeon caring for the pregnant patient would not expect to see much change in maternal vital signs with significant hemorrhage. However, the fetus, often called the "5th vital sign," will suffer the effects of the uteroplacental constriction and can serve as a warning of impending circulatory collapse.

Additionally, the anatomy of the hollow pelvis and the growing uterus lead to a condition where after approximately 20 weeks (when the fundus is at the umbilicus), the supine position leads to inferior vena cava compression by the uterus pressing upon the sacral promontory which leads to decreased preload, blood pressure, and ultimately decreased uteroplacental perfusion with subsequent fetal compromise.

The respiratory system's anatomical changes in pregnancy are similar to those seen in a pneumoperitoneum. From an anesthesia perspective, aspiration risk is increased and the oropharynx is edematous leading to difficulty with airway management. There is elevation of the diaphragm by 4 cm with a resulting increased anterior-posterior diameter of 2 cm and a 25% decrease in functional residual capacity.[8] Physiologically, by the 3rd trimester, the gravida has a compensated respiratory alkalosis and tidal volume has increased by 40%.[9]

As the maximum plasma expansion occurs, erythrocyte 2-3-diphosphoglycerate is maximally increased, and fetal oxygenation is optimized so long as maternal $PaO_2$ remains above 60 mmHg.[10] These changes in pregnancy have significant fetal benefits, but leave the mother with decreased $O_2$ reserve leading to rapid hypoxia when respiratory distress occurs as well as diminished buffering capacity in the setting of tissue hypoxia and acidemia.

All organ systems are changed during pregnancy from ureteral dilation to changes in the gastroesophageal junction to laxity of ligaments. However, an all-inclusive listing of these changes is beyond the scope of this chapter. The reader is referred to a text of maternal-fetal physiology for further details.

## 36.2
## Pathophysiology of Ballistic Trauma and the Gravid Uterus

In general, the surgeon is wise to surgically evaluate the victim of ballistic trauma, particularly with penetration of the peritoneum. However, in the stable gravida with a dead or previable fetus (generally less than 24 weeks gestation in tertiary care centers) and an entry wound below the umbilicus where gestational age allows the uterus to offer shielding, close observation may be justified. However, blast injuries lead to varying degrees of tissue damage. As detailed elsewhere[11] and in other areas of this book, solid abdominal organs, retroperitoneal colon, and small bowel mesentery appear to be injured by the long-duration shear waves generated by the gross displacement of the abdominal wall in primary blast injuries. If she survives the primary blast injury (the effect of the blast wave at the interface of air and body), and secondary blast injuries (i.e. – fragments) are few, the main concern for the maternal-fetal unit is disruption of the uteroplacental interface, or placental abruption. This is the most common outcome leading to fetal death in most literature reviews of trauma in pregnancy.[12] It can be catastrophic for the fetus as well as the mother if not treated promptly, and will classically present with vaginal bleeding, abdominal pain, uterine tenderness, and contractions, but there may be none of these even in a massive abruption.

Generally, the main determinants of the magnitude of secondary blast injury are the level of energy transfer, the sensitivity of the injured tissues, and the extent and nature of contamination.[13] In ballistic trauma to the gravid uterus, preterm labor is often seen, and although incompletely understood is likely due to cytokines and inflammation at the missile entry site as well as blood within the myometrium. Spontaneous abortion of previable infants is also a likely outcome in these cases.[14]

## 36.3
## Initial Care

Care in the field can set the stage for success or failure in the hospital. Experience gained in Operation Iraqi Freedom and Operation Enduring Freedom has shown that patients without acidemia, hypothermia, and hypotension upon presentation to the field hospital

**Fig. 36.2** Gestational age can be estimated by abdominal palpation. Most neonates will do well even with modest resources when the uterus is less than 8 cm from the xyphoid process. With full obstetric, neonatal, and surgical support, fetal survival is attainable with gestational age as low as 24 weeks (4 cm above the umbilicus) (Courtesy of Jillian P. Staruch)

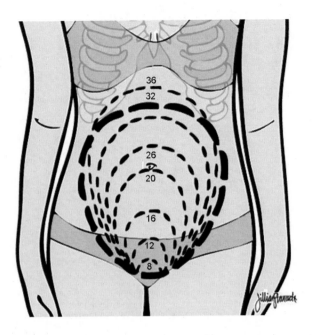

fare better than those with physiologic derangement,[15,16] although the importance of correcting this triad of poor prognosis has been seen only equivocally in civilian studies. The initial triage of the pregnant ballistic trauma patient can be challenging given that she is physiologically set to withstand significant bleeding and it is clear that significant hemorrhage can occur prior to maternal vital sign changes.[8,11,17] This notwithstanding, general trauma guidelines should be followed with notable additions as follows: While the patient is on a backboard, the board should be tilted 15 (usually to the left given the IVC passage on the right side of the spine) when gestational age is greater than 20-weeks (obtained by history-or a rough approximation of gestational age in weeks can be made by abdominal palpation as shown in Fig. 36.2). Two large-bore intravenous catheters are placed and supplemental oxygen should be given. A fluid bolus of lactated ringers should be given. While consideration is given to the unborn child, it must be remembered that at no time should the mother's life be placed in jeopardy for the sake of it.

## 36.4
## In-Hospital Management

Figure 36.3 shows an outline of trauma management of the gravida with a ballistic injury to the abdomen. Treatment decisions, due to the nature of trauma itself where even apparently minor maternal trauma can have lethal effects on the unborn child, need to be highly individualized depending on the status of the mother as well as the fetus in harmony with solid obstetric and surgical principles. The diagnostic evaluation of the gravid patient

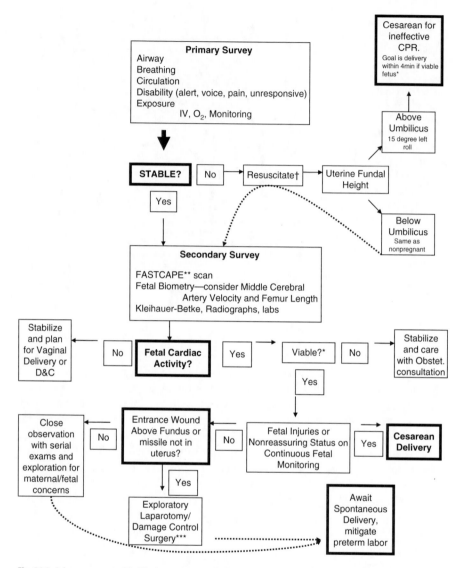

**Fig. 36.3** Management of ballistic trauma in the gravida. †Resuscitation may include exploratory laparotomy for obvious intraperitoneal injury and perimortem cesarean. *Viability depends on local resources. Generally, if fundus is at or less than 8 cm from xyphoid process, the majority of infants will do well after delivery even in areas with limited resources. **Focused assessment with sonography for trauma plus cardiac activity and placental evaluation. ***Degree of surgery depends on local resources and patient stability. Cesarean delivery only if uterus interferes with adequate surgical care of the mother (Adapted from Iliya et al.[47])

suffering from ballistic trauma must not be curtailed due to her pregnancy. All evaluations needed to adequately triage the patient are completed, although studies such as diagnostic peritoneal lavage are done supraumbilically or open.

Trauma scores are of limited value in the acute management of the trauma patient,[18,19] but are of some prognostic value with higher scores predicting fetal death and more severe maternal morbidity. Studies are small, and often retrospective. One small study of 20 patients reported that the injury severity score (ISS), blood loss, presence of disseminated intravascular coagulation and abruption were all associated with fetal mortality after all trauma.[20] Another in Washington State using a retrospective database found that the ISS was not predictive of fetal death. However, this study also showed that even minor injuries with an ISS of 0 (one-third of the cohort) led to adverse pregnancy outcomes, such as preterm labor, in one-half of them.[21]

The primary survey is identical to nonpregnant women with consideration given to early airway control with intubation, given decreased respiratory reserve and aspiration risk. If rapid sequence intubation is utilized, lower pseudocholinesterase levels in pregnancy require lower dosage of succinylcholine. Chest tube placement should be two intercostal spaces higher due to an elevated diaphragm. Finally, recall the need for lateral tilt of 15° to the left. If the board cannot be tilted, an assistant should displace the uterus to the patient's left.

The secondary survey includes evaluation of the fetus along with detailed evaluation of maternal well-being. Consideration for continuous fetal monitoring should be made. This "5th vital sign" can alert the surgical team to impending maternal compromise as fetal signs of distress nearly always occur prior to maternal distress. The Focused Assessment with Sonography for Trauma (FAST) exam has proven useful in the trauma survey and can be employed in pregnant women as well,[22] with the exception that the Pouch of Douglas cannot be visualized abdominally unless it is early in gestation. While performing the FAST, a survey of the uterus for signs of fetal life and placental location is valuable and adds little additional time. FASTCAPE can aid in remembering to look for Cardiac Activity and Placenta Evaluation. Two important and different questions can be answered at once: What is the cause of shock? What is the gestational age and status of the fetus? If the placenta is damaged, fetal status is certainly at risk. Placental location for surgical approach is easily noted during the ultrasound as well.[23] Additionally, the femur length may be easily measured and has good correlation with fetal gestational age if the history is unclear or cannot be obtained.[24,25]

More challenging is diagnosis of abruption – important due to its high rate of intrauterine fetal demise and high likelihood in cases of significant shear forces (i.e., primary blast injuries from an improvised explosive devise). In a recent review of placental abruption[26] two papers were detailed. In one,[27] researchers performed a retrospective cohort study of 57 cases of abruption, analyzed the images, and determined that the appearance of abruption in the acute phase was hyperechoic to isoechoic on ultrasound when compared with normal placenta in those same patients. After the hematomas resolved, they became hypoechoic within 1 week and sonolucent within 2 weeks. However, there were some cases where only a thickened heterogeneous placenta could be seen. This underscored the fact that abruptions on ultrasound have protean images. The placenta may "jiggle" when sudden pressure is applied with the transducer, the so-called "jello" sign.[26] In another retrospective cohort study, researchers found that the sensitivity, specificity, and positive and negative predictive values of ultrasonography for placental abruption were 24%, 96%, 88%, and 53%, respectively.[28] With this data, ultrasound will fail to detect at least one-half of cases of abruption. However, when the ultrasound seems to show an abruption, the likelihood that there is indeed an abruption is extremely high. Other relatively fast pieces of information can be obtained such as measurement of middle cerebral artery (MCA) Doppler velocimetry, and fetal position and number. MCA Doppler velocimetry has been shown to be a good predictor of fetal anemia at birth.[29-31] Increased MCA velocity may reveal compromise before abnormalities are seen on cardiotocography, and in the hands of an experienced practitioner may be of value in the assessment of fetal well-being.

The decision to operate or not depends on the overall clinical picture. Early recognition and treatment of intraperitoneal injuries are crucial. When in doubt, exploratory laparotomy is the best choice, however nonoperative management in select patients is acceptable.[32-34] When the fetus has died, the wound is below the fundus of the uterus, and the mother is otherwise stable, nonoperative management with delivery of the fetus vaginally is preferred. Many protocols utilizing CT scans have proven useful in management of penetrating wounds of the abdomen. CT offers significant advantages over any combination of diagnostic tests and has a very high negative predictive value that allows patients to be safely managed nonoperatively. The advent of dynamic helical CT has improved the definition and resolution of the projectile trajectory and intra-abdominal structures. Without optimal CT, nonoperative management of abdominal gunshot wounds (AGSW) is not advisable.[35]

The triple-contrast CT scan for penetrating abdominal injuries has proven very reliable in several studies. Sensitivity and specificity of triple-contrast CT scanning approaches 97% and 98%, respectively.[36-39] The rate of nontherapeutic laparotomy was low in these studies at 8%–11%. However, other studies have called into question the need for triple-contrast since even small amounts of air can be seen on single-agent (intravenous) CT scan with specificity approaching 96%.[40] Therefore a negative CT scan with only IV contrast should be sufficient with the addition of serial examination. In a terrorist attack with multiple casualties, in battle, or in areas with limited resources, the ability to proceed with single-agent CT scan is invaluable. This was certainly the case in the authors' experiences in Operation Iraqi Freedom. Concern for teratogenic and growth-restricting doses of radiation is not unwarranted, however the 5–10 rads delivered to the fetus during CT scanning of the abdomen/pelvis has not been shown to have adverse fetal outcomes. The American College of Obstetricians and Gynecologists has published guidelines with additional detailed recommendations regarding radiation exposure associated with diagnostic imaging in pregnancy.[41]

If surgical exploration is chosen, the uterus should be carefully inspected without twisting or excessive traction. In severe trauma, the need for surgery is evident. When the pregnant patient is showing signs of shock, expect large volume fluid, blood, and blood product replacement to be required.[6] Sound operative decision-making, open abdomen management, and occasionally damage control surgery are the keys to success.[42,43] Delivery of the fetus is rarely indicated, particularly when the infant is already dead. This maneuver will add on average 1,000 mL of blood loss with little maternal benefit. However, in the case of low rectal injury for example, or the general need for retroperitoneal exposure, or decreased preload from caval compression when the mother is in extremis, delivery of the unborn child at any gestational age and an empty uterus may assist in treating the mother.[11,42] Perimortem cesarean has been reported to be beneficial, although not proved, in a recent review of the literature.[42] The goal is for delivery of the infant to occur within 4 min of maternal cardiac arrest in order to improve both neonatal and maternal outcomes.[44,45] Finally, if the uterus is injured, direct repair or complete removal is warranted.[46]

## 36.5
## Summary

The leading cause of maternal mortality, not related to pregnancy complications, is trauma.[1,2] Care of the pregnant patient suffering from ballistic trauma is arguably the most challenging of trauma patients to attend. Two lives are at times competing for survival, and decisions for one can have profound effects on the other. Knowledge of the anatomical and physiological changes associated with advancing pregnancy will assist the surgeon in appropriate management. The basics of the tested and proven trauma surveys with slight modifications, as well as knowledge of the mechanism(s) of injury, will provide the best possible outcome for both patients. One should not delay diagnostic studies due to the patient's pregnancy, and early cardiotocographic monitoring of the fetus will be useful in most situations. Cesarean delivery should not be routine, even if laparotomy is required, unless fetal distress is present or evacuation of the uterus will aid the mother in resuscitation and recovery from her wounds. The best outcomes in perimortem cesarean occur when delivery is accomplished within 4 min of cardiopulmonary collapse.

## References

1. National Vital Statistics Reports. 2005;53(17).
2. Fildes J, Reed L, Jones N, Martin M, Barrett J. Trauma the leading cause of maternal death. *J Trauma*. 1992;32(5):643-645.
3. El Kady D. Perinatal outcomes of traumatic injuries during pregnancy. *Clin Obstet Gynecol*. 2007;50(3):582-591.
4. Franger AL, Buchsbaum HJ, Peaceman AM. Abdominal gunshot wounds in pregnancy. *Am J Obstet Gynecol*. 1989;160:1124-1128.
5. Clark S, Cotton D, Lee W, et al. Central hemodynamic assessment of normal term pregnancy. *Am J Obstet Gynecol*. 1989;161:1439.
6. Clark SL, Cotton DB, Hankins GDV, Phelan JP. *Critical Care Obstetrics*. 3rd ed. Cambridge, MA: Blackwell Scientific; 1997.
7. Lee W, Rokey R, Miller J, Cotton DB. Maternal hemodynamic effects of uterine contractions by M-mode and pulsed-Doppler echocardiography. *Am J Obstet Gynecol*. 1989;161:974-977.
8. Gonik B. Intensive care monitoring of the critically Ill pregnant patient. In: Creasy RK, Resnik R, eds. *Maternal Fetal Medicine*, Trauma in Pregnancy. 4th ed. Philadelphia: W.B. Saunders; 2001:913-918.

9. DeSwiet M. Pulmonary disorders. In: Creasy RK, Resnik R, eds. *Maternal Fetal Medicine*, Physiologic adaptations to pregnancy. 4th ed. Philadelphia: W.B. Saunders; 2000:923.

10. Brille-Brahe NE, Rorth M. Red cell 2-3-diphosphoglycerate in pregnancy. *Acta Obstet Gyn Scan*. 1979;58:19.

11. Buchsbaum HJ. Penetrating injury of the abdomen. In: *Trauma in Pregnancy*. Philadelphia: W.B. Saunders; 1979:82-100.

12. Pearlman MD, Tintinalli JE. Evaluation and treatment of the gravida and fetus following trauma during pregnancy. *Obstet Gyn Clin N Am*. 1991;18(2):371-381.

13. Garner J, Brett SJ. Mechanisms of injury by explosive devices. *Anesthesiol Clin*. 2007;25:147-160.

14. Weiss H, Songer T, Fabio A. Fetal deaths related to maternal injury. *JAMA*. 2001;286(15):1863-1868.

15. Fox CJ, Gillespie DL, Cox ED, et al. The effectiveness of a damage control resuscitation strategy for vascular injury in a combat support hospital: results of a case control study. *J Trauma*. 2008;64:S99-S107.

16. Holcomb JB, Jenkins D, Rhee P, et al. Damage control resuscitation: directly addressing the early coagulopathy of trauma. *J Trauma*. 2007;62:307-310.

17. Van Hook JW. Trauma in pregnancy. *Clin Obstet Gynecol*. 2002;45(2):414-424.

18. Corsi PR, Rasslan S, de Oliveira LB, Kronfly FS, Marinho VP. Trauma in pregnant women: analysis of maternal and fetal mortality. *Injury*. 1999 May;30(4):239-243.

19. Vasquez DN, Estenssoro E, Canales HS, et al. Clinical characteristics and outcomes of obstetric patients requiring ICU admission. *Chest*. 2007;131(3):718-724.

20. Ali J, Yeo A, Gana TJ, et al. Predictors of fetal mortality in pregnant trauma patients. *J Trauma*. 1997;42:782-785.

21. Schiff MA, Holt VL. The injury severity score in pregnant trauma patients: predicting placental abruption and fetal death. *J Trauma*. 2002;53:946-949.

22. Ma O, Mateer J, DeBenhke D. Use of ultrasonogrpahy for the evaluation of pregnant trauma patients. *J Trauma*. 1996;40(4):665-668.

23. Phelan HA, Roller J, Minei JP. Perimortem cesarean section after utilization of surgeon-performed trauma ultrasound. *J Trauma*. 2007;62:1-3.

24. Honarvar M, Allahyari M, Dehbashi S. Assessment of gestational age based on ultrasonic femur length after the first trimester: a simple mathematical correlation between gestational age (GA) and femur length (FL). *Int J Gynaecol Obstet*. 2000;70(3):335-340.

25. Johnsen SL, Rasmussen S, Sollien R, Kiserud T. Fetal age assessment based on femur length at 10-25 weeks of gestation, and reference ranges for femur length to head circumference ratios. [Comparative study. Journal article. Research support, Non-U.S. Gov't]. *Acta Obstet Gynecol Scand*. 2005;84(8):725-733.

26. Oyelese Y, Ananth CV. Placental abruption. *Obstet Gynecol*. 2006;108(4):1005-1016.

27. Nyberg DA, Cyr DR, Mack LA, Wilson DA, Shuman WP. Sonographic spectrum of placental abruption. *AJR Am J Roentgenol*. 1987;148:161-164.

28. Glantz C, Purnell L. Clinical utility of sonography in the diagnosis and treatment of placental abruption. *J Ultrasound Med*. 2002;21:837-840.

29. Mari G, Deter RL, Carpenter RL, Rahman F, Zimmerman R, Moise KJ. Non-invasive diagnosis by Doppler ultrasonography of fetal anemia due to maternal red-cell alloimmunization. *N Engl J Med*. 2000;342:9-14.

30. Rightmire DA, Nicolaides KH, Rodeck CH, Campbell S. Fetal blood velocities in Rh isoimmuniza[ophy]tion: relationship to gestational age and to fetal hematocrit. *Obstet Gynecol*. 1986;68:233-236.

31. Dukler D, Oepkes D, Seaward G, Windrim R, Ryan G. Noninvasive tests to predict fetal anemia: a study comparing Doppler and ultrasound parameters. *Am J Obstet Gynecol*. 2003;188:1310-1314.

32. O'Shaughnessy MJ. Conservative obstetric management of a gunshot wound to the second-trimester gravid uterus: a case report. *J Reprod Med*. 1997;42:606-608.

33. Buchsbaum HJ, Staples PP. Self-inflicted gunshot wound to the pregnant uterus: report of two cases. *Obstet Gynecol*. 1985;65:32S.
34. Goff BA, Muntz HG. Gunshot wounds to the gravid uterus: a case report. *J Reprod Med*. 1990;35:436-438.
35. Ginzburg E, Carillo EH, Kopelman T, et al. The role of computed tomography in selective management of gunshot wounds to the abdomen and flank. *J Trauma*. 1998;45:1005-1009.
36. Chiu WC, Shanmuganathan K, Mirvis SE, Scalea TM. Determining the need for laparotomy in penetrating torso trauma: a prospective study using triple-contrast enhanced abdominopelvic computed tomography. *J Trauma*. 2001;51:860-869.
37. Shanmuganathan K, Mirvis SE, Chiu WC, et al. Penetrating torso trauma: triple-contrast helical CT in peritoneal violation and organ injury: a prospective study in 200 patients. *Radiology*. 2004;231:775-784.
38. Shanmuganathan K, Mirvis SE, Chiu WC, et al. Value of triple-contrast spiral CT in penetrating torso trauma: a prospective study to determine peritoneal violation and the need for laparotomy. *AJR Am J Roentgenol*. 2001;177:1247-1256.
39. Munera F, Morales C, Soto JA, et al. Gunshot wounds of abdomen: evaluation of stable patients with triple-contrast helical CT. *Radiology*. 2004;231:399-405.
40. Velmahos GC, Constantinou C, Tillou A, Brown CV, Salim A, Demetriades D. Abdominal computed tomographic scan for patients with gunshot wounds to the abdomen selected for nonoperative management. *J Trauma*. 2005 Nov;59(5):1155-1160. discussion 1160-1161.
41. American College of Obstetricians and Gynecologists Committee Opinion #299: Guidelines for diagnostic imaging during pregnancy; 2004.
42. Aboutanos SZ, Aboutanos MB, et al. Management of a pregnant patient with an open abdomen. *J Trauma*. 2005;59:1052-1056.
43. Moise K, Belfort M. Damage control for the obstetric patient. *Surg Clin North Am*. 1997;77(4):835-852.
44. Katz VL, Balderston K, DeFreest M. Perimortem cesarean delivery: were our assumptions correct? *Am J Obstet Gynecol*. 2005;192:1916-1921.
45. Katz VL, Dotters DJ, Droegemueller W. Perimortem cesarean delivery. *Obstet Gynecol*. 1986;68:571-576.
46. Awwad JT, Ghassan BA, Muhieddine AS, Mroueh AM, Karam KS. High-velocity penetrating wounds of the gravid uterus: review of 16 years of civil war. *Obstet Gynecol*. 1994;83(2):259-264.
47. Iliya FA, Hajj SN, Buchsbaum HJ. Gunshot wounds of the pregnant uterus: report of two cases. *J Trauma*. 1980;20:90-92.

# Managing Ballistic Injury in the NGO Environment

# 37

Ari K. Leppäniemi

## 37.1
## Introduction

There are tens of thousands of nongovernmental organizations (NGOs) operating today in most countries, with their scope varying from large, Northern-based charities to community-based self-help groups in the South. The World Bank defines NGOs as "private organizations that pursue activities to relieve suffering, promote the interests of the poor, protect the environment, provide basic social services or undertake community development." With increasing globalization, NGOs have become more influential in world affairs, and it has been estimated that over 15% of total overseas development aid are channeled through NGOs. These organizations are not directly affiliated with any national government, but often have a significant impact on the social, economic, and political activity of the country or region involved.

The most prevalent form of conflict in the post-cold war era is the occurrence of local or regional low-intensity conflicts, such as civil wars, guerrilla warfare, terrorism, and counter-insurgency operations. In the 12-year post-cold war period 1990–2001, there were 57 different major armed conflicts in 45 different locations. All but three of the major conflicts were internal – the issue concerned control over the government or territory of one state. Other states contributed regular troops to one side or the other in 15 of the internal conflicts. As the historian Samuel Huntington has pointed out, communal conflicts between states or groups from different civilizations, or fault line conflicts, are likely to increase in the future. They tend to be protracted by nature, and when they are intrastate, they tend to last on average six times longer than interstate wars. Because of their protracted character, the fault line wars tend to produce a large number of casualties and refugees (see Table 37.1 for casualty figures).

With increasing erosion of nation-states, especially among the developing countries, many states are sliding into anarchy and ungovernability caused by scarcity of resources,

A.K. Leppäniemi
Department of Surgery, Emergency Surgery Division,
Helsinki University, Meilahti Hospital, Helsinki, Finland
e-mail: ari.leppaniemi@hus.fi

A.J. Brooks et al. (eds.), *Ryan's Ballistic Trauma*,
DOI: 10.1007/978-1-84882-124-8_37, © Springer-Verlag London Limited 2011

**Table 37.1** Casualty figures from fault-line wars in the early 1990s

| |
|---|
| 50,000 in the Philippines |
| 50,000–100,000 in Sri Lanka |
| 20,000 in Kashmir |
| 0.5–1.5 million in Sudan |
| 100,000 in Tajikistan |
| 50,000 in Croatia |
| 50–200,000 in Bosnia |
| 30,000–50,000 in Chechnya |
| 100,000 in Tibet |
| 200,000 in East Timor |

The number of injured victims being multiple times higher than those killed

overpopulation, refugee migration, tribalism, disease, environmental degradation, uncontrolled crime, and the empowerment of private armies, security firms, and international drug cartels.

Future wars will be associated with a large number of factors that have a major impact on the conditions of the affected people living in the conflict areas, and include population expansion, poverty, the AIDS epidemic, shortage of water and agricultural land, post-cold war availability of arms, megacities, drug trafficking (de facto governments), violent transnational groups and countries protecting them, rapid communications and travel, and recruitment of child-soldiers.

With increasing frequency of less-defined states between peace and war and risk of collapsing infrastructure, including medical facilities in the affected countries, the type of medical challenges to the local and international community is likely to involve more frequently humanitarian and peace-keeping type of missions, as well as providing surgical care for the war wounded under less-than-optimal conditions. It can be even more difficult when an internal war is combined with a total collapse of the country's infrastructure (failed states) and mass movements of people, as witnessed recently in western and central Africa. The care of the wounded under these extreme conditions has to be limited to the very basic with maximal use of the limited resources.

A major conventional war could require mobilization of surgical teams with relatively little experience in managing mass casualties. This creates an enormous challenge to peacetime training of the medical personnel. In spite of recent progress of minimally invasive surgical techniques, a surgeon in a twenty-first century conflict must have the capability to adequately assess the wounded patient and perform major conventional surgery under adverse conditions with very limited resources using different techniques and approaches depending on the available resources and overall situation.

There are several organizations directly participating in the patient care of wounded civilians and soldiers in conflicts around the world, especially in developing countries. One of the best-known delivering medical care to victims of war on a large scale and with established and published management guidelines is the International Committee of the Red Cross (ICRC). Based on the mandate of the ICRC to bring protection and assistance to the victims of international and non-international armed conflicts and internal disturbances and tensions, it deploys surgical teams for the treatment of victims of armed conflicts. Surgical care is promoted by placing teams in preexisting hospitals or establishing independent ICRC surgical hospitals. First aid posts near the conflict areas usually serve these hospitals.

This review is based on published reports of surgical care from ICRC and other NGO hospitals and the personal experience of the author while working as field surgeon in an ICRC hospitals in Khao-I-Dang on the Thai–Cambodian border, in Lokichokio in northern Kenya–South Sudan and in Peshawar, Pakistan.

## 37.2
## NGO Hospital Environment and Facilities

A health care system is one of the earliest casualties of the social and economic disruption of a country in conflict. Hospital doctors and nurses may not be able to perform their normal duties, they may not be paid or able to reach the hospital, or they might be discriminated against for working. Medical teams from humanitarian agencies who step in trying to work in these conflicts may do so in danger. There is little or no discipline among those who have the weapons, and one side of the conflict may target the agencies because they are perceived as aiding the other. With the prolongation of the conflict, the local health care facilities have little chance of reestablishing themselves, and there will be increasing demands on the NGO hospital to take care of the non-combat-related medical problems of the affected population. Occasionally, the organized management of patients is made more difficult by accompanying relatives and friends who may be armed and try to hasten treatment with threats.

The majority of NGO field hospitals can be compared with civilian hospitals, which are isolated in an area of conflict. They differ from typical military hospitals because they are not a part of echeloned care, but work, at the same time, as hospitals of first contact and referral hospitals, implying that both primary surgery, secondary surgery, and basic reconstructive surgery are conducted in the same hospital (Fig. 37.1). This poses great challenges to personnel working under these conditions because they must have broad knowledge and experience in all areas of surgical care, including wound surgery, amputations, fracture management, craniotomies, thoracotomies, vascular procedures, laparotomies, management of burns, and basic plastic surgical techniques.

Although there is great variation in the level of equipment, most NGO-run hospitals have limited availability of blood, no ventilatory equipment, minimal laboratory services, and only plain radiography. Because of the limitations and special conditions in these field hospitals, the planning of surgery is of utmost importance, and the restrictions encourage the use of simple methods of treatment and improvisation to provide adequate care. In addition, the geographical, climatic, cultural, and social environment imposes limitations and constraints, making adaptation to the environment essential. Local skills and materials

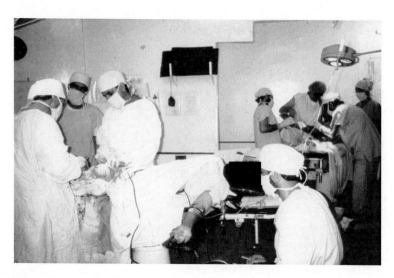

**Fig. 37.1** Operation room in the ICRC hospital in Peshawar, Pakistan, with two teams working parallel performing acute and planned surgery, respectively

should be used as much as possible. Sanitation and nutrition should be adapted to local needs and customs. The effects of endemic diseases such as malaria should be taken into account, especially in the early postoperative phase in a febrile patient. And finally, the surgical treatment should be conducted with the aim of minimizing blood loss and the need for blood transfusions, as well as optimizing the chances of postoperative recovery without the facilities for intensive care, total parenteral nutrition, and use of sophisticated and expensive medication.[1,2]

## 37.3
## Patient Characteristics in an NGO Hospital

A large number of wounded patients brought to an NGO field hospital are civilians, defined as women and girls, boys (under 16 years of age), and men of 50 or more. Of the 18,877 patients injured by bullets, bombs, shells, mortars, or mines and admitted to ICRC hospitals in 1991 through 1998, about 28% were civilians. The proportion of civilians injured by fragments and mines is larger than those injured by bullets, most probably because weapons that fragment can easily injure more than one person, and because mines remain after the conflict, both increasing the likelihood of civilian injuries. Overall, in most published reports from ICRC hospitals, fragments account for the majority of wounds, followed by bullets and mines.

Many of the wounded civilians, especially in developing countries, may not be optimal candidates for surgery because of preexisting malnutrition, chronic infections, and parasites.

The vast majority of wounded patients treated in NGO hospitals suffer from extremity injuries, with lower extremities being injured more often than upper extremities. The proportion of potentially life-threatening injuries of the head, neck, and torso is about 10–30%, but can be as low as 5% if there is lack of appropriate surgical attention and evacuation facilities in the field *because many of these patients die before receiving care.*

## 37.4
## Prehospital Care

Under conditions where most NGO hospitals work, the prehospital care is poorly organized if at all. The often-chaotic conditions, collapse of infrastructure, and mass movements of population prevent or pose enormous challenges in creating a functional and adequate prehospital care system. Sometimes, when an ICRC hospital has been located inside a border of a neighboring country not participating in the conflict, first aid posts in or near the conflict areas have served the hospitals.

In most cases, patients are brought to the hospital by relatives and friends using all available means of transport. The delay from the moment of wounding can be anything from a few minutes to several days. Because it has an effect of the method of treatment, it is important to try to find out the time of injury in spite of occasional difficulties of gaining adequate information due to language problems or because the information might be politically or militarily sensitive.

## 37.5
## Triage

In most mass casualty situations encountered in NGO hospitals, the conventional military type of triage process of categorizing patients according to the urgency of treatment can be applied.

Sometimes, however, the extent of work requires modification of the conventional approach, as described by Robin Coupland while working in ICRC hospital in Kabul, Afghanistan in 1992.[3]*

I was a team surgeon in one of four teams when we received roughly 600 new casualties over a period of 6 days. Most were civilians from the vicinity of the hospital. About 250 with small soft tissue wounds were sent home with antibiotic tablets after having received tetanus prophylaxis. They had instructions to return if they developed problems; few did. This was in keeping with a non-operative policy for small soft tissue wounds, but the extreme circumstances did not allow the patients to remain in hospital for observation. We were able to admit all patients with larger wounds to dress the wound and give fluids intravenously, benzylpenicillin, tetanus prophylaxis, and analgesia. Owing to fatigue and the

*From reference 3, page 1693, with permission.

proximity of the battle we were able to operate only for some hours each day and those with abdominal wounds had priority. The perioperative mortality was high. Those who were rushed into the operating theater because of the severity of their wounds usually died during or soon after surgery because the admission procedure had become so disrupted that many arrived on the operating table having received insufficient intravenous fluid replacement. After surgery more died through lack of postoperative supervision. Much valuable surgical time and energy was wasted. The patients with abdominal wounds who survived were those who required laparotomy for perforation and not for bleeding. The few patients admitted with thoracic wounds whose condition was not stabilized by fluid resuscitation and chest drainage died before they could reach the operating theater. Most patients with severe wounds of the limbs that required amputation or wound excision had to wait 3 or 4 days for their surgery; only those with massive multiple wounds died in the meantime.

Based on this experience in Kabul, three lessons were learned:[3]*

1. Intravenous fluids and antibiotics buy time for most patients.
2. Patients with severe life threatening injuries die despite treatment unless resources, the number of nursing staff, and the organization of the hospital infrastructure are adequate.
3. When the hospital infrastructure is disrupted, surgical resources are easily wasted by operating on patients whose prognosis is hopeless – underlining the importance of realistic triage for treatment – and the death rate is unacceptably high among those who should survive.

Thus, under extreme conditions, the traditional approach to triage and major surgical intervention can be challenged by an epidemiological approach, where less emphasis is placed on the more spectacular aspects of surgical care that benefit only a few, in favor of some effective care reaching many more with emphasis on adequate first aid and delayed surgery directed at casualties who would die of infective complications if surgery was not performed.

*Airway protection, fluid resuscitation, arrest of accessible hemorrhage, and tube thoracostomy could prevent early deaths. Later deaths could be avoided by prevention of infective complications with antibiotics, wound excision, correct amputation, and laparotomy for perforation alone.*

## 37.6
## Surgery in an NGO Hospital

### 37.6.1
### General Comments

The majority of surgical procedures carried out for wounded patients in NGO hospitals include wound surgery in different stages, amputations, and treatment of open fractures and abdominal surgery. Table 37.2 lists surgical procedures performed in one ICRC hospital.

In most cases, a NGO hospital is the sole provider of surgical care in the conflict area with no possibility of transferring patients to better-equipped hospitals for secondary surgical procedures, such as reconstructive plastic surgical procedures or correction of badly

---

*From reference 3, page 1693, with permission.

**Table 37.2** Surgical procedures performed by a New Zealand Red Cross surgical team in the ICRC hospital in Kabul during a 6 month period in 1990 ($n = 1,017$)

| | |
|---|---|
| Debridement | 240 |
| Wound revision | 364 |
| Delayed primary closure | 145 |
| Split skin graft, flaps | 30 |
| Amputation | 37 |
| External fixation | 31 |
| Steinman pins | 16 |
| Laparotomy | 70 |
| Closure of colostomy | 10 |
| Hemothorax | 26 |
| Craniotomy | 24 |
| Maxillofacial, eyes | 14 |
| Vascular | 8 |
| Laminectomy | 2 |

healed fractures. In addition, the local conditions to which patients return after being discharged may be challenging in terms of access to rehabilitation, prosthetic equipment, and disposable items, such as urine bags, colostomy equipment, and even gauze material. Finally, the social security network and means of surviving economically after a bilateral lower extremity amputation, for example, can in some societies and under times of conflict be almost non existent. All these factors have to be considered when surgical intervention is performed for victims of armed conflicts in a NGO environment, and the surgical procedure chosen must be the most appropriate for that patient under those circumstances.

## 37.6.2
## Damage Control

Successful damage control surgical approach requires access to adequate postoperative care facilities with expertise and equipment for invasive and aggressive hemodynamic monitoring, ventilatory management, correction of coagulation factors, and other procedures usually performed in a well-equipped intensive care unit (ICU). On most occasions, the NGO environment does not have the resources to establish an effective ICU, which would make a traditional damage control approach for patients with severe physiological derangement undergoing just the necessary procedure to stop hemorrhage and control contamination inappropriate. As discussed above in the triage section, most of the severely ill patients treated under extreme conditions die anyway, stressing the importance of adequate triage, concentrating the use of scarce resources to patients with a reasonable chance of survival under those conditions.

## 37.6.3
### Diagnostic Equipment

Under the most primitive conditions, physical examination is the only available method of assessing the patient after appropriate history from the patient or accompanying persons. In most NGO hospitals, however, basic laboratory and radiological equipment for plain X-rays are available, although the reading of the X-ray results has to be carried out by the clinician without the support of a trained radiologist. Occasionally, simple surgical procedures, such as diagnostic peritoneal lavage with macroscopic assessment of the lavage fluid, can be performed to aid decision making.

## 37.6.4
### Antibiotics

All war wounds are contaminated with bacteria and eventually will become infected. Although non-surgical treatment might be appropriate in some cases, antibiotics are not an alternative to proper wound surgery in grossly contaminated or old wounds in the presence of dead tissue because gas gangrene and tetanus are real threats in patients with inadequately managed wounds. Nevertheless, antibiotic prophylaxis with penicillin and adequate measures for tetanus prophylaxis should always accompany the surgical management of war wounds.

In patients with head wounds, penicillin should be combined with another antibiotic that, in resource-limited situations, could be chlorampenicol or trimethoprim-sulphametoxazole.

Bowel injuries are very common in penetrating abdominal war wounds, and a sufficiently broad-spectrum antibiotic with activity against anaerobic bacteria or an additional antibiotic with such activity should be given as early as possible to all abdominal casualties. A cephalosporin–metronidazole combination would probably be most effective, but with limited financial and logistical resources, other cheaper antibiotics such as crystalline penicillin or chloramphenicol could be well justified.

## 37.6.5
### Anesthesia

A range of anesthetic methods can be used for surgery of war wounds, and the method of choice depends on many variables, including the available expertise, equipment and drugs, circumstances, urgency, and postoperative monitoring capabilities. A trained anesthesiologist is an integral part of most NGO hospital teams, but occasionally the surgeon has to be his own anesthetist, using methods that are familiar, safe, and applicable in conditions where the surgeon is operating and can not dedicate his full time to monitor the anesthesia.

Anesthetic methods that can be administered with relative safety by doctors not formally trained in anesthesia, but with some previous practical experience, include topical anesthesia (eyes, mucosal surfaces), local infiltration anesthesia, digital and axillary nerve blocks, spinal or epidural anesthesia, and ketamine anesthesia with spontaneous ventilation.

## 37.6.6
## Blood Transfusions

Frequently, during war, the requirement to produce large quantities of blood often exceeds the ability to collect, prepare, and distribute sufficient quantities of donated blood. This is even truer in the NGO environment, where blood products are seldom available in large quantities. In a study of the use of blood products in ICRC hospitals, the average units per patient transfused were 2.9. The quantity of blood required for every 100 patients was 44.9 units. The low consumption of blood is probably related to long evacuation times, the availability of blood, and the strict ICRC criteria for transfusion.

Until oxygen-carrying blood substitutes are added to the everyday use in civilian hospitals and would be logistically and economically manageable under field conditions, there will be a constant shortage of blood products available to surgeons working in field hospitals. With appropriately measured surgical interventions, strict indications for blood transfusions, and meticulous attention to surgical technique to reduce blood loss, the blood transfusion requirements can be kept as low as possible and save the available blood for those benefiting most from it.

## 37.6.7
## Surgical Management

The principles of management of war wounds in NGO hospitals differ little from the general guidelines followed in regular military hospitals and will not be reviewed here in detail. The basic principles of wound excision, delayed primary closure, external fixation of fractures, etc. apply to most NGO conditions as well. There are, however, some adjustments required in managing ballistic trauma in a typical NGO hospital and environment; these will be emphasized below.

In addition to the previously mentioned lack of echeloned care and possibility of transferring patients to receive secondary surgical treatment in better-resourced facilities, the most typical feature is the common encounter of old (days, or even weeks) or neglected wounds. Their surgical management must be flexible to take into account the wound changes this delay produces. The wound may require more aggressive surgery because of putrefaction or gangrene. Alternatively, the wound assessment may reveal that the wound has started to heal and so a less-aggressive surgical approach may be taken. Intraoperative blood loss when excising an old wound may be great because the surgeon is working through edematous and inflamed tissue, and it can be difficult to identify viable muscle and vital anatomic structures under these circumstances.[4]

Under some conditions, another characteristic of an NGO hospital environment is the admission of patients who have had a front-line treatment by local providers, including suturing of wounds, splinting of fractures, or even a front-line laparotomy. These patients sometimes arrive with pus, feces, urine, or bile leaking from wounds, incisions, or drain sites. After rehydration, antibiotics, and correction of anemia, a second operation might reveal grossly infected tissues, and in case of a relaparotomy, missed perforations, leaking anastomoses or repairs, and retained surgical compresses.

## 37.7
## Wound Surgery

The majority of wound surgery is performed on limbs, and the application of a pneumatic tourniquet before the removal of field dressing can be helpful in initial surgery of the distal limb wounds to minimize blood loss and create a bloodless operative field, especially in patients with traumatic amputations.

Longitudinal skin incisions are usually most appropriate in extremity wounds and the surgical wound should always be larger than the initial wound, although as little skin as possible is removed. After managing the skin lesion, the wound is thoroughly exposed and debrided layer by layer by dissecting individual muscles and tendons bluntly and excising their damaged parts until healthy tissue is encountered. When a muscle group is injured, only those individual muscles that are partially divided are visible in the wound. Those muscles, completely transected, contract away from the wound. Their devitalized ends must be exposed by adequate skin incisions and dissection to achieve complete removal of dead muscle tissue. With through-and-through wounds, the skin incisions and dissection are based on both entry and exit wounds and, if possible, should meet.

Those foreign materials that could cause severe infection, such as mud, pieces of shoe, or cloth, must be meticulously removed. When the wound includes a fracture, that part of the bone must be exposed. Small and unattached bone fragments are removed and curettage is performed to remove exposed medullary bone back to firm marrow.

The fascial compartments, especially below the knee, are prone to the compartment syndrome (Fig. 37.2), and the surgeon should be prepared to perform an open fasciotomy at the time of wound excision, if needed.

After securing hemostasis with sutures and other surgical means, the wound is liberally washed with saline and then left open by packing it not too tightly with dry gauze in sufficient quantities so that blood and serum will be taken up. Gauze moistened with normal saline can be applied over exposed joints and tendons.

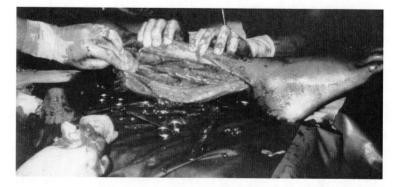

**Fig. 37.2** Compartment syndrome following a gunshot wound of the leg with necrotic muscle being excised from all compartments (ICRC hospital in Khao-I-Dang, Thailand)

Exceptions to the delayed primary closure method include wounds of the face, scalp, dura, joint capsules, and serous cavities, which are closed at initial wound surgery.

After wound excision the operative dressing is left for 4 or 5 days and removed in the operating theater with the patient under general anesthesia. The state of the dressings is no indicator of the state of the wound, especially in a field hospital in a hot country. If the muscle adheres to the adjacent gauze and contracts away as the dressing is gently peeled off – sometimes with the help of saline irrigation – and the wound is clean with a reddish healthy surface, the wound excision has been adequate and it can be closed without tension using appropriately placed interrupted sutures (Fig. 37.3). A large wound may require split skin grafting, which usually requires a longer period before the graft will be accepted.

If the patient's general condition is not improving after initial surgery, if there is temperature, excessive pain, and purulent discharge to the dressings, the wound requires

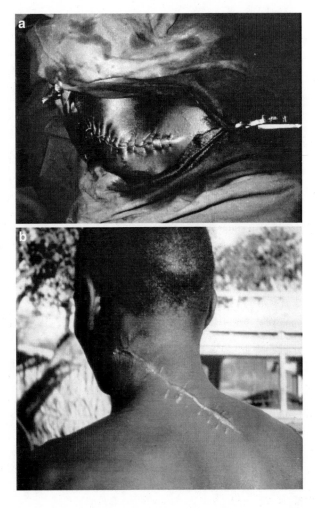

**Fig. 37.3** High-energy gunshot wound through the neck treated with wound excision, followed by delayed primary closure 5 days later (**a**) and seen at 2 months (**b**) (Lokichokio, Kenya)

reassessment in the theater and removal of remaining dead tissue, followed by open treatment with gauze dressings.

If the wound fails to heal after several days or even weeks, or if there is visible bone, more soft tissue usually has to be removed. A degree of healing will have occurred around the wound, which remains a cavity containing nonviable tissue, bone fragments, or protruding ends of fractured long bones. The treatment includes reincising the skin, curettage of the cavity, and excision of the dead bone ends. When reexcision is complete, digital examination confirms a smooth cavity free of bone ends and fragments, and it will slowly heal by secondary intention, and ultimately callus will form across it.[4]

## 37.8
## Amputations

Irreparable damage to the soft tissues or arteries of the extremities and significant bone loss are usually best treated with amputation with the primary intention of saving life by preventing infection and gas gangrene. Antipersonnel mines are, by design, intended to disable rather than kill, and the victim receives a typical pattern of injuries in which the foot, which triggers the weapon, is blown off, mud or earth, fragments of mine, shoe, or foot are blown up into genitals, buttocks, and the contralateral arm and leg. When the lower tibia is shattered by explosive injury, there is considerable proximal soft tissue damage, with the muscles of the anterior, lateral, and deep anterior fascial compartments being severely contused and contaminated.

Preservation of a functional knee joint is of paramount importance for the rehabilitation of lower limb amputees, even more so in developing countries where resources are limited for the manufacturing and maintenance of prosthesis. The level of amputation is determined by the extent of the original injury, but if a below-knee amputation stump becomes severely infected postoperatively, the consequence will often be an above-knee amputation, which is much more devastating.

Depending on the level of traumatic amputation and the degree of the soft tissue damage, the surgical amputation may resemble a thorough excision of the original wound or a formal amputation with planned skin and muscle flaps. Guillotine amputations should be avoided. With the help of a pneumatic tourniquet in the proximal limb, only damaged skin is removed and devitalized and contaminated muscle is excised. The optimal lengths of amputations are[1]:

- Tibia: 12–14 cm from the tibial tuberosity (minimum 5 cm)
- Femur: 25–28 cm from the top of the greater trochanter (minimum 10 cm)
- Arm: 6–8 cm above the elbow (minimum 2.5 cm of ulna beyond the anterior axillary fold)
- Forearm: 6–8 cm above the wrist (minimum 2.5 cm of ulna beyond the prominence of the biceps tendon when the elbow is flexed)

It is rare to be able to perform a below-knee amputation with a long posterior myocutaneous flap, and equal skin flaps are usually the sole option. After transfixing the principal vessels with sutures, hemostasis must be secured after release of the tourniquet.

The amputation stump is left open and delayed closure is performed after 4–6 days. Because of the retraction of the skin and swelling of the muscle, the stump might need trimming before closure can be achieved. A suction drain can be placed under the skin flaps during delayed closure.

In an analysis of 111 below-knee amputations performed mostly for mine injuries in the ICRC hospital in Peshawar, Pakistan in 1989, the closure was performed after an average of 6.4 days, with re-amputation above the knee being required in only one case due to wound sepsis. The best results were obtained when the stump closure was performed within 1 week after the amputation. Overall, 84% of the stumps healed without problems, and there were no patients with gas gangrene or tetanus.

## 37.9
## Fractures and Vascular Injuries of the Extremities

A wound with bone injury is treated with the same principles as any other ballistic wound, with careful removal of devitalized tissues including bone fragments. Fractures can be stabilized with skeletal traction, plasters, or external fixation, and the wounds are left open for delayed primary closure.

The optimal method of fracture stabilization depends on the circumstances, available equipment, surgical expertise, type and location of the fracture, degree of soft tissue injuries, and the presence of associated injuries. In general, external fixation is preferred in long bone fractures with large soft tissue injuries in adults, traction can be used with children, and plaster in cases with less degree of soft tissue injury.

In analysis of more than 200 high-velocity missile injuries treated in ICRC hospitals in Afghanistan and northern Kenya, the conclusion was that in an environment where facilities are limited and surgeons have only general experience, very careful initial wound excision is the most important factor determining outcome. Femoral fractures were treated either by traction or external fixation with identical positional outcome in both groups, but the patients treated with external fixation remained in the hospital longer than those treated with traction. In tibial fractures, the external fixator was only of extra benefit in those of the lower third when compared with simple plaster slabs, unless more-complex procedures such as flaps or vascular repair were to be performed. In complex humeral fractures, external fixation resulted in long stays in the hospital and a large number of interventions when compared with simple treatment in a sling.[5]

Because of the limited diagnostic equipment in most NGO hospitals, the diagnosis of extremity vascular injuries is based on a high index of suspicion, location of the missile track, local signs of major hemorrhage, and careful assessment of the circulatory status of the injured limb. If distal pulses remain absent after adequate fluid resuscitation, or if other signs indicating major vessel damage are present, rapid surgical exploration at the injury site for possible vascular injury is warranted. In addition to arterial transection or laceration, a possible arterial contusion has to be recognized and repaired early. Occasionally, a major vascular injury is presented as a false aneurysm or arterio-venous fistula.

The repair of vascular injuries is performed according to the established principles described elsewhere. In general, direct repair is preferred in small lacerations, but narrowing has to be avoided or prevented by using a vein patch. End-to-end anastomoses should be reconstructed without tension. Large segment damage of a major artery requires repair with a saphenous vein graft. Before completing any arterial repair, free forward bleeding and adequate back flow from the distal segment has to be established, and, if needed, distal embolectomy performed with a Fogarty balloon catheter. A repaired artery should be flushed with heparinized saline (5,000 international units per 100 mL of saline) injected into the distal arterial tree, but no heparin should be given after operation. Injuries to major concomitant veins should be repaired if possible. All vascular repairs should be covered with viable muscle, although the wound itself is left open. Stabilization of associated fractures should not create tension to a vascular anastomosis.

Under circumstances with long evacuation times, vascular repair is not always possible and appropriate, and an amputation to save life over limb can be a better option. Among 23 consecutive patients with combat wounds from the Afghan conflict treated at the ICRC hospital in Peshawar, the mean delay from injury to treatment was 34 h. The overall amputation rate was 65%, but only 22% for patients revascularized within 12 h from injury in contrast to the 93% amputation rate in patients undergoing surgery more than 12 h after injury.

## 37.10
## Abdominal Injuries

The proportion of external war wounds located in the anterior abdomen, flanks, and back is 10–20%, and the proportion of casualties with abdominal injuries is 11–14%. Small bowel, colon, and the liver are the most commonly injured organs. The ICRC wound database carries basic information of more than 25,000 war-wounded persons admitted to ICRC hospitals in different locations. Of the 7,479 patients with sufficient data, 15% had abdominal wounds, and 8% had wounds of the buttocks or pelvis. Of these, 335 had only abdominal wounds and 195 had only pelvic wounds. Of these 530 wounds, 257 (49%) did not penetrate the peritoneum or cause abdominal organ injury.

In the NGO environment, a substantial number of patients with abdominal injuries may arrive relatively late, even days after the injury. Among the 70 patients undergoing laparotomy for abdominal trauma in the ICRC hospital in Kabul from 1989 to 1990, 48 patients arrived within 12 h from injury, and the remaining 22 arrived 1–4 days later.

The value of mandatory laparotomy for all abdominal casualties can be questioned when some of the patients arrive several days after injury, resulting in natural triage with the more severely injured unlikely to reach the hospital alive. Among 17 patients with abdominal injuries treated at the ICRC hospital in Quetta in 1985, 12 were managed operatively, most of them suffering from intestinal perforations and operated on within 48 h from the injury. In five patients (29%), penetrating foreign bodies could be demonstrated radiologically to be intraperitoneal. As these injuries were several days old and the patients had no clinical signs of continuous bleeding or infection, they were managed nonoperatively with good results.

Experience from another ICRC hospital at the Thai–Cambodian border showed that when the influx of wounded overwhelms the capacity for timely surgical management of all patients, those with severe injuries and little chance of survival, such as severe thoracoabdominal injuries requiring thoracolaparotomy (Fig. 37.4) should not have priority unless several surgical teams are available and one team can be sequestered for several hours in an attempt to save some of these patients.

It is of note, however, that even under the most primitive circumstances such as described by De Wind from an Ugandan mission hospital, good results can be achieved with determined efforts. Out of 19 patients with penetrating abdominal and/or thoracic injuries, only two patients (11%) died; one from irreversible shock due to extensive blood loss and the other from multiple intestinal perforations and extensive contamination leading to death on the operating table.

In summarizing his extensive experience from treating abdominal war wounds in ten ICRC hospitals, Robin Coupland concluded:

(a)  assuming competent surgical care, energy transfer from the missile to tissue is the most important factor determining the mortality associated with abdominal war wounds.

(b)  outside a conventional military context, the focus of surgical resource and competence should always be on the majority with intestinal perforation only, who need surgery to save life but not necessarily on an urgent basis and who have a good chance of survival.

(c)  in modern wars, civilian casualties predominate and military forces are likely to be used in a United Nations context, and the wounded cannot travel along a conventional chain of evacuation.

(d)  a surgeon receiving wounded who have had a front-line laparotomy where the level of surgical competence or ethics is in doubt, should consider a routine second-look laparotomy to prevent death for those who have been subjected to an incompetent laparotomy and who have not yet become seriously ill through prolonged sepsis.[6]

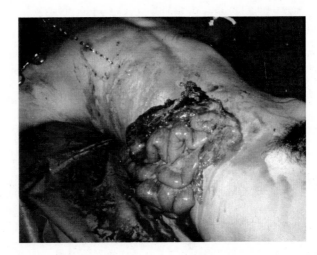

**Fig. 37.4** A soldier with multiple intrathoracic and intra-abdominal organ injuries (after detonating a mine with a jeep), exsanguinating on the operating table (Khao-I-Dang, Thailand)

A midline laparotomy incision is widely used due to its speed, wide exposure, and flexibility. The general conduct of trauma laparotomy depends on the surgeon's experience and preferences and should always be conducted with the time factor and overall triage situation in mind. Upon entry into the abdomen, all four quadrants should be rapidly packed to control bleeding. The importance of reducing blood loss and the need of blood transfusions while working under austere conditions can not be overemphasized. After packing, all four quadrants should be rapidly inspected for ongoing major hemorrhage. Once all major sites of hemorrhage have been identified, they should be controlled. Bleeding from venous injuries, which can initially be overlooked, can usually be controlled by packing, allowing time for volume restoration. This is also true of many arterial injuries and injuries of the liver.

After controlling major hemorrhage, gross contamination from hollow viscus injury is prevented by closing bowel injuries temporarily with clamps or sutures. Careful inspection of the small bowel and the colon, including mobilization of the retroperitoneal portions of the colon, should be performed.

After major bleeding and gross contamination have been taken care of, the abdomen can be examined in greater detail one quadrant at a time, not forgetting the lesser sac and rectum. All injured organs are repaired and the abdominal cavity is irrigated with warm saline and closed with a single-layer mass closure. Skin is closed separately; grossly contaminated skin incision wounds should be left open (see Chaps. 23 and 29).

The techniques of individual organ repair are summarized below. Under field conditions, simple, quick, reliable, and established war surgical methods of organ repair should be applied. The majority of patients have multiple gastrointestinal tract perforations and relatively minor (non-bleeding) liver injuries. Among 70 patients undergoing laparotomy for abdominal trauma in the ICRC hospital in Kabul from 1989 to 1990, the most commonly injured organs were the colon and rectum (35 patients), the small bowel in 33 patients, the liver in 17 patients, and the stomach in ten patients. There were no major vascular or pancreatic injuries.

A short list of the main principles in managing individual abdominal organ injuries in the NGO environment is presented below. Obviously, the circumstances, the skill and experience of the surgeon, and the condition of the patient have to be taken into consideration during the intraoperative decision-making process.

- Liver: non-bleeding injuries need no sutures; save blood, avoid extensive procedures; careful debridement of devitalized tissue and selective hemostatic suturing or ligation of bleeders; use perihepatic tamponade for severe bleeding from multiple lacerations; use intrahepatic balloon tamponade (not suturing entry and exit holes) for bleeding through-and-through injuries; anticipate bile leak by inserting a perihepatic drain.

- Extrahepatic bile ducts: cholecystectomy for gallbladder injuries; suture repair and/or T tube drainage for partial common bile duct injuries without tissue loss; in extensive common bile duct injuries Roux-en-Y hepaticojejunostomy or with less experience, a Roux-en-Y cholecystojejunostomy or ligation of the distal common bile duct and temporary external biliary drainage with subsequent reconstruction at a later stage.
- Spleen: non-bleeding injuries need no sutures; splenectomy for severe injuries; drain the splenic bed.

- Stomach: two-layer suture closure; explore posterior wall; decompress with a nasogastric tube.
- Duodenum: Kocher mobilization, two-layer suture closure, decompress with a nasogastro-duodenal tube with extra side holes, always insert external, periduodenal drainage; for injuries with tissue loss, Roux-en-Y duodenojejunostomy; repair of extensive injuries secured with pyloric exclusion.
- Pancreas: enter lesser sac if pancreatic injury suspected, Kocher mobilization of the duodenum and head of pancreas; distal pancreatectomy with splenectomy for distal main duct injury; other injuries treated with hemostatic sutures and external drainage only.
- Small bowel: suture repair in two layers; resection and primary end-to-end anastomosis in extensive injuries with multiple closely located perforations or devascularizing injury.
- Intraperitoneal colon: excision of devitalized tissue and primary repair if colon wall looks healthy; otherwise colostomy, aim for colostomy closure within 2–4 weeks.
- Rectum: suture repair (if visible without extensive mobilization) and mandatory proximal colostomy.
- Kidney: hemostatic sutures; severe injuries require nephrectomy (confirm existence of contralateral normal-sized kidney).
- Ureter: primary repair over stent; ureteroneocystostomy for distal injuries; nephrectomy (confirm existence of contralateral normal-sized kidney) for severe renal pelvic or proximal ureteric injuries.
- Urinary bladder: two-layer suture closure with bladder decompression (transurethral or suprapubic catheter); perivesical drainage.
- Urethra: primary repair if possible; otherwise suprapubic cystostomy.
- Retroperitoneal hematoma and abdominal vascular injuries: explore a hematoma if expanding or large following penetrating injury; secure proximal and distal control of potentially injured vessels; repair vessel if possible, consider temporary shunting and planned re-operation or packing if impossible; second-look laparotomy if intestinal ischemia risk after repair.
- Diaphragm: closure in two layers with nonabsorbable sutures; treat pneumothorax.

In order to outline the most common procedures and the every day conditions in managing abdominal injuries in the NGO environment, some published reports from ICRC hospitals are summarized herein:

Of 17 patients with liver injuries treated in the ICRC hospital in Kabul, five required no surgical intervention, seven were managed with debridement and suture, and three by debridement and omental pack. Two patients exsanguinated during operation from extensive parenchymal disruption. Morris and Sugrue managed 33 small bowel and mesenteric injuries in the ICRC hospital in Kabul with suture repair, resection of the involved segment, and primary anastomosis, or combination of these two procedures without any complications.

Of 29 patients with colon injuries treated in the ICRC hospital in Kabul from 1989 to 1990, primary suture repair or resection and primary anastomosis was performed in 16 cases, including four transverse and five left-sided colon injuries, with no mortality, no abscesses, and no fistulas. A series from the ICRC hospital in Kabul during 1990 through 1992 reported 73 patients with colon injuries, of which all underwent primary repair (resection and anastomosis in 52 and suture repair in 21) with an overall mortality rate of 6%. One patient had a fecal fistula treated conservatively and one colostomy was performed as a precaution in a patient undergoing relaparotomy for intra-abdominal abscess.

Of five patients with renal injuries treated at the ICRC hospital in Kabul from 1989 to 1990, four were managed conservatively and one with a lower pole partial nephrectomy. In the ICRC hospital in Kabul, one patient with a posterior urethral injury was treated with railroading catheters, leaving urethral and suprapubic catheters in place, suturing down the prostate to the perineum, and paravesical drainage.

In the ICRC hospital in Kabul, Morris and Sugrue successfully managed three patients with injuries to the inferior mesenteric vessels by ligation, whereas two patients with injuries of the portal vein and iliac artery and vein, respectively, died.

## 37.11
### Thoracic Injuries

More than 90% of all chest injuries can be managed initially by conservative measures, including chest tubes, without thoracotomy. A properly placed chest tube is life saving and should be inserted as soon as possible. Indications for thoracotomy include massive bleeding, persistent bleeding or air leak, mediastinal injury, and major defect in the chest wall.

Entrance and exit wounds of the chest wall are excised, intercostal vascular bleeding is treated with suture ligation, and the pleura and deep muscle layer are closed to ensure an airtight seal, leaving the outer layers open for delayed primary closure.

In thoracoabdominal injuries, separate incisions should be used when possible. A chest tube should be inserted routinely in all thoracoabdominal wounds, especially those requiring laparotomy.[1]

## 37.12
### Head and Neck Injuries

A large part of penetrating ballistic head injuries are fatal, but at times low-energy bullets or fragments, especially if tangential or in the frontal lobe of the brain, can cause injuries that are not immediately fatal. The aims of surgical treatment in these injuries include evacuation of intracranial hematomas, debridement of dead brain tissue, and closure of the wounds to prevent infection.

A burr hole is placed close to the bone defect and the craniectomy is performed by enlarging the hole towards the area of damage with bone nibblers until healthy dura around the damaged part is encountered. If not opened by the missile, the dura is opened in a stellate manner; all bone fragments, accessible foreign bodies, and dead brain tissue is debrided with careful use of forceps, low-pressure suction, and irrigation. Hemostasis is secured with accurate use of cautery and other topical hemostatic measures. Watertight closure of the dura is important. If not possible, the dural defect can be closed with a fascial graft from the temporalis muscle or fascia lata. It is important to elevate the dura with sutures to the skull to prevent the formation of hematomas compressing the brain. Large depressed bone fragments should be elevated, or if removed during craniectomy, replaced in situ. The bone should be covered with skin using rotation flaps if needed. Chloramphenicol should be added to the antibiotic treatment.

A penetrating ocular injury should be suspected in every wound around the eye and upper part of the face. Unless it is obvious that disruption of the globe is total, the possibility of salvaging the eye should be considered, and every effort should be made to get the patient to an ophthalmologist, even after delay. Although rare, the development of sympathetic ophthalmia (angry red eye or the quiet iridocyclitis) after a penetrating eye injury is a real threat under difficult circumstances and requires prompt treatment. Extensive corneoscleral lacerations with either prolapse or loss of the intraocular contents require early excision of the eye by complete evisceration of the contents of the eye (Fig. 37.5).

In patients with facial wounds, establishing and securing the airway is most important, followed by control of hemorrhage (Fig. 37.6). Soft tissue injuries are carefully debrided and can usually be closed primarily including approximation of the subcutaneous tissue. Fixation of fractures with wiring requires some experience, but those of the mandible with associated soft tissue injuries are usually stabilized with external fixation.

Any penetrating neck wound deeper than the platysma requires surgical exploration, which usually is performed through an incision along the anterior border of the sternocleidomastoid muscle. Small pharyngeal or esophageal lacerations are debrided and sutured; larger injuries may require a cervical esophagostomy and closure at a later time. Small tracheal injuries can often be suture repaired, more severe injuries require a tracheostomy. In most cases, injuries to the carotid arteries require vascular repair. One-sided injuries of the internal jugular vein can be ligated.

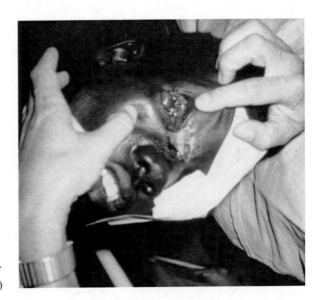

**Fig. 37.5** Penetrating eye injury leading to excision of the eye (Lokichokio, Kenya)

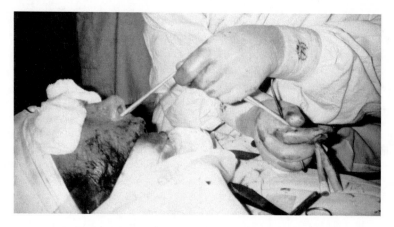

**Fig. 37.6** Mine blast injury of the face with posterior nasal hemorrhage controlled with Foley catheters and traction (Peshawar, Pakistan)

## 37.13
## Burns

Burns are not uncommonly encountered during conflicts. They require prompt correction of the hypovolemia, adequate pain control, and accurate estimation of the depth and extent of burn injury as a percentage of the total body surface. Subsequent fluid-replacement therapy calculations are based on the burn area. Under a typical NGO environment, closed treatment of the burn injury with a two-component dressing (inner dressing applying an antibacterial agent to the wound and an outer dressing absorbing the exudate and protecting the wound) is appropriate, although open treatment with topical antibacterial agents can also be used. One percent of silver sulphadiazine in a water-soluble cream base should be applied liberally to the wound and repeated twice daily. The definitive treatment includes excision of the dead tissue or eschar, followed by skin grafting.

### 37.13.1
### Postoperative Care and Casualty Transfer

Ideally, most war-wounded patients treated in the NGO hospital should undergo two operations: wound excision and other early surgery on admission and delayed primary closure about 5 days later. Unless contraindicated, patients should have normal oral intake of food started as soon as possible after the first operation. Even in patients with maxillofacial, cervical, or abdominal injuries, oral intake of liquids and subsequently food should be started as soon as possible. In unconscious patients, establishing a route for gastric or enteral feeding should be anticipated early if the patient has a favorable prognosis within a reasonable time and the hospital has other facilities to treat unconscious patients. One of the most important things in postoperative care is to avoid a vicious circle of repeated surgical interventions with the patient being nil-by-mouth every other day and rapidly getting malnourished, accompanied by poor wound healing and infectious complications, which emphasizes the importance of adequate wound surgery at the initial operation and adherence to the established principles of war surgery, especially to delayed primary closure of excised wounds and amputation stumps.

In patients with fractures treated with external fixation, the fixator can be replaced with plasters as soon as the wounds are healing, enabling the patients to be more easily discharged for further follow up. Sometimes there is no possibility to organize the follow up by local providers, and the recovery and rehabilitation phases have to be completed in the NGO system. In most cases, there are NGOs specialized in rehabilitation working in the same conflict area, and close cooperation between different agencies and organizations is of utmost importance in order to provide the patient with a best possible follow-up care available.

Although occasionally (and often with the help of the media), selected patients will be provided the opportunity for advanced reconstructive procedures abroad, most other patients with persisting postoperative problems have no place to go for more advanced treatment. Therefore, at every stage beginning with the triage and admission phases, the overall perspective has to be kept in mind and the patient's treatment planned and calibrated in a way to achieve the best possible long-term outcome in those particular circumstances. In some cases, this might require unconventional solutions and even unpleasant decisions made by the surgeon in charge of the patient's overall care, but profound understanding of surgical principles, good communication with the patient, relatives, and the hospital staff, familiarity with the available resources, measured optimism, determination, and common sense are the guidelines by which everybody working in the NGO environment can do the most good to most injured people who often have nowhere else to go.

## References

1. Dufour D, Kroman Jensen S, Owen-Smith M, Salmela J, Stening GF, Zetterström B. *Surgery for Victims of War*. Geneva: International Committee of the Red Cross; 1988.
2. Ryan J, Mahoney PF, Greaves I, Bowyer G, eds. *Conflict and Catastrophe Medicine. A Practical Guide*. London: Springer-Verlag Limited; 2002.
3. Coupland RM. Epidemiological approach to surgical management of the casualties of war. *BMJ*. 1994;308:1693-1697.
4. Coupland RM. Technical aspects of war wound excision. *Br J Surg*. 1989;76:663-667.
5. Rowley DI. The management of war wounds involving bone. *J Bone Joint Surg Br*. 1996; 78-B:706-709.
6. Coupland R. Abdominal wounds in war. *Br J Surg*. 1996;83:1505-1511.

## Further Reading

Bhatnagar MK, Smith GS. Trauma in the Afghan guerrilla war: effect of lack of access to care. *Surgery*. 1989;105:699-705.

Bowyer GW. Afghan war wounded: application of the Red Cross wound classification. *J Trauma*. 1995;38:64-67.

Bowyer GW. Management of small fragment wounds: experience from the Afghan border. *J Trauma*. 1996;40:S170-S172.

Coupland RM, Korver A. Injuries from antipersonnel mines: the experience of the International Committee of the Red Cross. *BMJ*. 1991;303:1509-1512.

Coupland RM, Samnegaard HO. Effect of type and transfer of conventional weapons on civilian injuries: retrospective analysis of prospective data from Red Cross hospitals. *BMJ*. 1999;319:410-412.

De Wind CM. War injuries treated under primitive circumstances: experiences in an Ugandan mission hospital. *Ann R Coll Surg Engl*. 1987;69:193-195.

Eshaya-Chauvin B, Coupland R. Transfusion requirements for the management of war injured: the experience of the International Committee of the Red Cross. *Br J Anaesth*. 1992;68:221-223.

Gosselin RA, Siegberg CJ, Coupland R, Agerskov K. Outcome of arterial repairs in 23 consecutive patients at the ICRC-Peshawar hospital for war wounded. *J Trauma*. 1993;34:373-376.

Huntington SP. *The Clash of Civilizations*. London: Simon & Schuster; 1997.

Husum H, Sundet M. Postinjury malaria: a study of trauma victims in Cambodia. *J Trauma*. 2002;52:259-266.

Leppäniemi A. Medical challenges of internal conflicts. *World J Surg*. 1998;22:1197-1201.

Morris D, Sugrue W. On the border of Afghanistan with the International Committee of the Red Cross. *N Z Med J*. 1985;98:750-752.

Morris DS, Sugrue WJ. Abdominal injuries in the war wounded of Afghanistan: a report from the International Committee of the Red Cross hospital in Kabul. *Br J Surg*. 1991;78:1301-1304.

Morris D. Surgeons and the International Committee of the Red Cross. *Aust N Z J Surg*. 1992;62:170-172.

Pesonen P. Pulse oximetry during ketamine anaesthesia in war conditions. *Can J Anaesth*. 1991;38:592-594.

Rautio J, Paavolainen P. Afghan war wounded: experience with 200 cases. *J Trauma*. 1988;28:523-525.

Simper LB. Below knee amputation in war surgery: a review of 111 amputations with delayed primary closure. *J Trauma*. 1993;34:96-98.

SIPRI Yearbook 2002. *Armaments, Disarmament and International Security*. Oxford: Oxford International Press; 2002.

Strada G, Raad L, Belloni G, Setti Carraro P. Large bowel perforations in war surgery: one-stage treatment in a field hospital. *J Colorectal Dis*. 1993;8:213-216.

Trouwborst A, Weber BK, Dufour D. Medical statistics of battlefield casualties. *Injury*. 1987;18:96-99.

# Part VII

## Critical Care

# Critical Care for Ballistic Trauma in Austere Environments

# 38

Christian B. Swift and Geoffrey S.F. Ling

*The opinions or assertions contained herein are the private views of the authors and are not to be construed as official or as reflecting the views of the Uniformed Services University, Department of the Army or the Department of Defense.*

## 38.1
## Introduction

Clearly recent wars and natural disasters have provided new insight on delivering critical care medicine in austere environments. Recent literature reviews and anecdotal experiences from clinicians providing care under such conditions support the view that sophisticated critical care can be provided worldwide even where advanced infrastructure with sophisticated technology is unavailable. While the orientation of this chapter is focused on deployed military settings, it could certainly be adapted for use in a civilian setting during periods of disaster management, catastrophes, and other incidents of mass casualty critical care (Fig. 38.1).

A collective review of current literature and anecdotal experience suggest that the fundamentals of successful critical care medicine in austere environments include: proper planning, careful management of resources, proper equipment, early evacuation of casualties, adherence to quality indicators, and employing the right people with the right skills through the use of an intensivist directed team model.[1-3] Furthermore, there is also the opportunity to advance clinical care by proper medical record keeping and properly conducting scientific research.

C.B. Swift (✉)
Internal Medicine Division, Department of Medicine, Madigan Army Medical Center, Tacoma, WA, USA
e-mail: christian.swift@amedd.army.mil

A.J. Brooks et al. (eds.), *Ryan's Ballistic Trauma*,
DOI: 10.1007/978-1-84882-124-8_38, © Springer-Verlag London Limited 2011

**Fig. 38.1** Critical Care, Camp
Bastion Afghanistan 2009

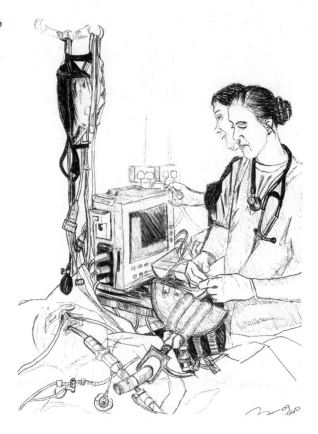

## 38.2
## Organizational Framework

US military organizations provide an excellent organizational framework to discuss the employment and delivery of critical care in austere environments. It is important to briefly review the echelons (levels) of care in US military medical care to understand the complexity and practicality of delivering critical care in the austere environment. US military medical care is divided into five echelons of care. Echelon I care is delivered on the battlefield, with care by the medic, a buddy or to oneself. Echelon 2 is the battalion aid station where a physician is located. A recent addition to Echelon 2 is the forward surgical team (FST). Echelon 3 is a combat support hospital. Presently, it is the highest level of care available in theater. Echelon 4 is an in-theater medical facility analogous to a modern full service medical center. Echelon 5 is a US based medical center.

The first critical care assets are found at Echelon 2 FSTs. FSTs primarily provide emergency life saving resuscitation and stabilization and are highly dependent upon rapid patient evacuation as a result of limited resources and personnel.[1] It is impractical to expect prolonged critical care at this echelon. Thus, to be effective, there must be adequate transportation assets to enable patients to be evacuated to a higher echelon of care. The Echelon III

CSH, however, provides advanced hospital level care to patients suffering from a wide variety of illness and at all severity levels. With medical resupply the CSH can indefinitely sustain care.[4] Importantly, CSHs are capable of providing more definitive care to include specialized surgery, such as cardiothoracic, vascular, burn, neurosurgery, etc. Because of this, critical care becomes especially important as the eventual level of clinical outcome depends not only on operative treatment but post-operative as well. Minimal organizational capabilities contained within the Echelon III facility include: command & control, security, communications, patient administration, nutritional care, supply and services, triage, emergency medical treatment, preoperative care, orthopedics, general surgery, operating rooms and central materiel and supply services, anesthesia, nursing services (to include intensive and intermediate care wards), pharmacy, clinical laboratory and blood banking, and radiology services.[4] Echelon III facilities represent the highest level of US military medical care in the forward deployed setting. As the CSH provides the necessary infrastructure for optimal critical care medicine, it will therefore be the focus of discussion for this chapter.

The US Army's delivery of critical care medicine has evolved and improved significantly from lessons learned in recent conflicts. Under current Medical Reengineering Initiatives (MRI), the US Army has re-designed their primary Echelon III facility, the Combat Support Hospital (CSH) into a more modular design that can be adapted to meet the needs of providing critical care in nearly any environment.[4] Per doctrine, the modular level III CSH can provide hospitalization for up to 84 patients (including 24 ICU patients) and provide 36 operating table hours (based on two OR tables) per day.[4] With its modular design, the CSH can be augmented with specialty teams, increased OR and inpatient capacity, etc. Within each 12-bed ICU, 24-h care is provided by a staff that includes: a head nurse, a wardmaster, clinical nurses, practical nurses, and respiratory therapists.[1] Because of the massive logistical coordination of personnel and equipment, a CSH can be ready to deploy to almost any austere environment within 72 h of validation.[4] Once in the austere environment, it generally takes 72 h to erect a stand-alone CSH that is complete and ready for operations, though components of the CSH such as the Emergency Room, OR, and ICU may be functional prior to the 72 h window.[4]

According to the US Army Field Manual (FM) 4–02.10, in reference to the CSH, "The ICUs (Intensive Care Units) manage surgical or medical patients, adult and/or pediatric, whose physiological status is so disrupted that they require immediate and continuous medical and/or nursing care. The staff is specially trained with the clinical and managerial skills necessary to deliver safe nursing care to patients with complex nursing and medical problems. The ICUs are also used as a preoperative stabilization area and post anesthesia recovery area for patients either awaiting surgery or recovering from surgery."[4]

## 38.3
## Organizational Characteristics

Grathwohl and Venticinque, 2008, determined the organizational characteristics of the intensive care unit in a CSH are imperative to improving outcomes and survival of critically injured patients.[2] From anecdotal experience and published literature, the intensivist-directed intensive

**Table 38.1** Intensivist-directed intensive care unit team (IDT)

| Specialty |
|---|
| 1. Critical care physician |
| 2. Rotating internist (nephrologist, cardiologist, etc. with experience in critical care) |
| 3. Staff surgeons |
| 4. Critical care nurses |
| 5. Respiratory therapist |
| 6. Dietician |
| 7. Discharge planning/patient evacuation representative |

care unit team (IDT) represents the most successful organizational model. The intensivist-directed intensive care unit team includes: a critical care physician, rotating internist (nephrologist or cardiologist with experience in critical care medicine), staff surgeon, critical care nurses, respiratory therapists, and various sub-specialists and ancillary staff[2] (see Table 38.1). The IDT team participates in daily multi-disciplinary rounds on all ICU patients, establishes daily patient goals, and provides continuous bedside management. From CSH ICU data, using the IDT model results in a significant reduction in mortality, decreased length of stay, and decreased resource utilization when compared to models using consultant intensivists or models without trained intensivists.[2] As a result of these findings, intensivists now deploy to CSHs in Iraq and Afghanistan to direct ICU teams and 2 intensivists are expected to be added to the organizational model of the US Army CSH under the next medical re-engineering initiative.[2]

From our experience of providing critical care at a US Army CSH deployed to Baghdad Iraq from 2005 to 2006, the IDT model worked exceptionally well. Involving more hospital staff during the a.m. multi-disciplinary ICU rounds made some improvements to the model discussed by Grathwohl and Venticinque. The theme from our experience seemed to be "the more the merrier." The halls of the ICUs were crowded with specialty surgeons (trauma, critical care, cardio-thoracic, urology, GYN, etc.), internists, anesthesiologists, nursing administration, discharge and patient transfer planners, patient administration personnel, dietary, chaplain, psychiatry, and many more. Patient progress, management, transfer, evacuation and ethical concerns were discussed in an open forum mediated by the hospital Deputy Commander for Clinical Services (DCCS). Everyone had input into the discussion and a consensus was always established based on a variety of resource limiting factors unique to the deployed ICU environment. The IDT team then managed the ICU patients according to the mutually established goals.

## 38.4
## Proper Planning

Traditional disaster preparedness (for mass critical care) focuses on rescue, stabilization, and transfer to a fixed facility with robust critical care capabilities.[1] This is not only impractical, but also unlikely to be possible in most mass-critical care cases, i.e. major disasters, acts of terrorism, etc. Many circumstances will most certainly necessitate the need for sustained critical care away from the traditional hospital setting.[1] It is likely that critical care services, either sustained or along transfer points will need to be provided in remote or field hospital settings.[1] A review of the literature and established initiatives by the US military and US National Disaster Medical System (NDMS) highlight the need to prepare and plan for a mobile field hospital, which is rapidly deployable.[1]

Venticinque and Grathwohl (2008) reviewed the lessons learned by critical care clinicians during recent disaster relief efforts and military operations and shed new light on important preparation considerations. A frequently encountered problem is the volume of patients with unexpected and concurrent medical conditions, as well as pediatric and obstetric issues.[1] From our experience, we routinely took care of patients that fell outside of the expected norm of a CSH operating in support of combat military operations. A majority of our patients were Iraqi civilians of all ages with a variety of penetrating and explosives related injuries. We also routinely took care of Iraqi civilians with a broad range of medical problems and often received patient transfers from Iraqi hospitals with surgical complications and sepsis. We also admitted a significant number of patients (Iraqi, US military and contractors) with the diagnosis of acute myocardial infarction (MI). When planning to provide critical care in austere and field hospital conditions one should be prepared to treat all types of trauma and a broad range of medical conditions, many of which may be outside of one's normal scope of practice. Significant emphasis must be placed on coordination of personnel, equipment, and supplies with the expectation that a fair amount of creativity and flexibility will be necessary for frequent problem solving.[1] Venticinque and Grathwohl summarize preparatory guidance noting that "comprehensive pre-disaster planning and logistic details are paramount" to success in these trying circumstances.[1]

One important planning consideration that needs highlighting is to minimize reliance upon locally provided electrical power. This is best accomplished through use of portable generators and back-up battery resources.[1] We had the good fortune to have both 110 V and 220 V generators and back-up generators, which powered the entire combat support hospital and support facilities. We seldom lost power and had enough backup generators and battery back up in all of our electronic medical equipment such that loss of power was never an issue. It may also be helpful to have transport ventilators available as back-up in the event of a prolonged power outage as ventilators are notoriously bad energy consumers.

Critical care preparation usually fits into the logistical considerations of the larger facility to which it is attached.[1] We were fortunate to have many of our logistical details taken care of by logistical planning staff, leaving us with only individual and unit-specific logistical concerns. Common considerations usually taken into account by logistical planning staffs include: power, O2, climate control, communications, sanitation, lodging, water, food, resupply, security, and an effective evacuation/aero-medical evacuation plan.[1] Items we found helpful that may be overlooked by the logistical planning staff include: hand sanitizer, portable pulse oxymetry probes, moveable endotracheal tube securing devices, oral care kits, variety of blood pressure cuff sizes, portable doppler, penlights, pneumatic compression devices, and enteral feeding pumps.

Although critical care can safely be provided for prolonged periods in the austere and field hospital environment, it is generally accepted that rapid evacuation to definitive care improves patient outcomes, decompresses bed space, and minimizes remote and field hospital ICU resource utilization.[1] We were fortunate to have a well-established aero-medical evacuation system and could reliably and routinely evacuate US military patients within 2 days. Our most significant difficulty was with transferring Iraqi military and civilian patients to local Iraqi medical facilities. We could not safely transfer these patients until they met basic clinical stability guidelines or we simply did not have adequate bed space or resources to properly care for them. Generally, to be stable for transfer, patients were: hemodynamically stable in the absence of vasopressors, had a "closed" abdomen, and were spontaneously breathing with a natural airway or tracheotomy tube. We would occasionally send patients with tracheotomies requiring temporary mechanical ventilator support to Iraqi medical facilities with a portable ventilator. We were also fortunate to have an Iraqi patient liaison working with us who would coordinate patient transfers to Iraqi medical facilities. From our experience, it is vital to establish a patient transfer agreement with area medical facilities to free up bed space and minimize resource utilization.

Proper training is obviously vital to delivering critical care in the austere environment. Critical care teams should train together on a regular basis to prepare for the variety of conditions they may encounter. It is impractical to believe that every member of the ICU team has received formal critical care training or works in critical care on a regular basis. It is therefore imperative that critical care practical and didactic team-oriented training with an emphasis on roles be offered on a continuous basis and be updated with lessons learned and evidence based practice recommendations. Knowing what skills and competencies to train for is highly variable depending on the environment the critical care team will work in. The 2008 article by Smith examines the major skill and cognitive competencies for deployed ICU nurses based on experiences from Operation Iraqi Freedom. Additionally, the competencies discussed by Smith have far reaching applications for critical care team members working in any remote critical care environment. Although the focus is on competencies for nurses, there is a broader application to the entire ICU team, including the physician managing the care and the respiratory therapist providing respiratory support. Although not all-inclusive, the competencies identified by Smith (see Tables 38.2 and 38.3) will serve as an excellent

**Table 38.2** Top ten cognitive competencies for the intensive care unit team[3]

1. Trauma triad of death
   (a) Acidosis
   (b) Coagulopathy
   (c) Hypothermia

2. Damage control resuscitation (end points of resuscitation, massive transfusion, postoperative damage control stabilization)

3. Critical care medications: (fentanyl, norepinephrine, dobutamine, epinephrine, hypertonic saline, mannitol, propofol, insulin, vasopressin, phenyephrine)

4. Managing neurotrauma (traumatic brain injury/spinal cord injury)
   (a) Preventing secondary brain injury
   (b) Intracranial pressure/cerebral perfusion pressure monitoring
   (c) Hypertonic saline management

**Table 38.2** (continued)

5. Ventilator management
   (a) Airway pressure release ventilation/inverse ratio
   (b) Transport ventilators
   (c) Arterial blood gas analysis
   (d) Ventilator liberation techniques/weaning
   (e) Pulmonary complications: inhalation injury, pulmonary contusion, acute respiratory distress syndrome/acute kidney injury/transfusion-related acute lung injury

6. En route care of ICU patient via rotary wing transport or ground ambulance transfer

7. Burn management
   (a) Assessing depth and% total body surface area of burn
   (b) Initial fluid resuscitation with correct documentation
   (c) Types of wound care and debridement techniques
   (d) Metabolic and temperature regulation

8. Advanced Assessment: minimally invasive hemodynamic monitoring, basic FAST and CXR interpretation, and tertiary survey

9. Post-anesthesia recovery

10. ICU quality indicators

Note the original table developed by Smith[3] has been modified to apply to the critical care team and has been abbreviated

**Table 38.3** Top ten skill competencies for the intensive care unit team[3]

1. Complex wound care management
   (a) Large soft tissue, disarticulations, amputations, fasciotomies, open abdomens, osteomies, and care of vacuum-assisted closure devices
   (b) Ankle-brachial indexing and assessing for compartment syndrome

2. Perform massive transfusion using Belmont or Level I rapid infuser

3. Monitor/manage intracranial pressure/cerebral perfusion pressure

4. Use portable monitors: cardiac, blood pressure lines, pulse oximetry, end-tidal CO2

5. Manage airway
   (a) Assist/perform endotracheal intubation/emergency surgical airway
   (b) Perform cricoid pressure/Sellick maneuver
   (c) Perform nasotracheal/endotracheal/tracheal suction
   (d) Perform tracheostomy care

6. Facilitate breathing
   (a) Perform ventilation using bag valve mask/ambu bag/positive pressure ventilation
   (b) Assist/perform chest tube (CT) insertion, manage CT drainage systems
   (c) Perform needle thoracotomy

7. Assist with emergency resuscitative procedures: thoracotomy, celiotomy

8. Monitor intra-abdominal pressure

(continued)

**Table 38.3** (continued)

| |
|---|
| 9. Package the patient on a litter for aero-medical/ground transport portable ventilator, suction apparatus, monitor, triple channel intravenous pumps, and other as needed transport equipment or supplies |
| 10. Routine ICU care and monitoring |

Note the original table developed by Smith[3] has been modified to apply to the critical care team and has been abbreviated

framework for developing a training plan for the critical care team and also for personal review.[3] It is significant to note that training should also focus on delivering en route critical care in fixed wing, rotary wing, and ground medical transport assets as members of the critical care team will likely be expected to accompany their patients during transfers.

## 38.5
## Equipment

All equipment utilized in the austere ICU must go through rigorous testing to ensure that it can function properly in a variety of extreme conditions. The Defense Medical Standardization Board (DMSB) develops and recommends criterion for consideration of new equipment that will be utilized by Department of Defense (DoD) medical assets (R. Morton, January 2009, Tripler Army Medical Center, personal communication). Table 38.4

**Table 38.4** CSH standard ICU equipment list[5]

| |
|---|
| 1. Blanket hypothermia |
| 2. Cleaner vacuum electric |
| 3. Defibrillator monitor recorder system |
| 4. Fluid warming system |
| 5. Generator oxygen medical system POGS |
| 6. Illuminator X-ray film |
| 7. Laryngoscope set |
| 8. Light floor LS-150 |
| 9. Light head general |
| 10. Light surgical field unit |
| 11. Monitor patient vital |
| 12. Otoscope & ophthalmoscope set |
| 13. Oximeter pulse finger |
| 14. Panel electrical distribution |

**Table 38.4**  (continued)

| |
| --- |
| 15. Patient warming system kit |
| 16. Pump intravenous infusion |
| 17. Refrigerator-freezer |
| 18. Resuscitation kit, mouth |
| 19. Sink unit surgical scrub |
| 20. Stimulator peripheral nerve |
| 21. Suction apparatus surgical programmable |
| 22. Table folding legs |
| 23. Thermometer kit clinical |
| 24. Ultrasonic unit, blood |
| 25. Ventilator volume portable |
| 26. Vital signs monitor |

provides a standard equipment list for an Army Combat Support Hospital intensive care unit.[5] For more detailed equipment information including technical data and model number information, visit the US Army Medical Material Agency (USAMMA) website at: http://www.usamma.army.mil/tara/med_equip_hdbk_index.cfm and select UA N309 Medical Material Set Post OP ICU Ward. The equipment list is current as of December 2008, and is updated frequently; check the index page for the most current information and additional durable and expendable medical equipment necessary for austere ICU operations.

The picture in Fig. 38.2 shows a typical ICU/trauma resuscitation bed set-up. This photo shows an example of how an ICU bed may be set up using standard equipment in a building/space of opportunity. A fair amount of creativity will be necessary when utilizing

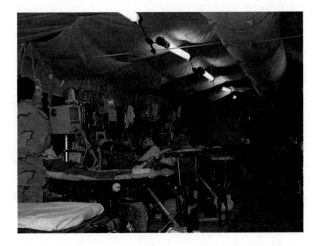

**Fig. 38.2**  A typical ICU/ trauma resuscitation bed set-up

whatever tent or building of opportunity space you have to work with to maximize workspace while simultaneously keeping equipment and supplies nearby.

## 38.6
## Adherence to Quality Indicators

Whenever possible, the general rule should be to follow the same routine ICU standards of care you would be held accountable to in a fixed medical facility with modern critical care capabilities.[1] Obviously modifications to routine practice standards will need to be made when considering such factors as: supply and equipment availability, triage decisions, environmental considerations, personnel availability, safety concerns, etc.[1] Venticinque and Grathwohl (2008) created a quality care checklist for the austere ICU that mirrors routine standards of care (see Table 38.5). The checklist provides a practical and reasonable solution to guide ICU care in the austere environment and should be checked against each

**Table 38.5** Quality care checklist for the austere ICU[1]

| |
| --- |
| • Infection control<br>  Strict adherence to hand hygiene?<br>  Field-placed venous access lines changed?<br>  Assess need for current central venous access?<br>  Appropriate antibiotics? |
| • Ventilated patients<br>  Head-of-bed elevation?<br>  Acute respiratory distress syndrome net<br>  protocol indicated/employed?<br>  Oral care protocol?<br>  Systematic ventilator liberation efforts?<br>  Sedation and analgesia protocol?<br>  Is paralysis justified?<br>  Measures to prevent skin breakdown? |
| • Deep vein thrombosis prophylaxis optimized? |
| • Stress ulcer prophylaxis required? |
| • Beta-blockade for patients with appropriate risk factors? |
| • Glycemic control best and safest for circumstance? |
| • Pain management<br>  Pain well controlled?<br>  Candidate for regional anesthesia? |
| • Trauma patients<br>  Traumatic brain injury guidelines followed?<br>  Tertiary survey completed? |

**Table 38.5** (continued)

| |
|---|
| • Nutrition optimization? |
| • Candidate for evacuation?<br>  Safe for transport?<br>  Air evacuation arrangements?<br>  Records ready? |

patient in the austere ICU every day. From our experience, adherence to ICU standards of care under the direction of an IDT was crucial in preventing common ICU complications.

## 38.7
## Research

To optimize the ability of busy clinicians to conduct research and ensure scientific rigor, the US Army and Air Force jointly established research teams at the CSHs. The team director is a physician with research experience. The co-director is a nurse with a PhD and is supported by research nurses and laboratory specialists. In 2006, the first research team was assigned to the Baghdad CSH in Iraq. Shortly thereafter, another research team was placed at the Balad CSH. It is anticipated that a similar team will be established soon at the Bagram CSH in Afghanistan. A human use institutional review board (HUC/IRB) at the Army Institute of Surgical Research (AISR) at Brooke Army Medical Center provides regulatory oversight and is the approval authority for appropriately designed clinical studies. The overall effort is managed by the AISR. This has enabled a number of research studies to be conducted. Most notably are those on the efficacy of tourniquets for traumatic amputation, factor VIIa for uncontrolled hemorrhage, early vascular surgical intervention and the benefit of 1:1 resuscitation with red blood cells: plasma (A. McClinton, January 2009, Army Institute of Surgical Research, personal communication; V. Thurmond, January 2009, Defense Center of Excellence for Psychological Health and Traumatic Brain Injury, personal communication).

## 38.8
## Database

An important aspect of clinical care is proper record keeping. Whenever realistically possible, records must be complete and compliant with patient privacy regulations, such the Health Insurance and Portability Act (HIPA). A well established database is an important element in optimizing patient care. This database also enables research to improve critical care delivery. Examples of the types of research that can and should be done are epidemiological, outcome, length of stay, etc. The database for OIF and OEF is the Joint Theater Trauma Registry (JTTR). For the Navy medicine, there is the Navy-Marine Casualty database.

The JTTR was initiated in 2002 as a demonstration. At the end of 2003, the JTTR was deployed to the war theaters. Very shortly thereafter, a JTTR team was created. It was led by a trauma surgeon supported by a small cadre of nurses. Their initial task was to begin populating the JTTR with records already available and to develop an enduring data entry system. Importantly, this effort was encouraged by the highest level of the Dept. of Defense, who mandated that all clinical records were to be integrated into this single database. This includes both physician and nursing records. To maintain relevance, a separate team led by a trauma registry expert was assigned to continually review the JTTR and improve it. At present, version 3 is active as this is the third software upgrade. A performance team led by another trauma surgeon was created to measure performance indicators, including long term patient outcomes. Thus, the entirety of each patient's clinical course is captured, including clinical care from point of injury through the echelons of care to discharge from the military medical system. In 2008, the JTTR was officially made operational (M. Spott, Army Institute of Surgical Research, personal communication, Jan, 2009; V. Thurmond, Defense Center of Excellence for Psychological Health and Traumatic Brain Injury, personal communication, Jan, 2009).

## 38.9
## Summary

Indeed high quality critical care medicine can be provided in the austere environment. Adherence to the fundamentals of austere critical care (proper planning and training, careful management of resources and equipment, early evacuation of casualties, adherence to quality indicators, and use of an intensivist directed team model) will optimize the austere ICU team's chance of success in any austere environment. The employment of research teams and sophisticated database systems in the austere ICU environment will continue to improve critical care outcomes in the austere ICU and provide planning guidance for future deployment of ICU teams to austere locations around the world.

## References

1. Venticinque SG, Grathwohl KW. Critical care in the austere environment: providing exceptional care in unusual places. *Crit Care Med.* 2008;36:S284-S292.
2. Grathwohl KW, Venticinque SG. Organizational characteristics of the austere intensive care unit: the evolution of military trauma and critical care medicine; applications for civilian medical care systems. *Crit Care Med.* 2008;36:S275-S283.
3. Smith KK. Critical care nursing in an austere environment. *Crit Care Med.* 2008;36:S297-S303.
4. Department of the Army, FM 4-02.10, Theater Hospitalization. Washington, DC: Government Printing Office. January; 2005.
5. US Army Medical Material Agency. UA N309, Medical Material Set Post OP ICU Ward, Fort Detrick, MD: US Army Medical Material Agency Equipment Publications Division. December; 2008.

# Transfer and Evacuation

**39**

Robert D. Tipping and Jonathan Vollam

Evacuation of a casualty starts from the point of wounding and ends with arrival at a definitive care facility. This is usually achieved by a sequence of transfers, with staging stops at intermediate care facilities where interventions may or may not be required. The most critically injured patients will require immediate lifesaving interventions, followed by evacuation to a facility where surgery to limit further injury may be performed. After a period of stabilization, onward transport to a definitive care unit will be required. These transfers are often time constrained since staff and transport resources, may be limited and once it has been decided that a casualty cannot be returned to his unit in the operational theater within a short time frame, there is no value, either to the patient or to the chain of command in keeping him in a forward location.

The operational area can be divided into three areas: forward, tactical, and strategic. The forward area contains the location of the original incident causing injury. Evacuation in this area may be under fire and is sporadic in nature, requiring rapid deployment of assets, which need to be almost instantly available to the chain of command. Depending on the distances involved, the terrain to be crossed, and the availability of assets, evacuation by road or air may be required. Initial evacuation may even be by foot, with the injured casualty being carried from point of wounding to the point of initial medical care.

The tactical area contains the forward area and involves those parts of the operational theater controlled by local commanders. Evacuation within this area frequently makes use of air assets, usually rotary wing although fixed wing aircraft may also be used for longer distance transfers. These transfers are generally slightly less time pressured and while capabilities will need to be rapidly available, crews will not require such an immediate state of readiness as those covering the forward areas. The control of assets in both the forward and tactical areas is frequently combined.

The strategic area is that part which is under the command of senior commanders in the country of origin. Transport within this area is almost universally by fixed wing air assets due to the distances involved. These transfers are also less time pressured but due to the length of time to get from the point of departure to where the casualty is, relatively high states of readiness are often required.

R.D. Tipping (✉)
Department of Anaesthetics and Critical Care, Royal Centre for Defence Medicine,
Birmingham, UK
e-mail: bobtipping@me.com, 489tippi@armymail.mod.uk

A.J. Brooks et al. (eds.), *Ryan's Ballistic Trauma*,
DOI: 10.1007/978-1-84882-124-8_39, © Springer-Verlag London Limited 2011

The decision as to which assets to use will be guided by their availability and the patients' needs; however, the terrain often limits the usefulness of ground assets and requires the use of air assets. In Afghanistan particularly, the mountainous nature of the terrain and the lack of metalled roads mean that road vehicles are limited in the speeds they can maintain and the level of comfort for the casualty is poor. Additionally, the distance from the likely point of wounding to the primary receiving hospital is considerable and so primary helicopter evacuation is frequently employed to reduce delays in advanced treatment.

The runway conditions at primary receiving hospitals are often poor with relatively short runways made of compacted earth, rocks, and sand. These runways are not suitable for most fixed wing aircraft and so it may be necessary to move a casualty to a more suitable airfield (with a long, tarmac runway) before transfer back to the country of origin. This will almost inevitably require another air transfer, using rotary wing assets.

The medical team accompanying these transfers will vary according to the level of dependency of the patient and the transfer times involved. Critically injured casualties will require full intensive care unit (ICU) – level care throughout their flight and this is usually accomplished by the use of specially trained and equipped teams. Within the UK military sphere, this role is performed by the Critical Care Air Support Teams (CCASTs) of the Royal Air Force (RAF) (Fig. 39.1). These teams will be described later in this chapter. Other countries have similar arrangements.

Patients with particular medical needs may require transfer for specialist interventions or advanced investigations not available in the primary receiving hospital. These patients

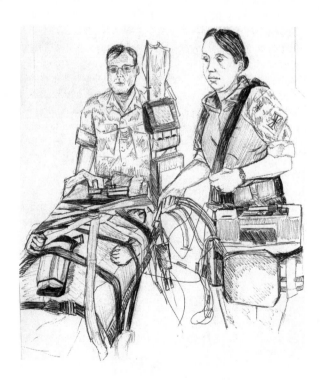

**Fig. 39.1** CCAST

are frequently critically ill and a CCAST level of care is required. Transfer may be to other medical units within the tactical area or outside the theater of operations to other countries with which the military may have arrangements (for example, neurosurgery). Transfers within the tactical environment may also be required to create space for actual or anticipated admissions. A lack of available hospital beds for possible casualties may lead to the undesirable postponement or cancelation of military operations. Where possible, patients should be transferred back to their country of origin. Some nations without specialist transfer teams have arrangements with coalition partners for the evacuation of their wounded so a CCAST may be required to transport a non-UK casualty to the patient's own country of origin.

## 39.1
## Transfer by Land

As can be seen from the preceding section, this is normally undertaken for short distances. Historically, land transport has been the primary method of evacuation but the larger distances and terrain of the modern battlefield mean that air assets are more commonly used when the security situation, terrain, or weather are favorable. Battlefield ambulances (BFAs) are modified off-road vehicles (generally the Land-Rover Defender). They are generally slow and uncomfortable on rough terrain but they are relatively plentiful. Armored personnel carriers (APCs) reduce the risk of being injured by small arms fire or improvised explosive devices (IEDs). They are not specifically designed with the medical role in mind but as most of the medical equipment is easily man-portable, they can be employed in areas where the security situation precludes the use of soft-skinned, non-armored vehicles. Air assets are only rarely deployed to areas where the enemy are still being actively engaged as they may come under attack from small arms and man-portable rocket and missile launchers when landing and taking off due to their large size, slow speed, and low altitude during these phases of flight however, aircraft can be armored to increase protection.

## 39.2
## Transfer by Air

This has the advantages of height, speed, and range. While the last two of these are almost universally beneficial, the first can present problems due to variations in the patients' physiology caused by the pressure changes with altitude. Fixed wing aircraft usually require prepared ground on which to land, significantly restricting their usefulness in the forward environment. Some military aircraft such as the Lockheed C130 Hercules are capable of landing on relatively short and unmade airstrips but they still need the ground to be relatively flat and free of obstructions. Fixed wing assets are of most value in tactical and strategic transfers since they are more comfortable and faster than helicopters; in addition, their capacity allows the transport of multiple patients. They have a greater range and their altitude capability allows them to fly above weather thereby reducing turbulence. Since air is less dense at altitude, there is also less drag and they can fly faster and more fuel efficiently increasing their operational range still further.

The inherent limitations, and benefits, of rotary wing assets mean that they are of most value in the forward zone. Helicopters are relatively fast (top speed around 100–150 mph) compared with land vehicles but slow compared with fixed wing assets (300–500 mph). This increase in speed must be offset against the response time to a call for assistance. The crew need to be prepared and briefed, the airframe may require adjusting or additional equipment may need to be loaded before the aircraft is ready to perform the role. There is a finite time required for the necessary checks before, during, and after take-off. This can be reduced by using allocated aircraft for the aeromedical role but must be factored into any calculations of the response time. They are altitude limited as they cannot be pressurized thus restricting their operational ceiling to 10–14,000 ft whereas fixed wing aircraft are capable of 30,000 ft or more. The maneuverability of helicopters and their lack of requirement for a runway make them ideal for forward operations. However, depending on the airframe used, capacity may be restricted which can limit their usefulness in a mass-casualty incident, especially if a large medical team is required to manage the patients. If helicopters are to be used in the forward zone, they will also need to be defended, both by having armed troops on board and by having a defensive aids suite to counter guided weapon attack such as shoulder launched missiles. Medical aircraft may also be accompanied by offensive air assets (particularly attack helicopters) for suppression of enemy ground fire.

## 39.2.1
## Critical Care Transfers

Critically ill patients require specialist intervention and care during transfer. While a critically injured patient may be identified in the forward area, the limitations of both time and capacity in the transfer vehicle often preclude the use of specialist transfer teams in the forward area. The capabilities of these specialist teams are best used in the tactical and strategic parts of the transfer chain. Critically injured patients do need initial stabilization and resuscitation and the skills and equipment to achieve these immediate life saving interventions (e.g., management of catastrophic bleeding, control of airway – with protection of the cervical spine – breathing and circulation) are delivered by paramedics and Emergency Department nurses who can be deployed forward to the point of wounding in Medical Emergency Response Teams (MERTs). If a doctor is used in the Team then it is designated a MERT((E)nhanced). While anesthetists are used in the MERT(E) role, these teams are usually staffed by Emergency Department doctors and General Practitioners with a special interest in Pre-Hospital Care. Furthermore, critical care providers are more used to the relatively controlled environment of the intensive care unit and so their skills are most efficiently used in these areas. If secondary care specialists are to be used in the MERT role, they need considerable extra training to prepare themselves for what would otherwise be an alien environment.

Critically injured patents transferred by air are escorted by specialist teams formed from within the Critical Care cadre of medical and nursing staff. In the UK military sphere, these are drawn from the Royal Air Force and formed into Critical Care Air Support Teams (CCASTs). These teams have a core structure of:

- An intensive care trained nurse (of either Officer or Non-Commissioned Officer (NCO) rank), called a Flight Nursing Officer (FNO) or a Flight Nurse (FN) who is the Team Leader
- A flight nursing attendant (FNA) who assists with patient interventions, transfer of the patient, and administrative duties
- A medical devices technician who maintains the equipment and also provides assistance with transfer of the patient and limited interventions
- A consultant anesthetist

This core team of four personnel has the capability to transfer one critically ill patient. The team is frequently augmented with a second nurse (FNO or FN) which increases the capability of the Team to two patients. The team will also often have a FNO, FN, FNA and/or an anesthetist under training as it is essential for personnel to gain experience of the CCAST environment before being tasked to undertake unsupervised missions. This is due to the administrative and clinical complexity of such missions. This team, in addition to their core training for their speciality, also undergo specific training relevant to their mission, whether that be the specific clinical challenges of transferring a patient long distances at altitude (with the consequent effects on the patient's physiology) or the practical considerations of travel on military aircraft (evacuation, safe use of aircraft systems, safe loading of patients and equipment, Dangerous Air Cargo regulations, etc.).

## 39.3
## Equipment

Equipment used in any critical care transfer should be robust, durable, and lightweight.[1] Transferring a patient from the field environment increases these demands: transfer equipment may need to operate at greater extremes of temperature and be able to withstand ingress of water and dust.[2] The international protection (IP) code system provides a universal rating guide to assessing this ability.[3] When removed from mains electricity it must be able to continue functioning on battery power. Whilst it may be possible to use an aircraft's power supply, the user must ensure, before departure, that it interfaces with the particular aircraft, does not affect the aircraft systems and a back-up system is in place. The RAF CCAST teams have a policy of running all equipment on batteries to ensure independence from aircraft power supplies. Any medical electrical equipment has the potential to create electromagnetic interference (EMI): the effect on the normal function of another piece of equipment in its proximity due to electrical or magnetic emissions transmitted from it. Similarly, the medical transfer equipment might be prone to interference from other nearby equipment including that integral to the aircraft, a problem of electromagnetic compatibility (EMC). This phenomenon is not limited to just the equipment itself; power cables can also radiate emissions and act as aerials.[2] All equipment must go though a period of airworthiness testing to ensure that any interference is identified and steps taken to remove this (for example, with shielding).

### 39.3.1
### Monitoring[1]

The minimum standards required for any transfer should be:

- Continuous presence of appropriately trained staff
- EKG
- Non-invasive blood pressure
- Arterial oxygen saturation
- End tidal carbon dioxide (EtCO$_2$) in ventilated patients
- Temperature

Whilst these standards are not disputed, it must be recognized that the aeromedical transfer environment creates its own specific difficulties. As well as the potential EMC effects described above, other environmental effects may have an impact. Although appropriately trained staff provide constant monitoring through observation, aircraft noise and vibration often make palpation and auscultation impossible; looking for color changes and changes to respiratory patterns become more challenging in poor lighting; and even the attendants' ability to hear audible alarms on equipment is compromised.[2] EKG, pulse-oximetry, and non-invasive blood pressures can be prone to artifact from aircraft movement and vibration, potentially activating alarms inappropriately, and paradoxically requiring attendants to rely on already hard-to-determine clinical signs.[2]

Many strategic aeromedical transfers are much longer that those experienced by road, indeed they will often be supplemented by road transfers in order for the patient to reach the departure airhead and move from the arrival airhead to receiving hospital. Transfer times for Royal Air Force CCAST transfers are often in excess of 10 h. Given these extended transfer times and the problems described above, there is a requirement for additional monitoring. Invasive blood pressure monitoring using a transduced indwelling arterial cannula is strongly advised; it negates some of the difficulties encountered by artifact on non-invasive monitoring and allows for arterial blood gas analysis. Notwithstanding EtCO$_2$ monitoring and pulse oximetry, blood gas analysis remains the gold standard.[2] It also has the added benefit of providing supplementary clinical data such as basic biochemistry. Hand held analysers are available on the market and should be seen as essential on transfers more than a few hours long. Central venous cannulation is required for administration of inotropes and can be transduced to provide clinical data in the form of central venous pressure. If not already provided from blood gas analysis, blood glucose analysis is simple to carry out using either a visual color coded strip, or more accurately with a small, handheld digital analyser.

Ideally, monitors should be able to measure and display EKG, pulse oximetry, non-invasive blood pressure, up to three invasive pressures, capnography, and temperature.[1] The result is the monitors' ever increasing demand for electrical power; capnography and non-invasive blood pressure place particularly high demands.[2]

## 39.3.2
## Batteries

As stated, RAF CCAST advocates and operates self-sufficiently in terms of electrical power; this limits the issues of EMI and EMC cited above and means that they do not rely on any external power source, which could be difficult to guarantee. This self-sufficiency, along with the requirement that equipment be lightweight, means that the type of batteries utilized is significant; the battery will largely determine the size and weight of any device, and its duration of function. When calculating the electrical (and therefore battery) power it should be anticipated that there will be delays, such as to aircraft departures, arrivals, and even emergency diversions. Secondary, or rechargeable, batteries are more commonly used especially in larger pieces of equipment with higher energy requirements such as patient monitors and ventilators. Smaller items of equipment may be designed to operate on primary, or disposable batteries and can operate for many hours. They are, however, usually less mission critical, have relatively low energy requirements and can usually be relied on to last many hours more than the transfer requires.

Rechargeable battery technology has advanced significantly in the last couple of decades, thanks largely to the popularity of personal electronic devices such as laptops and mobile phones. Improvements have in turn enhanced the capability of medical transfer equipment. The main battery options commonly available are lead-acid, nickel cadmium (NiCd), nickel metal hydride (NiMH), and lithium-ion (Li-ion), each with their own particular advantages and disadvantages. A principle consideration is that of weight and size, both for ease of movement on the ground with the patient and in reducing the "footprint" onboard the aircraft. For batteries, this is described in terms of energy density: the stored energy per unit mass or volume.[4]

The batteries with the highest energy density are Li-ion, commonly used in laptops. These would seem ideal as they provide a lot of stored energy for a relatively small and lightweight battery. Unfortunately, they pose a theoretical fire risk if abused and are treated as dangerous air cargo by many airlines[5]. Lead acid batteries have the lowest energy density, but are a tried and tested technology and have been in use for over a century. As this lower energy density suggests, they will be larger and heavier than other batteries and are thus not always the ideal choice for energy demanding medical equipment, and a possible handicap in transferring a patient. Of the remaining options, NiMH has a higher energy density than NiCd. The NiCd can suffer from memory effect, where its capacity is effectively "lost" over time. The newer generation NiMH batteries seem to have overcome the memory effect issue and are now taking much of market share traditionally held by NiCds.[4]

It should also be noted that most batteries work most efficiently within specific temperature ranges. Storage, charging, and use in extremes of either hot or cold are likely to reduce battery life and may increase likely re-charge times.[4] The extent of this will vary between battery types; ideally battery options would be varied dependant on environmental conditions. This is impractical, so attention must be paid to buy the most flexible option at the procurement stage. When not being used, most batteries will drop from their fully charged state. This self-discharge is obviously more significant the longer a battery is "sat on the shelf" and may be more pronounced in NiMH; for this reason batteries should be either regularly checked or stored on a trickle-charger. Ultimately, each manufacturer will give the most appropriate advice for its own particular brand and this should be followed as strictly as practicable; some manufacturers advising a re-conditioning processes to prolong the life of the battery.

### 39.3.3
### Oxygen and Ventilators

Supplemental oxygen should always be carried with the assumption that the patient's oxygen requirements will increase at altitude. Indeed it should also be assumed that the patient may deteriorate and thus require supplemental oxygen in excess of that required by altitude and consequent pressure changes alone. The safest approach is to assume that a ventilated patient will require ventilation at an inspired oxygen concentration ($FiO_2$) of 100%, and as with determining battery power consumption, delays should be anticipated. Sufficient oxygen must be carried; a diversion due to insufficient oxygen almost certainly indicates poor planning, carries a heavy financial burden and is rarely in the patient's interests.

As an oxidant, medical oxygen strongly supports combustion and may react violently with combustible materials.[6] Accordingly, oxygen cylinders are treated as dangerous air cargo and must be stored in accordance with carrier's instructions; the explosive potential of an oxygen cylinder was clearly demonstrated by depressurization of a civilian Boeing 747 in July 2008.[7]

Integral to calculating oxygen consumption, users must know the quantity of oxygen consumed by the particular ventilator used. This will vary depending on the technology utilized and whether gas or turbine driven; certain models of the latter are gas inefficient. At an $FiO_2$ of 100%, the volume of gas used beyond the delivered minute volume, i.e. wasted, can range anywhere from 1 to 11 L/min.[8] In terms of monitoring, transport ventilators should, as a minimum, have:

- Disconnection and high pressure alarms
- Ability to deliver positive end expiratory pressure (PEEP)
- Variable $FiO_2$
- Variable respiratory rate, inspiratory:expiratory (I:E) ratio, and tidal volume[1]

The ability of a transport ventilator to deliver pressure controlled ventilation, pressure support, and continuous positive airway pressure (CPAP) is desirable.[1] Audible alarms are essential but, as with alarms on patient monitors, accompanying personnel might not be able to hear them. Whilst problematic in an ambulance, engine noise will be even louder in an aircraft and constant vigilance by at least one qualified attendant should be viewed as mandatory. Some ventilators may require manual compensation for pressure changes due to altitude, or delivered tidal volumes will be significantly different to the set value.[2] Accompanying personnel must be aware of such issues. Equipment that automatically compensates for altitude and meets both desirable and minimum specification is obviously preferable and is widely available on the market.

## 39.4
## Patient Preparation

Preparing the patient for aeromedical transfer follows many of the same general principles required for a road transfer and these are covered in suitable detail by the Intensive Care Society Guidelines.[1] The patient should be moved onto a suitable transport ventilator at the earliest opportunity to allow the patient to "settle" and an arterial blood gas should be taken as a check prior to departure. The patient is then transferred to a transport stretcher or gurney. A useful addition to this is the use of a transfer vacuum mattress, a sealed mattress that is similar to a beanbag in texture and composition. This can be molded around the patient as air is pumped out of it, leaving a supportive rigid structure, which contours underneath and around the sides of the patient but leaves their front exposed. It has numerous benefits: it provides support in the case of spinal injury; it can help splint fractures, particularly of limbs; and it can effectively tie in loose lines. Care must be taken, however, to ensure that pressure areas are closely monitored; lines and cables must not press against exposed skin and in the case of longer transfers, the patient's position should regularly be changed.

Bedside medical devices such as monitors and infusion devices need to be systematically changed for an appropriate transfer equivalent. Loose lines and cables must be firmly secured with particular attention to the airway, IV lines, and NG tube. As a final step, the patient is secured to the stretcher using a harness. The RAF uses a specially designed 5-point harness for all aeromedical transfers. This is ideal for the strategic transfer of the critically-ill patient since it secures them for all stages of the evacuation: movement from Field Hospital to ambulance; ambulance to aircraft; and from aircraft to ambulance on arrival in the UK. Similar to the vacuum mattress it can also facilitate the securing of intravenous lines and cables. Consideration must be given to the noise likely to be endured by the patient in transit. On any aircraft there is a degree of background noise from the engines and this may be sufficient to interfere with verbal communication; the problem is particularly marked in helicopters and small aircraft. Protective foam plugs should be inserted into the patient's ears, prior to take-off.

When practicable, hypovolaemia should be reversed prior to departure as it is poorly tolerated by patients in transit.[1] Hypovolaemia can cause labile blood pressure on the application of acceleration and deceleration forces to the patient which occur on take-off and landing. For safe strategic transfer to the UK, patients should have no active bleeding and haemoglobin be deemed adequate for the journey; blood for transfusion can be transported for a limited duration and given if required. Sufficient intravenous access through which to give further resuscitation with crystalloid, colloids, or blood products, is mandatory. This is commonly in the form of two wide-bore cannulae.[1] Other physiological preparations should include: the correction of metabolic disturbances; the control of seizures; and addressing of raised intracranial pressure. Whilst these factors are usually addressed prior to moving the patient, the environmental conditions from which the patient is being evacuated may limit action. A casualty might need expedient evacuation to a place of safety, particularly in a combat situation, before these are achieved; a dedicated medical team such as MERT might also be better placed to provide treatment in transit. Similarly, RAF CCAST has the capability to provide treatment en route beyond that of a simple transfer facility; it can continue and initiate many aspects of medical management throughout aeromedical transfer. In the combat environment, aircraft assets may be a scarce resource and it can be in the patient's interests that they are utilized when available.

### 39.4.1
### Administration

In the pressure of preparing a patient it is easy to forget some simple but essential administrative details. Copies of medical documentation should be made from the medical facility from which the patient is departing, including medical and nursing notes and any radiological investigations; the latter can often be stored in an electronic form such as CD/DVD. In the tactical environment, all original documentation will usually be kept with the patient. A passport is still required for evacuation back to the UK where immigration procedures will still be in force. In the event of aircraft diversion to anywhere apart from the UK, difficulties with the host nation would undoubtedly ensue if a patient's passport was not available. Any belongings must, however, be rigorously checked for any items of dangerous air cargo; in the transportation of military casualties a search for live ammunition is pertinent. As with any patient transfer, arrangements for onward movements must be made including contact with the receiving hospital and advice on expected timelines.[1] Transport arrangements from the airhead of arrival should be confirmed; delays stretch oxygen and battery resources and potentially impinge on patient safety, at a time when the accompanying medical team are already likely to be fatigued.

### 39.5
### In-Flight Care

All aspects of care, drugs, and clinical observations should be recorded in-flight. As previously alluded to, many treatments can be initiated either before or during transfer. In the shorter, tactical, aeromedical transfer there will probably be insufficient time to undertake "nursing" care. Time is usually available in the longer strategic transfers. Pressure areas should be observed and the patient's position changed during transit; even if the patient does not have formal clearance from spinal injuries, at cruising altitude, most aircraft afford a suitably stable platform in which the patient can be safely log-rolled. Eye and mouth care are routine within a static intensive care facility and should be viewed no differently during strategic aeromedical evacuation. It may be difficult to access water in many aircraft, particularly military cargo airframes, where cleansing wipes provide a simple adjunct to meeting a patient's hygiene needs. Hand hygiene is still paramount; universal precautions should be utilized where possible and an alcohol based skin cleanser used to augment hand-washing. The minimum standard likely to be achieved in helicopters, where water is absent, is likely to be the wearing of disposable gloves.

## 39.5.1
## Administration

In the UK, a Strategic CCAST is maintained at a permanent 6 h' Notice to Move (NTM) readiness state. This means that the Team must be capable of being in the air within 6 h of notification of a mission. While this level of readiness is quoted within the Concept of Operations, there is usually more than 6 h' notice of a mission; however, on occasion, if an aircraft is already traveling to the required destination and is planned to leave within the six hour window, the team may be called upon to ready to move earlier. Tactical CCASTs may be on even shorter NTM restrictions as the operational tempo dictates. If the patient and the CCAST are co-located (as is frequently the case in established operations), the patient and equipment can be prepared and ready to board the aircraft in as little as 60–90 min from the notification of a mission.

Planning of CCAST missions frequently starts long before the patient is in a state to be transferred. If a patient is brought into the Emergency Department (ED) with obvious critical injuries, a Tactical CCAST may be notified that a transfer is likely to be required while the patient is still in the ED or the Operating Theatre. This transfer may be for specialist intervention (neurosurgery, cardiac surgery, specialist imaging) or evacuation. This gives the team the maximum time to prepare for the mission. Similarly, it takes time to task an aircraft for any mission and these administrative tasks can be started before the patient is ready for transfer. If a patient is obviously going to need a period of Intensive Care after their initial resuscitation in a field hospital then it is important to immediately start planning for their onward evacuation as intensive care beds are usually in very short supply in operational theaters and these patients use up large amounts of resources, both in equipment and in clinical time (each patient requires one-to-one nursing whilst on the intensive care unit). Both of these resources are often severely limited in the operational environment making rapid evacuation essential to maintain operational capability.

Some patients who initially require Intensive Care recover rapidly and their level of dependence can be rapidly reduced. While these patients still require evacuation to maintain operational capability (as very few are likely to be returned to duty within the operational theater without a period of convalescence for which there is no capacity in the operational environment), a CCAST may not be required for these patients. In this situation, evacuation may be undertaken by generalist Aeromedical Evacuation (AE) teams tailored to clinical need. Again, these teams may be based in the UK and sent out to collect a patient or based in the operational theater and then accompany the patient back to the UK before repositioning back to the operational theater. Personnel undertaking this role still require training in the management of the patient in the air but they will not require the Intensive Care training of the CCASTs to perform their duties.

The level of medical support to AE operations is determined by the clinical scenario prevailing at the time. If the patient has a medical (non-surgical) problem (such as angina or an uncomplicated pneumothorax) then it may be appropriate for a physician trained in aviation medicine to accompany the patient in addition to the FNO/FN and an FNA. Surgical patients are sometimes transferred with an anesthetic escort as their in-flight problems are most likely to be related to pain management and the physiological effects (usually respiratory) of altitude. It is very unusual to use a surgical specialist as an escort as the patient should already have had the necessary surgery before flight and further surgical procedures in flight are likely to be both clinically and practically inappropriate. The surgeon's skills are best kept in the operating theater and the Emergency Department where they can be most effectively used.

Frequently, if a patient is delayed in the deployed hospital for a few days, their level of dependency reduces to the extent that no medical escort is required as long as appropriate provision for management of their pain and possible respiratory embarrassment is made prior to emplaning. These patients can safely be managed by AE trained FNO/FNs and FNAs.

## 39.5.2
### Aviation Physiology

This chapter is not conceived as a treatise on Aviation Medicine so this section will only give a brief overview of the effects of changes in the composition of ambient air and the pressure and volume changes associated with an ascent to altitude.

For the purposes of this chapter, the atmosphere can be considered to have a constant relative composition of gases, namely:

- Nitrogen 78%
- Oxygen 20.9%
- Argon ~1%
- Carbon Dioxide 0.04%
- Neon, helium, methane, krypton, and hydrogen, all of which comprise less than 0.01%
- Water vapor

Water vapor is the only component whose percentage varies significantly over the altitude range concerned, being between 1% and 4% at the surface but averaging 0.4% over the whole atmosphere.

Pressure varies inversely with altitude, decreasing to approximately 50% at 18,000 ft and to a quarter at about 33,700 ft. Table 39.1 gives the pressures in kilopascals

**Table 39.1** Pressure changes with altitude

| Altitude (ft) | Altitude (m) | Pressure (kPa) | Pressure (mmHg) |
|---|---|---|---|
| 0 | 0 | 101.3 | 760 |
| 1,000 | 305 | 97.7 | 733 |
| 2,500 | 762 | 92.5 | 694 |
| 5,000 | 1,524 | 84.3 | 632 |
| 10,000 | 3,048 | 69.7 | 523 |
| 20,000 | 6,096 | 46.6 | 349 |
| 30,000 | 9,144 | 30.1 | 226 |
| 36,090 | 11,000 | 22.6 | 170 |

**Fig. 39.2** Variation in pressure of air, nitrogen, and oxygen with altitude

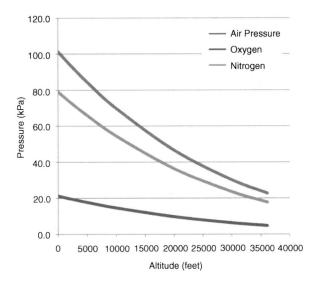

and millimeters of Mercury for various altitudes above sea level. For the remainder of this chapter, feet will be used to measure altitude as this is the unit generally used in aviation. Similarly, kPa will be used as the standard unit for pressure. The US uses mmHg to measure physiological pressures and these will be included for completeness where appropriate.

Using these data and the composition of dry air (not including water vapor), Fig. 39.2 shows graphically the change in pressure with varying altitude. Dalton's Law of Partial Pressures tells us that "the total pressure exerted by a gaseous mixture is equal to the sum of the partial pressures of each individual component in a gas mixture." That is to say that the pressure exerted by any component (its partial pressure) is the product of its relative concentration and the total pressure of the gas mixture. The variation of the partial pressures of Nitrogen and Oxygen in normal dry air is also shown in Fig. 39.2.

It can be seen that the reduction in partial pressure of oxygen rapidly becomes significant. An inspired oxygen concentration ($FiO_2$) of 21% roughly corresponds to an arterial oxygen tension ($PaO_2$) of 13.3 kPa (100 mmHg) due to a variety of physiological reasons that mean that not all the inspired oxygen reaches the alveolar capillaries. One reason for this is that inspired oxygen is humidified, either by evaporation from the respiratory epithelium or by humidification systems within the ventilator circuit in the intubated patient. This water vapor has a constant pressure of 6.3 kPa (47 mmHg) irrespective of altitude and should be removed from the total pressure prior to performing the partial pressure calculation. Thus inspired air has a partial pressure of $(101.3-6.3) \times 0.21 = 20$ kPa at sea level but has a partial pressure at 36,000 ft of $(22.6-6.3) \times 0.21 = 3.4$ kPa and not 4.8 kPa as might be expected from dry air. The relative increase in significance of this water vapor further impairs the body's ability to cope with increasing altitude and mandates supplementary oxygen for all but the most low level flights. Furthermore, any physiological derangement of the patient's respiratory function becomes far more significant at altitude. A patient who requires 60% oxygen at sea level in order to maintain a normal $PaO_2$ will require 90% oxygen at 10,000 ft.

The other major consideration caused by altitude is the change in the volume and pressure of gases trapped within the patient, for example, in a pneumothorax, a pneumocranium, or in a paralytic ileus. Boyle's Law states that for a fixed amount of gas at a constant temperature, the volume is inversely proportional to the pressure. Thus a volume of 200 mL at sea level will have increased to 400 mL at 18,000 ft (half atmospheric pressure). Similarly, if the volume is fixed (by being confined in an enclosed space), the pressure will double instead. Care must therefore be taken to ensure that all trapped air is ventilated before flight, by means of a nasogastric tube for the stomach, a chest drain for the thorax or even by craniectomy for a pneumocranium.

Tracheal mucosal blood flow has been shown to be compromised above a lateral wall pressure of 30 cmH$_2$O with cessation at 50 cmH$_2$O.[9] Even modest rises in cabin altitude cause increases in tracheal cuff pressure that could be clinically relevant.[10] Anecdotally, saline has been used to replace air in the cuff; this mitigates the problem to some extent but it can prove difficult to reach an exact pressure and even saline filled cuffs are prone to some pressure changes with some types of cuff exceeding 50 cm H2O above cabin altitudes of 7,000 ft.[11] While this might not be problematic in many fixed wing aircraft that maintain lower cabin pressures, helicopters are usually unpressurized and some RAF helicopters can theoretically operate up to 17,000ft.[12] A simple alternative method is to monitor cuff pressure on ascent and decent using a hand-held manometer; the cuff can be deflated and re-inflated gently as required.[13]

An alternative approach to limiting the effect of pressure changes is to maintain a lower cabin altitude by increasing the pressure within it. This is achieved by taking a feed from the compressors in the aircraft engines but it has the implication of reducing fuel economy. A sea level cabin altitude will also reduce the maximum operational ceiling for the aircraft as only a certain difference in pressure between the cabin and the outside air can safely be maintained. This reduced ceiling (to maybe 25,000 ft) reduces the possible speed achievable in flight and increases drag, further reducing fuel economy. Flight planning is affected as lower airspace is under different restrictions and some mountain ranges cannot be crossed at this altitude, requiring alternative routing. All these considerations may mean that a flight that could have been completed without refuelling may now require at least one stop for fuel thereby further increasing the length of the flight. Do not be surprised if the flight crew meets your request for sea level cabin altitude with some consternation!

Air is also contained within the sinuses of the face (predominantly the maxillary and frontal sinuses), the middle ear, teeth, and abscess cavities. Obstructed sinuses and eustachian tubes (due to a simple cold or similar upper respiratory tract condition) will not be able to equalize pressures via the usual routes on descent and cause excruciating facial and ear pain. On ascent the increased pressure relative to the outside environment is usually sufficient to overcome any obstruction (this is the cause of your ears "popping" in aircraft). People for routine aeromedical evacuation who cannot clear their ears should not be flown unless absolutely necessary. Vasoconstrictor nasal sprays such as xylometazoline can improve symptoms but their effect is slow and these should not be relied upon except in extreme cases. Dental pain may also occur in flight for due to expansion of air trapped between a deep cavity filling and the tooth substance on ascent.

As has been discussed above, these considerations primarily apply to fixed wing aircraft. Rotary wing aircraft cannot be effectively pressurized and so the likely altitude of flight must be considered when calculating oxygen requirements and considering pressure effects.

# References

1. Intensive Care Society. Guidelines for the transport of the critically ill adult. 2002.
2. McGuire N. Monitoring in the field. *Br J Anaesth*. 2006;97(1):46-56.
3. IEC. IEC 60529: Degrees of Protection Provided by Enclosures (IP Code), International Electrotechnical Commission. Ed 2.1, Geneva; 2001.
4. Dell RM, Rand DAJ. *Understanding Batteries*. Cambridge: Royal Society of Chemistry; 2001.
5. CAA. Dealing with In-flight Lithium Battery Fires in Portable Electronic Devices, Civil Aviation Authority Safety Regulation Group, CAA Paper 2003/4.
6. BOC. Medical gas Data Sheet (MED/004041/APUK/0208/2 M), BOC Medical; 2008.
7. ATSB. ATSB Transport Safety Report – Aviation Occurrence Investigation AO-2008-053, Canberra; Australian Transport Safety Bureau.
8. Josephs S, Lyons E, Branson R. Assessment of oxygen consumption from standard E cylinders by fluidic, turbine and compressor style portable mechanical ventilators. *Crit Care*. 2006;10(Suppl 1):63.
9. Seebolin RD, Van Hasselt GL. Endotracheal cuff pressure and tracheal mucosal blood flow: endoscopic study of the effects of four large volumes cuffs. *Br Med J*. 1984;288:965-968.
10. Henning J, Sharley P, Young R. Pressures within air-filled tracheal cuffs at altitude. *Anaesthesia*. 2004;59:252-254.
11. Smith R, McArdle B. Pressure in the cuffs of tracheal tubes at altitude. *Anaesthesia*. 2002;57:374-378.
12. RAF. Aircraft guide, www.raf.mod.uk. Accessed August 24, 2009.
13. Ruth M. Pressure changes in tracheal tube cuffs at altitude (correspondence). *Anaesthesia*. 2002;57:818-838.

# Critical Care Management: The Patient with Ballistic Trauma

# 40

Tim Nutbeam and Damian Douglas Keene

This chapter provides a practical, pragmatic approach to the critical care management of the patient with ballistic trauma. The chapter covers the practical aspects of receiving, assessing, and stabilizing these patients. It takes a systems based approach to ensure modern, evidence based, consensus derived care is provided throughout the patients stay. This chapter does not cover the provision of "critical care" in the pre-hospital environment, the transfer of these patients or critical care outreach systems.

The critical care management of these patients is a highly specialist field with many advances and novel therapies driven by the recent conflicts in Iraq and Afghanistan. Advances in pre hospital care, trauma resuscitation, and developments within damage control surgery have led to an increased survival rate for these patients – it also means that as critical care practitioners we are facing the challenge of dealing with multiply injured patients who previously would not have survived to reach the ICU.

Patients with ballistic trauma tend to differ from the standard ICU population seen in non-specialist civilian practise:

- Age: predominantly under 40
- Sex: predominantly male
- Co-morbidities: tend to be physiologically normal before wounding

These differences mean that attempts to predict admission, morbidity and mortality based on traditional ICU scoring systems may be misguided – some ICU's have defined admission criteria based upon injury pattern: penetrating thoracic injury, traumatic amputation, significant exposure to blast etc.

T. Nutbeam (✉)
Intensive Care, University Hospital Birmingham, Birmingham, UK
e-mail: timnutbeam@hotmail.com

A.J. Brooks et al. (eds.), *Ryan's Ballistic Trauma*,
DOI: 10.1007/978-1-84882-124-8_40, © Springer-Verlag London Limited 2011

## 40.1
## Receiving

### 40.1.1
### Before Arrival

These patients will come to the ICU in a variety of ways:

• Via the ED resuscitation room
• From the operating theater
• Transfer in (this may be internationally)

Regardless of route, admission of these patients should be preceded by a formal information handover at a senior level (normally consultant to consultant). This handover should occur as soon as it is confirmed that the patient will need intensive care treatment, and must be updated if the patient's condition or transfer arrangements change. This handover should include the following information as a minimum: type (mechanism) and time of wounding, injuries identified and suspected, significant past medical history, treatment initiated, interventions performed, current physiological status and transfer details.

This information will enable the receiving unit to prepare for the patients arrival and ensure the necessary personnel are available. It is necessary to ensure that the following will be informed and available on arrival of the patient:

• Specialist nursing staff
• Intensive care medical staff
• The receiving surgical team (if not with the patient in theater)
• Expert subspecialty teams: neurosurgery, cardiothoracics, plastic surgery, maxillofacial, etc.

In addition it may be necessary to clear emergency theaters, inform hematologist/bloodbank, involve microbiology services etc.

## 40.2
## Handover

Once again this process should occur at as senior level as resources permit. The handover should follow a standard pre-determined template: this reduces both errors and omissions. Both a nursing and medical handover should occur, which should cover the same information as the formal information handover above.

In addition all medical and transfer notes, the results of any investigations and any imaging should be formally handed over at this stage.

## 40.3
## Assessing

A rigid system of assessment will minimize errors:

1. A thorough systematic primary ABCDE type survey: this should identify all immediate life threatening pathology – this should be dealt with at this stage.
2. A full secondary/tertiary survey. This will include full examination of the patients back (log-roll), removal of cervical collars, splints etc. for full assessment of each body region. Particular attention must be paid to the axillae, groin, and buttocks where wounds are often missed.

The FAST 1, sternal intra osseous access leaves a characteristic "target" of wounds that may be found as part of this secondary survey – this is not part of the wounding pattern (see Fig. 40.1).

A full neurological examination should be performed at this stage, however many of these patients are ventilated and paralyzed so this examination should be performed at the earliest opportunity.

3. A systematic review of the:

- Nursing and medical notes
- Any operating theater/transfer charts
- The results of any investigations performed
- Imaging performed and planned
- Any surgical procedures performed and planned

Despite a full systematic assessment at this stage further injuries and pathology may be identified later in the patient's ICU stay. Repeated systematic review and assessment by experienced senior staff will lead to early identification of these injuries. A thorough understanding of the mechanism of injury will enable the experienced clinician to predict (and search for) injuries missed in the initial assessment.

During this assessment phase any instability in the patient should be identified, diagnosed, and appropriately managed.

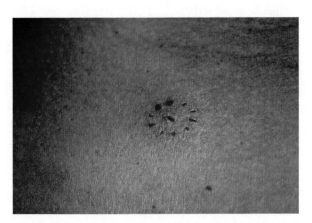

**Fig. 40.1** FAST 1' Imprint

## 40.4
## Stabilizing and Planning

By this stage any immediate life threatening injuries should have been identified and dealt with, the patient should be stable or have returned to the operating theater.

Once stability has been achieved:

*Line Changes*

All lines inserted in the pre-hospital environment or in a combat zone, should be assumed to be contaminated, these lines should be removed and fresh lines in new sites using full aseptic techniques should be inserted.

*Drains*

The position and patency of all drains should be assessed and if necessary re-secured.

*ET Tubes*

These have a tendency to become dislodged even during the shortest of transfers. A chest x-ray should be ordered to confirm the position of the tube. With aero-medical transfers, on arrival it is necessary to replace saline in tube cuffs with air (prolonged use of saline in cuffs may cause balloon rupture).

## 40.5
## Review of Medical Therapies

Rationalize ongoing medical treatments, ensure Tetanus immunoglobulin/booster has been administered, antibiotic prophylaxis has been initiated and that any medications related to previous medical conditions have been prescribed. Ensure appropriate and adequate sedation (including "breakthrough" analgesia) is prescribed and readily available.

## 40.6
## Additional Investigations

Imaging and specialist investigations should be planned at this stage. These need to be sorted into clinical priority based on the potential impact of their results on clinical decisions. Investigations which do not impact on clinical decisions are not necessary at this stage and can be organized later in the patients stay.

In all female patients of child bearing age a $\beta$-HCG should be performed and if positive, consideration given to anti-D immunoglobulin. The obstetric team should be involved and a staging scan performed.

## 40.7
## Operative Interventions

Relevant surgical specialists should hold a planning meeting with the ICU team. Interventions should be prioritized and organized in a logical manner. A plan for immediate and future visits to theater should be agreed: time must be allowed to correct the likely physiological effects of each intervention (see damage-control surgery).

## 40.8
## Involvement of Specialist Teams/Allied Therapies

Multiple specialist teams should be involved at an early stage, these will be dependant upon the patients pattern of wounding but is likely to include:

- Microbiologists
- Hematologists and blood bank
- Nutritionists/dieticians
- Physiotherapists and occupational therapists
- Plastics/Tissue viability specialists
- Pain team

## 40.9
## Family

Initial discussion with family members can be difficult and should only be approached by an appropriately trained medical and nursing team. Military patients may have trained family liaison officers who can aid you with this process.

Before discussion with family and friends it is essential to confirm their identity and relationship to the patient. It is also necessary to ensure that they were not involved in/responsible for the wounding.

This discussion is an opportunity to glean any additional information regarding the patients past medical history, normal physiological reserve, allergies, and medications.

The family members should be informed of the patient's current condition, likely prognosis, and treatment initiated and planned. Information should be delivered in clear language at an appropriate intellectual level. Those present should be encouraged to ask questions, informed of visiting arrangements, and given appropriate contact details.

It is important that all discussions are witnessed and clearly documented.

## 40.10
## Ongoing Assessment

Regular repeated assessment will identify missed injuries, detect new pathology, and allow the ICU practitioner to deliver optimal, progressive patient care. The examination should be performed under the direct supervision of the consultant responsible for the patient (if not the consultant themselves). Standard UK practise encourages a full assessment and examination twice in any 24 h time period, normally as part of a formal multi disciplinary ward round. In addition to this the patient should have a full assessment and examination on any of the following triggers:

- Acute change in physiology/patient condition
- On return from theater
- Before and following any major procedure (chest drain insertion, percutaneous tracheo-stomy, etc.)

The assessment should consist of a full clinical examination (this is best performed following a standard format to avoid omissions), and a review of the chart, blood, and investigation results. Each therapy, treatment, or invasive monitor/drain should be considered in turn – is it still necessary? Does it need to be changed, modified, or adjusted? Involvement of specialties and the multi-disciplinary team will enable thorough, holistic care.

The formal assessment process will aid your decision making and planning: is the patient fit enough for the treatments you had planned, do they require further stabilization prior to theater? The assessment process should end with a plan to progress the patients towards certain targets before the next formal review.

The family should be kept updated of decisions made, treatments planned, and their likely effect. Discussions should be held away from the bedside unless the patient has capacity to participate in which case they should always be held at the bedside.

## 40.11
## Damage Control Surgery and the ICU

Over the last 20 years there has been a shift in surgical trauma practise away from a single definitive surgical intervention towards damage control surgery. This stemmed from the realization that many trauma patients were dying, not as a result of surgical failure but as a result of the hypothermia, acidosis, and coagulopathy (the lethal triad) associated with extended operating times. Fig. 40.2.

The time on ICU is an opportunity to optimize the patient for their next surgical procedure. This will involve: reversal of the lethal triad, full reassessment of the patient (including imaging and investigations), and multi-speciality planning of the next operative stage in the patient's management.

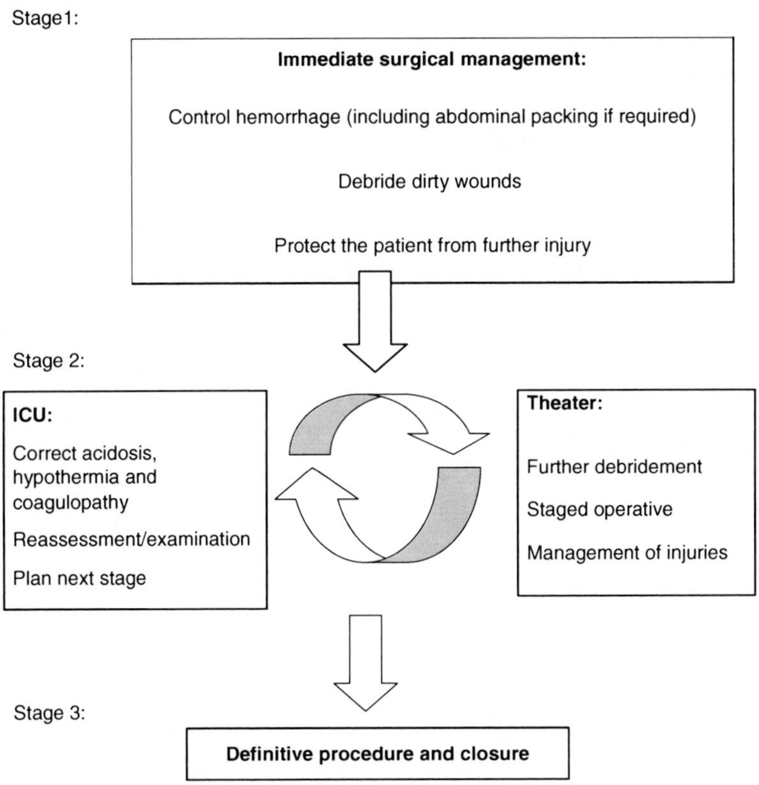

Stage 1:

Stage 2:

Stage 3:

**Fig. 40.2** The ICU is an essential part of the damage control cycle

## 40.12
## The "Lethal Triad" and Its Reversal

The lethal triad consists of hypothermia, acidosis, and coagulopathy. It is process which starts at the point of wounding and is likely to progress through surgical intervention and unless aggressively corrected continue to progress on the ICU. As each aspect of the triad affects the other two, they all must be corrected to stabilize the patient. This triad should be fully reversed before planned returns to theater. However, in the case of acute rapid deterioration with a potentially correctable surgical cause an un-optimized patient may have to return to theater.

## 40.13
## Hypothermia

*Cause:* Patients with polytrauma loose heat through convection, conduction, evaporation, and radiation. In many cases the bodies normal balance between heat production and heat loss is diminished. Heat loss begins at the point of wounding, and progresses through pre hospital care, the ED, and the patient's time in the operating theater.

Trauma patients at particular risk of hypothermia include:

- Those wounded in a cold environment
- Prolonged pre-hospital times
- Severe hypovolaemia
- Penetrating trauma to the abdomen or extremities
- Very young or very old
- High spinal injuries
- Burns

*Effects:* Enzymatic systems are designed to work optimally at the bodies "normal" core temperature. As the core temperature falls the efficiency of these enzymes falls dramatically. Hypothermia leads to inhibition of the clotting cascades and an increased risk of myocardial ischemia. Trauma patients are much more likely to die if they are hypothermic.

*Prevention and Reversal:* A majority of trauma patients arriving on the ICU will be hypothermic. Core body temperature should be continuously monitored throughout the patient's resuscitation. Prevention and reversal methods include:

External Rewarming:

- Removal from cold environment
- Removal of cold wet clothing/dressing
- Blankets
- Increasing ambient temperature (28°C)
- Placing heat packs in groin, armpits, etc.
- Convective warming blankets

Active rewarming (in addition to passive rewarming techniques):

- Use of body temperature resuscitation fluids
- Warmed humidified air oxygen mixes
- Gastric, pleural, peritoneal, and bladder warmed fluid lavage (not in injured or packed cavities!)
- Extracorpeal bypass/haemofiltration techniques

## 40.14
## Acidosis

*Cause:* Hypovolemic shock leads to a shift from aerobic to anaerobic metabolism. This directly leads to the production of lactate and a resultant acidosis.

*Effects:* Acidosis has a direct affect on cellular function and affects almost all body systems. The immediately lethal effects are: cardiac depression (decreased vasomotor tone and cardiac contractility), and hyperkalemia.

*Prevention and Reversal:* The acidosis can be reversed by increasing oxygenation of end organs and peripheral tissues. This will involve: adequate monitored fluid resuscitation (ensuring an adequate Hb is maintained), introduction of ionotropic support (if required) and adequate oxygenation. Persistent acidosis from causes other than direct hypovolaemia (e.g., renal failure) will require directed supportive therapy (e.g., haemofilitration).

## 40.15
## Coagulopathy

*Cause:* Coagulopathy in the trauma patient can arise from a multitude of causes:

- Loss of clotting factors, platelets etc. through continuing exsanguination
- Direct haemodilution of clotting factors, platelets, etc.
- Acute coagulopathy of trauma
- Hypothermia
- Acidosis

*Effects:* Uncontrollable hemorrhage from any injured tissue.

*Prevention and Reversal:* Any acidosis and hypothermia should be corrected as detailed above. The use of non-blood fluids should be minimized. Blood products should be administered in a 1:1:1 ratio (blood, fresh frozen plasma, platelets). Control surgical bleeding (this can not be done without surgery). You should involve specialist hematology services early and regular assessment and reassessment of the clotting profile (consider using a thromboelastograph) should guide your management.

## 40.16
## Infection and Microbiology

Trauma patients like any critically unwell patients are susceptible to infection. This can be from a more "classical" source such as line sepsis and Ventilator Associated Pneumonia (VAP) or as a direct result of wounds. Blast injury is likely to introduce infection directly into the tissues as foreign material will have microorganisms present on the surface. It is not only direct introduction that increases risk of infection, breaching of the skin and underlying tissue necrosis allows invasion and colonization of microorganisms causing local infection that can lead to sepsis. Even after the initial operative interventions wounds are likely to remain open for several days awaiting delayed primary closure.

It is important to remember than any microbiological intervention needs to be as directed as possible. Not only will the presumed area of infection, i.e., chest, alter antimicrobial prescribing but also the local environment where the injury occurred. Fungi can also colonize wounds which can cause significant local tissue necrosis.

If a patient develops sepsis it is important to treat them as per the surviving sepsis bundle guidelines;

---

Bundle Element 1: Measure serum lactate.

Bundle Element 2: Obtain blood cultures prior to antibiotic administration.

Bundle Element 3: Administer broad-spectrum antibiotic within 3 h of ED admission and within 1 h of non-ED admission.

Bundle Element 4: In the event of hypotension and/or serum lactate >4 mmol/L:

a. Deliver an initial minimum of 20 mL/kg of crystalloid or an equivalent

b. Apply vasopressors for hypotension not responding to initial fluid resuscitation to maintain mean arterial pressure (MAP) >65 mmHg

Bundle Element 5: In the event of persistent hypotension despite fluid resuscitation (septic shock) and/or lactate >4 mmol/L:

a. Achieve a central venous pressure (CVP) of ≥8 mmHg

b. Achieve a central venous oxygen saturation (ScvO2) ≥70% or mixed venous oxygen saturation (SvO2) ≥65%

www.survivingsepsis.org

---

It is vital that a source is identified. This may require the patient returning to theater so that wounds can be inspected and any further debridement carried out. The initial antimicrobial cover should be broad spectrum as directed by local microbiology policy until positive cultures are obtained. Strong consideration needs to be given to the possibility of invasive fungal infection particularly if there is ongoing pyrexia despite adequate wound debridement and antibiotics. Histological evidence of invasion of healthy tissue rather than infection in already necrotic regions is important, there is debate whether treatment is required if this is absent. The biggest complication of fungal infection is increased tissue loss and therefore increased impact on rehabilitation.

In blast there may be multiple victims unfortunately human tissue can become fragmentation, this carries the risk of viral transmission particularly of Hepatitis B and C. The role of post exposure prophylaxis and testing is contentious as the risk is difficult to judge and depends on the percentage of population infected (and therefore country of incident).

Wounds may continue to be a source of sepsis despite recent debridement and therefore must be regularly assessed if there is any change in the patients' condition.

Positive cultures of organisms from one individual may be useful in directing treatment of other casualties injured in the same incident, if the source is believed to be due to organisms present on fragmentation. Consideration should always be given to the deliberate impregnation of an explosive device with foreign pathogens.

Frequency of line changes is a contentious issue and common sense always needs to be applied. In the first instance of a diagnosis of sepsis changing of CVP lines is indicated: lines should be changed and tips sent for culture. The risk of sepsis from arterial line infection is perceived to be low due to the high velocity of blood flowing past the catheter. As sites for arterial lines can be limited due to multiple limb injuries/amputations (with femoral sites occasionally being the only possibility) the requirement to change the line is reduced if there is no evidence of local infection.

There is no hard and fast rule for frequency of CVP or arterial line changes in the absence of signs of local or systemic infection. The most important aim should be to remove central lines as soon as the patient can be managed with peripheral access.

## 40.17
## Ventilation, ARDS Net Guidelines, and Weaning

Not only are there occult chest injuries with ballistic trauma, there can also be concealed injury to the underlying lung tissue. This can be seen with blast injuries and presents as "Blast Lung," a direct consequence of the action of blast wave from an explosive device on the lung tissue. Effects can be seen up to 48 h post injury and it is therefore important to consider this diagnosis if there is any deterioration in respiratory gas exchange. Pulmonary contusions can be seen in ballistic trauma due to energy transfer when high velocity rounds hit protective vests. Both present in a similar fashion to ARDS and this is one of the differential diagnoses along with Transfusion Related Acute Lung Injury (TRALI).

The management is similar and is dependent on the clinical severity:

- Supplemental oxygen
- Judicious use of fluids
- Low tidal volume (6–8 mL/kg)
- Low Peak Airway Pressures
- Permissive Hypercapnia (Allowing a decrease in tidal volume)

These approaches reduce the probability of further injury to the lung tissue. It is important to note air emboli and particularly pneumothoraces are seen in blast lung.

An important consideration when weaning these patients is the likelihood of injury to the cervical spine. This is highly unlikely with gunshot wounds, but is important in blast injuries. Clearing of the c-spine of the unconscious is a controversial issue. UK practise differs widely and protocols need to balance the risk of injury against that of immobilization. One solution is that while sedated those at risk of c-spine injury with a radiologically normal c-spine on CT can be immobilized with straps and blocks and the collar removed. This is particularly important in those with possible head injury as the collar raises ICP. The patient will be log rolled until the c-spine is clinically cleared. MRI to look for ligamental injury is usually not possible as metal fragments cannot be ruled out and external fixators may be in situ. A spinal bed is required if there is a significant radiological change in the thoracic or lumbar spine.

Once fully awake and alert the c-spine can be cleared clinically following NEXUS guidelines.

## 40.18
## Sedation and Pain Control

Patients may require long periods of sedation: this can be with any adequate agent. It is important to remember that pain will be a significant factor so analgesia should be present alongside sedation i.e., midazolam and morphine. When weaning patients it may be necessary to continue opiate infusions to maintain analgesia: this should be titrated to have a minimal delay on extubation.

Patients with traumatic amputations or significant nerve injuries will require multimodal analgesia, this should be anticipated and pain teams involved early. Thought should be given to the early use of pregabalin or gabapentin for control of neuropathic pain even if sedated as their effects are delayed.

Regional blocks with indwelling nerve catheters may be present and provide good continuous pain relief in limb injuries, thus reducing the need for systemic analgesia. Catheters can be left in situ as long as the insertion site shows no signs of local infection. If a patients' pain has reduced in the affected limb thought needs to be given to short term surgical plans before removing the catheter. Further debridement/skin grafting may be needed and the block could be easily re-established.

## 40.19
## Renal

Renal support in the form of Central Veno-Venous Haemofiltration (CVVH) may be required in those with acute renal failure. This could be secondary to initial hypovoleamic shock or rhabdomyolysis, e.g., from crush injury following structural collapse when explosive devices have been used.

Renal failure may also occur due to sepsis and multi organ failure. CVVH can be of use in severe sepsis to reduce circulating inflammatory markers and reduce their systemic effects. It is also possible to actively warm using CVVH in the hypothermic patient.

## 40.20
## Abdominal Compartment Syndrome

Abdominal compartment syndrome (ACS) results from penetrating or blunt trauma although there may not be any specific underlying abdominal injury. A diagnosis should be considered in those who have had a profound period of hypotension and have a falling urine output and rising CVP. The effects of ACS are summarized below;

- *Cardiovascular* Decrease in cardiac output due to fall in venous return, despite rise in CVP
- *Respiratory* Ventilatory compromise due to splinting of diaphragm
- *Renal* Decreased urine output, acute renal failure
- *Neurological* Raised Intracranial Pressure due to rise in CVP

It is diagnosed if the intra abdominal pressure is over 30 cmH2O, normal pressure being negative or zero. Pressure can be measured easily using a foley catheter in the bladder or via a Nasogastric tube attached to a simple water manometer. Treatment involves a laparotomy to decompress the abdomen then leaving the abdomen open as a laparostomy to allow room for tissue swelling to occur.

## 40.21
## Nutritional and Metabolic Care

Early nutritional support is extremely important as the calorific requirements of patients will be raised as the body enters a hypermetabolic state post injury. This effect is exaggerated in those with significant burn injuries. In sedated patients or those unable to maintain adequate calorie intake commencement of nasogastric feeding is required; a standard regimen can initiated whilst waiting for dietician input. It is important to recognize if feed is not being absorbed and take measures to correct it. This can be with the use of prokinetics, such as metoclopramide and low dose erythromycin. If this is unsuccessful early naso-jejunal tube placement needs to be considered.

Gastric protection such as IV Ranitidine should be used whilst intubated until adequate feeding has been initiated.

## 40.22
## Psychological Support

As the last memory of a patient may be at the time of injury, it is important to have familiar faces and voices to hand when considering stopping sedation. They are likely to be severely disorientated especially if the effects of sedation are still present. It may be necessary to repeatedly explain and reassure them.

If injuries are secondary to blast there may be a degree of hearing loss or eye injury adding to the patients' distress when initially woken. In these patients the early presence of familiar family and friends is vital.

The care of these patients may be distressing for all involved. They often relive their experiences vocally, and suffer from profound paranoia and flashbacks. Psychological support should be freely available for all involved in their care.

## 40.23
## Summary

The management of the severely injured trauma patients can be daunting for all involved, especially in units with minimal trauma exposure. It must not be forgotten that the basic management of all ITU patients is fundamentally the same, following an ABC approach, with early and often aggressive interventions being performed as needed.

In trauma patients it is fundamental that a close relationship between the ICU and the surgical team is maintained at every stage of the patients care. Multiple trips to theater should not be seen as a failure but as providing a high standard of evidence based care.

## Recommended Reading

ARDS NET. Ventilation with lower tidal volumes as compared with traditional tidal volumes for acute lung injury and the acute respiratory distress syndrome. *N Engl J Med*. 2000; 342:1301.

ARDS NET. Higher versus lower positive end-expiratory pressures in patients with the acute respiratory distress syndrome. *N Engl J Med*. 2004;351:327.

Clasper JC. Lower limb amputations – A consensus. *J R Army Med Corps*. 2007;153(3): 172-174.

Davis PR, Byer M. Accidental hypothermia. *J R Army Med Corps*. 2006;152:223-233.

Dellinger RP, Carlet JM, Masur H, et al. Surviving sepsis campaign guidelines for management of severe sepsis and septic shock. *Crit Care Med*. 2004;32:858-873.

DePalma RG, Burris DG. Champion HR. blast injuries. *N Engl J Med*. 2005;352:1335.

Dutton R, McCunn M, et al. Factor VIIa for correction of traumatic coagulopathy. *J Trauma-Inj Inf Crit Care*. 2004;4:709-719.

Ferrara A, MacArthur J, et al. Hypothermia and acidosis worsen coagulopathy in the patient requiring massive transfusion. *Am J Surg*. 1990;160:515-519.

Geeraedts L, Kamphusigen P, Kaasjager H. The role of recombinant factor VIIa int he treatment of life-threatening haemorrhage in blunt trauma Injury. *Int J Care Injured*. 2005;36: 495-500.

Hess J, Lawson J. The coagulopathy of trauma versus disseminated intravascular coagulation. *J Trauma-Inj Inf Crit Care*. 2006;60(6):s12-s19.

Hess J, Brohi K, et al. The coagulopathy of trauma: A review of mechanisms. *J Trauma-Inj Inf Crit Care*. 2008;65(4):748-754.

Hodgetts TJ, Mahoney PF, Kirkman E. Damage control resuscitation. *J R Army Med Corps*. 2007;153(4)):299-300.

Hoffman A, Henning JD. Military intensive care part 2. Current practice. *J R Army med Corps*. 2007;153(4)):286-287.

Implement the resuscitation bundle - within the first 6 hours of care. Surviving sepsis campaign. http://www.survivingsepsis.org/Bundles/Pages/SepsisResuscitationBundle.aspx; Accessed June 2009

Kress JP, Pohlman AS. Daily interruption of sedative infusions in critically Ill patients undergoing mechanical ventilation. *N Engl J Med*. 2000;342:1471.

Lynn M, Jeroukhinov I, et al. Updates in the management of severe coagulopathy in trauma patients. *Intensive Care Med*. 2002;28:S241-S247.

Malone D, Hess J, Fingerhut A. Massive tranfusion practices around the globe and a suggestion for a common massive tranfusion protocol. *J Trauma-Inj Inf Crit Care*. 2006;60(6):s91-s96.

Moore E. Staged laparotomy for the hypothermia, acidosis, and coagulopathy syndrome. *Am J Surg*. 1996;172(5):405-410.

Morris CGT, McCoy E. Clearing the cervical spine in unconscious polytrauma victims, balancing risks and effective screeing. *Anaesthesia*. 2004;59:464-482.

O'Grady NP, Alexander M, Dellinger EP, et al. Centers for disease control and prevention (2002): Guidelines for the prevention of intravascular catheter-related infections centers for disease control and prevention. *MMWR*. 2002;51:1-29.

Rivers E, Nguyen B, Havstad S, et al. Early goal-directed therapy in the treatment of severe sepsis and septic shock. *N Engl J Med*. 2001;345:1368-1377.

Schien M, Wittmann DH, Aprahamian CC. The abdominal compartment syndrome: The physiological and clinical consequences of elevated intra-abdominal pressure. *J Am Coll Surg*. 1995;180:745-753.

Schrier R, Wang W. Acute renal failure and sepsis. *N Engl J Med*. 2004;351:159-169.

Shirley PJ. Critical care delivery: The experience of a civilian terrorist attack. *J R Army Med Corps*. 2006;152:17-21.

Ware LB, Matthay MA. The acute respiratory distress syndrome. *N Engl J Med*. 2000;342:1334.

Yehuda R. Post-traumatic stress disorder. *N Engl J Med*. 2006;354:1052.

# Critical Care Nursing at Role Four

# 41

Clare Dutton

Many people may say that nursing the military critical care patient is no different to nursing any critical care patient. In many instances that is correct but the experiences we have gained nursing military casualties over the last few years has highlighted a number of challenges that had not previously been experienced by many of the nursing and medical staff.

This personal view will take the reader through our experiences and the ways we have met these challenges and how we are taking things forward.

Critical Care support in the operational environment is aimed at resuscitation and stabilization of the casualty, then transfer to a role four facility such as ours as quickly as possible and as clinically indicated for definitive care.

Patients arrive at Royal Centre for Defence Medicine, Selly Oak Hospital Birmingham UK following a long transfer with the Critical Care Air Support Team sometimes between 12 and 24 h post incident.

Patients are usually sedated and ventilated for transfer, although many of them do not require long term ventilation (unless they have sustained blast or other injuries to the chest). Following initial assessment of ventilation, sedation may be stopped although this may be delayed until the patient has had their wounds assessed in theater (operating room [OR]). One of the main reasons for continuing ventilation is the frequency of patients returning to the OR as this can be as often as alternate days for a prolonged period depending on the amount of tissue damage.

Generally this patient population is fit and strong and can compensate cardiovascularly during their transfer although many will have received massive transfusions and may still require a large amount of fluid resuscitation on admission, partly due to the large amount of leaky open wounds. On arrival, bloods are taken for FBC, U&E's, clotting, and cross match, and the majority of the multiple injured casualties will go to theater within hours of arriving at RCDM.

We have set up a working group involving Intensive Care, the Dieticians, Burns and Plastics, and military surgeons, with the aim to introduce early low volume feeding commencing in the Operational environment in all military patients with Polytrauma and especially those with massive tissue loss. An enteral feeding tube should have been passed in

C. Dutton
Critical Care Division, MDHU(N), Friarage Hospital, Northallerton, UK
e-mail: claredutton@hotmail.com

A.J. Brooks et al. (eds.), *Ryan's Ballistic Trauma*,
DOI: 10.1007/978-1-84882-124-8_41, © Springer-Verlag London Limited 2011

the Operational environment and low volume feeding and prokinetics commenced at the earliest opportunity. This is currently stopped during flight, but restarted as soon as possible at Selly Oak Hospital. The majority of our military casualties are fit young men, who have been consuming a high calorie diet, but have little fat reserves due to the strenuous nature of their jobs. A proactive approach is required working closely with the dieticians to ensure weight loss is minimal. Experience has shown that these patients easily fall through the net due to regular trips to theater – e.g., tubes coming out and then not being re-inserted till the next day- patients could potentially go days without being fed.

When the patient arrives on the unit we make every effort to wash and roll them as soon as possible. The flight is very long and the patient is lying in one position and is usually hot and sweaty when they arrive so this is the perfect opportunity for the nurse to be able to make a thorough assessment of the patient and pick up on any potential problems before they develop further. Mouth and eye care are regularly carried out, teeth cleaned with toothpaste and mouthwash. Injured limbs are elevated in slings or supported on pillows and patients where able sat up to at least 30° in line with the unit ventilator care bundles. Patients generally have all invasive lines changed on admission and tips sent for culture. MRSA screen, urine, and sputum specimens are also sent.

Majority of military casualties have complex injuries and require careful positioning to prevent skin breakdown, with many having open wounds and multiple drains. Where possible the patients are nursed on a nimbus mattress and rolled regularly or if on a spinal bed, then patients are turned two hourly and log rolled at least once per shift. These patients can often require four to five people to turn them, even when not being log rolled this is mainly to support limbs during the move. It does however mean they are very labor intensive.

The Pain team led by a consultant nurse have a lot of input into the patient's management when they are moved off ITU to the ward and have introduced a specific military pain management pathway. The team also includes a military ITU nurse.

It can be very challenging manage our patients waking from ventilation. One day they are in a hostile environment many of them under fire the next they are waking up in Selly Oak Hospital. This has manifested itself in patients still thinking they are in Iraq or Afghanistan and still under attack, therefore they can be very aggressive and fearful for there lives. We have had patients trying to get under their beds and one who thought he had a bomb in his bladder because he had a catheter in. This has provided the staff both military and civilian with many challenges. Damage to genitals is of great concern to many young soldiers and is often one of the first questions they will ask.

We try not to re sedate them unless they are a danger to themselves. Much of the time it requires a huge amount of input from the nurses and doctors sitting with the patients explaining over and over where they are and what has happened to them.

To assist with this we have introduced patient diaries that are started in the Operational theater and follow the patient on their journey to Selly Oak and are then continued by nurses and family members until they are awake and orientated. Reading messages from friends and colleagues deployed with them can sometimes help them to piece together what has happened. When the soldier is fit enough to move from Critical Care to the ward he/she will be followed up by a member of the military ITU team. This is predominantly to discuss care given in Critical Care and also to go through the diary and answer any questions raised. The diaries contain no clinical information.

Relatives are obviously very shocked and sometimes angry when they arrived, often having to travel long distances to be with there loved one. Many of them have seen all the negative press over the last few years and can be unhappy that their relative is being treated in a civilian hospital. They do receive a huge amount of support from the Defence Welfare, military liaison officers, and the staff on the unit. Nursing is carried out by both military and civilian nursing staff. This integration is important and many people may question why military nurses are not looking after military casualties continually. It is important to ensure continuity of care so that if the military staff were deployed on mass the care would remain with no impact on the patient. As military nurses we have an appreciation of the circumstances surrounding the soldier's admission and are therefore able to discuss this with the family.

All trauma patients are challenging to nurse both mentally and physically, but the nature of the injuries sustained by the military casualties and the age group makes it emotionally challenging for all the team. In the early days many of the staff found it very difficult to look after this group of patients but now there is an overriding sense of pride in the standard of care given to our military casualties.

# The Role of Nutrition in the Treatments of Injured Military Personnel

# 42

Susan Duff, Susan Price, and Jennifer Gray

## 42.1
## Introduction

The importance of nutrition within a patient's treatment has evolved and developed as new research is published. Historically, nutrition was considered as an additional part of a patient's treatment. However with increasing evidence and research (within the NHS civilian population group) the role of nutrition has changed to that of an integrated and essential part of a patient's treatment to promote recovery and aiding in their rehabilitation.

Nutrition at Role Four has developed with the military patients and with the changing injury's they have sustained. Patients are transferred to University Hospitals Birmingham NHS Foundation Trust (UHBFT) with multiple and severe injuries that may require multiple complex surgeries and procedures. It is important to optimize their nutritional intervention early to aid recovery.

Currently military patients present with various injuries including gunshot wounds, burns, head injuries, blast injuries, traumatic amputations, and polytrauma. These injuries increase the body's metabolic demands, and increase a patient's nutritional requirements. Ensuring an adequate provision of nutrients has been shown to lower the incidence of metabolic abnormalities, reduce septic morbidity, improve survival rates, and can decrease length of hospital stay.[1]

The information that follows in this chapter provides a summary of the nutritional care that military personnel received at the UHBFT in 2009. Due to limited published research for injured military personnel conclusions have to be drawn from research undertaken with civilian patients with similar injuries. However due to the differences in body composition,

S. Duff(✉)
Nutrition and Dietetic Department, University Hospitals Birmingham
NHS Foundation Trust, Birmingham, UK
e-mail: susan.duff@uhb.nhs.uk

A.J. Brooks et al. (eds.), *Ryan's Ballistic Trauma*,
DOI: 10.1007/978-1-84882-124-8_42, © Springer-Verlag London Limited 2011

nutritional status of military personnel prior to injury and the severity of the injuries, extrapolating data used in civilian patients has its limitations.

## 42.2
## Nutritional Screening

### 42.2.1
### Critical Care

All military patients on critical care are screened by a Dietitian. Sedated and ventilated patients are assessed for the most appropriate route of feeding and then if appropriate started on enteral feed.

For extubated patients who are tolerating small amounts of oral diet but have repeated episodes of being placed nil by mouth (NBM) for the operating theater or wound dressing changes, or patients whose appetite or food intake is poor, or not meeting their nutritional requirements, enteral feeding as an overnight (10–14 h) feed is often used to supplement their oral (food) intake.

For those patients where enteral or oral nutrition is not indicated, parenteral nutrition (PN) will be considered.

### 42.2.2
### Wards

On transfer to a ward at UHBFT nursing staff complete a nutrition screening tool on all patients to identify those patients at high risk of malnutrition. The Malnutrition Universal Screening Tool (MUST) is completed on admission and repeated weekly during a patient's in-patient stay.[2]

Screening on admission to the ward highlights any patient presenting malnourished or patients at risk of becoming malnourished. There is also close liaison between the critical care Dietitian and the ward Dietitian. Weekly screening highlights individuals whose clinical condition or body mass is changing during their in-patient stay, allowing nutritional problems to be highlighted early. The aim is to prevent or treat malnutrition early thus reducing the complications of malnutrition.[2]

The MUST tool involves taking nutritional measurements, body mass and height, and recording a patient's body mass index (BMI); it also takes into account previous weight loss and the acute disease effect to provide a classification of malnutrition. BMI in this patient group is used as a guide only due to differing body composition of military personnel compared with the general population. The screening tool is unique[2] as it provides surrogate measures that can be taken if a patient cannot be weighed, e.g., mid upper arm circumference (MUAC) or ulnar length if their height is not able to be measured. MUST provides an overall score that categorizes patients as low, medium, or high risk of malnutrition allowing the nursing staff to set up an appropriate nutritional care plan. Patients highlighted as high risk are referred to the Dietitian for a full dietary assessment and advice.

## 42.3
## Nutritional Assessment

To be able to provide military patients with an individualized nutritional plan a detailed dietetic assessment needs to be undertaken. Nutritional advice is not given on one individual result but multiple factors (listed below) are taken into account before nutritional advice is provided. These factors are then regularly monitored throughout a patient's hospital stay and the nutritional advice is adapted to meet their changing needs.

## 42.4
## Anthropometric Measurements

Military personnel on deployment may have a change in body composition prior to injury. Weight loss can be as a result of decreased fat stores and changes in lean body (muscle) mass. As a result, after an injury military patients may have depleted fat and glycogen stores to mobilize as an energy source. This can lead to an increase in muscle catabolism and further body mass loss. Unfortunately no published data is currently available to assess the change in body mass for UK military personnel on deployment but work in this area has been undertaken.

A range of the anthropometric measurements detailed in Table 42.1 are taken but the measurements taken depend on the patients injuries.

**Table 42.1** Anthropometric measurements used at UHBFT

| Measurement | Rational |
|---|---|
| Weight | Provides a limited amount of information when used on its own but used in combination with an individual's height can provide an indication whether a patient is under or overweight and monitoring weight allows trends to be tracked to assess whether an individual is losing or gaining weight. Weight should be taken within a day of admission[3] and repeated on a weekly basis[2] |
| Edema, plaster casts and fluid balance | All have to be taken into account to assess the accuracy of a measured weight. e.g., severe peripheral edema can account for up to 10 kg of weight gain in some patient's[4]<br>Data collected by the British Association for Parenteral and Enteral Nutrition (BAPEN) on the weight of different plaster casts and frames can be subtracted from a patient's measured weight to provide a more accurate weight[2]<br>Patient's who have undergone amputations:calculations by Osterkamp[5] can used to ensure nutritional requirements are not under and over estimated |
| Mid arm muscle circumference (MAMC) | Is calculated using mid upper arm circumference (MUAC) and triceps skinfold (TSF) measurements. This measurement is used as an estimation of muscle mass and can show changes in protein stores during a patient's hospital stay[6] |
| Hand grip dynamometry | Is used to assessment a patient's grip strength. This provides an assessment of functional changes in muscle strength[7] and often responds more quickly to a patient's nutrition support than MAMC which shows a more gradual increase as patient's nutrition improves[8] |

## 42.5
## Nitrogen Balance

In critically ill and very catabolic patients measuring urinary urea nitrogen, in a 24 hour urine collection, allows nitrogen losses to be estimated taking into account nitrogen lost from skin, sweat, aspirates, fistula losses, dialysate fluid, and faeces. Nitrogen balance is used to assess and monitor trends in total body protein and trends in catabolism.

## 42.6
## Biochemistry

The Dietitian will use biochemical parameters (see Table 42.2) as part of their nutritional assessment and it contributes towards the Dietitian's recommendations for the type of feed, nutritional supplement, and fluid volume required.

## 42.7
## Temperature

A patient's temperature is monitored as ongoing pyrexia often indicates an infection or sepsis and as a result will cause an increase in the energy and fluid requirements of the patient.

## 42.8
## Medications

A patient's current medication is monitored as some may have an impact on a patient's nutrition:

- Sedation or opioid analgesics such as morphine and fentanyl slows gastric emptying[14] and if a patient's bowels are not opening regularly nausea and vomiting may result, leading to a reduction of food intake, or decreased tolerance of enteral feed.
- Antibiotics, in some patients, can give gastrointestinal symptoms such as nausea, vomiting, or diarrhea, and this may result in a reduction in food intake.
- Some sedation agents e.g., propofol, provide an additional source of calories and when used for prolonged periods of time need to be taken into account when adjusting a feeding regimen.
- Anticonvulsant medication such as oral phenytoin (not intravenous) requires a 2 hours break in enteral feed pre- and post phenytoin administration. This is due to the calcium and protein in enteral feed binding to the phenytoin, reducing the absorption of the drug. Therefore patients on oral phenytoin should only be fed over a maximum of 20 hours.[15] Water can be run if needed during the 4 hours break from feed.

**Table 42.2** Biochemical Parameters used to aid nutritional assessment at UHBFT

| Parameter | Role |
|---|---|
| Urea and Electrolytes (U + E's) | Daily estimations of sodium, potassium, and urea along with fluid balance charts and clinical observations allow assessment of hydration |
| Creatinine | Increasing creatinine can reflect changes in muscle mass in individual's with stable renal function |
| Albumin | Albumin is a poor indicator of nutritional status as it is often low as a result of non-nutritional changes such as trauma, burns, sepsis, and recent surgery. Albumin levels can be affected by a patient's hydration status |
| | During periods of high stress the liver reduces its synthesis of albumin. Albumin results are always interpreted with the C-reactive protein (CRP) result to distinguish between malnutrition and the effects of illness. Low albumin levels can also indicate the body's impaired ability to cope with major illness/surgical intervention or sepsis[9] and have been shown to indicate an increased morbidity and mortality[10,11] |
| White blood cells (WBC) | Changes in WBC levels reflect the changes in an individual's infection and inflammation state. This is taken into account when calculating nutritional requirements as prolonged infection and/or inflammation can have a negative impact on a patient's nutritional status if their nutritional requirements are not being met. WBC results are monitored and interpreted in conjunction with temperature and CRP results |
| C-reactive protein (CRP) | CRP is used as an indicator to detect the presence of inflammation and is essential in the interpretation of protein results.[12] Trends in CRP are used to monitor acute phase responses and this information is used when assessing a patient's nutritional requirements |
| Phosphate ($PO_4$), Calcium ($Ca^{2+}$), and Magnesium ($Mg^{2+}$) | These electrolytes are checked with U + E's prior to commencement of feeding and should be monitored daily in patients at risk of re-feeding syndrome e.g. malnourished patients or patients starved for 5 days or more.[2] (see re-feeding syndrome below) |
| Glucose | Hyperglycaemia is common in critically ill patients due to an increase in catecholamine, glucagon, cortisol, and growth hormone levels. Maintaining a tight blood glucose control may improve the mortality and morbidity of critically ill patients[13] |

## 42.9
## Nutritional Intake

For all patients on an oral diet a detailed 24 hour dietary recall is taken to allow the Dietitian to estimate the patient's current energy and protein intake. If a patient is unable to provide this, detailed food record charts are requested. A patient's food intake is then compared to their estimated nutritional requirements, so a nutritional plan can be devised. An assessment of a patient's food intake also highlights their individual food preferences, as well as any allergies or intolerances. If a patient is enterally fed, the Dietitian compares what is documented on fluid charts to establish if a patient is receiving their prescribed feeding regimen.

## 42.10
## Nutritional Requirements

A patient's nutritional requirements are calculated on an individual basis and will vary depending on, if they are in an acute or recovery phase of their injury, the severity and type of the injury and their nutritional status prior to injury. The body's individual response to trauma differs but there are three documented phases; the ebb phase, the flow phase, and the anabolic or recovery phase.[16]

## 42.11
## Ebb Phase

The ebb phase occurs just after injury and can last up to 24 hours. The body's metabolic rate decreases to preserve energy and allow the individual to react to the injury. Energy reserves are mobilized, glycogen from the liver is converted to glucose and free fatty acids are released from tissues. As this phase occurs just after an injury and the effects are short lived it is unusual for the Dietitian at Role Four to review the patient during this phase.

## 42.12
## Flow Phase

The ebb phase is followed by the flow phase which can last from several days to several months depending on the type and severity of injury. The body's metabolic rate and temperature increase to deal with the stress of the injury. There is a large increase in hormones (catecholamines, glucogon, cortisol) and cytokine levels that results in catabolism and increase tissue breakdown to provide energy for the body to use.[16] This phase leads to a rapid loss of muscle, and can be identified in military patients by a significant and often visible decrease in body mass. The Dietitian will provide nutritional recommendations during this catabolic phase. The aim of nutritional intervention is to provide an adequate energy intake to minimize muscle and weight loss while not overfeeding the critically ill patient [26].

## 42.13
## Anabolic Phase

The anabolic or recovery phase occurs as catabolism declines and is often seen at a ward or rehabilitation level. Patients normally have an increase in appetite and food intake and at this time the aim of nutritional intervention is to gradually improve a patient's nutritional status, promoting the regain of weight and muscle mass lost during the ebb and flow phase.

In addition to the injury, during periods of starvation the body again adapts by using itself as an energy source. An injury, in addition to starvation, increases the rate in which glycogen stores are mobilized from the liver and muscle, gluconeogenesis releases amino acids from muscle, and fatty acids are broken down to produce ketone bodies used by the brain.[16] During this time micronutrients, mineral, and electrolytes are used. Early initiation of nutritional support is recommended to minimize these losses and to minimize body and muscle loss.

## 42.14
## Calculating Nutritional Requirements

### 42.14.1
### Energy Requirements

At Role Four a patient's energy requirements are calculated using Schofield equations.[17] This prediction equation calculates a patient's basal metabolic rate (BMR) which accounts for between 45% and 70% of total energy expended per day. The Schofield equations use age, weight, and gender to calculate BMR. An activity factor and stress factor are then added to the BMR to provide an estimated energy requirement.

Clinical judgement and interpretation of a patient's condition are used by the Dietitian when estimating a patient's nutritional requirements. Examples of stress factors added to BMR are given in Table 42.3.

### 42.14.2
### Protein Requirements

The Department of Health[25] recommends the average healthy adult needs 0.75 g of protein per kilogram (kg) of body weight per day (d). However large nitrogen losses are known to occur in patients with sepsis, major trauma, and burns. When the body is

**Table 42.3** Examples of stress factors that can be added to BMR

| Injury | Stress factor added |
|---|---|
| Head injury (acute) | 30%[18,19] |
| Head injury (recovery) | 30–50%[18,19] |
| Long bone fracture | 10%[20] |
| Polytrauma | 30–50%[21] |
| Burns | 1% increase in stress factor for every 1% full thickness burn[17,22] |
| Surgery | 5% for uncomplicated surgery through to 25% for an extensive and complicated surgery[23,24] |

catabolic nitrogen balance post injury is difficult to achieve and the aim is to minimize muscle mass losses. Some evidence suggests the body is unable to utilize excess nitrogen when a patient is critically ill therefore it is not recommended to exceed 1.25 g protein/kg/day (0.2 g N/kg/day).[26] Up to 1.87 g protein/kg/day (0.3 g N/kg/day) can be given during the anabolic phase.[22]

## 42.14.3
## Fluid Requirements

For maintenance fluid requirements in patients aged 16–60 years 35 mL/kg is used as a guide[4]. If a patient is pyrexial, 2–2.5 mL/kg is added for each °C rise in temperature above 37°C. Fluid charts, U+E's, fluid losses via drains, aspirates, exudate, and fluid restrictions are all monitored and taken into account when adjusting a patients fluid intake.

## 42.14.4
## Electrolytes

Electrolytes are calculated or the Department of Health[25] lower reference nutrient intake (LRNI) to reference nutrient intake (RNI) range can be used to provide a target intake. Patients with severe burns or trauma will require a higher intake of electrolytes but this will be assessed on an individual basis, taking into account their clinical condition and whether losses are occurring e.g., from fistulae, exudate, or diarrhea. Military patients can be depleted in electrolytes and monitoring of serum biochemistry can identify when they need to be corrected.

## 42.14.5
## Trace Elements

Burns patients have increased requirements for trace elements due to increased losses in urine, plasma exudate, skin, and eschar. At UHBFT patients with a greater than 30% burn receive an 8 day supply of IV supplementation of copper, zinc, and selenium. Ideally this is administered via a central line, but a peripheral line can be used. In burns of between 20% and 30% oral supplementation of copper, zinc, and selenium is given. A patient's trace element levels are regularly monitored.

## 42.14.6
## Nutritional requirements

A patient's nutritional requirements are regularly re-calculated as their clinical condition changes thought out their treatment. After estimated nutritional requirements have been calculated a nutritional plan can be prepared. Enteral feeding rates can be calculated, or recommendations for oral diet and oral nutritional supplements type and volume can be made.

## 42.15
## Aim of Nutritional Intervention

Feeding of critically ill patients is a current topic of debate. Appropriate nutritional feeding is seen as supportive therapy and benefits such as reduced rates of nosocomial infection, reduction in length of critical care and hospital stay, and improved wound healing and reduction in muscle wasting can result. Adequate feeding prevents a reduction in respiratory muscles and prevents an increased weaning time from mechanical ventilation. Also the early introduction of enteral feeding is commonly quoted as being important in decreases in complications and infection rates.[27,28]

Traditionally there has been a tendency to attribute large stress factors to ongoing illness when calculating energy requirements based on recommendations from 1979 that hospital patients had higher requirements than their healthy counterparts and increased energy expenditure and hypermetabolism increased depending on severity of illness and degree of stress the body was under.[29] However, as more research has become available, it has been recognized that these stress factors have generally tended to overfeed patients. There has been a body of evidence produced showing that overfeeding patients can be just as problematic as underfeeding, particularly in the critical care setting.

The consequences of overfeeding a critically ill patient can be increased physiological stress leading to azotemia, hepatic steatosis, hypercapnia (which may lead to prolonged weaning from mechanical ventilation), hyperglycemia, hyperlipidemia, and fluid overload.[27,30]

Ventilator settings, renal replacement therapy, and insulin therapy can be altered to correct for hypercapnia, azotemia, and hyperglycemia, respectively. However underfeeding will cause loss of lean body mass, including cardiac and respiratory muscles, prolonged weaning from mechanical ventilation, delayed wound healing and increased infections.[31-33] The current practice at UHBFT is to aim to feed patients in critical care to their energy requirements and meet protein requirements while not over or underfeeding.

Enteral nutrition is used when oral intake on nutritional support is not practical, inadequate, or unsafe.[26] It is used as it provides a physiological and immunologically beneficial way of feeding patients. Feeding regimens are designed to fit patient's requirements, e.g., 24 hours feeding is used when patients are sedated and ventilated or critically ill to provide nutrition at a steady lower rate of feed to provide better fluid balance and blood glucose control. On the wards a 16 – 18 hours feed may be recommended or a supplemental overnight feed may be used to encourage oral intake during the day.

Early nutrition support has also been associated with a reduction in the body's catabolic response to injury, providing improved clinical outcomes including decreased complication rates, improved wound healing and promoting graft and donor site healing by assisting cell renewal and growth.[34]

For critically ill patients, enteral nutrition should ideally be initiated within 12–48 hours after injury for all patients unlikely to meet their full nutritional requirements within 3 days.[32] For major burns enteral nutrition should be started as soon as possible and ideally within 6 hours of burn injury. This has been proven to be beneficial[35] with the aim of having established enteral feeding by 72 hours.[36] Early enteral feeding in critically ill patients has been shown to be beneficial[37,38] as it prevents excessive muscle protein breakdown, improves immune function, and reduces mortality and morbidity in traumatic brain injury patients.[1,39] Early enteral feeding in polytrauma patients has shown a reduction in infection rate, shorter hospital stay, and an improved outcome.[40]

Prolonged ileus and stress ulcers in burns patients have been largely eliminated by early enteral feeding. Some evidence suggests that in burn patients early enteral feeding may decrease hypermetabolism, decrease catabolic hormones, and improve nitrogen balance. Enteral nutrition also prevents bacterial translocation, while maintaining gastrointestinal function and structure is maintained, reducing incidence of diarrhea and length of hospital stay.[41-44]

Therefore starting early enteral feeding at a low rate (up to 50 mls/h of standard feed) has been proposed for injured military personnel on deployment prior to their transfer back to the UK to bring the early nutritional intervention in line with NHS civilians in the UK.

The aim of nutritional intervention is to maintain normal body mass or in critically ill patients minimize weight loss, preserve lean body mass, and promote optimal wound healing and skin graft take. Without appropriate nutrition, depletion of muscle mass is accelerated with some patients losing up to 1.5 kg/day.[16]

The aim of nutritional support is to:

1. Maintain nutritional status in normally nourished patients
2. Minimize body and muscles mass losses in catabolic patients and to improve a patient's nutritional status, once the patient is not catabolic
3. Improve nutritional status in malnourished patients
4. Ensure adequate macro and micronutrients intake to meet an individual's requirements
5. Maintain fluid balance

## 42.16
## Enteral Feeding

Possible indications for enteral nutrition[26] are:

- Unconscious patient e.g., head injury or sedated and ventilated patient
- Increased nutritional requirements e.g., amputations, multiple fractures, burn injury
- Neuromuscular swallowing disorder e.g., brain injury
- Specific treatment to correct malnutrition e.g., weight loss of greater than 10%, muscle wasting
- Inadequate or little or no food intake for more than 5 days or predicted poor food intake for next 5 days

## 42.17
## Tubes

In critical care at UHBFT there are three main types of tubes used for short term enteral feeding:

## Nasogastric Tubes (NGTs)

These are the most commonly used for artificially feeding patients. Fine bore polymethane tubes 12FG are recommended for use rather than wide bore Ryles type tubes made from PVC. The 12FG contains the same internal diameter as a Ryles tube. This allows for gastric aspirates to be drawn easily and for medication to be given without blocking the tube.

If a Ryles tube is placed once feeding is established and the patient is absorbing their feed, for patient comfort the tube can be changed to an 8FG tube. Ryle's tubes should be changed before 14 days as the PVC can plasticize in a reaction with gastric contents causing the tube to become brittle, increasing gastric ulceration and erosion.[45,46] Wide bore Ryles tubes are also linked with rhinitis, pharyngitis, oesophageal strictures, increased reflux, as well as discomfort and difficulty in swallowing for patients.[47] The use of polymethane tubes overcomes the need for Ryles tubes to be changed.

## Orogastric Tubes (OGTs)

OGTs are placed in sedated and ventilated patients with a suspected or confirmed skull fracture, head injuries, and for some maxillofacial traumas. Before a patient is extubated a plan needs to be formulated for the patient to meet their nutritional requirements, as an OGT will not be tolerated by a conscious patient. OGT are normally replaced with an NGT, passed with care by the medical team, to meet a patients nutritional requirements until oral diet can be established.

## Nasojejunal Tubes (NJTs)

NJTs are placed beyond the ligament of Treitz to allow feed to be delivered below the stomach into the jejunum. They are used in critically ill patients who have problems with delayed gastric emptying,[48] post operative gastric stasis and gastroparesis. Patients after gastrointestinal surgery or with liver or pancreatic damage often require post pyloric feeding. Insertion of NJT can take place during laparotomy's or endoscopically. At UHBFT most tubes are placed endoscopically and a single or double lumen tube can be used. A double lumen NJT allows for feeding down NJ port and the NG port allows for gastric aspiration.

Potential complications of NJTs are abdominal distension, migration of NJT into stomach (less likely if the tube is in jejunum rather than duodenum) and this can cause reflux, increased risk of aspiration, and vomiting.

Pharmacy advice should be sought on the most appropriate route of administering medication as some medication may need to be absorbed in the stomach rather than the post pyloric.

On the wards 8FG NGTs are placed and if gastric emptying was a problem then an NJT single lumen or double lumen tubes would be placed endoscopically.

### 42.17.1
### Position of Feeding Tube

Confirming the feeding tube is in the correct position is essential. There have been five deaths reported in 2007 to the National Patient Safety Agency (NPSA)[49] due to misplaced

NGTs delivering feed into the patient's lungs. Unconscious, sedated and ventilated, or patients without a swallow reflex are at high risk from tubes being incorrectly positioned in the trachea or bronchus. Proton pump inhibitors, $H_2$ antagonists and antacids, and 24 hours feeding will all affect the pH of the stomach. Therefore UHBFT's enteral feeding guidelines recommend all fine bore feeding tubes are x-rayed on insertion in critically ill or head injury patients and the position is confirmed and documented in the patient's notes before feed is commenced.

Confirming NGT position on the wards is completed by using the pH method and is recommended by the Medical and Healthcare Products Regulatory Agency.[50] This involves aspirating a small amount of fluid from the tube and using pH paper, ensuring the pH is 5 or below. Blue litmus paper should not be used[49,50] nor should the tube position be checked by the "whoosh test"–pushing air down the NGT–as this does not differentiate between the tube being in the patient's stomach, esophagus, or lungs.[49]

An NJT position can be verified with an abdominal x-ray.

### 42.17.2
### Enteral Feed

Whole protein polymeric feeds are used to meet a patient's requirements:

- Standard feeds (1 kcal/ml) e.g., Nutricia Nutrison Standard, Abbott Osmolite, Fresenius Kabi Fresubin Original are used to meet requirements when patients can tolerate larger volumes.
- High energy feeds (1.5 kcal/ml) are used with patients who need to meet requirements without providing large volumes of fluid or patients on overnight feeds, e.g., Nutricia Nutrison Energy, Abbott Ensure Plus, Fresenius Kabi Fresubin Energy.
- High energy, high protein feeds (1.5 kcal/ml) provides further protein and is used for patients with high protein requirements (i.e., polytrauma or burns patients), e.g., Fresenius Kabi Fresubin HP Energy.
- Low electrolyte feeds, can also be used when patients are not on renal replacement therapy and need a strict fluid restriction or need a low electrolyte feed, e.g., Nutrica Nutrison Concentrated, Abbott Nepro.

The standard and high energy feeds all come in a high fiber version. This is used for patients that are prone to constipation, for example patients on high amounts of pain relief or patients that are bedbound and immobile.

### 42.17.3
### Immune Modulated Enteral Feeds

Currently there is no evidence to support the use of feeds supplemented with arganine, dietary nucleotide, or fish oils. More evidence is needed in this area before these types of feeds should be used with patients.[40,51-54] These are currently not used at UHBFT.

Glutamine is a conditionally essential amino acid in trauma and burns patients and is needed to provide fuel for rapidly dividing cells. Studies have shown that enteral glutamine can improve biochemical markers (increased plasma glutamine and prealbumin levels), improve wound healing rates, morbidity, and length of stay, and suggest that it helps maintain mucosal integrity in patients who have severe burns.[32,55] The European Society for Parenteral and Enteral Nutrition (ESPEN) guidelines[32] suggest its use for burns and trauma patients in which it has been proven to be beneficial. In critically ill general surgical and head injured patients supplementation of glutamine is not recommended. At present it is not standard practice to supplement glutamine at UHBFT but it can be given. Studies recommend using for a minimum of 5 days to a maximum of 14–30 days depending on inflammatory markers (CRP, WCC).

### 42.17.4
### Monitoring an Enteral Feed

There have been no clinical trials assessing monitoring of enteral feeding but Dietitians follow the NICE[26] recommends:

- Ensuring short and long term goals are met
- Ensuring feed prescribed is delivered
- Monitoring body mass or other anthropometrics measures
- Monitoring biochemistry and hematology
- Monitoring fluid balance, taking into account effects of temperature on fluid requirements
- Ensuring the correct tube position prior to feeding and ensuring tube fixed in place appropriately
- Monitoring for gastrointestinal symptoms, e.g., nausea, vomiting, diarrhea, constipation
- Assessing changes in patient's clinical condition and adjusting their nutritional requirements and feeding regimen as appropriate
- Monitoring drug therapy

### 42.18
### Complications of Enteral Nutrition

### 42.18.1
### Re-feeding Syndrome

Before enteral feeding is commenced a patient should be assessed for risk of re-feeding syndrome. This is unlikely in military patients but common can be amongst UK civilians and in host nationals. Some military patients however can present with depleted electrolytes (potassium, magnesium, and phosphate) so individual monitoring and correction is important.

**Table 42.4** Current practice for supplementing low electrolytes at UHBFT

| Electrolyte | Corrected by using |
| --- | --- |
| $K^+$ | Sando K or IV $K^+$ replacement |
| $PO_4$ | Phosphate polyfusor if levels of $PO_4$ are below 0.32 mmol/L; if greater than 0.32 mmol/L but below normal range, effervescent phosphate tablets can be given |
| $Mg^{2+}$ | IV magnesium sulfate if below 0.5 mmol/L; oral supplementation should not be used as it is poorly absorbed and gives gastrointestinal side effects in large doses |

Re-feeding syndrome is described by Soloman and Kirby[56] as "the metabolic and physio-logical consequences of the depletion, repletion, component shifts and interrelationships of the following: phosphate, potassium, magnesium, glucose metabolism, vitamin defi-ciency and fluid restriction."

Patients at risk of re-feeding syndrome can be identified as those who have had very little or no nutrition for greater than 5 days, along with severely being malnourished patients. If a patient is suspected to have re-feeding syndrome, feed should be started slowly, NICE[26] recommend at 10 kcal/kg for the first 24 hours. Electrolytes listed below need to be checked and corrected as appropriate. A patient's feed rate is not increased if electrolyte levels are depleted.

Electrolytes potassium ($K^+$), phosphate ($PO_4$), calcium ($Ca^{2+}$), and magnesium ($Mg^{2+}$) should be checked prior to feeding and daily until levels are stable. Replacement should be provided for patients who have depleted levels. At UHBFT the current practice for supple-mentation is listed in Table 42.4.

All levels should be checked daily after they are corrected and levels should be moni-tored regularly until a patient is tolerating and meeting their full nutritional requirements.

## 42.19
### Aspiration/Delayed Gastric Emptying

Vomiting, regurgitating, and reflux can result in aspiration into the lungs which can in some cases lead to increased risk of pneumonia. Aspiration risk can be reduced by ensur-ing patient's head is at $30-45°$ and by ensuring tube position is confirmed by checking the pH before every use.

Delayed gastric emptying can be caused by sedation, opiate use and raised intracranial pressure (ICP). It may also be as a result of the body's response to critical illness or trauma by conserving plasma volume and providing essential organs with sufficient oxygen and nutrients. This can lead to a reduced blood flow to non-essential organs such as the gut.

It is common practice to aspirate NGT or OGTs every 4 hours to assess gastric empty-ing when patients are on critical care. At UHBFT an aspirate greater than 200 ml is indica-tive of delayed gastric emptying.[57,58] If aspirates are repeatedly above 200 ml the patient is not absorbing or tolerating feed, then feed rate should be reduced and prokinetics started.

Currently at UHBFT metoclopramide IV 10 mg three times per day and oral erythromycin 125 mg four times per day are used to promote gastric emptying. If NG aspirates remain elevated post-pyloric feeding should be considered.

### 42.19.1
### Diarrhea

Diarrhea is often referred to as being a result of the enteral feeding. It is more commonly a result of antibiotic use or clostriduim difficile overgrowth.[59,60] The sorbitol content of some liquid medications can also cause loose stools. Adjusting the fiber content of a patient's feed or reducing feed rate and running the feed over a longer time period can help provide symptomatic relief. Any alteration in feed type or rate requires an assessment by the Dietitian to ensure that the patient is still meeting their nutritional requirements.

### 42.19.2
### Blocked Tubes

The blocking of tubes often occurs as a result of failure to flush the enteral feeding tube at the end of the feed delivery or inadequate water flushing after medications administered. This can be prevented by adequate and timely water flushes or by using medications in syrup or suspension form rather than crushable tablets. However even after liquid medications adequate water flushing is required also.

Blocked tubes can be unblocked by using warm water and 50 ml catheter tip enteral syringe in a push/pull plunge technique. The tube can be rolled between fingers to move blockages. The UHBFT enteral feeding guidelines does not recommend the use of fruit juices or carbonated drinks (e.g., cola or lemonade) to unblock tubes as these products are likely to curdle the feed further.[61]

### 42.19.3
### Medications

When patients are nil by mouth, medication is often administered through feeding tubes. The opening or crushing of a tablet prior to administration changes the medication to an unlicensed medication. Pharmacy advice is sought and where possible syrups or suspensions should be used. Medications that are modified release, enteric coated, hormonal, cytoxic, or steroidal should never be crushed or opened and an alternative should be sought.

### 42.19.4
### Fluid Balance

All patients should have their fluid balance monitored to prevent dehydration and hypernatremia or prevent a patient from becoming fluid overloaded. If a patient has a raised sodium and urea, dehydration is likely even in patients with severe edema, additional oral or NG water can help reduce these levels. A raised urea with a normal sodium level can occur if a patient is dehydrated and losing both sodium and fluid, e.g., in a patient with diarrhea. Urinary sodium can be measured in patients with large fluid losses, e.g., burns patients, to check for depletion.

## 42.20
## Oral Nutrition

For ward patient, or patients extubated on critical care, oral nutrition support is encouraged. Patients that have been enterally fed have their feeding regimen altered to an overnight or 12–14 hours regimen and a light diet is trialled to ensure they can tolerate oral diet. If a patient has a tracheostomy or any swallowing difficulties such that coughing or choking on oral intake, a referral is made to the Speech and Language Therapist (SLT). SLT complete a Dysphagia Screening Test and advise on the most appropriate texture of food and fluids to prevent aspiration.

As a patient's food intake improves the volume of feed via their enteral feeding tube is reduced. Enteral feeding is stopped when a patient can meet their nutritional requirements consistently using food and oral nutritional supplements.

Military patients transferred directly to the wards and who do not require enteral feeding or SLT input are started on the high protein menu. Advice is given to patients on eating foods that are energy, protein and nutrient dense to promote recovery. Patients are encouraged to initially eat and drink with the aim of building up to three meals and three snacks per day as tolerated. Larger portions of hospital meals, a cooked breakfast, and meal vouchers are provided to ensure patients are meeting their nutritional requirements. If a patient cannot meet their nutritional requirements solely from food, nutritional supplements are recommended. Patients are advised on the type and number of supplements to drink depending on the calculated deficit between their food intake and their nutritional requirements.

Military patients often want to optimize their food intake and learn of the importance of nutrition and the role food plays in preventing muscle and weight loss. The Dietitian has found increased compliance to nutritional recommendation when patients are aware of their nutritional requirements and detailed discussions are held with patients on how they can meet their requirements through diet, nutritional supplements and/or enteral feeding.

The supplements that are used at UHBFT range from:

- High calorie supplements (e.g., Nutrica Fortisip Compact 300 kcal, 12 g protein per bottle)
- High protein supplements (e.g., Nutrica Fortimel 250 kcal, 20 g protein per bottle or Nestle Build-up milkshakes 200 kcal, 15 g protein per drink)
- High calorie and high protein supplements (e.g., Nutrica Fortisip Extra 300 kcal, 20 g protein per bottle)
- Energy only supplements (e.g., Nutrica Calogen 405 kcal/90 mL)

While in hospital many factors can affect an individual's food intake making it difficult for them to meet their nutritional requirements. Loss of appetite, early satiety, tiredness, pain, nausea, vomiting or diarrhea, dislike of hospital meals, and multiple periods of being made NBM for theater or test and investigations all have an impact on a patients nutrition.

Advice is given to the individual patients, nursing and medical staff on ways to improve their oral intake through food and nutritional supplements. However if a patient continues to struggle to reach or maintain their nutritional requirements via food and supplement intake an overnight NGT feed will be commenced until their nutritional requirements can be met orally, with the aim of promoting a patient's recovery, wound healing, and preventing weight loss.

## 42.21
## Parenteral Nutrition (PN)

Enteral feeding is not suitable for all patients and clinical decisions should be made on an individual patient basis. Possible contraindications to enteral nutrition and indications for PN are[26,61,62]:

- Gut failure, e.g., severe obstruction, perforation, prolonged gastrointestinal ileus, dysmotility, fistulae, or severe malabsorption
- Intestinal failure for greater than 5 days
- NBM following major surgery
- Proximal high out-put or enterocutaneous fistula
- Intractable vomiting
- Gastrointestinal tract is insufficient or inaccessible

PN is only indicated when it is not possible to meet a patients nutrition enterally as a result of the gastrointestinal tract is not functioning or inaccessible. A patient will undergo a nutritional assessment as described previously and a recommended prescription of PN will be made for the Doctors to prescribe.

Patients with PN need to be monitored closely for complications. These can include metabolic complications such as fluid overload, hyperglycaemia, electrolyte abnormalities, deranged liver function tests, hypertriglyceridemia, cholestasis, and hepatic steatosis.[16,26] The complications of a PN line insertion (which is commonly a central venous or long term peripheral indwelling line) should also be considered such as air embolism, pneumothorax, central venous thrombosis, cardiac arrhythmias, and nerve injury as well as catheter related sepsis.[63] Weaning from PN should start as soon as an enteral route can be established to meet the patient's nutritional requirements. Close monitoring is required.

## 42.22
## Monitoring of Nutritional Intervention

With any nutritional intervention (oral, enteral, or parenteral) monitoring is just as important as the nutritional assessment. The discussed items in the nutritional assessment section are monitored at each review by the Dietitian. Monitoring is used to assess the effectiveness of the nutritional support ensuring dietary aims are being met. Timely and effective monitoring can reduce or minimize incidence of complications, reduce electrolyte and metabolic disturbances, and ensure that a patients nutritional requirements are being met.[64]

## 42.23
## Conclusion

Nutrition plays a vital part in promoting the recovery of military personnel at all stages of their injury from acutely ill thought to rehabilitation on the ward and in rehabilitation centers. The aim of nutritional intervention is to preserve muscle mass and physical strength, promote wound and graft healing, and promote recovery from injuries. Optimizing a patient's nutrition, help reduce their risk of complications and aid patient progress forward for their ongoing intensive rehabilitation.

Research is ongoing to determine the changes in nutritional status, nutritional care, nutritional requirements, and body composition of injured military personnel and the impact this has on their rehabilitation. Conclusions are often drawn from research undertaken with civilian patients with similar injuries. Further research has been proposed to improve nutrition for military patients.

**Acknowledgments**   This chapter is based on an article originally published in JR Army Med Corps 2008;154:284−291. Material is used with permission.

## References

1. Krakau K, Hansson A, Karlsson T, et al. Nutritional treatment of patients with severe traumatic brain injury during the first six months after injury. *Nutrition.* 2007;23:308-317.
2. Elia M (Chairman and editor). *Screening for Malnutrition: A Multidisciplinary Responsibility. Development and use of the Malnutrition Universal Screening Tool (MUST) for Adults.* Redditch: BAPEN 2003.
3. NHS Quality Improvement Scotland. *Clinical Standards − Food, Fluid and Nutritional care Standards in Hospitals.* Ediburgh: NHS Quality Improvement Scotland; 2003.
4. Todorovic V, Micklewright A, eds. The Parenteral and Enteral Nutrition Group of the British Dietetics Association. *A Pocket Guide to Clinical Nutrition.* 3rd ed. 2004.
5. Osterkamp LK. Current perspective on assessment of human body proportions of relevance to amputees. *J Am Diet Assoc.* 1995;95:215-218 L.
6. Bishop CW, Bowen PE, Ritchley SI. Norms for nutritional assessment of American adults by upper arm anthropometry. *Am J Clin Nutr.* 1981;34:2530-2539.
7. Gale CR, Martyn CN, Cooper C, Sayer AA. Grip strength, body composition, and mortality. *Int J Epidemiol.* 2007;36:228-235.
8. Jeejeebhoy KN, Detsky AS, Baker JP. Assessment of nutritional status. *JPEN.* 1990;14:193S-196S.
9. Scott A, Skerrant S, Adma S. *Nutritional for the Critically Ill: A Practical Hand Book.* London: Arnold; 1998.
10. Feldman M. The myth of serum albumin as a measure of nutritional status. *Gastroenterology.* 1990;99:1845-1857.

11. ASPEN Board of Directors and the Clinical Guidelines Task Force. Guidelines for the use of parenteral and enteral nutrition in adult and paediatric patients. *JPEN* 2002;26:Suppl.

12. Gabay C, Kushner I. Acute phase proteins and other systemic responses to inflammation. *N Engl J Med*. 1999;340:448-454.

13. Van den Berghe G, Wouters PJ, Bouillon R, et al. Outcome benefit of intensive insulin therapy in the critically ill: Insulin dose versus glycemic control. *Crit Care Med*. 2003;21:359-366.

14. Bosscha K, Nieuwenhuijs VB, Vos A, et al. Gastrointestinal motility and gastric tube feeding in mechanically ventilated patients. *Crit care med*. 1998;26:1510-1517.

15. Au Yeung SC, Ensom MH. Phenytoin and enteral feedings: Does evidence support an interaction? *Ann Pharmacother*. 2000;34:896-905.

16. Thomas B, Bishop J, eds. *Manual of Dietetic Practice*. 4th ed. Oxford: Blackwell publishing; 2007.

17. Schofield WN. Predicting basal metabolic rate, new standards and review or previous work. *Hum Nutr Clin Nutr*. 1985;39:5-96.

18. Bruder N, Dumont JC. Francois. Evolution of energy expenditure and nitrogen excretion in severe head-injured patients. *Crit Care Med*. 1991;19:43-48.

19. Weekes E, Elia M. Observation on the patterns of 24 hour energy expenditure changes in body composition and gastric emptying in head injuries patients receiving nasogastric tube feeding. *JPEN*. 1996;20:31-37.

20. Paillaud H, Bories P, Le Parco J, et al. Nutritional status and energy expenditure in elderly patients with recent hip fractures during 2 month follow-up. *Br J Nutr*. 2000;83:97-103.

21. Brandi LS, Santini L, Bertolini R, et al. Energy expenditure and severity of injury and illness indices in multiple trauma patients. *Crit care med*. 1999;27:2684-2689.

22. Elia M. Artificial nutrition support. *Med Int*. 1990;82:3392-3396.

23. Barak N, Wall-Alonso E, Sitrin MD. Evaluation of stress factors and body weight adjustments currently used to estimated energy expenditure in hospitalised patients. *JPEN*. 2002;26: 231-238.

24. Cortes V, Nelson LD. Errors in estimating energy expenditure in critically ill surgical patients. *Arch Surg*. 1989;124:287-290.

25. Department of Health (DH). Dietary reference values for food energy and nutrients for the United Kingdom. Report to the panel on dietary reference values of the committee on medical aspects of food policy. Report on health and social subjects 41. London: HMSO, 1991.

26. National Institute for Health & Clinical Excellence. Nutrition Support in Adults. Clinical Guideline 32. London : NICE, 2006.

27. Alberda C, Snowden L, McCargar L, et al. Energy requirements in critically ill patients: How close are our estimates? *Nutr Clin Pract*. 2002;17:38-42.

28. Miles JM. Energy expenditure in hospitalised patients: Implications for nutritional support. *Mayo Clin Proc*. 2006;81:809-816.

29. Long CL, Schaffel N, Geiger JW, et al. Metabolic response to injury and illness: Estimation of energy and protein needs from indirect calorimetry and nitrogen balance. *JPEN*. 1979;3: 452-456.

30. Klein CJ, Stanek GC, Wiles III. Overfeeding macronutrients to critically ill adults: Metabolic complications. *J Am Diet Assoc*. 1998;98:795-806.

31. Frost P, Bihari D. The route of nutritional support in the critically ill: Physiological and economical considerations. *Nutrition*. 1997;13:58s-63s.

32. Kreymann KG, Berger MM, Deutz NEP, et al. ESPEN guidelines on enteral nutrition: Intensive care. *Clin nutr*. 2006;25:210-223.

33. Verity S. Nutrition and its importance to intensive care patients. *Intensive Crit Care Nurs*. 1996;12:71-78.

34. Perel P, Yanagawa T, Bunn F, et al. Nutrition support for head-injured patients. *Cochrane Collab* 2008;2.

35. McDonald WS, Sharp CW, Deitch EA. Immediate enteral feeding in burn patients is safe and effective. *Ann Surg*. 1990;213:117-183.

36. Raff T, Hartmann B, Germann G. Early intragastric feeding of seriously burned and long-term ventilated patients: a review of 55 patients. *Burns*. 1997;23:19-25.

37. Marik PE, Zaloga GP. Gastric versus post-pyloric feeding: a systemic review. *Crit Care*. 2003;7:R45-R51.

38. Heyland DK, Novak F, Drover J, et al. Canadian clinical practice guidelines for nutrition support in mechanically ventilated, critically ill adult patients. *JPEN*. 2003;27:355-373.

39. Sacks GS, Brown RO, Teague D, et al. Early nutrition support modifies immune function in patients with severe head injuries. *JPEN*. 1995;19:387-392.

40. Hasenboehler E, Williams A, Leinhase I, et al. Metabolic changes after polytrauma imperative for early nutritional support. *World J Emerg Surg*. 2006;1:29-43.

41. Chiarelli A, Enzi G, Casadei A, et al. Very early nutrition supplementation in burned patients. *Am J Clin Nutr*. 1990;51:1035-1039.

42. McClave SA, Snider HL, Spar DA. Preoperative issues in clinical nutrition. *Chest*. 1999;115:648-705.

43. Saito H, Trocki O, Alexander JW, et al. The effect of route of nutrient administration on the nutritional state, catabolic hormone secretion and gut mucosal integrity after burn injury. *JPEN*. 1987;11:1-7.

44. Wasiak J, Cleland H, Jeffery R. Early versus late enteral nutrition support in adults with burn injury, a systemic review. *J Hum Nutr Diet*. 2007;20:75-83. Cochrane collaboration 2008.

45. Dewar H. Nasogastric Tube Audit: Standard setting and review of specifications. *J Hum Nutr Diet*. 1997;10:313-315.

46. Ibaney J, Perafiel A, Marse P, et al. Incidence of gastroesophageal reflux and aspiration in mechanically ventilated patients using small bore nasogastric tubes. *JPEN* 1999;24:103-106.

47. Navinski N, Yehuda Y, Serour F. Does the size of nasogastric tube affect gastroeosophageal reflux in children? *J Paediatr Gastroenterol Nutr*. 1999;29:448-451.

48. Arnold W, De Legg M, Schwaitzberg S Enteral access – the foundation of feeding in nutritional considerations in the intensive care unit. Ed: Shikora SA, Mackindale RG, Schwaitzberg SB. Chapter 13. Kendall Hunt, Iowa, USA; 2002: 139–151.

49. National Patient Safety Agency Summary up-date: Advise to the NHS for reducing harm caused by the misplaced of nasogastric tubes NPSA, London; 2007.

50. Medical and Healthcare products regulatory Agency (MHRA) Safety Alert – Enteral feeding tubes (nasogastric) June 2004, MDA/2004/MHRA, Department of health. London.

51. Heys SD, Walker LG, Smith I, et al. Enteral nutritional supplementation with key nutrients in patients with critical illness and cancer: A meta-analysis of randomised controlled clinical trials. *Ann Surg*. 1999;229:467-477.

52. Garcia-De-Lorenzo A, Zarayaga A. Critical evidence for enteral nutritional support with glutamine: a systemic review. *Nutrition*. 2003;19:805-811.

53. Caparros T, Lopez J, Gran T. Early enteral nutrition in critically ill patients with a high protein diet enriched with arganine, fibre and antioxidants accompanied with a standard high protein diet The effect on nosocomial infections and outcomes. *JPEN*. 2001;25:299-309.

54. Heyland DK, Novak F, Drover J, et al. Should immonutrition become routine in critically ill patients? A systemic review of the evidence. *J Am Med Assoc*. 2001;286:944-953.

55. Novak F, Heyland DK, Avenell A, et al. Glutamine supplementation in serious illness: a systematic review of the evidence. *Crit Care Med*. 2002;30:2022-2029.

56. Soloman SL, Kirby DF. The re-feeding syndrome: a review. *JPEN*. 1990;14:90-97.

57. McClave SA, Snider HL, Lowes LL, et al. Use of residual volume as a marker for enteral feeding intolerance: prospective blinded comparison with physical examination and radiographic findings. *JPEN*. 1992;16:99-105.

58. Davies AR, Fromes PR, French CJ, et al. Randomised comparison of nasojejunal and nasogastric feeding in critically ill patients. *Crit Care Med*. 2002;30:586-590.
59. Bowling TE, Silk DBA. Colonic responses to enteral tube feeding. *Gut*. 1998;42:147-151.
60. Bliss DZ, Johnson S, Savik K, et al. Acquisition of c-difficile and clostridium difficile - associated diarrhoea in hospitalised patients receiving tube feeding. *Ann Intern Med*. 1998;129: 1012-1019.
61. Pickering K. The administration of drugs via enteral feeding tubes. *Nurs Times Supp Nutr*. 2003;99:46.
62. Dudrick SJ, Maharaj AR, McKelvey AA. Artificial nutrition support in patients with gastrointestinal fistulas. *World J Surg*. 1999;23:570-576.
63. Pennington CR. *Current Perspectives on Parenteral Nutrition in Adults*. Maidenhaed: BAPEN; 1996.
64. Shikora SA. Approaches to nutritional support for battle casualties and trauma: Current military practice and lessons leaned from the civilian sector. *Mil Med*. 1995;160:312-317.

# Part VIII

## Reconstruction and Rehabilitation

# Role 4 and Reconstruction

# 43

Steven L.A. Jeffery and Keith Porter

## 43.1
## Introduction

The Royal Centre for Defence Medicine is made up of three organizations, the Defence Medical Services (DMS), University Hospital Birmingham Foundation Trust (UHBFT) and Birmingham University. It has three pillars: clinical, training, and research.

UHBFT provides the Role 4 clinical care to all military trauma patients requiring inpatient treatment following aeromedical evacuation, the only exception being ophthalmic trauma which is managed in conjunction with the Birmingham and Midland Eye Centre. Clinical care is provided by a multidisciplinary approach which is consultant based and overseen by the authors who are all very active in the totality of care provision to military patients.

From an agreed established level of 40 cases per month in 2002 this figure has grown considerably with an average work load of 114 cases per month in 2008. Approximately 40–50% of RCDM aeromeds originate from an operational theater.

There is considerable variation in the monthly numbers of casualties reflecting the operation tempo. Such variations demand clear uplift protocols. This is reflected in UHBFTs ability to meet demand by making available or opening additional intensive care capacity (up to five patients from a single flight) and additional theatre capacity. The demand for civilian patients requiring theater cannot be compromised, therefore, additional lists are generated at times of high demand. Patients frequently return to theater every 48 h constituting a sustained demand. A single patient early in 2008 required 33 h of operating time during five visits to theater over a 2 week period.

The demand on specialties at RCDM during 2008 is recorded in Table 43.1 (in patients) and Table 43.2 (out patients).

As can be seen the predominant demand is for musculoskeletal services. For this reason the remaining chapter will address the interface between Role 2E and Role 4. Integral to the onward progress of patients beyond Role 4 is the regular liaison at weekly ward rounds with consultant staff from Headley Court.

S.L.A. Jeffery (✉)
Burns and Plastic Surgery, The Royal Centre for Defence Medicine, Birmingham, UK
e-mail: slajeffery@rcsed.ac.uk

A.J. Brooks et al. (eds.), *Ryan's Ballistic Trauma*,
DOI: 10.1007/978-1-84882-124-8_43, © Springer-Verlag London Limited 2011

**Table 43.1** RCDM in patient episodes for 2008

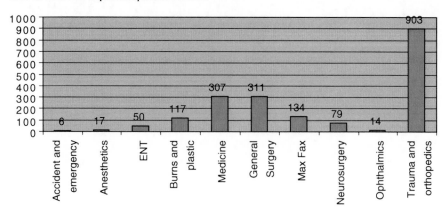

**Table 43.2** RCDM out patient episodes 2008

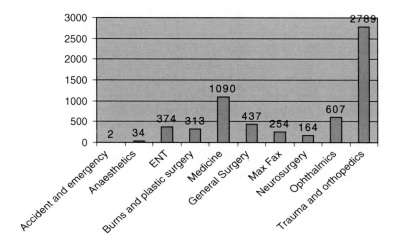

The treatment of the injured soldier on arrival back in the UK is both a privilege and a challenge. They bring back with them wounds which are often complex and are associated with unusual microbiology. There is often media interest in these patients, and the tabloid press are aware that stories about these soldiers will make "good copy," regardless of accuracy.

Treatment at Role 4 should attempt to get soft tissue and bony healing in as short a time period as possible, with the minimum of in-patient hospital stay, so the soldier can rapidly progress to rehabilitation.

## 43.2
## Prior to Arrival at Role 4

We have found that that it is useful if the following factors are addressed prior to the aero-medical transfer to Role 4.

## 43.2.1
## Analgesia

Adequate analgesia given to the patient for the duration of the transfer will help deliver a calm and compliant patient to Role 4. Insufficient analgesia during the transfer will produce a patient who is exhausted, irritable, non-compliant, and primed to expect agony during every subsequent procedure. Such a patient is afraid of experiencing such pain again, and will do anything to avoid it. This makes dressings, physiotherapy, and interventions such as line placements more fraught than they otherwise need to be. Pain produces profound physiological effects, which are not conducive to wound healing. These sequelae can be avoided if analgesia is planned before the aeromedical evacuation. We have found multimodal pain management to be very useful, including the following.

### 43.2.1.1
### Nerve Block Catheters

As long as correct placement is maintained, the pain experienced by the patient during transfer will be greatly reduced. It is important that the sensory and motor function of the limb affected is assessed and clearly documented prior to insertion of the catheter, to enable surgical planning on arrival at Role 4 and reducing the need for excessive surgical exposure. If there is insufficient documentation of the motor and sensory function prior to the administration of the nerve block catheter, this will require cessation of the local anesthetic infusion until such function can be determined. If the patient still complains of pain despite a nerve block catheter in situ, this may be because the catheter has dislodged *in transit*. If the patient has not had fasciotomies performed, increasing pain could be caused by developing compartment syndrome. Depending on this form of analgesia alone will therefore be insufficient and alternative analgesia such as PCA (see below) should be considered.

Once at Role 4, the catheter should be left in situ, however, until no longer needed for pain control. We have not found any problems in leaving such catheters in situ for several days.

### 43.2.1.2
### Patient Controlled Analgesia

If utilized, these must be left on during the transfer. If the patient continues to experience pain, attention must be paid to whether the cannula has "tissued," preventing circulation of the drug.

## 43.2.2
## Feeding

This should be initiated as soon as is possible, prior to aeromedical transfer. Minor injuries should be able to eat normally. It is difficult to be specific as to what the threshold should be, but more significant injuries will require enteral feeding. We are currently looking at whether criteria such as the Injury Severity Score (ISS) can predict the need for enteral feeding.

Feeding will enable the consumption of sufficient calories and nutrients to maximise the potential for healing, and will help prevent enteric complications such as bacterial translocation. The use of nasojejunal rather than nasogastric feeding will reduce the need to stop feeding prior to subsequent surgery. As patients with complex injuries often require many trips to theater, this can prevent the loss of many hours of feeding.

### 43.2.3
### Lines

Central and peripheral access lines which were inserted "pre-hospital" cannot be considered sterile and should therefore be replaced, as infection of these can be life-threatening.

### 43.2.4
### Debridement

At this stage, debridement, as part of the initial "damage control surgery," should be thorough, but not excessive. In this regard it is helpful to reflect upon the surgical debridement classification described by Granick and Chehade.[1] This is based on a view of injured tissue similar to that taken by Jackson for his burn wound model,[2] namely a zone of necrosis, a zone of injured (but still alive) tissue, and healthy tissue. Based on these zones, wound debridement can be classified into one of five categories: non-debrided wound (0), incomplete (1), marginal (2), complete (3), or radical (4) (Fig. 43.1).

Incomplete debridement implies that not all of the necrotic tissue has been removed, and is therefore inappropriate in this setting as such necrotic tissue left behind can be a focus for infection (Fig. 43.2).

Marginal debridement implies that all of the necrotic tissue has been debrided, but not the zone of tissue which, although injured, may survive. This is the most appropriate level

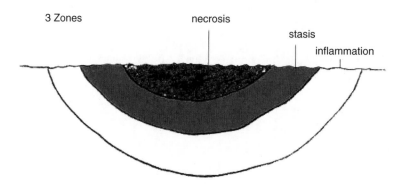

**Fig. 43.1** Jackson's burn model

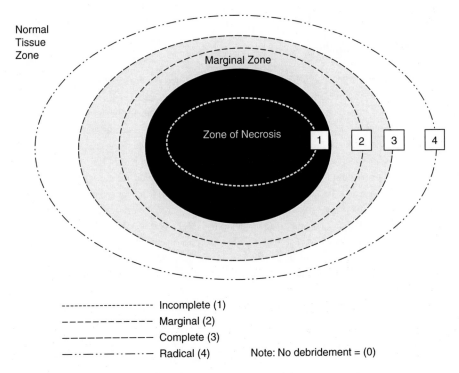

Normal Tissue Zone

Marginal Zone

Zone of Necrosis

| 1 | 2 | 3 | 4 |

---------------------- Incomplete (1)

– – – – – – – – – – Marginal (2)

– – – – – – – – – – Complete (3)

–··–··–··–··– Radical (4)          Note: No debridement = (0)

**Fig. 43.2** Classification of debridement

of debridement in this setting, as tissue which may survive should be left if at all possible.

Complete debridement implies the removal of all necrotic tissue, and also the injured tissue (which has the potential to survive), back to "normal" tissue. This level of debridement is not appropriate at this stage, as tissue which may survive will be unnecessarily removed.

Radical debridement is as above, with the addition of also removing a rim of "normal" tissue. This will ensure a perfect wound be prior to formal reconstruction, but is not appropriate at this stage.

Debridement should be performed before, not after, the application of external fixation. The use of tourniquets for debriding limb trauma should be routine. If the injury is proximal, a sterile disposable tourniquet should be applied by the surgeon once the skin has been prepped. If the patient is not sufficiently stable to allow for debridement of his wounds, for example, after major injury requiring emergency laparotomy, thoracotomy, or amputation, then they should be stabilized in ITU and taken back to the operating theater when sufficiently stable. Transfer to the UK should not be undertaken until this has happened. If the patient is not stable enough to return to the operating theater, then he is not stable enough to undergo a long flight, during which surgical intervention will not be possible.

## 43.3
## Bilateral Testicular Injuries

These injuries are fortunately rare, but are devastating for the patient and their family. In our experience severe bilateral testicular injury is associated with landmine/PPIED (Pressure Plate Improvised Explosive Device) detonation. The soldier is typically young and without children. Because of the potential for significant psychological disturbance, special consideration is required when debriding these injuries. Every effort should be made to preserve testicular tissue, to enable the potential for survival of both the sperm and the hormone producing components. Debridement should therefore be marginal. The testes should be cleaned thoroughly. Sharp debridement should be limited so that the maximum amount of testicular material is retained. There should be no attempt at radical or even complete excision of all necrotic tissue at this stage, as it is unlikely that the retention of incompletely debrided material will cause the patient significant harm in the period before secondary surgery can be performed in the UK. There should be no attempt to "bury" the testes (and hence any underdebrided necrotic tissue) under groin flaps etc. The testes should be dressed in such a way as to minimize desiccation (e.g. paraffin gauze), with the generous application of an antimicrobial agent (such as betadine ointment).

## 43.4
## Fasciotomies

There must be a low threshold for performing fasciotomies in military injuries to the limbs, particularly when associated with blast injury, fragmentation perforating the investing fascia or underlying fracture. The prolonged flight transfer time also should make the surgeon err on the side of performing a fasciotomy. In the military setting, trauma significant enough to warrant the insertion of nerve block catheters to control pain usually warrants a fasciotomy (Fig. 43.3).

There is no place in military trauma for incomplete, "limited," or "single incision" fasciotomies. In an injured leg, the anatomical landmarks can be difficult to ascertain, so a marker pen should be used to mark out the proposed incision: "draw twice, cut once." Do not perform fasciotomy incisions directly over the tibia: it can convert a closed fracture into an open one. Closed fractures should not need flap cover! Therefore do not worry about damaging the perforators that a plastic surgeon may use: he shouldn't need them. Never, ever primarily close fasciotomy incisions (Fig. 43.4).

## 43.4.1
## Dressings

Dressings should be securely applied, so that they do not slip during the aeromedical transfer. Junctional areas, such as the groin, neck, or axilla are difficult to dress with conventional

**Fig. 43.3** This fasciotomy has been placed too anteriorly, exposing the tibia

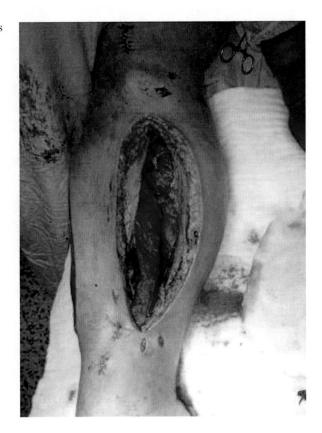

**Fig. 43.4** This poorly placed fasciotomy incision was then primarily closed (!). The leg required amputation

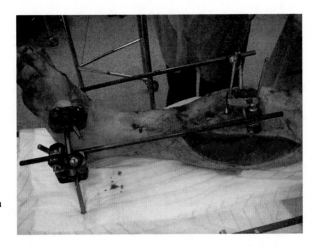

**Fig. 43.5** TNP dressings
following land mine injury

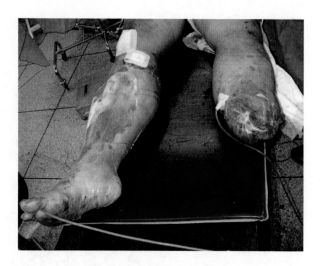

dressings. Topical Negative Pressure (TNP) dressings should be considered for such transfer, as they are much less likely to fall off *in transit*, and are also not prone to the "strike-through" associated with conventional dressings. This "strike-though" risks potentially contaminating the air frame (and every one else on board), as well as posing an infection control risk to the patient. It also results in dressings which smell, and this is often a source of embarrassment for the patient (Fig. 43.5).

## 43.5
## On Arrival at Role 4

### 43.5.1
### Lines

Central and peripheral arterial and venous lines, and nerve block catheters, do not need to be automatically replaced if they have been inserted in a Role 3 facility, where they would have been inserted aseptically. Likewise, nasojejunal / nasogastric tubes do not need to be replaced without good reason.

### 43.5.2
### Feeding

Patients should be weighed on arrival and a nutritional assessment obtained. Soldiers are often relatively malnourished prior to the injury; they have often been working very hard for many months and may have had little access to fresh fruit and vegetables during this time. If normal feeding is inadequate, enteral feeding should be initiated promptly. Soldiers are often reluctant to accept "a tube down the nose," but should be motivated by the knowledge that this is likely to lessen the length of their hospital stay.

### 43.5.3
### Family

It is important that the surgeon responsible for reconstructing a severely injured soldier gets to know the soldier's family. These are usually young soldiers, who may also have relatively young parents. These parents are understandably very anxious about the condition and prognosis for their child.

Such patients often require prolonged hospital admission. It is also very likely that there will be set-backs during this admission, as complications such as infection, wound dehiscence, or slow healing may occur. This will come as less of a shock to the soldier and his family if they are forewarned this is likely to happen. Although there may be one step back for every two steps forward, progress will still be made. These patients will often require prolonged follow up, so it is important that trust develops between the surgeon, the patient, and the family.

### 43.5.4
### First Theater Session

As long as sufficient details about the injuries are signaled ahead of the patient, theater sessions can be booked and planned for when the patient arrives back in the UK. It is our practice that the first dressing change always be done under general anesthesia in theater, unless the injury is minor. This first dressing change can usually wait until "social hours," unless the viability of a limb is threatened, there is gross undebrided contamination, or there is suspected sepsis e.g. abdominal. The general anesthesia will allow for the dressings to be removed without pain to the patient. It is important that at this stage the wounds are assessed by senior orthopedic and plastic surgeons as necessary, so that a plan can be made for the reconstruction of the injuries. This is best performed, if at all possible, during "day light" hours, when these senior members of staff are more likely to be available. At this first theater session at Role 4, the following steps should be performed:

### 43.5.4.1
### Debridement

Larrey, Napoleon's surgeon, described debridement as "one of the most important and significant discoveries in all of surgery."[3] At this stage, the level of debridement, as classified above, should be "complete." Sharp dissection will easily remove dead tissue. We have found that a hydrosurgery device hydrosurgery device is useful for removing ingrained mud, grit, and sand from the wounds, which can otherwise be difficult to remove entirely.

Beware that this material can be driven far up into the tissue planes, and can often be found far removed from the original injury. It is vital that all such potentially heavily contaminated material is removed if subsequent infections are to be avoided.

### 43.5.4.2
### Microbiology

Microbiological swabs must be taken of all wounds, and these swabs must be plated out that night. Likewise muscle which has been debrided should be sent for histological examination for fungal species.

### 43.5.4.3
### Bony Fixation

External fixation should be removed, and replace with either simple splintage or internal fixation.

### 43.5.4.4
### Photography

The wounds should be photographed. This will facilitate the formation of the surgical reconstruction plan, which should then be determined over the next day or two.

### 43.5.4.5
### Dressings

TNP dressings should be applied on significant wounds in order to reduce the tissue edema as well as the benefits as described previously. These dressings should not be thought of as a definitive treatment, but as a "bridging maneuver" between debridement and definitive closure.

If TNP is not used, a dressing with antimicrobial activity (such as silver) should be applied.

### 43.5.4.6
### Burns

In order to assess the depth of burn injury, particularly if creams such as flamazine or flammacerium have been used, we recommend the use of laser Doppler imaging (LDI).

### 43.5.4.7
### Soft Tissue Reconstruction

For military injuries, this should not be attempted until the patient is physiologically stable. This means that the patient should be apyrexial, have his nutrition well controlled, and be off all inotropic medication. Attempts at reconstruction before these goals have been met are likely to fail, with not only the wastage of potential donor site areas but the real chance of increasing the problems that the patient has to deal with, such as a dead, infected flap. The microbiological profile of the patient should also be known before any reconstructive attempts are made.

Likewise, reconstruction should only take place once the wound is ready. This means that there is no longer any necrotic tissue or potential sources of infection, and that the exudate levels are not excessive. This may take several debridements. If fungal infection is suspected, do not attempt flap reconstruction: certain fungi grow up the intima of blood vessels, thrombosing side branches and perforators, causing certain death of flaps and wastage of donor sites. Fungal infection is not uncommon in soldiers who have been injured in the Middle East or Asia, who have extensive wounds and who have been lying in contaminated ditch water after the injury. Such patients often show prolonged pyrexia before the fungus if finally recognized on histology. Wounds infected by fungus require repeated debridements because of extending necrosis.

Reconstruction relying on local perforating blood vessels should be used with caution in patients who have been exposed to an explosion, as it is likely (though yet unresearched with animal models) that the Primary blast wave immediately following an explosion is detrimental to these vessels, particularly where a vessel is fixed in position before becoming mobile (i.e. where they penetrate the fascia).

In the authors opinion rigid guidelines, such as those produced by associations such as the British Association of Orthopaedic Surgeons or the British Association of Plastic, Reconstructive and Aesthetic Surgeons, which dictate by which day wounds, particularly of open fractures, should be closed, should be ignored in these military injuries. They are inappropriate and may be dangerous if wounds are closed before they are ready.

These patients do not need to be kept as inpatients until they are 100% healed, if the rehabilitation center to which they will be sent can cope with relatively simple dressings. Before transfer to the rehabilitation center, it is helpful if a prosthetist can assess the amputee to cast stumps, so that they are ready for when the patient arrives. The prosthetist can also reassure the patient that the loss of one or more limbs is still compatible with an independent, meaningful life. It is particularly helpful if a previous patient, who has a similar combination of injuries, can come and visit the newly injured soldier to show him what can be achieved, and to give the injured soldier realistic expectations and goals.

Injured soldiers should be nursed together in the same open ward if at all possible. His will facilitate camaraderie, and the soldiers will essentially debrief each other. Being able to talk about their experiences with people who have had similar experiences is worth 20 psychologists. Nevertheless, significant or persistent issues such as "flash backs" or emotional lability warrant referral to a psychologist.

All patients with blast injuries must have an ENT review for perforated ear drums, and a neurological assessment for the consideration of Mild Traumatic Brain Injury.

It is useful to feed back to the surgeons at Role 2 or 3 on how their patients have fared. We do this by means of a weekly teleconference, where all patients who have been sent back to the UK over the preceding 2 weeks are discussed. This is an opportunity for learning points to be raised, but care must be taken that this does not develop into a "witch hunt." Any criticism should be constructive only, and praise should be given when possible.

## 43.6
## On Discharge

We have found it useful to hold a clinic monthly at the rehabilitation centre to check on patients and their healing fractures and wounds. Problems can then be identified earlier rather than later. Heterotopic Ossification should be considered if the patient's progress is slower than expected.

## References

1. Granick M, Chehade M. Surgical wound management. In: Granick M, Gamelli R, eds. *Informa.* 2007:17-29.
2. Jackson DM. The diagnosis of the depth of burning. *Br J Surg.* 1953;40:588-596.
3. Reichert FL. The historical development of the procedure termed debridement. *Bull Johns Hopkins Hosp.* 1928;42:93-104.

# Conflict Rehabilitation

John Etherington

## 44.1
## Introduction

The rehabilitation of patients who have suffered ballistic injury during conflict is a critical element of the patient pathway. The medical services have a duty of care to maximize the physical, psychological, and social outcome of military and civilian personnel injured during conflict. In addition, the commanders of military units need to demonstrate that their servicemen injured during operational duties will obtain optimal medical treatment – in order to maintain morale of the force and uphold the moral contract with society.

The ultimate aim is to take injured service personnel from point of wounding through surgical and medical management to rehabilitation and eventually return them to duty. As a consequence the outcome goals for service personnel after injury are considerably higher than those normally set within civilian practice.

Rehabilitation in this group of patients is complicated by a number of factors. There are frequently multiple injuries affecting many bodily systems including, cutaneous, musculo-skeletal, and neurological. Therefore, it is not possible to compartmentalize treatment in one area of therapy alone. Service personnel left with multiple injuries as a result of blast must therefore be assessed and treated for neurological as well as musculo-skeletal consequences of injury. Psychological factors will be a key component in the long-term success of rehabilitation. Exposure to psychological trauma prior to injury, near death experiences, loss of colleagues, loss of employability, and loss of perceived roles in society together with disfigurement will further complicate rehabilitation outcome. This confounds the assessment of surgical outcome when based on measures of the principle physical trauma alone. Patients with similar injuries from similar circumstances may have widely different outcomes because of the individual's emotional response to the traumatic event. Similarly, even mild brain injury unrecognized at the time of initial trauma can have devastating consequences on the final outcome as it impacts on psychological stability, the ability to learn new activities or return to work.

J. Etherington
Defence Medical Rehabilitation Centre, Headley Court, Epsom, Surrey KT186JN, UK
e-mail: johnethe@doctors.org.uk

A.J. Brooks et al. (eds.), *Ryan's Ballistic Trauma*,
DOI: 10.1007/978-1-84882-124-8_44, © Springer-Verlag London Limited 2011

## 44.2
## Principles of Conflict Rehabilitation

There are a number of principles that are key to the rapid and successful rehabilitation of patients injured in conflict. They are itemized below:

1  Early assessment
2  Use of a multi-disciplinary team (MDT)
3  Active case management
4  Exercise-based rehabilitation
5  Rapid access to further specialist opinion

## 44.3
## Early Assessment

Assessment of a patient needs to occur as soon after the point of wounding as possible to identify future needs, rehabilitation potential, and to initiate earliest stages of physical rehabilitation. Psychological factors can be identified at this point and peer support can be initiated if required. In the British Armed Forces there is a doctrine of forward rehabilitation using Deployed Medical Rehabilitation Teams (DMRT) in field hospitals or further forward to manage minor musculo-skeletal injuries but also to initiate rehabilitation in military or civilian in-patients. A rehabilitation plan can be constructed even prior to departure from the operational theater and therapy teams informed of the patient's needs prior to their arrival.

## 44.4
## Use of a Multi-disciplinary Team

The medical consultant-led MDT is vital to the management of these type of cases. The complexity and multi-system nature of these injuries means that they cannot be compartmentalized into single therapy responsibilities. A standard multi-disciplinary team would include:

• Medical staff
• Physiotherapy
• Occupational therapy
• Social work/welfare workers
• Exercise therapist
• Prosthetist
• Podiatrist/orthotist
• Mental health and psychology support

There must be regular multi-disciplinary team meetings with goal setting and treatment planning for each patient.

## 44.5
## Active Case Management

Active case management means that a patient's care pathway is planned from the point of wounding, through the moment they are ready for transfer from acute hospital services to the point where they are discharged back to their unit requiring no further treatment. Relying on external agencies in an optimistic view that everything will be sorted out is ineffective and frequently undermines the trust the patient has in the system. The key agency in facilitating the ongoing medical and social management of the patient is the rehabilitation MDT. There is a need to coordinate medical care (including ongoing surgical review), investigations, equipment requirements (e.g., wheelchairs), and social and welfare support. This may include, in severe cases the provision of plans for resettlement into supported living environments.

## 44.6
## Exercise-Based Rehabilitation

Exercise-based rehabilitation relies on the physical training of injured tissue and bodily systems to enhance function, improve well-being, and generate confidence. This relies on an understanding of tissue healing processes, exercise physiology, and the ability to modify exercise programs to suit patients with multiple concomitant injuries. In the British Armed Forces the exercise therapist is known as a Remedial Instructor. These are Service physical training instructors who have undergone a further 6 month training program in exercise-based rehabilitation. In the British military system the majority of exercise-therapy is delivered to groups of patients with similar levels and types of condition.

## 44.7
## Rapid Access to Further Specialist Opinion

Rapid access to further opinion is critical. After the initial trauma surgery there may be several follow-up surgical procedures required, including orthopedic, plastic, and reconstructive surgery. This may call on the technical skills of the original surgical trauma and orthopedics teams who referred the patient or alternatively input from specialist units with experience in for example neuro-urology and peripheral nerve injury. Psychiatric services and psychological support are essential.

## 44.8
## Rehabilitation Process

The rehabilitation process will vary between nations and local services and what is outlined below are based on the principles used in the British Armed Forces. This relies on doctrine developed as part of the Defence Medical Rehabilitation Programme. This has at its core the main specialist rehabilitation unit at the Defence Medical Rehabilitation Centre, Headley Court, Surrey. Supporting this are the Regional Rehabilitation Units (RRU), small scale rehabilitation centers, which in turn, are aided by Primary Care Rehabilitation Facilities (PCRF) – small physio-led departments.

The aim of the DMRP is to accelerate the rehabilitation process and return injured servicemen and women back to their primary role as quickly as possible. This is done by the consultant-led MDTs.

Rehabilitation at Headley Court is an interactive process with patients attending for 3-week periods of treatment, a period of recovery or consolidation, followed if necessary, by readmission to the same group or a different group providing a higher level of therapeutic exercise.

The rehabilitation program centers on three layers of treatment. The early stage involves a very specific prescription of exercise, tailored to patients particular needs and designed to achieve pre-set outcome goals. At the Intermediate stage there is a shift to a more functional approach to treatment with emphasis placed on improving confidence and general physical conditioning within the limitations of the patient's injury. The final stage of treatment is the Late stage, which is the ceiling of exercise, based rehabilitation, and prepares the patient for the physical demands of their military role.

This latter phase of treatment entails a demanding period of physical training and employment oriented tasks, as well as formal assessment to ensure the return to optimum physical and vocational capability.

The process is as follows:

- Patient tracking
- Patient assessment
- Goal-setting
- Treatment planning
- Delivery of exercise-based rehabilitation
- Case management
- Discharge – readmission process
- Discharge planning
- Vocational rehabilitation
- Reintegration into society
- Follow-up

### 44.8.1
### Patient Tracking

Effective rehabilitation depends on the ability to deliver the appropriate care package to the appropriate patient at the appropriate time. This cannot be achieved if there is an absence of rehabilitation facilities or capacity. This is a problem in highly developed, affluent societies, where rehabilitation is often a low medical priority but is a particular problem in areas of conflict where there are frequently limited medical facilities prior to the conflict, which are further compromised by war. Civilian societies tend to reduce rehabilitation capability in times of peace whilst life-prolonging facilities are built-up at their expense. This means that any society sending troops to war requires a military rehabilitation capability with capacity commensurate with the anticipated levels of casualties. Likewise appropriate medical intelligence is required to provide an accurate estimate of casualty numbers and rehabilitation resources required. It is difficult to maintain rehabilitation knowledge and skills without an appropriately trained cadre of military and civilian staff prior to any conflict.

Identification of casualties returning from conflict who require rehabilitation may be more problematic than first assumed. The most seriously injured will pass through a hospital to undergo definitive trauma surgery and may require intensive care. The patient will then be identified and a rehabilitation program set in motion. Less seriously injured patients may have only transient periods in a secondary care facility and to ease pressure on these facilities discharge to local physiotherapy services. The risk of this process is that apparently minor injuries with significant functional sequelae are passed to inexperienced services. There is anecdotal evidence that these cases may be at greater risk of severe psychological disturbance than the more severely injured. There is a tendency to underestimate the severity of some injuries and the psychological consequences of even minor trauma may be significant, particularly as the injury may have been sustained at the time of a colleague's death.

To avoid the loss of patients from rehabilitation services the British Armed Forces have developed a patient tracking system. All patients aero-medically evacuated from any part of the world will have a signal generated to initiate further medical treatment and to notify the tracking cell of the patient's presence in the evacuation system. Thereafter, the patient's journey through the pathway can be monitored and the appropriate medical service notified of the patient's whereabouts. Integral to this system is the monitoring of the patients' pathway by an experienced consultant medical officer to ensure they are being directed to the appropriate care.

## 44.8.2
### Patient Assessment

The initial and most important part of the rehabilitation process is the assessment of the patient. This involves detailed history and examination and here the medical team play a critical part in the rehabilitation process. It allows prescription of medication which at the earliest stage may include opiates and drugs for neuropathic pain. It also allows assessment of medical stability of the patient and early direction to the appropriate medical staff or secondary agencies. When is a patient fit for rehabilitation? There can be a number of rehabilitative activities carried out as early as ITU but for the patient to be able to make significant progress he or she must be medically stable, free from serious infection, and not undergoing frequent medical procedures which stop any continuity of treatment. Wound or skin contamination with organisms such as MRSA does not exclude treatment but will alter how the patient is managed logistically.

### 44.8.2.1
### Key Elements in the History

- Chronology
- Nature of wounding, single or multiple entry wounds
- Level of energy transfer
- History of impairment

Was impairment at the time of wounding or later in the course of the day, postoperative or during the period of recovery?

- History of loss of consciousness
- Time on intensive care
- Nature of surgical and medical interventions
- Patient perception
- Social history
- Home support
- Past medical history
- Current medication
- Pain quality and level
- History of psychological disturbance in particular nightmares, flashbacks, and intrusive thoughts
- Changes of mood
- Cognitive deficits; word finding difficulties, memory, concentration, and executive skills
- Sensory deficits including tactile, visual, and auditory

### 44.8.2.2
### Examination Skills

It is essential that the examiner has skills in both musculo-skeletal and neurological examination to define deficits, record impairments, and monitor change.

### 44.8.2.3
### Multi-disciplinary Assessment

A multi-disciplinary assessment is vital in any rehabilitation program. Assessments by medical physiotherapy, occupational therapy, social work, exercise therapy, and nursing staff inform the rehabilitation plan. After a multi-disciplinary assessment good communication in an MDT meeting will produce a problem list from which goals are set and a treatment plan derived.

Goal Setting is an important element of the rehabilitation program. Goals need to be set over the long (6 months), medium (2–3 months) and short term 3–4 weeks. They should be Specific, Measurable, Achievable, Realistic, and Timely (SMART). Critically they need to be set in discussion with the patient, although frequently patients – particularly service personnel – need to be given guidance so as to avoid setting unattainable goals in unrealistic time frames. Alternatively, their goals may be very general and therefore difficult to extrapolate a treatment plan from – 'I want to return to running'. Once long term goals are set the shorter time period goals can be worked out from this. Goals must be set in accordance with the patient's wishes and personal aim.

For example:

| | |
|---|---|
| Long term goal | In 6 months I will return to part-time sedentary work |
| Medium term goal | In 3 months I will be walking on my prosthetic for 1 km using one stick |
| Short term goal | At the end of this one month admission I will be wearing my new prosthesis for 3 h/day. |

It may be necessary to determine goals over even shorter periods, such as week, in order to demonstrate to the patient measurable improvement in their function when they are skeptical or dismissive of their progress in rehabilitation. Alternatively, patients may need short term goals in order to rein-in over enthusiastic activity detrimental to their rehabilitation. Patients may need encouragement and support to improve their performance but the more difficult cases to manage require a limitation to be placed on their activity – a common phenomenon in high achieving military or sporting personnel.

Goal setting should focus on occupational outcomes when dealing with people capable of returning to functional employment. A lack of focus on this aspect of rehabilitation will limit overall outcome in the working population in a variety of domains. Returning patients to work de-medicalises them and reaffirms their usefulness to society and family.

## 44.8.3
## Treatment Planning

Treatment goals are set after discussion between the therapy staff, doctors, and the patient. There is production of a joint treatment plan which includes the timelines for treatment, and indicates the external agencies to be involved including employers and social services. Decisions should be recorded on a MDT document and actions identified for individual therapists and doctors to perform.

## 44.8.4
## Delivery of Exercise-Based Rehabilitation

Patient involvement is critical to success and if necessary requires involvement with the patient's consent, of the family and their employer. Ideas, concerns, and wishes may need to be explored and an explanation of the treatment he is receiving and the prognosis improves patient's concordance.

Once rehabilitation has commenced MDT planning meetings are essential on a regular basis and progression recorded and discussed with the patient.

Regular review of the patient is essential and active discharge planning as soon as the patient is admitted. In the system we employ, rehabilitation is undertaken over short periods usually up to 4 weeks of admission. At discharge, there is readmission planning and a selection of goals to be carried out whilst the patient is at home which allows for continued progression even when not in the rehabilitation centre and improved progression on return.

Patients' exercise therapy is usually delivered in groups.

### 44.8.4.1
### Group Therapy

Each group is composed of patients suffering similar musculo-skeletal disabilities including spinal, lower-limb, and upper-limb injuries. In recent years there have been separate groups for patients with early stage rehabilitation after complex injury. All groups complete a varied daily program of 5 h exercised-based activity that includes: Class Therapy, Hydrotherapy, Postural Re-education, Walking/Running and Gait Re-education, Recreational Therapy, and individually tailored treatment programs.

Most rehabilitation relies on the training benefits of exercise. Therefore it is important to continue exercise programs long after the active rehabilitation program is finished.

Peer support is important in overcoming the psychological consequences of this trauma and group therapy is a major contributor to this. Being surrounded by injured patients from similar backgrounds with identical experiences improves recovery and aids concordance with treatment and stimulates competition. The patients' exercise therapy regime is designed, implemented, and supervised by Service Remedial Instructors.

The Group therapy programme centers on three layers of treatment. The 'Early' stage involves a very specific prescription of exercise, tailored to patients' particular needs and designed to achieve pre-determined outcome goals. At the 'Intermediate' stage there is a progression towards a more functional approach to treatment, with emphasis placed on improving confidence with the patient's injury and general physical conditioning within the patient's limitations. The final stage of treatment is the 'Late' stage, which is the ceiling of exercise-based rehabilitation and prepares the patient for the physical demands of a military role. As the DMRC has needed to take patients at earlier stages of recovery the complex trauma team RIs have had to focus exercise therapy at a more impaired group of patients.

### 44.8.4.2
### Physiotherapy

Physiotherapy forms a key component of the rehabilitation service provided for patients with severe physical injury and each patient requires a comprehensive assessment.

Treatments typically take place on a one to one basis. Core skills include manual therapies such as mobilization, manipulation, soft and deep tissue massage, and scar tissue mobilization. Physiotherapists will provide orthotics, correct gait abnormalities and muscle imbalances, provide stretches, exercise therapy, and progression. They may also use acupuncture and a number of electrotherapy modalities particularly for pain relief.

They will contribute to the decision as to whether further admission would be beneficial or further rehabilitation could be better provided in the RRUs or PCRFs.

### 44.8.4.3
### Social Work

Specialist medical Social Workers play a key role in the rehabilitation process and should have expertise in health related issues that individuals or families may be experiencing following trauma or illness. They provide advice and support to the multidisciplinary team to aid the successful rehabilitation of injured Service personnel, offering the following services:

- Assessment and Counseling
- The Social Worker will guide the patient and their family along the process of adjustment, providing support, and assisting the individual and his/her relative to plan for change.
- Care and Discharge Planning
- They are responsible for planning and implementing a discharge care plan where required
- Provision of Resources
- They will provide information about resources such as care facilities, resettlement, retraining opportunities, housing, welfare benefits, and access to legal advice.
- Advocacy
- Social Workers will represent the patient or families view at clinical meetings and advise on difficult choices. Advocacy may also be required with outside agencies such as Housing Departments or the government departments in relation to welfare benefits.
- Resettlement
- When a patient has to consider leaving the military as a result of their injuries the Social Worker, in conjunction with the Occupational Therapist, will advise them on opportunities for retraining and refer them to the Military Resettlement Officers. Vocational assessment can be arranged and patients will be assisted, to apply to retraining colleges.

### 44.8.4.4
### Occupational Therapy

Occupational Therapy enables patients to be as independent as possible in self-care, their chosen occupations, or leisure.

They provide the following services:

- Education and Practical Advice about the nature of the patient's illness or injury and how to deal with its effects on their everyday lives. Advice is given on areas such as work, personal care, and leisure activities.
- Activities of Daily Living
- Assessment and treatment of problems in daily living including personal care, and preparing meals. This may involve home visits to advise on equipment or adaptations that are required to improve safety and aid independent living.
- Provision of Equipment
- Assessment for, and provision of specialized equipment to solve the problems of a temporary or permanent disability e.g., wheelchairs adapted cutlery, bath boards, pressure garments, and cushions.
- Community Living Skills
- Assessment and training in community living skills such as traveling on public transport, shopping, and accessing local community facilities. Driving assessments can be arranged and advice is provided on equipment and adaptations to enable individuals to return to driving.
- Emotional Support
- Practical support and teaching of coping strategies to help patients adjust to their limitations, and explore their worries and concerns regarding their disability.
- Cognitive Rehabilitation
- Assessment and treatment of the functional impact of cognitive problems such as memory, concentration, and speed of thinking in patients who have sustained a brain injury.
- Work Skills
- Assessment of work skills and provision of advice on strategies and adaptations that can be implemented to improve work retention. Through a graded program of work hardening, individuals are gradually introduced back to their trade. If they are unable to work, recommendations are made regarding future employment, training, or rehabilitation.

### 44.8.4.5
### The Nursing Team

A named nurse is responsible for devising a plan of nursing care with the patient and for supporting the patient through his rehabilitation. The team requires specialist nurses in orthopedics, neurological rehabilitation, amputee care, spinal injury care, multiple sclerosis, sexual dysfunction, mental health nurse, and continence care. Of particular importance is tissue viability nursing for the multiple wounds, split skin grafts, reconstructive flaps, and burns seen in these patients. Nursing staff assist patients with activities of daily living in order to promote and encourage independence.

Dietician support is useful for enhancing the nutritional status of patients who have been in a highly catabolic state for many weeks and who need nutritional support during a period of intense physical activity. PEG feeding may be required in more dependent patients.

### 44.8.5
### Case Management

At all times, the rehabilitation program should focus on reintegration of the patient into society at work or home. There requires coordination of external agencies involved in this, including Social Services, the Health Service, the employer, and housing agencies. On-going specialist medical investigations and treatments may be required, for example urodynamics to inform bladder management in the spinal cord injured patients or bone infection management. The consultant which leads the MDT is responsible for the case management of these cases and must ensure the rehabilitation process is a smooth as possible.

### 44.8.6
### Discharge: Readmission Process

The scheme below demonstrates a program for serial admissions to a complex trauma rehabilitation team. Patients are admitted for approximately 4 weeks at a time. Within 10 days the goals for that period are stated, agreed, and written in the MDT summary. At discharge Readmission goals are set for the patient to achieve while they are away and for the first 10 days of their admission. At the end of the first admission long term Outcome goals are set to determine what is expected to be the clinical outcome after 6 months. In this way a series of admissions are conducted with greater periods of time away on sick leave, or later, back at work (Fig. 44.1).

### 44.8.7
### Discharge Planning

The MDT must work closely with the patient, their family, and outside agencies to co-ordinate a package of care that meets the needs of the patient. This often involves liaising

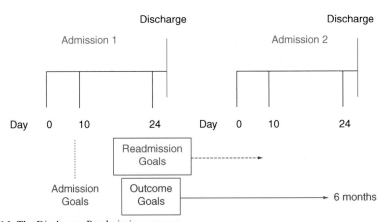

**Fig. 44.1** The Discharge: Readmission process

with Health Authorities, Social Services, and other external organizations to negotiate the appropriate level of support for the individual. But the main focus of our rehabilitation program is on return to work and to do this we have developed a team of vocational Occupational Therapists who liaise between the MDT, the patient, their line manager, and the chain of command to ensure that the maximum number of patients return to military employment or if not – back to civilian work. Where appropriate the patient will be sent back to their workplace for a period of work assessment; if this is not possible patients will be supported with further neurological and/or vocational rehabilitation.

Reintegration into society may be difficult and will depend on a number of factors including, the physical, mental, and cognitive status of the patient, the family support the individual receives, and the support from society itself. This may be compounded by views on an un-popular war. Transition from the military into civilian care can be complicated by reluctance on the part of commissioning authorities to take on additional financial responsibilities. To that end the ministry of defence has developed a contract with an external charitable agency to help transfer patients into civilian life through transitional living facilities, whilst temporarily retaining the soldier on a salary and paying the therapy costs.

## 44.9
## Measuring Outcome

Outcomes can be measured in a number ways:

- Success of the team in accurately predicting goals, using goal attainment scaling
- Repeated measurements of standardized physical tests e.g., 6 min walk test, multi-stage fitness tests
- Patient Reported Outcome Measures e.g., SF 36
- Validated questionnaire-based therapist completed outcome measures e.g., SIGAM, AMP Q
- Return to work data

The use of outcome measures allows self-monitoring and audit against standards of performance. In the polytrauma population at DMRC there have been measurable improvements in SF36 within and between admissions, improvements in Hospital Anxiety and Depression scale (HAD) scores, and improvements in independence in activities of daily living. Of a group of 19 cases 17 required assistance in ADL on admission, at discharge 16 were fully independent. Thirteen could not drive but by discharge 15 were driving some form of vehicle.

Return to work is a valuable source of information on outcome. Of an un-selected group of brain injury patients over a 12 month period 57% returned to some form of work in the military a further 3% to civilian employment. Of 58 military amputees who had completed their rehabilitation 6, approximately 10% had been medically discharged leaving 90% in military employment. For transtibial amputees the time from point of wounding to return to work was a mean of 7.5 months.

One of the problems with many civilian designed outcome measures is the ceiling effect seen in the military population. The Special Interest Group in Amputee Medicine (SIGAM) has produced a single-item scale comprising six clinical grades (A–F) of amputee mobility. Unfortunately, although it is international standard most military patients are in the higher functional scores of it on admission prior to fitting! There will be a need to produce validated outcome measures for military populations.

## 44.10
## Specialist Rehabilitation Issues: Amputee Rehabilitation

### 44.10.1
### Considerations

Rehabilitation of the patient who has sustained an amputation as a result of a ballistic injury requires special consideration. The majority of cases of amputation in the developed world affects the older population, over the age of 50 with diabetic or vascular causes of limb loss. The population affected by war injury is younger, has higher levels of physical function and expectation of recovery. The majority of research and experience therefore does not pertain to this patient group. The increase in disabled sport, particularly in response to the Paralympic movement, has demonstrated the high level of functional outcome attainable from these patients and has set the bar higher for clinical success. Managing expectation of the amputee can be one of the greatest challenges in this situation.

Nevertheless, the improvements in the technical provision of prosthetic components have revolutionized the prognosis for patients with amputations. In particular socket-suspension system developments have significantly improved comfort and practical function.

## 44.11
## Principles of Prosthetic Fitting

There are seven elements to a prosthetic prescription depending on the level of amputation.[1]

### 44.11.1
### The Structure

In developed medical societies the usual structure is the endoskelatal form of prosthesis, which consists of metal or composite materials (e.g., carbon fiber) strut attached to the end fittings which may be covered by a cosmesis. The structure holds the socket in the correct linear and angular orientation.

## 44.11.2
## Socket

Transmits the forces between the stump (residual limb) and the prosthesis;

- Vertically for weight-bearing in the stance phase and some suspension in the swing phase
- Horizontally and rotational about the long axis. To stabilize the socket and energize the prosthesis.

The socket shape is usually a modification of the stump shape as it has to take into account the contained skeleton, the consistency of the soft tissues, the stump volume, and pressure sensitive areas.

## 44.11.3
## Suspension

This may come from the socket shape and material or additional belts. More commonly in this patient population the use of silicon suspensory sleeves with ratchet or vacuum suspension systems is the gold standard. These systems give the patient more freedom of movement, greater comfort, are tolerated well, and are considerably more robust than earlier models. Their selection is usually based on personal preference and tolerance.[2] They allow good suspension particularly for high performance amputees where stump shape or scarring is less than optimal. They may increase sweating, but this frequently adapts, can be corrected by better fitting or can be treated with aluminum based deodorants or botulinum injection.

## 44.11.4
## The Ankle and Foot

Are usually considered as one unit and have to transfer forces between the prosthesis and the ground but also have to modify this transfer in the gait cycle. This may be provided by a mechanical uni-axial joint providing movement in one plane only or a flexible bush allowing multi-axial movement, an assembly of spring components producing multi-axial movements or compression wedges at the heel. High performance limbs for running may use a spring system like the carbon fiber Flex-run® or Cheetah® systems.

## 44.11.5
## Knee Joint

These joints may be uniaxial or polycentric and whereas there are many knees, including the simplest locked systems only released for sitting – the patient population in this situation usually require high performance prosthetics. The vast majority of knees will need to be free during walking.

- Stance phase. Simply aligning the ground reaction forces in front of the knee joint causes the latter to extend and stop – giving a stable knee joint for stance. However mechanical stabilizers – using hydraulic knee systems or 4 bar polycentric systems (or a combination) can allow weight to be behind the knee making walking easier.
- Swing phase. Pneumatic and hydraulic swing phase controls allow a resistance to the swing phase which varies with speed and therefore are self-adjusting for various gait velocities.

The most significant innovations of recent years for the above knee amputee have been in the technology of behind the knee systems. The introduction of microprocessor controlled knees such as the C Leg® or the Rheo® system has revolutionized knee control particularly where stability is a critical issue, such as the bilateral trans-femoral amputee.

These systems use a knee-angle sensor to measure the angular position and angular velocity of the flexing joint. There are moment sensors, using multiple strain gauges, to determine exactly where the force is being applied to the knee from the foot and the magnitude of that force. Measurements are taken up to 50 times a second. A microprocessor receives signals from each sensor and determines the type of motion and phase of gait of the amputee. The microprocessor directs a hydraulic cylinder to control the knee motion accordingly. The C-Leg® is powered by a lithium-ion battery which is housed inside the prosthesis below the knee joint.

These systems can provide a close approximation to an amputee's natural gait and increases their walking speeds. Variations in walking speed are detectable by the sensors and communicated to the microprocessor, which can alter the swing through stance phases of the prosthesis. The knee system will allow the amputee to walk down stairs with a step-over-step approach, rather than the one step at a time approach used with mechanical knees and it can deliver additional stability in other contexts – including recovery from stumbles.

The microprocessor limbs have disadvantages – battery time can be limited dependent on usage, it is susceptible to water damage and they are not suitable for running. This can make them unsuitable for patients with expectations of high functional performance. It takes time to adjust and program the microprocessor and train the patient in its use. The major restraint on prescription is cost – with a prosthesis using these systems frequently costing in excess of £15,000. Clearly, this outside the price range of most developing nations and it is frequently not funded by health commissioners, even in the UK.

Nevertheless, they can deliver significant benefits to the patient. The increased stability can dramatically help the bilateral trans-femoral amputee, particularly in the early stages of mobilization. Patients ambulating with a microprocessor-controlled knee significantly increased their physical activity during daily life, outside the laboratory setting and expressed an increased quality of life.[3]

## 44.11.6
### Hip Joint

In the event of hip disarticulation or trans-pelvic amputations a hip joint is required. Fortunately this is a relatively rare phenomenon as the functional limitation on such patients may be severe. The hip joint will need to be mounted onto the anterior inferior surface of the socket, using the 'Canadian Principle' in order to allow the patient sit. It may be uni-axial, polycentric or may incorporate one of the microprocessor joints described for use in the knee. Given the severity of the injury, initial mobilization is relatively straight-forward as the shallow nature of the hip disarticulation socket means that the patient, for all practical purposes, 'sits' on the socket when walking.

### 44.11.7
### Miscellaneous Units

Axial units will allow rotation about the long axis of the prosthesis against resistance – provide greater freedom of action and reduce the torque applied between the socket and stump. This is of particular use in high functional end patients for example in those who wish to play golf where a rotational motion would aid the swing.

The successful provision of a prosthetic limb to an amputee relies on close interdisci-plinary working with all members of the aforementioned rehabilitation team. In addition, the prosthetists, prosthetic workshop technicians, and physiotherapists must work closely to provide equipment which fits, is suitable for purpose, and provide instruction on appro-priate limb usage. The modular nature of the newer prosthetics means that once the equip-ment is identified the assembly is relatively straight-forward. The skill is in the provision of a comfortable well aligned socket.

Stump volume rapidly changes in the earliest stages of rehabilitation and may continue to decrease for up to 2 years after amputation. Early use of compression socks such as the Juzo® compression sock will aid this and reduce healing time. Nevertheless, the rapid loss of stump volume will lead to a need to use additional socks to ensure a comfortable fit with the pros-thesis. When the volume has changed sufficiently to require a socket change it is vital that this is done rapidly so that time is not lost from rehabilitation and the patient does not become frustrated or disillusioned with progress. This can be expensive and time consuming for prosthetics departments as sockets in this context may need to be changed within 6 weeks. The speed of socket replacement can be increased and the cost reduced by the use of com-puter-aided design/computer-aided manufacturing (CAD/CAM) technology, which can scan a stump and carve a positive mold – from which sockets can be cast- within minutes.

### 44.12
### Neurological Rehabilitation

Ballistic injury can affect any aspect of the peripheral and central nervous system. From a rehabilitation perspective the trauma produces quite different consequences depending on the site of injury – most devastating are the consequences of traumatic brain injury. This section will deal with the principles behind the treatment of these central nervous system injuries.

In the recent conflicts in which the British Armed Forces have been involved the num-ber of severe traumatic brain injuries requiring rehabilitation have been relatively small.

Ballistic injury from conflict comprises only approximately 20% of the total workload of the neurological rehabilitation team, compared to 80% of the complex trauma team's activity. There may be many reasons for this finding including; improved cranial/cerebral protection by helmets and other force protection equipment or the fatal nature of many of the injuries which would present to a rehabilitation team. At present there is no data to confirm either of these hypotheses.

The neurological rehabilitation team at DMRC provides comprehensive assessment, rehabilitation, and management of neurological illness and injury for a range of conditions including brain injury, stroke, and multiple sclerosis. The majority of cases are acquired brain injury as a result of road traffic accidents and assault – the same principles apply for treatment whether there has been a closed or open injury to the brain.

The aim is to provide an intensive program of rehabilitation including vocational assessment, which is delivered by a specialized and experienced multi-disciplinary team. The staff team comprises a Military Consultant in Rehabilitation Medicine, other medical staff, Physiotherapists, Occupational Therapists, Speech and Language Therapists, therapists delivering cognitive rehabilitation, Psychologists, Social Workers, a Group Therapist, and a full Nursing team. The neurological patients benefit from the advantage of having access to the musculoskeletal rehabilitation facilities and related specialists on site including splinting, orthotics, and hydrotherapy. The structured program of therapy addresses the physical, cognitive, communication, psychosocial, vocational, and daily life issues. Involving families and carers in the patient's recovery is essential where possible, although it has to be recognized that military patients not uncommonly come from families where there is poor contact and support. Many soldiers join the army to escape from family conflict – this can make management of the consequences of traumatic brain injury very difficult.

The principles of management are identical to other areas of rehabilitation- there are differences in the length of treatment required, brain injury patients require longer and the pace of treatment slower. It is good practice to assign a key worker to each patient to co-ordinate their treatment and to liaise with the patient and their family, about any areas of concern.

Brain injury rehabilitation requires another of specialist therapies including neuro-psychology speech and language therapy. The whole team contributes to the process of cognitive rehabilitation.

Cognition encompasses all those elements used in learning and thinking, which enable us to make sense of the world. These elements include: arousal, concentration, ability to ignore distractions, learning, memory, visual processing, speed of thinking, planning, self-monitoring, goal setting, initiation, self-awareness.

Cognitive deficits frequently overshadow physical deficits as the cause of difficulties in social adaptation, independent living, family life, and vocational activity. Without appropriate intervention, cognitive deficits can lead to frustration, anxiety, depression, and social withdrawal.

Cognitive rehabilitation is provided at the DMRC by specialist Occupational Therapists. It focuses on the regaining of those cognitive skills, which are lost or altered as a result of neurological trauma or illness. The aim of treatment is to improve the patient's abilities in everyday life situations. The process includes gaining skills through direct retraining, learning to use compensatory strategies and education about cognitive skills.

### 44.12.1
### Mild Traumatic Brain Injury

Recently there has been increased interest in the concept of mild traumatic brain injury. This has fallen out of the observation that a number of soldiers, particularly from US deployments, have displayed cognitive deficit after exposure to blast, in the absence of evidence of other ballistic trauma, and a causative relationship inferred. This has generated a significant degree of medical controversy, not least because of confusion over terminology. A severe brain injury may leave a patient with major cognitive impairment and other impairments – but the outcome is highly un-predictable. For example, there is a poor correlation between Glasgow Coma Scale at time of injury and prognosis. It is possible that a severe acute injury leaves a patient with only mild functional impairment; conversely a minor injury can produce socially devastating consequences. For many years our unit has been treating patients with mild functional impairment from a variety of levels of injury. The concept of MTBI is variably used to describe a minor trauma or a minor consequence of trauma. There is a move away from the terminology towards using post concussional syndrome which more properly describes its etiology and presentation.

Patients exposed to severe blast who sustain multiple musculo-skeletal injuries are clearly at risk of having sustained a brain injury as a result on axonal shearing or possibly delayed resuscitation or anesthetic accident. It is policy for us to screen these patients for cognitive impairment and other issues which may represent underlying brain injury. Of 37 polytrauma cases screened so far as part of our MTBI program 54% have features which would be compatible with the WHO criteria for MTBI. However, closer examination of the history and diagnostic criteria in these patients confirms MTBI in only 11%. Mental health issues were relatively infrequent with only 5% meeting the criteria for PTSD. There are a number of potentially confounding issues in the assessment of these patients, the use of pain relief medication with cognitive side-effects, adjustment reaction, and post-traumatic stress disorder – all of which may produce similar symptoms and cognitive impairment. A recent study from the US has implicated PTSD and depression as important mediators of the relationship between mild traumatic brain injury and physical health problems.[4] Although the findings are controversial there are obvious confounding factors with US troops as result of their prolonged, intense deployments and the reported incidence of PTSD. In a British study, symptoms associated with post-concussional syndrome were associated with exposure to blast and also other risk factors and exposures such as aiding the wounded.[5]

### 44.13
### Lessons Learnt in Rehabilitation from Recent Conflicts

### 44.13.1
### Attempt Limb Salvage

There are frequently debates at the time of ballistic trauma on whether a limb can be salvaged. This author of this chapter cannot advise on the optimum surgical treatment in such cases, clearly the preservation of life is the principal aim of damage control surgery.

However, it is a reasonable approach to try and preserve an injured limb if possible and allow further surgical interventions and the rehabilitation teams to try and maximise function and minimise pain over a period of time before a judgement is made by the patient some months or years later. Clearly limbs of limited use or causing pain can be removed at a later date if the patient so decides. From discussion with a number of our patients it is felt that removal of a limb of equivocal future utility at the first surgical procedure, because it would allow the patient to adjust earlier to his disability, does not appear to be a sound argument. Most patients are glad to have the opportunity to make an informed decision for themselves at a later date. The literature is inconclusive about whether limb salvage or amputation is more effective interms of hospital stay, pain and functional outcome.[6]

## 44.13.2
## The Ideal Stump

The technology now available for fitting limbs in this patient population allows a wide degree of flexibility in stump length, quality and scarring. Healed split skin grafts will usually tolerate the silicon sleeves and suspension systems well. The optimum length of a stump in the lower limb is frequently discussed. In the trans-tibial amputation an optimal range would be 12–16 cm when measured from the medial joint line and in trans-femoral 14–21 measured from the crotch, or 23–30 cm measured from the tip of the greater trochanter. Ideally, the optimal stump length should be proportional to the overall stature of the patient. An 'ideal' length of 16 cm in someone with short legs may not leave enough ground clearance to fit in the total length of the modular components in the prosthesis. This may be particularly critical in the high performance amputee where the prosthetic componentry may need to be longer. In a trans-tibial amputee an approximate guide is for 8 cm of stump length per metre height. Anything shorter than 7 cm in a trans-tibial is very difficult to fit. In the trans-femoral patient a gap of 15 cm above the medial tibial plateau is described as ideal for fitting a knee joint system in place whilst retaining a sufficient lever arm.

Often of greater difficulty is the management of a bulbous stump. A stump with a distal circumference greater than that measured at the level of the patella tendon can be difficult to fit. Post-operative edema can be reduced with stump shrinkers and early mobilisation with PAM- aids (Pneumatic aid to mobilization). But excess muscle bulk is the main source of concern. This more commonly occurs in a posterior flap rather than a skew flap technique which produces a more conical shape which allows better prosthetic fitting. However, these are decisions for the cold light of day rather than the battlefield and over-long or badly scarred stumps can be revised at a later date.

## 44.13.3
## Through-Knee (Disarticulation) Can Be a Very Effective Amputation

There is considerable bias against the use of knee disarticulation as a surgical option in trauma. This is based on poor experience of the procedure in civilian practice and reflects real concerns but ones which are not always applicable to military practice.[7] The Gritti-

Stokes procedure, involving reattachment of the patella to the articular surface of the femoral condyles, has fallen out of fashion and a simple disarticulation can have many benefits. The main advantage of the through knee amputation is an end weight-bearing stump. Once the prosthesis has been fitted then the patient can make rapid progress to high-level weight-bearing activity and a level of function, including running, in excess of that expected from a trans-femoral amputation. Fitting requires time and a high level of prosthetic skill. Disadvantages are mainly cosmetic, as the knee system will sit at a level below that of the contralateral knee. On sitting the knee joint on the prosthetic limb will protrude further forward than the non-affected side. Lowering the centre of rotation of the joint may have a produce a minor biomechanical disadvantage but this is more than compensated by the stability and control gained from the long lever arm, deep socket and polycentric knee joint combined with hydraulic swing phase controls.

### 44.13.4
### Silicon Suspension Systems Allow Prosthetic Fitting of Most Stumps

The new systems of suspension give improved comfort, function and are sufficiently robust for servicemen to use on operational deployments. We have now had a small number of patients to return to operational roles, mainly in support jobs but also on forward infantry roles. The limbs are tolerated well and survive the extreme environments to which they are exposed. There have not been any stumps which we have been unable to fit. There is occasionally a requirement to add suspension systems, such as neoprene belts in high trans-femoral amputees, but stump length has not yet been a problem.

### 44.13.5
### Concomitant Injuries May Be the Factor Limiting Recovery Rather than the Amputation

The functional performance of the lower limb prostheses in many of our amputees is so good and the socket/stump interface so effective that the main limitation to mobilisation is frequently the concomitant injury. Fractures have a rate of healing considerably slower than prosthetic fitting and multiple fractures in a contralateral limb, particularly the foot can have a considerable slowing effect on the rehabilitation process. This frequently leads non-amputees with protracted rehabilitation due to delayed fracture union to request an early amputation. This requires careful counselling.

### 44.13.6
### Aggressive Treatment of Neuropathic and Phantom Pain Is Critical: Non-pharmacological Methods of Pain Control Are Important

Anecdotal evidence would suggest the importance of early, aggressive treatment with analgesics to prevent the development of neuropathic pain. This includes the use of opiates, and drugs such as gabapentin, amitriptylline and pregabalin. There should be no hesitation in using maximum doses of all this medication to obtain complete control of pain. Audit of our practice shows that, once in the rehabilitation setting the requirement for analgesic rapidly diminishes and very few of our patients require long standing medication for phantom pain control. Education, reassurance, peer support, and physical distraction all play apart in this. Wearing the socket and physical activity often dramatically improve the pain. Other modalities such as mirror therapy and acupuncture can be very effective in certain cases although carry over can be limited.

## 44.13.7
### Early Assessment of Peripheral Nerve Injury with Surgical Repair Will Reduce Pain and Limit Disability

It is important to avoid a nihilistic approach to peripheral nerve injury. Early expert assessment is important following primary repair and follow-up vital. Persisting pain following brachial plexus or peripheral nerve injury warrants consideration of surgical exploration and repair or grafting if needed. Monitoring progress of nerve re-growth allows interventions to be carried out rapidly if the graft or repair is failing. There may be a later requirement for tendon transfer to return function, which further demands the need for expert follow-up.

## 44.13.8
### The Psychological Component to Rehabilitation Has an Influence on Outcome

It is evident that the psychological status of the patient has a major influence on physical outcome. Self efficacy is associated with good outcomes in spinal rehabilitation and probably this complexity of injury also. Depression, persistent adjustment reactions, and PTSD are all detrimental to recovery. What is remarkable is the low level of psychological morbidity detectable in these patients. Peer support is probably an important factor in this. In an audit of 30 patients using the Hospital Anxiety and Depression scale (HAD) 77% reported normal levels of anxiety on admission, 20% mild, and 3% moderate. 87% were within normal limits for depression, 7% mild, 2% moderate, and 2% severe. On average these scores improved by discharge. Many patients have mild psychological morbidity in the early stages of their rehabilitation but the long term outcomes are unknown.

## 44.13.9
### Concomitant Traumatic Brain Injury Is a Major Prognostic Determinant of Amputee and Polytrauma Outcome

In assessing outcome from polytrauma and amputation there is a tendency to dwell on the surgical and physiological factors which determine outcome. Additional injury – particularly brain injury may not be apparent at audit review but could have a major effect on physical outcome including donning and doffing the prosthesis, ability to understand rehabilitation instruction, balance, and return to work.

## 44.14
## Conclusion

Patients returning from areas of conflict with severe injuries deserve the highest quality of rehabilitation available. This requires a skilled, consultant-led, multidisciplinary team with rapid access to modern rehabilitation technologies. It requires systems in place to identify and track the patient through the care pathway and needs a focus on a high expectation of functional and work-related outcome.

## References

1. Marks LJ, Michael JW. Clinical review – Science, medicine, and the future: artificial limbs. *Br Med J.* 2001;323(7315):732.
2. Coleman KL, Boone DA, Laing LS, Mathews DE, Smith DG. Quantification of prosthetic outcomes: elastomeric gel liner with locking pin suspension versus polyethylene foam liner with neoprene sleeve suspension. *J Rehabil Res Dev.* 2004;41(4):591-602.
3. Kaufman KR, Levine JA, Brey RH, McCrady SK, Padgett DJ, Joyner MJ. Energy expenditure and activity of transfemoral amputees using mechanical and microprocessor-controlled prosthetic knees. *Arch Phys Med Rehabil.* 2008;89(7):1380-1385.
4. Hoge CW, McGurk D, Thomas JL, Cox AL, Engel CC, Castro CA. Mild traumatic brain injury in U.S. Soldiers returning from Iraq. *N Engl J Med.* 2008;358(5):453-463.
5. Fear NT, Jones E, Groom M, et al. Symptoms of post-concussional syndrome are non-specifically related to mild traumatic brain injury in UK Armed Forces personnel on return from deployment in Iraq: An analysis of self-reported data. *Psychol Med.* 2008;23:1-9.
6. Saddawi-Konefka D, Kim HM, Chung KC. A systematic review of outcomes and complications of reconstruction and amputation for type IIIB and IIIC fractures of the tibia. *Plast Reconstr Surg.* 2008;122(6):1796-1805.
7. Met R, Janssen LI, Wille J, et al. Functional results after through-knee and above-knee amputations: does more length mean better outcome? *Vasc Endovasc Surg.* 2008;42(5):456-461.

# Part IX

## And Finally

# Have You Read MASH?

# 45

Peter F. Mahoney

"Have you read MASH?"[1]

"Seen the film- not read the book."

We're sitting on a concrete ledge- part of a blast wall- at the front of the hospital in Camp Bastion, Afghanistan. Just in front of us a group of about 15 people are conducting a high spirited, impromptu game of "almost American football." The players wear odd combinations of camouflage, scrub tops, and brightly colored theater caps.

It is hot, very hot. Sitting on the ledge is just about bearable. No breeze today.

"Book's better- really captures the madness."

The game continues. Visitors look bemused. Far in the distance two tiny specks appear.

"Who is coming in- MERT or SHOCKER?" (Figs. 45.1–45.2)

"SHOCKER."

"That'll be them then."

The specks get closer. They are two SHOCKER call signs- two US Combat Search and Rescue aircraft. The UK MERT (Medical Emergency Response Team) travel in a Chinook. They are out on a different mission. It is going to be a long day.

Fire trucks wait patiently.

The aircraft are on their approach. Dust clouds swirl on the landing zone.

"OK Guys- get into character"- the senior surgeon for the day ushers the players back into the hospital. Every one knows where they are going. Everyone knows their place on the trauma teams. Coffee cups are put down. Lead gowns and plastic aprons put on.

SHOCKERs land. Ambulances move through the dust cloud like ungainly beetles. Firecrews jog towards the aircraft doors. Aircraft engines continue to scream. Rotor blades blur.

"How many?"

"Looks like three stretchers. Can't tell if there are any walkers."

Ambulances leave the LZ and approach the hospital. Joggers on the hospital road stop and watch. This is the critical time- blue lights on and coming to us? - Or no lights and the sad final journey round the corner. This time all lights are on. Good.

P.F. Mahoney
Defence Professor Anaesthesia and Critical Care,
Royal Centre for Defence Medicine, Birmingham, UK
e-mail: prof.dmacc@rcdm.bham.ac.uk

A.J. Brooks et al. (eds.), *Ryan's Ballistic Trauma*,
DOI: 10.1007/978-1-84882-124-8_45, © Springer-Verlag London Limited 2011

**Fig. 45.1** Call Sign "Shocker",
Afghanistan 2009. Cpl Tony
Green

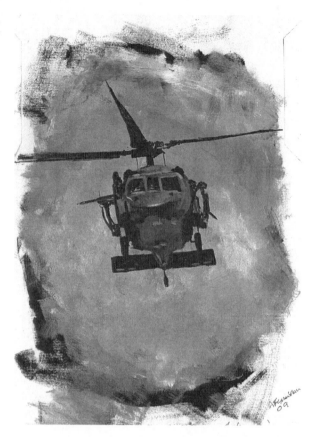

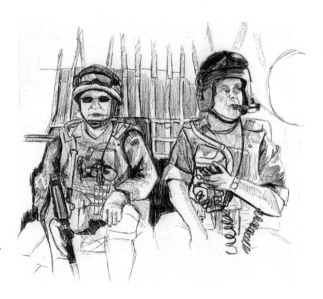

**Fig. 45.2** Medical Emergency
Response Team- MERT-
Afghanistan 2007

Ambulances arrive. The ED Consultant opens the rear doors of the first one.

"What do you have?"

"GSW, right chest- stable."

"Bay three."

A dusty young man is wheeled past. He gives a thumbs up. That's good. GSW, Gunshot wound chest can mean many things. The sound of "Bay three- take him to bay three" can be heard through the hospital doors. His trauma team will now be locked on to him. The other teams wait.

Next ambulance.

"What do you have?"

"Multiple facial frags- IED blast. Doin' OK tho."

That's also good. IED, Improvised Explosive Devices are unforgiving.

"Bay 5- take him to bay 5."

Weapons, ammunition, and armor are deftly removed before the casualties enter the hospital. We really don't want a grenade loose in there. The pile grows. Last ambulance. Doors open. The medic looks anxious. We all pick up on the non verbal signs.

"This one's real bad doc. Had to do CPR in the bird. Got him back but he ain't good."

A pair of ash white feet can be seen protruding from under the blanket. He is sooo pale!!

What will it be? Bay one or Right turn?

"Right turn- take him straight into theater."

The ambulance crews- never slouches- move with real urgency now. Off the back of the vehicle, onto the trestle- let's go. Through the doors of the hospital. Into the cool. The joys of aircon. Through the doors of resus. Down the department- past the bays. Turn right into the operating theater.

We're good at this. We've done it often enough. The trays and high volume infusers have already been moved from the bay into theater. The digital x ray is ready. Three anesthetists wait. Shock packs- two blood, two plasma in each- have already been collected from the laboratory. Lab tech is assessing the scene- a well casualty means get the blood back in the fridge. A sick one means get more ready. Lots more. The right turn has already answered that question.

"Get him across onto the table on my count: One two three roll (PATSLIDE® in) one two three across, one two three PATSLIDE® out"- and imaging plate in. Anesthesia has the helm now. ED can have it back in a moment but we need to get our tubes and lines sorted.

"Any access for induction?"

"Not yet."

"IO please." ED team place an Intra-Osseous needle. We're not fussy- we'll take tibia, humerus, or iliac crest depending on the injury pattern. Bombs don't respect our need for access. In really bad times we can go for suxamethonium into the tongue and ketamine up the nose but today we have an IO site.

"Give the K and sux." You don't need much ketamine for these guys- though it is worth giving the full sux dose.

"Tube's in- check for $CO_2$."

The vascular access team now move in. Right and left. 8.5 Fr large bore subclavians. Blood samples taken then each gets hooked up to a rapid fluid infuser- already primed.

"Let's get ten red and ten yellow in and see where we are."

One unit of product every 100 s. That what it takes. Like I said, we're good at this now. ED rapidly does the rest of the survey. Radiology gets the pictures- x ray and ultrasound.

10 min since coming through the doors.

"OK- what's the plan?"

This is not a place for turf wars. We don't own the space- the space belongs to the casualty. ED, Surgery, and Anesthesia make rapid choices. Care is staged depending on the injury and the physiology. These young people are sick- acidotic and coagulopathic. Add in massive rapid transfusion and cue a metabolic storm.

One of our ODPs has put together a massive transfusion support pack. Calcium, tranexamic acid, Factor VIIa, Dextrose, insulin, and an i-STAT. In the big traumas we have one person dedicated to drawing up drugs, measuring gases, and taking blood for the ROTEM. The ROTEM has really helped us- this is minute by minute management of coagulation.

Multiple teams get to work. Scrubbing. Debriding.

A colleague looks across from table 3.

"Anything for me?" Always looking for the casualty needing a nerve catheter. Gold plated pain care- one of the real mercies we can offer.

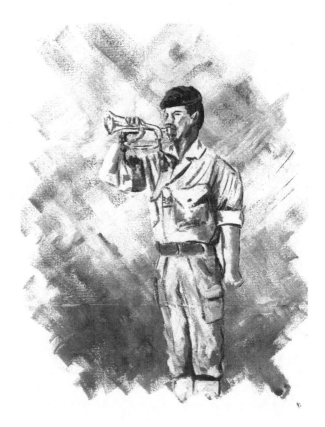

**Fig. 45.3** Bugler

"Maybe- lets get him to ICU and see how he does." Priority is to break this coagulopathy and do the surgery. Balance the needs of this with those of injured lungs. Complexity upon complexity. The text books are not written yet about all this.

Start of a long journey.

"Have you read MASH?"

**Acknowledgment**   Reproduced here with permission from The Royal College of Anaesthetists.

## Reference

1.  Hooker R. MASH (Mobile Army Surgical Hospital). William Morrow 1968.

# Index

A.J. Brooks et al. (eds.), *Ryan's Ballistic Trauma*,
DOI: 10.1007/978-1-84882-124-8, © Springer-Verlag Berlin Heidelberg 2011